Selected Papers on
Analysis of Algorithms

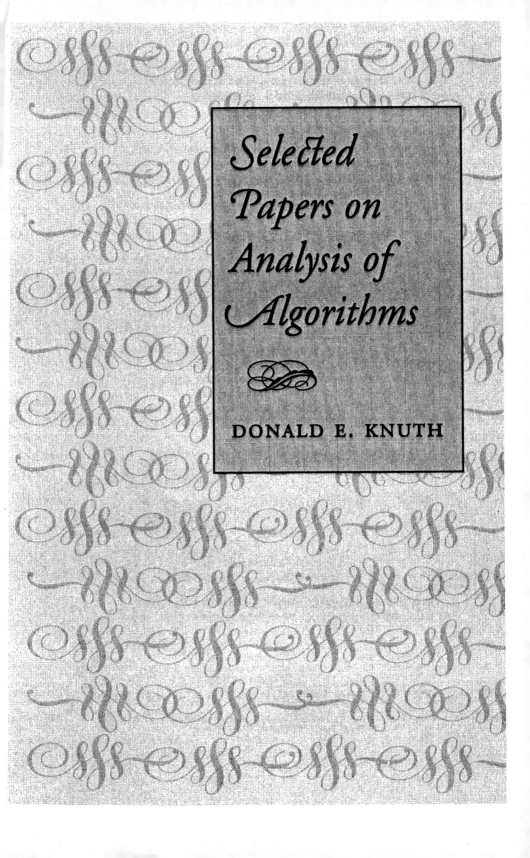

Selected Papers on Analysis of Algorithms

DONALD E. KNUTH

Copyright ©2000
Center for the Study of Language and Information
Leland Stanford Junior University
13 12 11 10 09 08 07   5 4 3 2 a

This printing incorporates all changes to the first printing that
were present in the author's master copy on 22 December 2006.

Library of Congress Cataloging-in-Publication Data

Knuth, Donald Ervin, 1938-
    Selected papers on analysis of algorithms / Donald E. Knuth.
    xvi,622 p. 23 cm. -- (CSLI lecture notes ; no. 102)
    Includes bibliographical references and index.
    ISBN13 978-1-57586-211-8 (cloth : alk. paper)
    ISBN10   1-57586-211-5 (cloth : alk. paper)
    ISBN13 978-1-57586-212-5 (pbk. : alk. paper)
    ISBN10   1-57586-212-3 (pbk. : alk. paper)
    1. Algorithms. I. Title. II. CSLI lecture notes ; no. 102.
QA9.58 .K65 2000
511'.8--dc21   00-023847
                                          CIP

Internet page
    http://www-cs-faculty.stanford.edu/~knuth/aa.html
contains further information and links to related books.

to Professor N. G. de Bruijn
for more than three dozen years
of inspiration and guidance

Contents

vii

Preface

"People who analyze algorithms have double happiness. First of all they experience the sheer beauty of elegant mathematical patterns that surround elegant computational procedures. Then they receive a practical payoff when their theories make it possible to get other jobs done more quickly and more economically."

I once had the pleasure of writing those words for the Foreword of *An Introduction to the Analysis of Algorithms* by Robert Sedgewick and Philippe Flajolet (Addison–Wesley, 1996), and I can't think of any better way to introduce the present book. After enjoying such double happiness for nearly forty years, I'm delighted that I can finally bring together this collection of essays about the subject that I love most.

Very few people ever have a chance to choose the name for their life's work. But in the 1960s it was necessary for me to invent the phrase "analysis of algorithms," because none of the existing terms were appropriate for the kinds of things I wanted to do. I vividly recall a conversation that I once had at a conference of mathematicians: The man sitting next to me at dinner asked what I did, and I mentioned that I was interested in computer science. "Oh," he said, "numerical analysis?" "Um, not really." "Artificial intelligence?" "No." "Ah, then you must be a language man." I readily confessed that I was indeed quite interested in programming languages, but I couldn't easily explain the kinds of questions that really motivated me the most. I realized for the first time that all of computer science had essentially been divided up into three parts, in other people's minds, and that there would be no room for another kind of research unless it at least had a name.

"Analysis of algorithms" was, of course, an obvious name, because the idea is simply to study algorithms and to analyze them as carefully and quantitatively as possible. So I wrote to my editors at Addison–Wesley, proposing that the title of the book I was writing be changed

from *The Art of Computer Programming* to *The Analysis of Algorithms.*
"Oh no," they said; "that will never sell." Surely they were right,
in those days at least, because the word "algorithm" itself was barely
known. But I like to think that the spirit of algorithmic analysis is omnipresent in the books now called *The Art of Computer Programming.*

Most of the chapters in this book appeared originally as research
papers that solved basic problems related to some particular algorithm or
class of algorithms. But the emphasis throughout is on techniques that
are of general interest, techniques that should lead also to the solution
of tomorrow's problems. The way a problem is solved is generally much
more important than the solution itself, and I have therefore tried to
explain the principles of solution and discovery as well as I could. Thus
I believe the material in this book remains highly relevant even though
much of it was written many years ago. I have also appended additional
material to most of the chapters, explaining subsequent developments
and giving pointers to more recent literature.

Chapters 1, 2, and 3 present an overview of the field as it stood in
1970 and 1971. Chapter 4 explains "big-Oh notation" and its cousins,
which are crucial for describing most of the results of algorithmic analysis
in a convenient way. The remaining chapters are organized by technique
and subject matter rather than by date.

As Chapters 1 and 3 point out, analyses of algorithms tend to be of
two kinds, either "local" or "global." A local analysis applies to a particular algorithm for some problem, or to a small number of closely related
algorithms; such analyses are the subject of Chapters 5–27. A global
analysis, on the other hand, applies to all conceivable algorithms for a
problem, and attempts to find algorithms that are absolutely best from
certain points of view; such analyses are considered in Chapters 28–34.

Chapter 5 begins the study of local analyses by considering how to
take empirical measurements of a fairly arbitrary algorithm, using the
minimum number of measuring points. Chapter 6 discusses simple ran-
domization techniques that make it easy to estimate the running time
needed to search exhaustively through a possibly large tree of possibilities. Chapter 7 introduces and analyzes a technique called "ordered
hashing" that has proved to be useful in many applications. Chapter 8
is a short note pointing out that certain results obtained originally in the
study of hashing also yield the solutions of several other apparently unrelated problems. Chapter 9 analyzes the famous "alpha-beta" method
for evaluating positions that arise in games like chess.

Chapters 10–13 are essentially devoted to the granddaddy of all
nontrivial algorithms, Euclid's method for finding the greatest common

divisor of two given numbers, and the related subject of continued
fractions: Chapter 10 discusses generalized Dedekind sums, which are
important in number theory and the study of random number generation; such sums are evaluated using a variant of Euclid's algorithm.
Chapter 11 discusses the approximate behavior of Euclid's algorithm on
quadratic irrationalities; this topic is motivated by applications to factoring. Chapter 12 is devoted to a constant that arises directly in the
expected running time of Euclid's algorithm, and Chapter 13 derives
a surprising result about a precursor of Euclid's algorithm that uses
subtraction instead of division.

The next few chapters deal largely with generating-function techniques, namely with the use of power series whose coefficients represent
the solution to a problem; standard techniques of complex variable theory allow us to deduce the behavior of those coefficients. Chapter 14,
which was in fact my first published analysis of an algorithm, shows that
several questions about sorting large quantities of data can be fruitfully
answered by studying the appropriate generating functions. A more
difficult problem, related to the size of a stack needed to traverse a
random binary tree, is tackled in Chapter 15; the solution involves surprising connections to the functions $\Gamma(z)$ and $\zeta(z)$ of classical analysis.
Chapter 16 considers an elementary process whose behavior changes
drastically (from constant growth to growth of order n) when one of
the parameters of the problem passes through a critical point; again,
generating functions give us a chance to understand what is happening.

Chapter 17 analyzes the effectiveness of cache memory, using techniques from the study of Markov processes in probability theory. Chapter 18 uses recursive integral equations to deduce the behavior of a data
structure that continually grows and shrinks; although the algorithm is
extremely simple, its analysis turns out to be inherently complex. Chapter 19 discusses a general framework for studying data structures whose
elements are randomly inserted and deleted. Recursive integral equations of another type are important in Chapter 20, which deduces the
behavior of a simple algorithm for discovering prime factors. And Chapter 21 uses multidimensional integrals in yet another way, to deal with
connectivity properties of an evolving random graph as its components
gradually merge together.

Innocuous-looking recursive functions lead to surprises that are explored in Chapter 22. Combinatorial methods prove in Chapter 23 that
an algorithm in economics related to stable allocation of goods actually
has the same analysis as a simple variant of hashing. Stability of another
kind is the subject of Chapter 24, which makes important use of three

basic techniques of algorithmic analysis: late binding, tail inequalities, and the principle of negligible perturbation. Another variation of the latter principle, often called "coupling," is exploited in Chapter 25 to derive properties of a sorting method that had long resisted analysis. Chapter 26 illustrates yet another basic technique, which subsequent researchers have generalized and named the method of Mellin transforms.

My favorite chapter of all is probably Chapter 27, which presents a modern solution to the analysis of linear probing; linear probing was the algorithm that first got me hooked on algorithmic analysis in 1962. With great satisfaction I was able in 1997 to replace my original ad hoc approaches with general high-level symbolic methods that had been developed by a number of other researchers, thereby obtaining solutions to problems well beyond what I could possibly have dreamed of doing 35 years earlier. At the same time I learned that the analysis of linear probing is intimately related to the analysis of random graphs, which I had fortuitously been studying in another context. The writing of Chapter 27 gave me a warm realization that the field of algorithmic analysis has certainly come a long way.

Global questions of complexity analysis begin in Chapters 28 and 29, which record the interesting discussions of 1973 that led to today's standard terminology for NP-complete problems. Chapters 30 and 31 are brief explorations of topics related to the two most classic questions of optimum computation: sorting with fewest comparisons, and exponentiation with fewest multiplications.

Chapter 32 considers another problem with a long history, the question of laying out a graph so that the maximum distance between related vertices is minimized. For me this chapter is especially interesting not only because of the mathematical techniques it contains, but also because I tried extra hard to develop suitable techniques of technical writing so that the proofs of two rather difficult theorems could be presented in what I hope is a pleasant and understandable way. Another exposition of a construction related to NP-completeness appears in Chapter 33; this one is somewhat simpler.

Finally, Chapter 34 introduces theoretical underpinnings for the optimum transformation of coin flips into random variables that have any given probability distribution in a given number system.

I've been blessed with the opportunity to carry out this work in collaboration with outstanding coauthors: Ole Amble, N. G. de Bruijn, Michael R. Garey, Ronald L. Graham, Svante Janson, David S. Johnson, Arne T. Jonassen, E. B. Kaehler, Ronald W. Moore, Rajeev Motwani, Christos H. Papadimitriou, Boris Pittel, Arvind Raghunathan,

Gururaj S. Rao, Stephan O. Rice, Arnold Schönhage, Francis R. Stevenson, Luis Trabb Pardo, and Andrew C. Yao. Without their help I would have been unable to make much progress on the majority of the problems whose solutions are presented here. Indeed, I am dedicating this book to N. G. "Dick" de Bruijn, because his influence can be felt on every page. Ever since the 1960s he has been my chief mentor, the main person who would answer my questions when I was stuck on a problem that I had not been taught how to solve. I originally wrote Chapter 26 for his $(3 \cdot 4 \cdot 5)$th birthday; now he is 3^4 years young as I gratefully present him with this book.

I'm also grateful for the skills of Jim C. Chou, William J. Croft, David A. Halper, Lauri Kanerva, Kimberly A. Lewis, and William E. McMechan, who helped me put hundreds of pages of typographically difficult material into a consistent digital format. The process of compiling this book has given me an incentive to improve some of the original wording, to make all of the notations consistent with *The Art of Computer Programming*, to doublecheck almost all of the mathematical formulas and the reasoning that supports them, to correct all known errors, to improve the original illustrations by redrawing them with METAPOST, and to match the bibliographic information with original sources in the library. Thus the articles now appear in a form that I hope will remain useful for at least another generation or two of scholars who will carry the work forward.

This is the fourth in a series of books that Stanford's Center for the Study of Language and Information (CSLI) plans to publish containing archival forms of the papers I have written. The first volume, *Literate Programming*, appeared in 1992; the second, *Selected Papers on Computer Science*, appeared in 1996; the third, *Digital Typography*, appeared in 1999. Four additional volumes are in preparation containing selected papers on Computer Languages, Design of Algorithms, Discrete Mathematics, Fun and Games.

Donald E. Knuth
Stanford, California
February 2000

Acknowledgments

"Mathematical Analysis of Algorithms" originally appeared in *Proceedings of IFIP Congress 71* (Amsterdam: North-Holland, 1972), pp. 19–27. Copyright ©1972 by the International Federation for Information Processing. Reprinted by permission.

"The Dangers of Computer Science Theory" originally appeared in *Logic, Methodology and Philosophy of Science* **4** (Amsterdam: North-Holland, 1973), pp. 189–195. Copyright ©1973 by North-Holland Publishing Company. Reprinted by permission of Elsevier Science.

"The Analysis of Algorithms" originally appeared in *Actes du Congrès International des Mathématiciens* **3** (Paris: Gauthier–Villars Éditeur, 1971), pp. 269–274. Copyright presently held by the author.

"Big Omicron and Big Omega and Big Theta" originally appeared in *SIGACT News* **8**, 2 (April–June 1976), pp. 18–24. Copyright ©1976 by Association for Computing Machinery, Inc. Reprinted by permission.

"Optimal Measurement Points for Program Frequency Counts" originally appeared in *BIT* **13** (1973), pp. 313–322. Copyright ©1973 by Nordisk Tidskrift for Informationsbehandling. Reprinted by permission.

"Estimating the Efficiency of Backtrack Programs" originally appeared in *Mathematics of Computation* **29** (1975), pp. 121–136. Copyright ©1975 by American Mathematical Society. Reprinted by permission.

"Ordered Hash Tables" originally appeared in *The Computer Journal* **17** (May 1974), pp. 135–142. Copyright ©1974 by The British Computer Society. Reprinted by permission.

"Activity in an Interleaved Memory" originally appeared in *IEEE Transactions on Computers* **C-24** (1975), pp. 943–944. Copyright ©1975 by The Institute of Electrical and Electronics Engineers, Inc. Reprinted by permission.

"An Analysis of Alpha-Beta Pruning" originally appeared in *Artificial Intelligence* **6** (1975), pp. 293–326. Copyright ©1975 by North-Holland Publishing Company. Reprinted by permission of Elsevier Science.

"Notes on Generalized Dedekind Sums" originally appeared in *Acta Arithmetica* **33** (1977), pp. 297–325. Copyright ©1977 by the Institute of Mathematics, Polish Academy of Sciences. Reprinted by permission.

"The Distribution of Continued Fraction Approximations" originally appeared in *Journal of Number Theory* **19** (1984), pp. 443–448. Copyright ©1984 by Academic Press. Reprinted by permission.

"Evaluation of Porter's Constant" originally appeared in *Computers and Mathematics with Applications* **2** (1976), pp. 137–139. Copyright ©1976 by Pergamon Press. Reprinted by permission of Elsevier Science.

"Analysis of the Subtractive Algorithm for Greatest Common Divisors" originally appeared in *Proceedings of the National Academy of Sciences of the United States of America* **72** (1975), pp. 4720–4722. Copyright ©1975 by the author.

Chapter 1

Mathematical Analysis of Algorithms

[An invited address presented to the Congress of the International Federation for Information Processing in Ljubljana, Yugoslavia, August 1971. Originally published in Proceedings of IFIP Congress 71 (Amsterdam: North-Holland, 1972), 19–27.]

Typical techniques for analyzing the efficiency of algorithms are illustrated by considering two problems in detail, namely (a) the problem of rearranging data without using auxiliary memory space, and (b) the problem of finding the element of rank t when n elements are ranked by some linear ordering relation. Both problems lead to interesting applications of discrete mathematics to computer science.

1. Introduction

The general field of algorithmic analysis is an interesting and potentially important area of mathematics and computer science that is undergoing rapid development. The central goal in such studies is to make quantitative assessments of the "goodness" of various algorithms. Two general kinds of problems are usually treated:

Type A. Analysis of a particular algorithm. In a Type A analysis we investigate important characteristics of some algorithm, usually by doing a *frequency analysis* (to determine how many times each part of the algorithm is likely to be executed), or a *storage analysis* (to determine how much memory it is likely to need). For example, we often are able to predict the execution time of various algorithms for sorting numbers into order.

Type B. Analysis of a class of algorithms. In a Type B analysis we investigate the entire family of algorithms for solving a particular problem, and attempt to identify one that is "best possible." Or we place bounds on the *computational complexity* of the algorithms in the

1

class. For example, it is possible to estimate the minimum number $S(n)$ of comparisons necessary to sort n numbers by repeated comparison.

Type A analyses have been used since the earliest days of computer programming; each program in Goldstine and von Neumann's classic memoir [9] on "Planning and Coding Problems for an Electronic Computing Instrument" is accompanied by a careful estimate of the "durations" of each step and of the total program duration. Such analyses make it possible to compare different algorithms for the same problem.

Type B analyses were not undertaken until somewhat later, although certain of the problems had been studied for many years as parts of "recreational mathematics." Hugo Steinhaus analyzed the sorting function $S(n)$, in connection with a weighing problem [18]; and the question of computing x^n with fewest multiplications was raised by H. Dellac as early as 1894 [3]. Perhaps the first true study of computational complexity was the 1956 thesis of H. B. Demuth [4], who defined three simple classes of automata and studied how rapidly such automata are able to sort n numbers, using any conceivable algorithm.

It may seem that Type B analyses are far superior to those of Type A, since they handle infinitely many algorithms at once; instead of analyzing each algorithm that is invented, we obviously prefer to prove once and for all that a particular algorithm is the "best possible." But this observation is true only to a limited extent, since Type B analyses are extremely technology-dependent; very slight changes in the definition of "best possible" can significantly affect which algorithm is best. For example, x^{31} cannot be calculated with fewer than 9 multiplications, but it can be done with only 6 arithmetic operations if division is allowed.

In fact the first result in Demuth's pioneering work on computational complexity was that "bubble sorting" is the optimum sorting method for a certain class of automata. Unfortunately, Type A analyses show that bubble sorting is almost always the *worst* possible way to sort, of all known methods, in spite of the fact that it is optimum from one particular standpoint.

There are two main reasons that Type B analyses do not supersede Type A analyses. First, Type B generally requires us to formulate a rather simple model of the complexity, by abstracting what seem to be the most relevant aspects of the class of algorithms considered, in order to make any progress at all. These simplified models are often sufficiently unrealistic that they lead to impractical algorithms. Secondly, even with simple models of complexity, the Type B analyses tend to be considerably difficult, and comparatively few problems have been solved. Even the problem of computing x^n with fewest multiplications is far from being thoroughly understood (see [13, §4.6.3]), and the exact value of $S(n)$ is known only for $n \leq 12$ and $n = 20, 21$ (see [15, §5.3.1]). The sorting method of Ford and Johnson [8] uses fewer comparisons than any other technique currently known in 1971, yet it is hardly ever useful in practice since it requires a rather unwieldy program. Comparison counting is not a good enough way to rate a sorting algorithm.

Thus I believe that computer scientists might well look on research in computational complexity as mathematicians traditionally view number theory: Complexity analysis provides an interesting way to sharpen our tools for the more routine problems we face from day to day. Although Type B analyses are extremely interesting, they do not deserve all the glory; Type A analyses are probably even more important in practice, since they can be designed to measure all of the relevant factors about the performance of an algorithm, and they are not quite as sensitive to changes in technology.

Fortunately, Type A analyses are stimulating intellectual challenges in their own right; nearly every algorithm that isn't extremely complicated leads to interesting mathematical questions. But of course we don't need to analyze every algorithm that is invented, and we can't hope to have a precise theoretical analysis of any really big programs.

In this paper I shall try to illustrate the flavor of some current work in algorithmic analysis by making rather detailed analyses of two algorithms. Since I was asked to be "mathematical," I have chosen some examples that are interesting primarily from a theoretical standpoint. The procedures I shall discuss (namely, *in situ* permutation and selecting the tth largest of n elements) are not among the ten most important algorithms in the world, but they are not completely useless and their analysis does involve several important concepts. Furthermore they are sufficiently unimportant that comparatively few people have studied them closely, hence I am able to say a few new things about them at this time.

2. In Situ Permutation

As a first example, let us consider the problem of replacing a one-dimensional array $(x_1, x_2, \ldots, x_n)$ by $(x_{p(1)}, x_{p(2)}, \ldots, x_{p(n)})$, where p is a permutation of $\{1, 2, \ldots, n\}$. The algorithm is supposed to permute the x's in place, using only a bounded amount of auxiliary memory. The function p is one of the inputs to the algorithm; we can compute $p(k)$ for any k but we cannot assign a new value to $p(k)$ as the algorithm proceeds. For example, p might be the function corresponding to the transposition of a rectangular matrix, or to the unscrambling of a finite Fourier transform.

If $(p(1), p(2), \ldots, p(n))$ were stored in a read/write memory, or if we were allowed to manipulate n extra "tag" bits specifying how much of the permutation has been carried out at any time, there would be simple ways to design such an algorithm whose running time is essentially proportional to n. But we are not allowed to change p dynamically, nor are we allowed n bits of extra memory. Thus there seem to be comparatively few solutions to the problem.

The desired rearrangement of $(x_1, x_2, \ldots, x_n)$ is most naturally done by following the cycle structure of p (see [12, §1.3.3]). Let us say that j is a "cycle leader" if $j \leq p(j)$, $j \leq p(p(j))$, $j \leq p(p(p(j)))$, etc.; each cycle of the permutation has a unique leader, and so the following procedure due to J. C. Gower (see also Windley [20] and MacLeod [16]) carries out the desired permutation by doing each cycle when its leader is detected:

1	**for** $j := 1$ **step** 1 **until** n **do**	1
2	**begin comment** the permutation has been	n
3	done on all cycles with leader $< j$;	n
4	$k := p(j);$	n
5	**while** $k > j$ **do**	$n + a$
6	$k := p(k);$	a
7	**if** $k = j$ **then**	n
8	**begin comment** j is a cycle leader;	b
9	$y := x[j];\ \ l := p(k);$	b
10	**while** $l \neq j$ **do**	$b + c$
11	**begin** $x[k] := x[l];\ \ k := l;\ \ l := p(k)$ **end**;	c
12	$x[k] := y;$	b
13	**end** permutation on cycle;	b
14	**end** loop on j.	n

The first and most basic part of the analysis of any algorithm is, of course, to prove that the algorithm works. The comments in this program essentially provide the key inductive assertions that will lead to such a proof. On the other hand, the program seems to be beyond the present range of "automatic program verification" techniques, and to go a step further to "automatic frequency analysis" is almost unthinkable.

Let us now do a frequency analysis of the above program, counting how often each statement is executed and each condition is tested. There are 9 statements and 3 conditions, but we don't have to solve 12 separate problems because there are obvious relations between the frequencies.

"Kirchhoff's law," which says that the number of times we get to any given place in the program is the number of times we leave it, makes it possible to reduce the 12 individual frequencies to only 4, namely $n, a, b,$ and c, as shown in the column to the right of the program. Kirchhoff's law is especially easy to apply in this case, since there are no **go to** statements; for example, we must test the condition "$k > j$" in line 5 exactly $n + a$ times, if we execute line 4 n times and line 6 a times.

The next step in a frequency analysis is to interpret the remaining unknowns in terms of characteristics of the data. Obviously n, the number of times we do line 4, is the number of elements in the vector x. And b is the number of cycles in the permutation p. Furthermore we can see that each element of x is assigned a new value exactly once, either on line 11 or line 12, hence $c + b = n$ (a relation that cannot be deduced solely from Kirchhoff's law). Thus only one variable, a, remains to be interpreted; it is somewhat more complicated, the sum of "distances" from j to the first element of $(p(j), p(p(j)), \dots)$ that is $\leq j$.

To complete the analysis we should explore the behavior of these quantities a and b. It is customary to start by making a "worst case" analysis, which leads to an upper bound on the program's running time. If $(p(1), p(2), \dots, p(n)) = (2, \dots, n, 1)$, we have $a = (n-1) + (n-2) + \dots + 0 = \frac{1}{2}(n^2 - n)$, which is surely the worst case for a.

The same choice of p makes $b = 1$, which is the best case for b. If $(p(1), p(2), \dots, p(n)) = (1, 2, \dots, n)$, we get the worst case for b (and the best for a).

A more interesting problem arises when we try to consider the *average* case. First we must decide what is meant by the average case; this is often the chief stumbling block in making a Type A analysis, since "typical" input distributions are not always easy to specify. For the problem at hand we may say that each of the $n!$ permutations p is equally likely.

A special transformation of permutations is often useful when cycle properties are being considered (see Foata [7] and Knuth [12, §1.3.3], [15, §5.1.2]), since it changes cycle properties into ordering properties. Consider for example the permutation $(p(1), \dots, p(9)) = (8, 2, 7, 1, 6, 9, 3, 4, 5)$; in cycle form this is $(184)(569)(2)(73)$ because $p(1) = 8$, $p(8) = 4$, $p(4) = 1$, $p(5) = 6$, $p(6) = 9$, $p(9) = 5$, $p(2) = 2$, $p(7) = 3$, and $p(3) = 7$. The cycle form can be written in exactly one way such that

(a) the leader comes first in each cycle;
(b) the leaders of different cycles are in decreasing order from left to right.

In our example this canonical representation is $(569)(37)(2)(184)$. And the parentheses are redundant in canonical form, since ")(" occurs just before each number that is smaller than all of its predecessors. Thus we obtain a one-to-one mapping of permutations onto permutations, such that cycle properties are mapped into ordering properties. In our example, $(8, 2, 7, 1, 6, 9, 3, 4, 5)$ maps into $(5, 6, 9, 3, 7, 2, 1, 8, 4)$.

Suppose $(p(1), p(2), \dots, p(n))$ is mapped by this process into the permutation $(q(1), q(2), \dots, q(n))$. We can easily reinterpret the quantity b in terms of this transformation: b is the number of cycles in p, so it is the number of "left-to-right minima" in q, namely the number of indices j such that $q(j) = \min\{q(i) \mid 1 \leq i \leq j\}$. This quantity has been analyzed in detail in [12, §1.2.10], where the number of permutations with k left-to-right minima is shown to be $\left[{n \atop k}\right]$, a Stirling number of the first kind. The average value of b is shown there to be H_n, and the variance is $H_n - H_n^{(2)}$, where

$$H_n = 1 + \frac{1}{2} + \cdots + \frac{1}{n} \qquad \text{and} \qquad H_n^{(2)} = 1 + \frac{1}{4} + \cdots + \frac{1}{n^2}$$

are harmonic numbers of degrees 1 and 2.

We can also analyze the quantity a, although that problem is somewhat deeper. When the loop variable j in the algorithm takes on the value $q(i)$, the auxiliary variable k will take on the successive values $q(i + 1)$, $q(i + 2)$, ... because of the way we obtained q from p; we continue until reaching a value $q(i + r) < q(i)$. There is an exception to this rule, namely if k is set equal to the leader of the cycle: Then either $i + r > n$ or $q(i+r)$ is the leader of the *next* cycle; but in the latter case, again $q(i + r) < q(i)$.

Consequently we can represent a in the following way. Let the quantities y_{ij} be functions of q defined for all $1 \leq i < j \leq n$ as follows:

$$y_{ij} = \begin{cases} 1, & \text{if } q(i) < q(k) \text{ for } i < k \leq j; \\ 0, & \text{otherwise.} \end{cases}$$

Then

$$a = \sum_{1 \leq i < j \leq n} y_{ij};$$

indeed, for fixed i, $\sum_{i < j \leq n} y_{ij}$ is the number of times line 6 of the program is performed when the loop variable j is equal to $q(i)$.

For example, if $(p(1), \dots, p(9)) = (8, 2, 7, 1, 6, 9, 3, 4, 5)$ we have seen that $(q(1), \dots, q(9)) = (5, 6, 9, 3, 7, 2, 1, 8, 4)$; hence $y_{12} = y_{13} = y_{23} =$

$y_{45} = y_{78} = y_{79} = 1$, and all other y's are zero. Line 6 is performed $(2, 1, 0, 1, 0, 0, 2, 0, 0)$ times when $j = (5, 6, 9, 3, 7, 2, 1, 8, 4)$ respectively.

Let $\overline{y}_{ij}$ be the average value of y_{ij}, as $(q(1), \ldots, q(n))$ ranges over all permutations. This is simply the number of permutations with $y_{ij} = 1$, divided by $n!$, so it is the probability that $q(i) = \min\{q(k) \,|\, i \le k \le j\}$, namely $1/(j-i+1)$. It follows that $\overline{a}$, the average value of a, is given by

$$\overline{a} = \sum_{1 \le i < j \le n} \overline{y}_{ij} = \sum_{1 \le i < j \le n} \frac{1}{j - i + 1}$$

$$= \sum_{2 \le r \le n} \frac{n + 1 - r}{r};$$

in the last equation we have replaced $j - i + 1$ by a new variable r that occurs $n + 1 - r$ times in the original sum. Hence

$$\overline{a} = (n+1) \sum_{2 \le r \le n} \frac{1}{r} - \sum_{2 \le r \le n} 1 = (n+1)(H_n - 1) - (n-1) = (n+1)H_n - 2n.$$

The variance of a can be calculated too; the derivation is instructive but quite complicated, so the details will only be summarized here. We need the average value of

$$\left(\sum_{1 \le i < j \le n} y_{ij} \right)^2 = \sum_{1 \le i < j \le n} y_{ij}^2 + \sum_{\substack{1 \le i < j \le n \\ 1 \le k < l \le n \\ (i,j) \ne (k,l)}} y_{ij} y_{kl}$$

$$= \sum_{1 \le i < j \le n} \overline{y}_{ij}$$

$$+ 2 \sum_{1 \le i < j < k < l \le n} (y_{ij}y_{kl} + y_{ik}y_{jl} + y_{il}y_{jk})$$

$$+ 2 \sum_{1 \le i < j < k \le n} (y_{ij}y_{jk} + y_{ik}y_{jk} + y_{ij}y_{ik})$$

$$= \overline{a} + 2(A + B + C + D + E + F)$$

where the letters $A, \ldots, F$ represent the sums $\sum y_{ij}y_{kl}, \ldots, \sum y_{ij}y_{ik}$. When the indices $i < j < k < l$ are fixed, it is not difficult to prove that the average value of $y_{ij}y_{kl}$ is $1/(j-i+1)(l-k+1)$; similarly, the average of $y_{ik}y_{jl}$ is $1/(l-i+1)(l-j+1)$, the average of $y_{il}y_{jk}$ is $1/(l-i+1)(k-j+1)$, the average of $y_{ij}y_{jk} = y_{ik}y_{jk}$ is $1/(k-i+1)(k-j+1)$, and the average of $y_{ij}y_{ik} = y_{ik}$ is $1/(k-i+1)$. We are left with several triple and quadruple summations to perform; it is not difficult to carry out a few of the sums, reducing them to

$$B = \binom{n}{2} - 2Z, \quad C = Y - Z - 2\binom{n}{2} + 3X,$$

$$D = E = Z - X, \quad F = \binom{n}{2} - 2X,$$

where

$$X = \sum_{1 \le i < j \le n} \frac{1}{j - i + 1},$$

$$Y = \sum_{1 \le i < j \le n} H_{j-i},$$

$$Z = \sum_{1 \le i < j \le n} \frac{1}{j - i + 1} H_{j-i}.$$

We have already summed X by replacing $j-i+1$ by r, and the same device works for Y and Z. After applying well-known formulas for dealing with harmonic numbers (see [12, §1.2.7]), we therefore obtain

$$X = (n+1)H_n - 2n,$$

$$Y = \frac{1}{2}(n^2 + n)H_n - \frac{3}{4}n^2 - \frac{1}{4}n,$$

$$Z = \frac{1}{2}(n+1)(H_n^2 - H_n^{(2)}) - nH_n + n.$$

This determines B, C, D, E, and F. The quantity A is harder to deal with; we have

$$A = \sum_{1 \le i < j < k < l \le n} \frac{1}{(j - i + 1)(l - k + 1)}$$

$$= \sum_{\substack{r \ge 2 \\ s \ge 2 \\ r+s \le n}} \frac{1}{rs} \binom{n - r - s + 2}{2}$$

$$= \sum_{\substack{2 \le r \le t-2 \\ 4 \le t \le n}} \frac{1}{t} \left(\frac{1}{r} + \frac{1}{t-r} \right) \binom{n-t+2}{2}$$

$$= 2 \sum_{\substack{2 \le r \le t-2 \\ 4 \le t \le n}} \frac{1}{rt} \binom{n-t+2}{2}$$

$$= \sum_{\substack{2 \le r \le t-2 \\ 4 \le t \le n}} \frac{1}{rt} \left((n+2)(n+1) - t(2n+3) + t^2 \right)$$

$$= (n+2)(n+1)U - (2n+3)V + W$$

if we let $r = j - i + 1$, $s = l - k + 1$, $t = r + s$. Then

$$U = \frac{1}{2}(H_n - 1)^2 - \frac{1}{2}H_n^{(2)} + \frac{1}{n},$$
$$V = (n-1)H_{n-2} - 2n + 4,$$
$$W = \frac{1}{2}\left((n^2 + n - 2)(H_{n-2} - 1) - \frac{1}{2}(n-1)(n-2) + 1 - 3(n-3) \right).$$

Putting the whole mess together, and subtracting $\bar{a}^2$ from the average of a^2, gives the exact value of the variance,

$$\sigma^2 = 2n^2 - (n+1)^2 H_n^{(2)} - (n+1)H_n + 4n.$$

(This is a calculation that should have been done on a computer. People are now working on computer systems for symbolic computations such as this.)

Taking asymptotic values, we can summarize the statistics as follows:

$$a = \left(\min 0, \quad \text{ave } n \ln n + O(n), \quad \max \tfrac{1}{2}(n^2 - n), \right.$$
$$\left. \text{dev } \sqrt{2 - \pi^2/6} \, n + O(\log n) \right);$$
$$b = \left(\min 1, \quad \text{ave } \ln n + O(1), \quad \max n, \quad \text{dev } \sqrt{\ln n} + O(1) \right).$$

The total running time of the algorithm is therefore of order $n \log n$ on the average, although the worst case is order n^2; the comparatively small standard deviation indicates that worst-case behavior is very rare.

This completes our frequency analysis of the given algorithm for *in situ* permutation. What information have we learned? We have found that the algorithm almost always takes about $n \log n$ steps, and that lines 5 and 6 are the "inner loop," which consumes most of the computation time.

The analysis of one algorithm often applies to another algorithm as well. For example, the quantity a we have just studied appears also in the analysis of an algorithm to compute the inverse of a permutation [12, Algorithm 1.3.3J].

Our analysis can also be extended to measure the advisability of incorporating various refinements into the algorithm. For example, suppose that we introduce a new counter variable called *tally*, which is initially set to n. In line 11, and also in line 12, we will insert the statement '*tally* := *tally* − 1'; then at the end of line 12 we can insert a new test, '**if** *tally* = 0 **then go to** *exit*', where *exit* ends the program. This modification (see MacLeod [16]) will terminate the algorithm more quickly, since it stops the j loop when the largest leader has been found. At the cost of 1 more variable, 1 execution of the statement '*tally* := n', n executions of '*tally* := *tally* − 1', and $b \approx \log n$ tests '**if** *tally* = 0', we save some of the work in lines 2–7 and we need no longer test "**if** $j > n$" to see whether the j loop is exhausted. How much is saved? The number of iterations of lines 4 and 7 is clearly reduced from n to $q(1)$, where $(p(1), p(2), \ldots, p(n))$ maps into $(q(1), q(2), \ldots, q(n))$ as above; so the average saving there is $\frac{1}{n}(n-1+\cdots+1+0) = \frac{1}{2}(n-1)$. The number of iterations of line 6, the main loop, is reduced by $\sum_{2 \leq i < j \leq n}[q(1) < q(i)] \, y_{ij}$, an average saving of

$$\sum_{2 \leq i < j \leq n} \frac{1}{(j-i+1)(j-i)} = \sum_{2 \leq r \leq n} \frac{n-r}{r(r-1)} = n - 1 - H_{n-1}.$$

So this change improves the average running time slightly. Another $\frac{1}{2}(n-1)$ iterations of line 6 can be saved by making use of the fact that j is always a cycle leader when $j = 1$. Neither of these improvements decreases the asymptotic running time as $n \to \infty$, however, because they leave the coefficient of $n \log n$ unchanged.

The application to rectangular matrix transposition suggests that we might also design a similar algorithm in which the inverse function p^- is given as well as p. Then we could look for a cycle leader by first testing $p(j)$, then $p^-(j)$, $p(p(j))$, $p^-(p^-(j))$, etc., until finding a value $\leq j$. It turns out that the average number of operations performed is the same as in our first algorithm, but the worst case is reduced to $O(n \log n)$. (I learned this fact from John Hopcroft; it solves a problem stated by MacLeod [16].)

It is amusing to derive the latter $n \log n$ bound by obtaining the *exact* maximum number $f(n)$ of steps needed to rule out each of the non-leaders, while processing an n-cycle, if we assume that both $p^k(j)$ and $p^{-k}(j)$ are fetched simultaneously in one step. Consider first placing the element 1, then 2, then 3, etc., into an initially empty cycle so as to obtain the worst case; we obtain the recurrence

$$f(1) = 0,$$
$$f(n) = \max_{1 \le k < n} \big(\min(k, n - k) + f(k) + f(n - k)\big).$$

The solution to this recurrence is quite interesting; it turns out to be $f(n) = \sum_{0 \le k < n} \nu(k)$, where $\nu(k)$ is the number of 1s in the binary representation of k. If $a_1 > a_2 > \cdots > a_r$, we have

$$f(2^{a_1} + 2^{a_2} + \cdots + 2^{a_r}) = \frac{1}{2}\big(a_1 2^{a_1} + (a_2+2)2^{a_2} + \cdots + (a_r+2r-2)2^{a_r}\big).$$

The fact that this function satisfies the recurrence can be proved by letting $g(m, n) = f(m+n) - m - f(m) - f(n)$, and showing that $g(2m, 2n) = 2g(m, n)$, $g(2m + 1, 2n) = g(m, n) + g(m + 1, n)$, $g(2m, 2n + 1) = g(m, n) + g(m, n+1)$, $g(2m+1, 2n+1) = 1 + g(m+1, n) + g(m, n+1)$; hence by induction $g(m, n) \ge 0$ when $m \le n$, with equality when $m = n$ or $m = n - 1$. (Asymptotic properties of $f(n)$ have been studied by Bush [2], Mirsky [17], Drazin and Griffith [5].)

So much for Type A analyses of *in situ* permutation; what can be said about the computational complexity of this problem? I don't really know; it seems reasonable to conjecture that every algorithm for *in situ* permutation will require at least $n \log n$ steps on the average, but I don't know how to prove it.

In the first place there is a difficulty in defining the idea of a "step"; the frequency analysis above assumes that $p(k)$ can be calculated in one step, and that $x[k]$ can be fetched or stored in one step, for arbitrary k between 1 and n. A complexity analysis must, however, consider the limit as $n \to \infty$; an algorithm that works optimally for all $n \le n_0$ could be set up with something like $n_0!$ branches, and that would be uninteresting. But as $n \to \infty$, we need at least $\log n$ steps just to *look at* the number k when we are dealing with $p(k)$ or $x[k]$, so the program above really takes $n(\log n)^2$ steps instead of $n \log n$, as $n \to \infty$. On the other hand, no programmer really believes that the given algorithm really takes $\log n$ steps each time $x[k]$ is fetched or stored, since the time is bounded for any reasonable value of n that arises in practice. In other words, we want a complexity measure that models the situation for practical ranges of n, even though the model is unrealistic as $n \to \infty$, and in spite of the fact that we require the algorithm to be valid for arbitrarily large n.

A second difficulty is how to phrase the constraint of "bounded auxiliary memory." If we assume that the x's are integers, and if we allow arithmetic operations to be carried out, we could replace each $x[k]$ by $2x[k]$ and use the units digits as n extra tag bits. If operations on the x's are forbidden, yet auxiliary integer variables like j, k, l are allowed as in the algorithm above, we could still get the effect of n extra bits of memory by doing arithmetic on an integer variable whose value ranges from 0 to $2^n - 1$; on the other hand, it isn't obvious that any algorithm with running time $O(n)$ could be designed even when such a trick is used.

These considerations suggest a possible model of the problem. Consider a device with n^c states, for some constant c. Each state deterministically specifies a "step" of the computation by (a) specifying numbers i and j with $1 \leq i \leq j \leq n$, such that $x[i]$ is to be interchanged with $x[j]$; and (b) specifying n states $(q_1, \ldots, q_n)$ and a number k, such that the next step is $q_{p(k)}$. Can such a device do the rearrangement in $O(n)$ steps, or are $n \log n$ steps needed? (See the Appendix for a precise formulation of this question.)

3. Selecting the tth Largest

Now let us turn to another problem, this time somewhat less academic. C. A. R. Hoare [10] has given a method for finding the tth largest of n elements, by making repeated comparisons, and F. E. J. Kruseman Aretz has shown (see [19]) that Hoare's method makes approximately $(2 + 2 \ln 2)n$ comparisons when finding the median element in the case $t = (n + 1)/2$. Our goal is to do a partial frequency analysis of the algorithm, determining the exact average number of comparisons that are made, as a function of t and n.

I shall state the algorithm informally, since I am not attempting to make a frequency analysis of each step. Let $(x[1], \ldots, x[n])$ be the given elements, and assume that they are distinct. We start by selecting an arbitrary element y and comparing it to each of the $n - 1$ others, rearranging the other elements (as in "quicksort") so that all elements $> y$ appear in positions $x[1]$, ..., $x[k - 1]$ while all elements $< y$ appear in positions $x[k + 1]$, ..., $x[n]$. Thus, y is the kth largest. If $k = t$, we are done; if $k > t$ we use the same method to find the tth largest of $(x[1], \ldots, x[k - 1])$; and if $k < t$ we find the $(t - k)$th largest of $(x[k + 1], \ldots, x[n])$. A very interesting formalization and proof of this procedure has recently been given by Hoare [11].

Let $C_{n,t}$ be the average number of comparisons made by Hoare's selection algorithm, when the elements are in random order. We have

$$C_{1,1} = 0;$$

$$C_{n,t} = n - 1 + \frac{1}{n}(A_{n,t} + B_{n,t}), \quad \text{for } 1 \le t \le n \text{ and } n \ge 2,$$

where

$$A_{n,t} = C_{n-1,t-1} + C_{n-2,t-2} + \cdots + C_{n-t+1,1},$$
$$B_{n,t} = C_{t,t} + C_{t+1,t} + \cdots + C_{n-1,t}.$$

This is not the kind of recurrence that we would ordinarily expect to be able to solve, but let us make the attempt anyway. The first step in problems of this kind is to get rid of the sums, by noting that

$$A_{n+1,t+1} = A_{n,t} + C_{n,t} \quad \text{and} \quad B_{n+1,t} = B_{n,t} + C_{n,t};$$

these identities allow us to eliminate the A's and B's, getting a "pure" recurrence in the C's:

$$(n+1)C_{n+1,t+1} - nC_{n,t+1} - nC_{n,t} + (n-1)C_{n-1,t}$$
$$= (n+1)n - n(n-1) - n(n-1) + (n-1)(n-2)$$
$$+ A_{n+1,t+1} - A_{n,t+1} - A_{n,t} + A_{n-1,t}$$
$$+ B_{n+1,t+1} - B_{n,t+1} - B_{n,t} + B_{n-1,t}$$
$$= 2 + C_{n,t} - C_{n-1,t} + C_{n,t+1} - C_{n-1,t}.$$

In other words

$$C_{n+1,t+1} - C_{n,t+1} - C_{n,t} + C_{n-1,t} = 2/(n+1). \tag{$*$}$$

What an extraordinary coincidence that $n + 1$ was a common factor on each of the C variables remaining! This phenomenon suggests that we may actually be able to solve the recurrence after all.

Checking the derivation shows that formula $(*)$ is valid for $1 < t < n$; we need to look at the boundary conditions next, when $t = 1$ or $t = n$:

$$C_{n,1} = n - 1 + \frac{1}{n}(C_{1,1} + C_{2,1} + \cdots + C_{n-1,1});$$

$$(n+1)C_{n+1,1} - nC_{n,1} = (n+1)n - n(n-1) + C_{n,1};$$

$$C_{n+1,1} - C_{n,1} = 2n/(n+1) = 2 - 2/(n+1).$$

The latter recurrence is easily solved, $C_{n,1} = 2n - 2H_n$. By symmetry, $C_{n,n} = 2n - 2H_n$ also. Now the recurrence

$$(C_{n+1,t+1} - C_{n,t}) - (C_{n,t+1} - C_{n-1,t}) = 2/(n+1)$$

implies that

$$C_{n+1,t+1} - C_{n,t} = \frac{2}{n+1} + \frac{2}{n} + \cdots + \frac{2}{t+2} + C_{t+1,t+1} - C_{t,t}$$

$$= 2(H_{n+1} - H_{t+1}) + 2 - 2/(t+1),$$

and this relation can likewise be iterated:

$$C_{n,t} = 2 \sum_{2 \le k \le t} (H_{n-t+k} - H_k + 1 - 1/k) + C_{n+1-t,1}.$$

Thus, finally, we have the solution

$$C_{n,t} = 2\big((n+1)H_n - (n+3-t)H_{n+1-t} - (t+2)H_t + n + 3\big),$$

valid for $1 \le t \le n$. In the special case when we are calculating the median of $n = 2t - 1$ elements, the average number of comparisons comes to

$$4t(H_{2t-1} - H_t) + 4t - 8H_t + 4$$

$$= (4 + 4\ln 2)t - 8\ln t + 1 - 8\gamma + O(t^{-1}).$$

A Type B analysis of this problem is essentially the question "What is the smallest number of comparisons needed to select the tth largest of n elements?" There are really two questions, depending on whether we want to minimize comparisons in the worst case or in the average case.

When $t = 1$, the questions are easily answered: We always need at least $n - 1$ comparisons to determine the largest element. For if we consider each comparison as a match in a knockout tournament, every player except the champion must lose at least one game. This argument can be extended also to the case $t = 2$, to show that an algorithm to determine the second best player must use at least $n - 2 + \lceil \log_2 n \rceil$ comparisons, a result first stated by J. Schreier in 1932 and first proved rigorously by S. S. Kislitsyn in 1964. (See [15, §5.3.3].)

When $t = 3$ the minimum number of comparisons in the worst case is still not known; and the minimum *average* number of comparisons is not even known when $t = 2$.

Some very interesting asymptotic results on the complexity of selection have recently been obtained. Blum, Floyd, Pratt, Rivest, and Tarjan [1] have shown that at most about $5.2n$ comparisons are needed in the worst case to determine the tth largest of n elements, for all t and n. R. W. Floyd [6] has discovered that the *average* number of comparisons needed for selection can be reduced to $n+\min(t, n+1-t)+o(n)$. In particular, he has developed an algorithm that selects the median of n elements while making an average of only $\frac{3}{2}n + O(n^{2/3}\log n)$ comparisons; and he has proved that at least $\frac{5}{4}n + o(n)$ comparisons are always necessary on the average, no matter what algorithm is used.

4. Summary

I have tried to indicate the nature of algorithmic analysis by describing two nontrivial problems in detail. Perhaps the complexities of these examples have obscured the main points I wanted to make, so I will attempt to summarize what I think is most important.

1. Analysis of algorithms is an interesting activity that contributes to our fundamental understanding of computer science. In this case, mathematics is being applied to computer problems, instead of applying computers to mathematical problems.

2. Analysis of algorithms relies heavily on techniques of discrete mathematics such as the manipulation of harmonic numbers, the solution of difference equations, and combinatorial enumeration theory. Most of these topics are not presently being taught in colleges and universities, but they should form a part of many computer scientists' education.

3. Analysis of algorithms is beginning to take shape as a coherent discipline. Instead of using a different trick for each problem, we are able to use some reasonably systematic techniques. (Numerous examples of these unifying principles may be found by consulting the entries under "Analysis of algorithms" in the indexes to [12], [13], and [15].) Furthermore, the analysis of one algorithm often applies to other algorithms.

4. Many fascinating problems in this area are still waiting to be solved.

5. Appendix

The complexity of *in situ* permutation can be studied by defining a special kind of automaton. Let us say that a Rearrangement Device M_n for rearranging n elements is a quadruple $(\Sigma, \delta, q_0, q_f)$, where Σ is a finite set of states including an initial state q_0 and a final state q_f, and where δ is a transition function mapping Σ into $[1 \mathbin{..} n]^3 \times \Sigma^n$. Given a permutation $(p(1), \ldots, p(n))$ and an array of elements $(x[1], \ldots, x[n])$, the device operates as follows, starting in state q_0: Upon reaching a state $q \neq q_f$, where $\delta(q) = (i, j, k, q_1, \ldots, q_n)$, the device interchanges $x[i]$ with $x[j]$ and goes to state $q_{p(k)}$. After some finite number $T(M_n, p)$ of steps, the final state q_f should be reached, and the device halts; at this time it is supposed to have rearranged the x's according to p.

For example, the program in Section 2 above essentially corresponds to a rearrangement device with $n^3 + n^2 + n + 1$ states

$$\Sigma = 0 \times [1 \mathbin{..} n + 1] \cup 1 \times [1 \mathbin{..} n]^2 \cup 2 \times [1 \mathbin{..} n]^3,$$

where $q_0 = (0, 1)$, $q_f = (0, n + 1)$, and

$$\delta(0, j) = (1, 1, j, (1, j, 1), \ldots, (1, j, n));$$

$$\delta(1, j, k) = \begin{cases} (1, 1, k, (1, j, 1), \ldots, (1, j, n)), & \text{if } k > j; \\ (1, 1, j, (2, j, j, 1), \ldots, (2, j, j, n)), & \text{if } k = j; \\ (1, 1, 1, (0, j + 1), \ldots, (0, j + 1)), & \text{if } k < j; \end{cases}$$

$$\delta(2, j, k, l) = \begin{cases} (k, l, l, (2, j, l, 1), \ldots, (2, j, l, n)), & \text{if } k \neq l; \\ (1, 1, 1, (0, j + 1), \ldots, (0, j + 1)), & \text{if } k = l. \end{cases}$$

Notice that the auxiliary variables j, k, and l have been encoded as part of the states.

The analysis above shows that $T(M_n, p) \sim nH_n$ for almost all p on this device, although some permutations will require order n^2.

I conjecture that no Rearrangement Device is substantially better than this. A more precise conjecture is the following: Given any constant c there is a constant K such that all Rearrangement Devices M_n with at most n^c states satisfy

$$\frac{1}{n!} \sum_p T(M_n, p) \geq Kn \log n.$$

This research was supported in part by the National Science Foundation.

References

[1] Manuel Blum, Robert W. Floyd, Vaughan Pratt, Ronald L. Rivest and Robert E. Tarjan, "Time bounds for selection," *Journal of Computer and System Sciences* **7** (1973), 448–461.

[2] L. E. Bush, "An asymptotic formula for the average sum of the digits of integers," *American Mathematical Monthly* **47** (1940), 154–156.

[3] H. Dellac, "Question 49," *L'Intermédiaire des Mathématiciens* **1** (1894), 20.

[4] H. B. Demuth, *Electronic Data Sorting* (Ph.D. thesis, Stanford University, 1956), 92 pages. Partially reprinted in *IEEE Transactions on Computers* **C-34** (1985), 296–310.

[5] M. P. Drazin and J. Stanley Griffith, "On the decimal representation of integers," *Proceedings of the Cambridge Philosophical Society* **48** (1952), 555–565.

[6] R. W. Floyd, "Notes on computing medians, percentiles, etc.," unpublished memorandum (1971).   See Robert W. Floyd and Ronald L. Rivest, "Expected time bounds for selection," *Communications of the ACM* **18** (1975), 165–172; "Algorithm 489: The algorithm SELECT — for finding the ith smallest of n elements," *Communications of the ACM* **18** (1975), 173.

[7] Dominique Foata, "Étude algébrique de certains problèmes d'analyse combinatoire et du calcul des probabilités," *Publications de l'Institut de Statistique de l'Université de Paris* **14** (1965), 81–241.

[8] Lester R. Ford, Jr., and Selmer M. Johnson, "A tournament problem," *American Mathematical Monthly* **66** (1959), 387–389.

[9] H. H. Goldstine and John von Neumann, *Planning and Coding Problems for an Electronic Computing Instrument* **1** (Princeton, New Jersey: Institute for Advanced Study, 1 April 1947), 89 pages. Reprinted in von Neumann's *Collected Works* **5** (New York: Pergamon, 1963), 80–151.

[10] C. A. R. Hoare, "Algorithm 65: FIND," *Communications of the ACM* **4** (1961), 321–322.

[11] C. A. R. Hoare, "Proof of a program: FIND," *Communications of the ACM* **14** (1971), 39–45.

[12] Donald E. Knuth, *Fundamental Algorithms*, Volume 1 of *The Art of Computer Programming* (Reading, Massachusetts: Addison–Wesley, 1968).

[13] Donald E. Knuth, *Seminumerical Algorithms*, Volume 2 of *The Art of Computer Programming* (Reading, Massachusetts: Addison–Wesley, 1969).

[14] Donald E. Knuth, "The analysis of algorithms," *Actes du Congrès International des Mathématiciens* **3** (Paris: Gauthier-Villars, 1971), 269–274. [Reprinted as Chapter 3 of the present volume.]

[15] Donald E. Knuth, *Sorting and Searching*, Volume 3 of *The Art of Computer Programming* (Reading, Massachusetts: Addison–Wesley, 1973).

[16] I. D. G. MacLeod, "An algorithm for in-situ permutation," *Australian Computer Journal* **2** (1970), 16–19.

[17] L. Mirsky, "A theorem on representations of integers in the scale of r," *Scripta Mathematica* **15** (1949), 11–12.

[18] H. Steinhaus, *Mathematical Snapshots*, second edition (Oxford University Press, 1950), 38–39.

[19] M. H. van Emden, "Increasing the efficiency of quicksort," *Communications of the ACM* **13** (1970), 563–567.

[20] P. F. Windley, "Transposing matrices in a digital computer," *The Computer Journal* **2** (1959), 47–48.

Addendum

Substantial advances have been made since 1971 in the complexity analysis of the selection problem; see the 1998 edition of [15, §5.3.3]. But the conjecture about Rearrangement Devices in the appendix above remains unsolved, and the true asymptotic complexity of *in situ* permutation is still not known.

Chapter 2

The Dangers of Computer Science Theory

[An invited address presented to the International Congress on Logic, Methodology and Philosophy of Science in Bucharest, Romania, September 1971. Originally published in Logic, Methodology and Philosophy of Science 4 (Amsterdam: North-Holland, 1973), 189–195.]

The text of my sermon today is taken from Plato [*The Republic*, vii:531e], who said, "I have hardly ever known a mathematician who was able to reason." If we make an unbiased examination of the accomplishments made by mathematicians to the real world of computer programming, we are forced to conclude that, so far, the theory has actually done more harm than good. There are numerous instances in which theoretical "advances" have actually stifled the development of computer programming, and in some cases they have even made it take several steps backward! I shall discuss a few such cases in this talk.

Last week at the IFIP 71 Congress in Ljubljana, I presented a lecture that had quite a different flavor: I spoke pro-Computer-Science, and I extolled the virtues of the associated mathematical theory. Today, however, I must consider the Methodology and Philosophy of Computer Science, and so I feel it necessary to right the balance and to give an anti-Computer-Science talk. (I hope that by showing the other side of the coin I will not prejudice the sales of the books I have written.)

Perhaps the most famous example of misdirected theory has occurred in connection with random number generation. Many of you know that sequences of pseudorandom numbers are often generated by the rule

$$x_{n+1} = (ax_n) \bmod m$$

for some multiplier a and some modulus m. For many years such sequences were used successfully, with multipliers a chosen nearly at random. The numbers passed empirical tests for randomness, but no theoretical reason for this was known except that number theory was

19

able to predict that the sequence has a very long period before it begins to repeat. Finally, the first theoretical advance was made: A proof was found (see Greenberger [8]) that the serial correlation between adjacent members of the sequence, averaged over the entire period, is bounded by

$$\left| r(x_i, x_{i+1}) \right| < \frac{4}{a} + \frac{16a + 28}{m}.$$

As you know, a correlation coefficient of $+1$ or -1 indicates a strong dependency, while a random sequence should have 0 correlation. According to this new theorem, if we choose the multiplier to be

$$a \approx \sqrt{m}$$

we can guarantee a small overall serial correlation.

As I said, this was the first nontrivial theorem about the multiplicative congruential sequences; because of it, people changed the random number generators they were using, and the result was catastrophic (see Greenberger [9]). A multiplier near $\sqrt{m}$ is always bad when *other* tests for randomness are considered. For example, the correlation is indeed nearly zero when averaged over the entire period, but the theory did not take into account the fact that the correlation is nearly $+1$ over half the period and -1 over the other half! It turns out that almost all multipliers are *better* than those near $\sqrt{m}$. Yet the horrible sequence

$$x_{n+1} = (2^{16} + 3)x_n \bmod 2^{31}$$

is still being supplied by IBM as the standard random number generator for use on its System/360 computers.

Such misapplications of theory have been with us since the beginning. From a historical point of view I believe that the very first work on what is now called the theory of computational complexity was the Ph.D. dissertation of Demuth [4], who made a theoretical study of the problem of sorting numbers into order. From a mathematical standpoint, Demuth's thesis was a beautiful piece of work; he defined three classes of automata, and he found reasonably tight bounds on how fast each of these classes of machines is able to sort. But from a practical standpoint, the thesis was of no help.

In fact, one of Demuth's main results was that in a certain sense "bubble sorting" is the optimum way to sort. During the last three years I have been studying the sorting problem in great detail, and I have therefore analyzed about 30 different sorting methods including the bubble sort. It turns out that the other 29 methods are always better in practice, in spite of the fact that Demuth had proved the optimality of bubble sorting on a certain peculiar type of machine.

Unfortunately, people still play the same game today with computational complexity theory: Instead of looking for the best way to solve a problem, we first think of an algorithm, and then we look for a sense in which it is optimum!

Traditionally the problem in finding an optimum sorting method is to minimize the number of comparisons between data elements while the sorting takes place. The best method currently known, in the sense that it takes fewer comparisons than any other known scheme, was invented by L. R. Ford and S. M. Johnson [6]. But their approach has fortunately never been used by programmers, because the complex method used to decide what comparisons to make costs much more time than the comparisons themselves.

The three most commonly known methods of sorting with magnetic tapes are the *balanced merge* (Mauchly [12]), the *cascade merge* (Betz and Carter [3]), and the *polyphase merge* (Gilstad [7]). Cascade merging with n tapes is based on an $(n-1)$-way merge, $(n-2)$-way merge, ..., 2-way merge, while polyphase is apparently an improvement since it uses $(n-1)$-way merging throughout. But David Ferguson [5] noticed that cascade merging is surprisingly better than polyphase on a large number of tapes: Given N records to sort on n tapes, the following asymptotic formulas for the tape read/write time are valid when N and n are large:

$$\text{balanced merge,} \quad N \log N / \log(n/2);$$
$$\text{cascade merge,} \quad N \log N / \log(\pi n/4);$$
$$\text{polyphase merge,} \quad N \log N / \log 4.$$

This is all very fine in theory but almost worthless in practice. In the first place, the number n of tapes must be large. But tapes are very unreliable; I have never seen more than about six tape units simultaneously in working condition! More seriously, these formulas are valid only as N goes to infinity, yet all N records must fit on one finite reel of tape. Commercial tape reels are never more than 2400 feet long, and this means that other factors suppressed in the above formulas actually are more important than the leading terms. For practical sizes of N it turns out therefore that polyphase is superior to cascade, contrary to the formulas.

Incidentally, Professor Karp of Berkeley has proved a beautiful theorem, showing that cascade merging is optimum in the sense that it minimizes the number of phases, over all possible tape merging patterns. But unfortunately this theoretical notion of a "phase" has no physical significance; it is not the sort of thing anyone would ever want to minimize.

Such experiences lead me to quote from Webster's dictionary of the English language (pre-1960), where we find that the verb "to optimize" means "to view with optimism."

A few months ago I computed the effect of tape rewind time, which is excluded in the formulas above, and I discovered to my great surprise that the old-fashioned balanced merging scheme was actually better than both polyphase and cascade on six tapes! Thus the theoretical calculations, which have been so widely quoted, have caused an inferior method to be used.

An overemphasis on asymptotic behavior has often led to similar abuses. For example, some years ago I was preparing part of an operating system where it was necessary to determine whether or not a given record called a "page" was in the high-speed computer memory. I had just learned the very beautiful method of balanced binary trees devised by the Russian mathematicians Adelson-Velsky and Landis [1], which guarantees that only $O(\log n)$ steps are needed to find a particular page if n pages are present. After I had devised a complicated program using their method, I remembered that the computer I was using had a special search instruction that would do the same job by brute force in n cycles. Since this instruction operated at hardware speed, and since the memory size guaranteed that n would never exceed 1000, the brute force method was much faster than the sophisticated $\log n$ method.

Now I should say a few words about *automata theory*. For many years the theory of automata was developing rapidly and solving problems that were ostensibly related to computers; but real programmers could not care less about those theorems because Turing machines were so different from real machines. However, one result was highly touted as the first contribution of automata theory to real programming, an efficient algorithm that was discovered first by the theoreticians: The Hennie–Stearns construction [11] shows that a k-tape Turing machine can be simulated elegantly by a 2-tape machine with only a logarithmic increase in the execution time. This means, for example, that sorting can be achieved on two tapes in $O(N(\log N)^2)$ steps, significantly beating the methods of order N^2 previously known for two tapes. But once again the theory did not work in practice; the Hennie–Stearns construction involves writing in the middle of a magnetic tape, which is rather difficult, and it allows a lot of unused blank space to appear on the tapes.

As I mentioned before, a single tape is only 2400 feet long; so the asymptotic formulas do not tell the story. When the Hennie–Stearns method is actually applied to a tape full of data, almost 40 hours are required, compared with only about 8 hours for the asymptotically slow method.

The theory of automata is slowly changing to a study of random-access computations, and this work promises to be more useful. Last week in Ljubljana, S. A. Cook presented an interesting theorem, stating in essence that any algorithm programmable on a certain kind of pushdown automaton can be performed efficiently on a random-access machine, no matter how slowly the pushdown program runs. When I first heard about his theorem last year, I was able to use it to find an efficient pattern-matching procedure; this was the first time in my experience that I had learned something new about real programming by applying automata theory. (Unfortunately I found out that Morris [13] had independently discovered the same algorithm a few weeks earlier, without using automata theory at all.)

Is there *any* area (outside of numerical analysis) where mathematical theory has actually helped computer programmers? The theory of languages springs to mind; surely the development of programming languages has been helped by the highly sophisticated theory of mathematical linguistics. But even here the theory has not been an unmixed blessing, and for several years the idea of top-down parsing was unjustly maligned because of misapplied theory. Furthermore, many problems in mathematical linguistics have been shown to be unsolvable, in certain levels of generality, and this has tended to make people afraid to look for solvable subproblems. People often forget that every problem they solve is a special case of some recursively unsolvable problem!

Another difficulty with the theory of languages is that it has led to an overemphasis on syntax as opposed to semantics. You all know the old joke about the man who was searching for his lost watch under the lamppost. His friend came up to him and said, "What are you doing?"

"I'm looking for my watch."

"Where did you lose it?"

"Oh, over there, down the street."

"But why are you looking for it here?"

"Because the light is much better here."

For many years there was much light on syntax and very little on semantics; so simple semantic constructions were unnaturally grafted onto syntactic definitions, making rather unwieldy grammars, instead of searching for theories more appropriate to semantics.

Of course you know that the theory of languages has by now become ultrageneralized so that it bears little relation to its practical origins. This is not bad in itself, although sometimes it reminds me of a satirical article published a few years ago by Austin [2]; paraphrasing his article, we should not be surprised to find someday a paper entitled "On triply-degenerate prewaffles having no proper normal subwaffle with the pseudo-A_4 property, dedicated to R. J. Drofnats on his 19th birthday." Sometimes theories tend to become very baroque! The tendency of modern mathematics to be "modern" in the sense of "modern art" has been aptly described in an extraordinary article by Hammersley [10], which should be required reading for everyone.

At this point I would like to quote from some lectures on *Pragmatism* (Chapter 2) given by the philosopher William James at the beginning of this century:

> When the first mathematical, logical, and natural uniformities, the first *laws* were discovered, men were so carried away by the clearness, beauty and simplification that resulted, that they believed themselves to have deciphered authentically the eternal thoughts of the Almighty.

You see that computer science has been subject to a recurring problem: Some theory is developed that is very *beautiful*, and too often it is therefore thought to be *relevant*.

An article has recently been published by Christopher Strachey of Oxford University, entitled "Is Computing Science?" [14]. He presents two tables, one that ranks topics now considered part of computer science in order of their relevance to real programming and another that ranks those same topics in order of their present state of theoretical development. As you might suspect, the two rankings are in opposite order.

Perhaps this is the way things should be. Maybe theories are more beautiful and more worthy of development if they are further from reality. Some of the examples I have mentioned suggest in fact that it is dangerous even to *try* to develop any theory that is relevant to actual computer programming practice, since the record shows that such theories have usually been misapplied.

Well, I must confess that I have had my tongue in my cheek, in many of the remarks above. When I first prepared this talk, sitting in beautiful Cișmigiu Park, I was not intending to write it down for the published proceedings, and I couldn't resist the temptation to have some fun giving an unexpected "methodology" lecture. I have stated the case against computer science theory as well as I could; but, as many of you probably suspect, I do not really believe everything I said. It is true that theory has often been irrelevant and misapplied; but so what? We get enjoyment and stimulation from abstract theories, and the mental concepts we learn to manipulate as we study them often give us practical insights and skills. On the other hand, practical considerations do not necessarily lead to awkward mathematical problems that are inherently impure or distasteful. In fact I have been spending many years preparing a series of books in an attempt to show that a great deal of beautiful mathematics is directly helpful to computer programmers. My experience has been that theories are often more structured and more interesting when they are based on real problems; somehow such theories are more exciting than completely abstract theories will ever be.

This research was supported in part by the National Science Foundation and the National Research Council. My wife and I wish to thank our Romanian hosts, Dragoş and Constanţa Vaida, for their extraordinary hospitality.

References

[1] G. M. Adel'son-Vel'skiĭ and E. M. Landis, "Один алгорифм организации информации," *Doklady Akademii Nauk SSSR* **146** (1962), 263–266. English translation, "An algorithm for the organization of information," *Soviet Mathematics — Doklady* **3** (1962), 1259–1263.

[2] A. K. Austin, "Modern research in mathematics," *The Mathematical Gazette* **51** (1967), 149–150.

[3] B. K. Betz and W. C. Carter, "New merge sorting techniques," *Preprints of Summaries of Papers Presented at the 14th National Meeting* (Association for Computing Machinery, 1959), Paper 14.

[4] H. B. Demuth, *Electronic Data Sorting* (Ph.D. thesis, Stanford University, 1956), 92 pages. Partially reprinted in *IEEE Transactions on Computers* **C-34** (1985), 296–310.

[5] David E. Ferguson, "More on merging," *Communications of the ACM* **7** (1964), 297.

[6] Lester R. Ford, Jr., and Selmer M. Johnson, "A tournament problem," *American Mathematical Monthly* **66** (1959), 387–389.

[7] R. L. Gilstad, "Polyphase merge sorting — an advanced technique," *Proceedings of the Eastern Joint Computer Conference* **18** (1960), 143–148.

[8] Martin Greenberger, "An *a priori* determination of serial correlation in computer generated random numbers," *Mathematics of Computation* **15** (1961), 383–389.

[9] Martin Greenberger, "Method in randomness," *Communications of the ACM* **8** (1965), 177–179.

[10] J. M. Hammersley, "On the enfeeblement of mathematical skills by 'Modern Mathematics' and by similar soft intellectual trash in schools and universities," *Bulletin of the Institute of Mathematics and Its Applications* **4**, 4 (October 1968), 66–85.

[11] F. C. Hennie and R. E. Stearns, "Two-tape simulation of multi-tape Turing machines," *Journal of the Association for Computing Machinery* **13** (1966), 533–546.

[12] John W. Mauchly, "Sorting and collating," in *Theory and Techniques for the Design of Electronic Digital Computers* **3** (Philadelphia, Pennsylvania: Moore School of Electrical Engineering, 1946), Lecture 22. Reprinted in *The Moore School Lectures* (Cambridge, Massachusetts: MIT Press, 1985), 271–287.

[13] J. H. Morris, Jr., and Vaughan R. Pratt, "A linear pattern-matching algorithm," Technical Report No. 40 (Berkeley, California: University of California, Computation Center, 1970). [See Donald E. Knuth, James H. Morris, Jr., and Vaughan R. Pratt, "Fast pattern matching in strings," *SIAM Journal on Computing* **6** (1977), 323–350.]

[14] Christopher Strachey, "Is computing science?" *Bulletin of the Institute of Mathematics and Its Applications* **6**, 1 (April 1970), 80–82.

Chapter 3

The Analysis of Algorithms

*[An invited address presented to the International Congress of Mathematicians in Nice, France, September 1970. Originally published in Actes du Congrès International des Mathématiciens **3** (Paris: Gauthier-Villars, 1971), 269–274.]*

Some general aspects of algorithmic analysis are illustrated by discussing Euclid's algorithm. Euclid's method is extended in such a way that the greatest common divisor of two n-digit numbers can be found in $O(n(\log n)^5(\log \log n))$ steps as $n \to \infty$.

The advent of high-speed computing machines, which are capable of carrying out algorithms so faithfully, has led to intensive studies of the properties of algorithms, opening up a fertile field for mathematical investigations. Every reasonable algorithm suggests interesting questions of a "pure mathematical" nature; and the answers to these questions sometimes lead to useful applications, thereby adding a little vigor to the subject without spoiling its beauty. The theory of queues, which analyzes a very special class of algorithms, indicates the potential richness of the theories that can be obtained when algorithms of all types are analyzed in depth.

The purpose of this paper is to illustrate some general principles of algorithmic analysis by considering an example that is interesting for both historical and mathematical reasons, the calculation of the greatest common divisor (gcd) of two integers by means of Euclid's algorithm. Euclid's procedure [2], which is one of the oldest nontrivial algorithms known, may be formulated as follows, given integers $U \geq V \geq 0$:

E1. If $V = 0$, stop; U is the answer.

E2. Let R be the remainder of U divided by V, so that $U = AV + R$, $0 \leq R < V$. Replace U by V, then replace V by R, and return to step E1. □

1. "Local" Analysis

Analyses of algorithms are generally of two kinds, "local" and "global." A local analysis consists of taking one particular algorithm (like Euclid's) and studying the amount of work it does as a function of the inputs; a global analysis, on the other hand, considers an entire family of algorithms and investigates the "best possible" procedures in that class, from some point of view. In both types of analysis we can consider either the "worst case" of the algorithms, namely the work involved under the least favorable choice of inputs, or the "average case," the expected amount of work under a given input distribution. More generally, we may be able to obtain the distribution of work, given the distribution of inputs. "Work" may be measured in terms of the number of times each step of the algorithm is performed, or the amount of data that must be remembered, etc.

The first local analysis of Euclid's algorithm was published in 1844 by G. Lamé [10], who showed that step E2 will never be performed more than five times the number of digits in the decimal representation of V. His analysis was based on the fact that the method is least efficient when U and V are consecutive Fibonacci numbers.

The *average* behavior of Euclid's algorithm is much more difficult to determine than the worst case, and it has been established only in recent years. Let $T(U, V)$ be the number of times step E2 is performed. J. D. Dixon proved [1] that, for all ϵ and $C > 0$, the probability that

$$\left| T(U,V) - (12\pi^{-2}\ln 2)\ln U \right| \geq (\ln U)^{1/2+\epsilon} \quad \text{is} \quad O\big((\ln N)^{-C}\big),$$

given that $1 \leq V \leq U \leq N$. His proof is based on careful refinements of Kuzmin's study of continued fractions [9], showing that partial quotients are nearly independent if they are far apart in the sequence.

At about the same time, H. Heilbronn introduced a new approach [6] to the study of continued fractions and Euclid's algorithm. Let

$$T(V) = \lim_{N \to \infty} \frac{1}{N} \sum_{U=V+1}^{V+N} T(U,V) = \frac{1}{V} \sum_{U=V+1}^{2V} T(U,V)$$

be the average number of iterations when V is fixed. Heilbronn showed in effect that

$$nT(n) = \left\lfloor \frac{3n}{2} \right\rfloor + 2\sum \left[\left(\frac{n}{y+t} - t' \right) \frac{1}{y} \right],$$

where $\lfloor x \rfloor$ is the greatest integer $\leq x$, $\lceil x \rceil$ is the least integer $\geq x$, and the sum is over all positive integers y, t, t' such that $\gcd(t, y) = 1$, $t \leq y$, and $tt' \equiv n$ (modulo y). Evaluating this sum, he essentially found that $T(n) = (12\pi^{-2} \ln 2) \ln n + O(\sigma_{-1}(n)^2)$. Indeed, somewhat more seems to be true, although proof is still lacking; there is extensive empirical evidence [8, §4.5.3] that $\sum_{1 \leq k \leq V, \gcd(k,V)=1} T(V + k, V)/\varphi(V) = (12\pi^{-2} \ln 2) \ln V + 1.47 + o(1)$ as $V \to \infty$.

2. "Global" Analysis

Is Euclid's algorithm the "best" way to calculate greatest common divisors? Analyses of other gcd algorithms (see [8]) show that, under certain conditions, Euclid's method is inferior; and the average behavior of an interesting new algorithm proposed by V. C. Harris [4] is still unknown.

In searching for a "best" method, one way to measure the work is to consider the amount of time taken to perform the algorithm with pencil and paper, or with a conventional computer. Various abstract automata have been defined by which the latter notions can be made precise (see [5] and [7, §2.6]). When we apply such models to Euclid's algorithm, it is not difficult to see [8, exercise 4.5.3–45] that the amount of work to calculate the gcd of two n-digit numbers is essentially proportional to n^2, for both the average case and the worst case; thus the running time is comparable to that of familiar pencil-and-paper methods for multiplication and division. On the other hand, extremely fast methods of multiplication and division have recently been discovered; A. Schönhage and V. Strassen have proved [13] that an m-digit number can be multiplied by an n-digit number in only $O(n \log m \log \log m)$ units of time, when $n \geq m > 1$.

It is therefore natural to ask whether the gcd of two n-digit numbers can be calculated in fewer than order n^2 steps. Section 3 of this paper shows that this is indeed possible, in $O(n^{1+\epsilon})$ steps for all $\epsilon > 0$, by suitably arranging the calculations of Euclid's algorithm. Obviously at least n steps are necessary in any event (we must look at the inputs), so this result provides some idea of the asymptotic complexity of gcd computation.

3. High-speed GCD Calculation with Large Numbers

If step E2 is performed t times, let $A_1, \ldots, A_t$ be the partial quotients obtained. It is well known that $U = K_t(A_1, \ldots, A_t)D$ and $V = K_{t-1}(A_2, \ldots, A_t)D$, where $D = \gcd(U, V)$ and K_t is the continuant polynomial defined by $K_{-1} = 0$, $K_0 = 1$, $K_{t+1}(x_0, x_1, \ldots, x_t) =$

$x_0 K_t(x_1, \ldots, x_t) + K_{t-1}(x_2, \ldots, x_t)$. We shall call $[A_1, \ldots, A_t, D]$ the *Euclidean representation* of U and V. After k iterations of step E2 we have $U = U_k = K_{t-k}(A_{k+1}, \ldots, A_t)D$, $V = V_k = K_{t-k-1}(A_{k+2}, \ldots, A_t)D$. Euler [3, §359] observed that $K_t(x_1, \ldots, x_t)$ is the set of all terms obtainable by starting with $x_1 \ldots x_t$ and striking out pairs $x_i x_{i+1}$ zero or more times. From this remark, it follows immediately that

$$K_{s+t}(x_1, \ldots, x_{s+t}) = K_s(x_1, \ldots, x_s)K_t(x_{s+1}, \ldots, x_{s+t})$$
$$+ K_{s-1}(x_1, \ldots, x_{s-1})K_{t-1}(x_{s+2}, \ldots, x_{s+t}), \quad (*)$$

an identity that forms the basis of Heilbronn's work cited above; it was used on several occasions by Sylvester [14] and given in more general form by Perron [12, pages 14–15].

For convenience we shall write nonnegative integers N in binary notation, using lN binary digits where $lN = \lceil \log_2(N+1) \rceil$. It is easy to prove that $K_t(A_1, \ldots, A_t) \leq (A_1 + 1) \ldots (A_t + 1)$, hence

$$lK_t(A_1, \ldots, A_t) \leq lA_1 + \cdots + lA_t + 1;$$

and Lamé's theorem implies that $lA_1 + \cdots + lA_t \leq lK_t(A_1, \ldots, A_t) + t = O(\log U)$ in Euclid's algorithm. Thus we need essentially as much space to write down the Euclidean representation $[A_1, \ldots, A_t, D]$ as we do to write U and V themselves in binary form, except for a constant factor. We shall show that it is possible to convert rapidly between these two representations of U and V.

Theorem 1. *Let $S(n) = n(\log n)(\log \log n)$ and $n = lA_1 + \cdots + lA_t$. There is an algorithm that, given the respective binary representations of $A_1, \ldots, A_t$, computes the binary representation of $K_t(A_1, \ldots, A_t)$ in $O(S(n) \log t)$ steps.*

Proof. Consider four continuants associated with $(A_1, \ldots, A_t)$, namely $K = K_t(A_1, \ldots, A_t)$, $K^\bullet = K_{t-1}(A_1, \ldots, A_{t-1})$, $^\bullet K = K_{t-1}(A_2, \ldots, A_t)$, and $^\bullet K^\bullet = K_{t-2}(A_2, \ldots, A_{t-1})$. The four continuants associated with $(0, A_1, \ldots, A_t)$ are the same, in another order, so we add zeros if necessary until t is a power of 2. Now let $L, L^\bullet, {}^\bullet L, {}^\bullet L^\bullet$ and $R, R^\bullet, {}^\bullet R, {}^\bullet R^\bullet$ be the continuants associated with $A_1, \ldots, A_t$ and $A_{t+1}, \ldots, A_{2t}$ respectively. By $(*)$, $K = LR + L^\bullet \, {}^\bullet R$, $K^\bullet = LR^\bullet + L^\bullet \, {}^\bullet R^\bullet$, $^\bullet K = {}^\bullet LR + {}^\bullet L^\bullet \, {}^\bullet R$, $^\bullet K^\bullet = {}^\bullet LR^\bullet + {}^\bullet L^\bullet \, {}^\bullet R^\bullet$. Choosing C so that we can evaluate the L's in $CS(lA_1 + \cdots + lA_t)k$ steps, the R's in $CS(lA_{t+1} + \cdots + lA_{2t})k$ steps, and the 8 multiplications and 4 additions in $CS(lA_1 + \cdots + lA_{2t})$ further steps by the Schönhage–Strassen algorithm, we can evaluate the K's in at most $CS(lA_1 + \cdots + lA_{2t})(k+1)$ steps. $\square$

Let $U = 2^m U' + U''$ and $V = 2^m V' + V''$, where $0 \le U'', V'' < 2^m$. D. H. Lehmer [11] has suggested that the partial quotients for (U, V) be found by first obtaining some of those for U' and V', stopping at A_s, where s is maximal such that $(U'+1, V')$ and $(U', V'+1)$ have $A_1, \ldots, A_s$ in common. Then $A_1, \ldots, A_s$ are partial quotients for (U, V) also. We shall call $(A_1, \ldots, A_s)$ the "Lehmer quotients" for (U', V'). Sometimes the Lehmer quotients don't amount to anything; for example, when V' divides U' we have $s = 0$. But we can prove that three additional Euclidean iterations will always give a useful reduction.

Lemma 1. Let $U = 2^m U' + U'' \ge V = 2^m V' + V''$, where $0 \le U'' < 2^m$ and $0 \le V'' < 2^m$. Let $[A_1, \ldots, A_t, D]$ be the Euclidean representation of (U, V), and let $(A_1, \ldots, A_s)$ be the Lehmer quotients for (U', V'), where $t \ge s + 3$. Then we have $U_{s+3} < U/\sqrt{U'}$.

Proof. Let $P_k = K_{k-1}(A_2, \ldots, A_k)$ and $Q_k = K_k(A_1, \ldots, A_k)$; also let $\theta = V/U$, $\theta' = V'/(U' + 1)$, $\theta'' = (V' + 1)/U'$. The well-known pattern by which P_k/Q_k converges to θ, schematically

$$\frac{P_k}{Q_k} < \frac{P_k + P_{k+1}}{Q_k + Q_{k+1}} < \frac{P_k + 2P_{k+1}}{Q_k + 2Q_{k+1}} < \cdots < \frac{P_{k+2}}{Q_{k+2}} < \theta < \frac{P_{k+2} + P_{k+1}}{Q_{k+2} + Q_{k+1}} < \frac{P_{k+1}}{Q_{k+1}}$$

when k is even and the same with '$<$' replaced by '$>$' when k is odd, shows that if θ' and θ'' are two real numbers whose continued fractions differ first at $A'_{s+1} \ne A''_{s+1}$, then P_{s+1}/Q_{s+1} lies between θ' and θ''. Hence

$$\frac{1}{2} Q_{s+3}^2 \ge Q_{s+1}(Q_{s+2} + Q_{s+1}) > \frac{1}{|\theta - P_{s+1}/Q_{s+1}|} > \frac{1}{\theta'' - \theta'}$$
$$> \frac{1}{2} U',$$

using the well-known relation $|\theta - P_k/Q_k| > 1/Q_k(Q_{k+1} + Q_k)$. And by (*), we have $U_{s+3} = K_{t-s-3}(A_{s+4}, \ldots, A_t) < U/Q_{s+3}$.   □

Lemma 2. Under the assumptions of Lemma 1 and its proof, we also have $Q_s < \sqrt{U'}$.

Proof. The well-known relation $|\theta - P_k/Q_k| \le 1/Q_k Q_{k+1}$ yields

$$Q_s^2 < Q_s Q_{s+1} \le \frac{1}{\max(|\theta' - P_s/Q_s|, |\theta'' - P_s/Q_s|)} < \frac{1}{\theta'' - \theta'}$$
$$\le U'.   □$$

Lemma 3. *There is an algorithm that, given $U \geq V \geq 0$ with $lU = n$, finds all the Lehmer quotients for (U, V) in at most $O(S(n)(\log n)^3)$ steps.*

Proof. For large n the algorithm first applies itself recursively to the leading $\frac{1}{2}n$ binary digits of U and V, finding r partial quotients; then it computes

$$U_r = (-1)^r \big(K_{r-2}(A_2, \ldots, A_{r-1})U - K_{r-1}(A_1, \ldots, A_{r-1})V \big),$$
$$V_r = (-1)^r \big(K_r(A_1, \ldots, A_r)V - K_{r-1}(A_2, \ldots, A_r)U \big)$$

in $O(S(n) \log n)$ steps by the method of Theorem 1. We can find the next quotient A_{r+1} in $O(S(n) \log n)$ further steps (see [8, Algorithm 4.3.3R]), so by Lemma 1 the algorithm performs a bounded number of Euclidean iterations until reaching U_{r+k} with at most $\frac{3}{4}n$ digits. Now the same process is repeated on the $\frac{1}{2}n$ leading digits of U_{r+k} and V_{r+k}; after a bounded number of further Euclidean iterations, we have reduced U to fewer than $\frac{1}{2}n$ digits, and we have found quotients $A_1, \ldots, A_p$. At this point $p \geq s$, because $(*)$ implies that $U < 2U_p Q_p$ and we have $Q_s < \sqrt{U}$ by Lemma 2.

   Finally the value of s is located in approximately $\log_2 p = O(\log n)$ iterations, using the well-known "binary search" bisection technique; each iteration tests some k to see whether or not $k < s$ or $k \geq s$. Such a test can rely on the fact that P_k/Q_k and P_{k+1}/Q_{k+1} are both "good" when $k < s$, while they are not both "good" when $k \geq s$, where P_k/Q_k is called good when it is $< V_k/(U_k + 1)$, for k even, or $> (V_k + 1)/U_k$, for k odd. The running time $L(n)$ of this algorithm as a whole now satisfies $L(n) \leq 2L(\frac{1}{2}n) + O(S(n)(\log n)^2)$.   □

Theorem 2. *There is an algorithm that, given $U \geq V \geq 0$ with $lU = n$, determines the Euclidean representation $[A_1, \ldots, A_t, D]$ in $O(n(\log n)^5 \log \log n)$ steps as $n \to \infty$.*

Proof. Begin as in Lemma 3 to reduce n to $\frac{3}{4}n$ in $L(\frac{1}{2}n) + O(S(n) \log n)$ steps, then apply the same method until $V_t = 0$. The running time $G(n)$ of this algorithm satisfies the recurrence

$$\begin{aligned} G(n) &= G(\tfrac{3}{4}n) + O(S(n)(\log n)^3) \\ &= G(\tfrac{9}{16}n) + O(S(n)(\log n)^3) + O(S(\tfrac{3}{4}n)(\log n)^3) \\ &= \cdots = O(S(n)(\log n)^4). \end{aligned}$$ □

   In particular, we can find the gcd of n-digit numbers in $n^{1+\epsilon}$ steps, as $n \to \infty$, for all $\epsilon > 0$. The method we have used is rather complicated, but no simpler one is apparent to the author. In general, the idea of reducing n to αn for $\alpha < 1$ often leads to asymptotically efficient algorithms.

References

[1] John D. Dixon, "The number of steps in the Euclidean algorithm," *Journal of Number Theory* **2** (1970), 414–422.

[2] Euclid, *Elements* (c. 300 B.C.), Book 7, Propositions 1 and 2.

[3] Leonhard Euler, *Introductio in Analysin Infinitorum* (Lausanne: 1748). Reprinted in his *Opera Omnia*, series 1, volume 8.

[4] V. C. Harris, "An algorithm for finding the greatest common divisor," *Fibonacci Quarterly* **8** (1970), 102–103.

[5] J. Hartmanis and R. E. Stearns, "On the computational complexity of algorithms," *Transactions of the American Mathematical Society* **117** (1965), 285–306.

[6] Hans Heilbronn, "On the average length of a class of finite continued fractions," in *Number Theory and Analysis* (Papers in honor of Edmund Landau), edited by Paul Turán (Plenum, 1969), 87–96. Reprinted in Heilbronn's *Collected Papers* (1988), 518–525.

[7] Donald E. Knuth, *Fundamental Algorithms*, Volume 1 of *The Art of Computer Programming* (Reading, Massachusetts: Addison–Wesley, 1968).

[8] Donald E. Knuth, *Seminumerical Algorithms*, Volume 2 of *The Art of Computer Programming* (Reading, Massachusetts: Addison–Wesley, 1969).

[9] R. Kuzmin, "Sur un problème de Gauss," *Atti del Congresso internazionale dei matematici* **6** (Bologna: 1928), 83–89.

[10] Gabriel Lamé, "Note sur la limite du nombre des divisions dans la recherche du plus grand commun diviseur entre deux nombres entiers," *Comptes Rendus hebdomadaires des séances de l'Académie des Sciences* **19** (Paris: 1844), 867–870.

[11] D. H. Lehmer, "Euclid's algorithm for large numbers," *American Mathematical Monthly* **45** (1938), 227–233.

[12] Oskar Perron, *Die Lehre von den Kettenbrüchen* (Leipzig: 1913).

[13] A. Schönhage and V. Strassen, "Schnelle Multiplikation großer Zahlen," *Computing* **7** (1971), 281–292.

[14] James J. Sylvester, "On a fundamental rule in the algorithm of continued fractions," *Philosophical Magazine* **6** (1853), 297–299. Reprinted in his *Collected Mathematical Papers* **1** (1904), 641–644.

Addendum

Shortly after seeing a preprint of this paper, Arnold Schönhage discovered a somewhat simpler algorithm that requires only $O(S(n)\log n)$ steps. ["Schnelle Berechnung von Kettenbruchentwicklungen," *Acta Informatica* **1** (1971), 139–144.]

Lamé's theorem was widely believed for many years to be the first upper bound on the running time of Euclid's algorithm to be rigorously proved, but several instances of earlier work were resurrected in an interesting paper by Jeffrey Shallit, "Origins of the analysis of the Euclidean algorithm," *Historia Mathematica* **21** (1994), 401–419.

See also the addendum to Chapter 12, for a discussion of long-forgotten early work on $T(u, v)$ by Gustav Lochs.

Chapter 4

Big Omicron and Big Omega and
Big Theta

[Originally published in SIGACT News 8, 2 (April–June 1976), 18–24.]

Most of us have gotten accustomed to the idea of using the notation
$O(f(n))$ to stand for any function whose magnitude is upper-bounded
by a constant times $f(n)$, for all large n. Sometimes we also need a
corresponding notation for lower-bounded functions, namely for those
functions that are *at least* as large as a constant times $f(n)$ for all large n.
Unfortunately, people have occasionally been using the O-notation for
lower bounds, for example when they reject a particular sorting method
"because its running time is $O(n^2)$." I have seen instances of this in
print quite often, and finally it has prompted me to sit down and write
a Letter to the Editor about the situation.

The classical literature does have a notation for functions that
are bounded below, namely $\Omega(f(n))$. The most prominent appearance of this notation is in Titchmarsh's magnum opus on Riemann's
zeta function [8], where he defines $\Omega(f(n))$ on page 152 and de-
votes his entire Chapter 8 to "Ω-theorems." See also Karl Prachar's
Primzahlverteilung [7, page 245].

The Ω notation has not become very common, although I have noticed its use in a few places, most recently in some Russian publications
that I consulted about the theory of equidistributed sequences. Once I
suggested to someone in a letter that he use Ω-notation "since it had
been used by number theorists for years"; but later, when challenged to
show explicit references, I spent a surprisingly fruitless hour searching
in the library without being able to turn up a single reference. I have recently asked several prominent mathematicians if they knew what $\Omega(n^2)$
meant, and more than half of them had never seen the notation before.

Before writing this letter, I decided to search more carefully, and to
study the history of O-notation and o-notation as well. Cajori's two-
volume work on the history of mathematical notations does not mention

35

any of these. While looking for definitions of Ω I came across dozens of books from the early part of this century that defined O and o but not Ω. I found Landau's remark [6, page 883] that the first appearance of O known to him was in Bachmann's 1894 book [1, page 401]. In the same place, Landau said that he had personally invented the o-notation while writing his handbook about the distribution of primes; his original discussion of O and o is in [6, pages 59–63].

I could not find any appearances of Ω-notation in Landau's publications; this was confirmed later when I discussed the question with George Pólya, who told me that he had been Landau's student and was quite familiar with his writings. Pólya knew what Ω-notation meant, but never had used it in his own work. (Like teacher, like pupil, he said.)

Since Ω notation is so rarely used, my first three trips to the library bore little fruit, but on my fourth visit I was finally able to pinpoint its probable origin: Hardy and Littlewood introduced Ω in their classic 1914 memoir [4, page 225], calling it a "new" notation. They used it also in their major paper on distribution of primes [5, pages 125 and following], but they apparently found little subsequent need for it in later works.

Unfortunately, Hardy and Littlewood didn't define $\Omega(f(n))$ as I wanted them to; their definition was a negation of $o(f(n))$, namely a function whose absolute value exceeds $Cf(n)$ for infinitely many n, when C is a sufficiently small positive constant. In all the applications I have seen so far in computer science, a stronger requirement (replacing "infinitely many n" by "all large n") is much more appropriate.

After discussing this problem with people for several years, I have come to the conclusion that the following definitions will prove to be most useful for computer scientists:

$O(f(n))$ denotes the set of all $g(n)$ such that there exist positive constants C and n_0 with $|g(n)| \leq Cf(n)$ for all $n \geq n_0$.

$\Omega(f(n))$ denotes the set of all $g(n)$ such that there exist positive constants C and n_0 with $g(n) \geq Cf(n)$ for all $n \geq n_0$.

$\Theta(f(n))$ denotes the set of all $g(n)$ such that there exist positive constants C, C', and n_0 with $Cf(n) \leq g(n) \leq C'f(n)$ for all $n \geq n_0$.

Verbally, $O(f(n))$ can be read as "order at most $f(n)$"; $\Omega(f(n))$ as "order at least $f(n)$"; $\Theta(f(n))$ as "order exactly $f(n)$." Of course, these definitions apply only to behavior as $n \to \infty$; when dealing with $f(x)$ as $x \to 0$ we would substitute a neighborhood of zero for the neighborhood of infinity (that is, $|x| \leq x_0$ instead of $n \geq n_0$).

Although I have changed Hardy and Littlewood's definition of Ω, I feel justified in doing so because their definition is by no means in wide use, and because there are other ways to say what they want to say in the comparatively rare cases when their definition applies. I like the mnemonic appearance of Ω by analogy with O, and it is easy to typeset. Furthermore, these two notations as defined above are nicely complemented by the Θ-notation, which was suggested to me independently by Bob Tarjan and by Mike Paterson.

The definitions above refer to "the set of all $g(n)$ such that ...", rather than to "an arbitrary function $g(n)$ with the property that ..."; I believe that this definition in terms of sets, which was suggested to me many years ago by Ron Rivest as an improvement over the definition in the first printing of my Volume 1, is the best way to define O-notation. Under this interpretation, when the O-notation and its relatives are used in formulas, we are actually speaking about sets of functions rather than single functions. When A and B are sets of functions, $A + B$ denotes the set $\{a + b \mid a \in A \text{ and } b \in B\}$, etc.; and "$1 + O(n^{-1})$" can be taken to mean the set of all functions of the form $1 + g(n)$, where $|g(n)| \leq Cn^{-1}$ for some C and all large n.

The phenomenon of *one-way equalities* arises in this connection. For example, we write

$$1 + O(n^{-1}) = O(1)$$

but not

$$O(1) = 1 + O(n^{-1}).$$

The equal sign here really means $\subseteq$ (set inclusion), and this asymmetry has bothered many people who propose that we not be allowed to use the $=$ sign in this context. My feeling is that we should continue to use one-way equality together with O-notations, since it has been common practice of thousands of mathematicians for so many years now, and since we understand the meaning of our existing notation sufficiently well.

We could also define $\omega(f(n))$ as the set of all functions whose ratio to $f(n)$ approaches infinity, by analogy to $o(f(n))$. Personally I have felt little need for these o-notations; on the contrary, I have found it a good discipline to obtain O-estimates at all times, since it has taught me about more powerful mathematical methods. However, I expect someday I may have to break down and use o-notation when faced with a function for which I can't prove anything stronger.

There is a slight lack of symmetry in the definitions of O, Ω, and Θ given above, since absolute value signs are used on $g(n)$ only in the case of O. This is not really an anomaly, since O refers to a neighborhood of zero while Ω refers to a neighborhood of infinity. (Hardy's book on divergent series uses O_L and O_R when a one-sided O-result is needed. Hardy and Littlewood [5] used Ω_L and Ω_R for functions respectively $< -Cf(n)$ and $> Cf(n)$ infinitely often. Neither of these conventions has become widespread.)

The notations above are intended to be useful in the vast majority of applications, but they are not intended to meet all conceivable needs. For example, if you are dealing with a function like $(\log\log n)^{\cos n}$ you might want a notation for "all functions that oscillate between $\log\log n$ and $1/\log\log n$ where those limits are best possible." In such a case, a local notation for the purpose, confined to the pages of whatever paper you are writing at the time, should suffice; we needn't worry about standard notations for a concept unless that concept arises frequently.

I would like to close this letter by discussing a competing way to denote the order of function growth. My library research turned up the surprising fact that this alternative approach actually antedates the O-notation itself. Paul du Bois-Reymond [2] used the relational notations

$$g(n) \prec f(n) \qquad \text{and} \qquad f(n) \succ g(n)$$

already in 1871, for positive functions $f(n)$ and $g(n)$, with the meaning we can now describe as $g(n) = o(f(n))$ (or as $f(n) = \omega(g(n))$). Hardy's interesting tract on orders of infinity [3] extends this idea by using also the relations

$$g(n) \preceq f(n) \qquad \text{and} \qquad f(n) \succeq g(n)$$

to mean $g(n) = O(f(n))$ (or, equivalently, $f(n) = \Omega(g(n))$, since we are assuming that f and g are positive). Hardy also wrote

$$f(n) \asymp g(n)$$

when $g(n) = \Theta(f(n))$, and

$$f(n) \eqsim g(n)$$

when $\lim_{n\to\infty} f(n)/g(n)$ exists and is neither 0 nor ∞; and he wrote

$$f(n) \sim g(n)$$

when $\lim_{n\to\infty} f(n)/g(n) = 1$. (Hardy's $\eqsim$ notation may seem peculiar at first, until you realize what he did with it; for example, he proved the following nice theorem: "If $f(n)$ and $g(n)$ are any functions built up recursively from the ordinary arithmetic operations and the exp and log functions, we have exactly one of the three relations $f(n) \prec g(n)$, $f(n) \asymp g(n)$, or $f(n) \succ g(n)$.")

Hardy's excellent notation has become somewhat distorted over the years. For example, Vinogradov [9] writes $f(n) \ll g(n)$ instead of Hardy's $f(n) \preceq g(n)$; thus, Vinogradov is comfortable with the formula

$$200n^2 \ll \binom{n}{2},$$

while I am not. In any event, such relational notations have intuitively clear transitive properties, and they avoid the use of the one-way equalities that bother some people. Why, then, should they not replace O and the new symbols Ω and Θ?

The main reason why O is so handy is that we can use it right in the middle of formulas (and in the middle of English sentences, and in tables that show the running times for a family of related algorithms, and so on). The relational notations require us to transpose everything except the function we are estimating to one side of an equation. (See [7, page 191].) Simple derivations like

$$
\begin{aligned}
\left(1 + \frac{H_n}{n}\right)^{H_n} &= \exp(H_n \ln(1 + H_n/n)) \\
&= \exp(H_n(H_n/n + O(\log n/n)^2)) \\
&= \exp(H_n^2/n + O((\log n)^3/n^2)) \\
&= \exp((\ln n + \gamma)^2/n + O((\log n)^3/n^2)) \\
&= (1 + O((\log n)^3/n^2))e^{(\ln n + \gamma)^2/n}
\end{aligned}
$$

would be extremely cumbersome in relational notation.

When I am working on a problem, my scratch paper notes often contain ad hoc notations, and I have been using an expression like "$(\leq 5n^2)$" to stand for the set of all functions that are $\leq 5n^2$. Similarly, I can write "$(\sim 5n^2)$" to stand for functions that are asymptotic to $5n^2$, etc.; and "$(\preceq n^2)$" would therefore be equivalent to $O(n^2)$, if I made appropriate extensions of the $\preceq$ relation to functions that may be negative. This would provide a uniform notational convention for all sorts of things, for use in the middle of expressions, giving more than just the O and Ω and Θ proposed above.

In spite of this alternative, I much prefer to publish papers with the O, Ω, and Θ notations; I would use other notations like "$(\sim 5n^2)$"

only when faced with a situation that needed it. Why? The main reason is that O-notation is so universally established and accepted, I would not feel right replacing it by a notation "$(\preceq f(n))$" of my own invention, however logically conceived; the O-notation has now assumed important mnemonic significance, and we are comfortable with it. For similar reasons, I am not abandoning decimal notation although I find that radix 8 (say) is more logical. And I like the Ω and Θ notations because they now have mnemonic significance inherited from O.

Well, I think I have beat this issue to death, knowing of no other arguments pro or con the introduction of Ω and Θ. On the basis of the issues discussed here, I propose that members of SIGACT, and editors of computer science and mathematics journals, adopt the O, Ω, and Θ notations as defined above, unless a better alternative can be found reasonably soon. Furthermore I propose that the relational notations of Hardy be adopted in those situations where a relational notation is more appropriate.

References

[1] Paul Bachmann, *Die analytische Zahlentheorie*, Volume 2 of *Zahlentheorie* (Leipzig: B. G. Teubner, 1894).

[2] Paul du Bois-Reymond, "Sur la grandeur relative des infinis des fonctions," *Annali di Matematica pura ed applicata*, series 2, **4** (1871), 338–353.

[3] G. H. Hardy, "Orders of Infinity: The 'Infinitärcalcül' of Paul du Bois-Reymond," *Cambridge Tracts in Mathematics and Mathematical Physics* **12** (1910; Second edition, 1924).

[4] G. H. Hardy and J. E. Littlewood, "Some problems of Diophantine approximation," *Acta Mathematica* **37** (1914), 155–238.

[5] G. H. Hardy and J. E. Littlewood, "Contributions to the theory of the Riemann zeta function and the theory of the distribution of primes," *Acta Mathematica* **41** (1918), 119–196.

[6] Edmund Landau, *Handbuch der Lehre von der Verteilung der Primzahlen* (Leipzig: B. G. Teubner, 1909), two volumes.

[7] Karl Prachar, *Primzahlverteilung* (Berlin: Springer, 1957).

[8] E. C. Titchmarsh, *The Theory of the Riemann Zeta-Function* (Oxford: Clarendon Press, 1951).

[9] I. M. Vinogradov, *The Method of Trigonometrical Sums in the Theory of Numbers*, translated from the 1947 Russian edition by K. F. Roth and Anne Davenport (London: Interscience, 1954).

Addendum

The three definitions proposed here have in fact become widely adopted. A contrary opinion about Ω notation has, however, been presented by P. M. B. Vitányi and L. Meertens, "Big Omega versus the wild functions," *Bulletin of the European Association for Theoretical Computer Science (EATCS)* **22** (1984), 14–19; reprinted in *SIGACT News* **16**, 4 (Spring 1985), 56–59.

Chapter 5

Optimal Measurement Points for Program Frequency Counts

*[Written with Francis R. Stevenson. Originally published in BIT **13** (1973), 313–322.]*

Armen Nahapetian has recently devised a procedure for reducing the number of measurements needed to determine all the execution frequencies in a computer program. We show that his procedure is optimal, by interpreting it in a new way.

Introduction

Perhaps the most fundamental way to measure the speed of an algorithm in a reasonably machine-independent manner is to count how frequently each part of the algorithm is executed. Theoretical tools for analyzing such frequency counts are discussed in [3], but in many cases the best available information comes from system programs that measure the frequencies empirically and report them back to the programmer. Indeed, recent experience with such programs [2] [4] [7] has been so favorable as to suggest that *all* compilers should routinely produce programs capable of making such measurements, and that frequency counts (possibly weighted by execution times) ought to be reported to all programmers.

Such a rash change in today's methods of programming might seem uncalled for, but in any event we clearly can benefit from knowing a simple way to perform the minimum number of measurements that will determine all frequencies. The purpose of this paper is to describe such a method.

The Reduction Algorithm

Consider the flow chart in Figure 1. The five boxes (which we shall call *vertices*) represent five steps of an algorithm, starting at step 1 and ending at step 5. The arrows (which we shall call *arcs*) represent possible flows of control as the algorithm is performed.

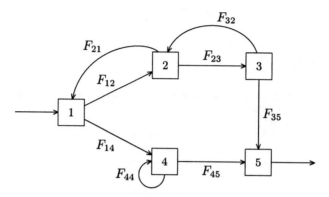

FIGURE 1. An example flow chart, for an algorithm that starts at box 1 and ends at box 5.

Suppose the corresponding algorithm has been executed in such a way that the arc from i to j was taken exactly F_{ij} times, for all arcs shown in Figure 1. Furthermore, suppose the algorithm was started f times at vertex 1, so that it also terminated f times at vertex 5. If we add an extra arc from 5 to 1, with frequency $F_{51} = f$, then "Kirchhoff's first law" holds at all vertices; that is, the amount of flow into a vertex equals the amount of flow out. Thus if F_x denotes the number of times vertex x was executed, Kirchhoff's first law tells us the following about the flows in Figure 1:

$$F_{51} + F_{21} = F_1 = F_{12} + F_{14} \, ;$$
$$F_{12} + F_{32} = F_2 = F_{21} + F_{23} \, ;$$
$$F_{23} \quad\quad\ \ = F_3 = F_{32} + F_{35} \, ;$$
$$F_{14} + F_{44} = F_4 = F_{44} + F_{45} \, ;$$
$$F_{35} + F_{45} = F_5 = F_{51} \, .$$

It is well known (see, for example, Section 2.3.4.1 of [3]) that Kirchhoff's first law allows us to determine exactly $n - 1$ of the arc flows F_{ij} from the other arc flows, when there are n vertices. If there are m arcs, we need measure only $m - n + 1$ arc flows to determine all the frequencies. For Figure 1 this is $9 - 5 + 1 = 5$ measurements (including the arc from 5 to 1).

But in practice, we do not care about the arc flows F_{ij}; only the vertex flows F_x are significant, and only the vertex flows can conveniently be measured. This raises the natural question, what is the minimum number of vertex flows that need to be measured in order to determine all others?

In order to analyze this problem, let us merge some of the vertices into a single combined vertex, in such a manner that the vertex flows F_x will appear directly along the arcs. For example, since $F_4 = F_{44} + F_{45}$, we can make F_4 appear directly if we merge vertices 4 and 5 (see Figure 2).

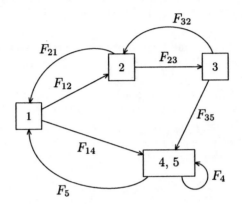

FIGURE 2. The first step of a reduction procedure applied to Figure 1.

In Figure 2, the arc $F_{51} = F_5$ has been shown explicitly, and the two arcs F_{44} and F_{45} have been combined into the single arc F_4. Similarly we can combine F_{12} and F_{14} into a single arc F_1 if we merge 2 with $\{4, 5\}$ as shown in Figure 3. Fortunately this also makes it possible to combine F_{32} and F_{35} into F_3. The only vertex flow that remains split is F_2, which is still divided into F_{21} and F_{23}.

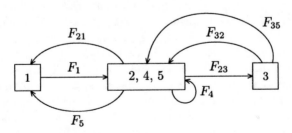

FIGURE 3. The second step.

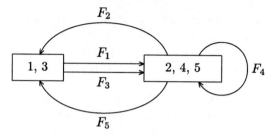

FIGURE 4. The reduced form of Figure 1, in which the original vertex frequencies now appear as arc frequencies.

Finally we merge 1 and 3 to create F_2 and obtain the directed graph shown in Figure 4. All the vertex flows of Figure 1 now appear as *arc* flows.

Each step of the reduction clearly preserves Kirchhoff's first law, so we can apply the known theory for arc flows to deduce that $5 - 2 + 1 = 4$ of the flows in Figure 4 need to be measured. In this case any one of the vertex frequencies except F_4 can be deduced from the remaining four, since the construction proves that

$$F_1 + F_3 = F_2 + F_5.$$

The reduction procedure we have used is based on the well-known "addition rule" used with signal-flow graphs [1] [5].

Proof of Minimality

It should be clear that the reduction procedure carried out for the particular flow chart in Figure 1 can be applied to any flow chart. We define an equivalence relation between vertices of a flow chart by saying that $x \equiv y$ whenever there is a vertex z such that arcs $z \to x$ and $z \to y$ exist from z to x and y respectively; or $x \equiv y$ if there is a finite sequence $x = x_0 \equiv x_1 \equiv \ldots \equiv x_n = y$ with $x_i \equiv x_{i+1}$ by the stated relation. Then the vertices of the reduced directed graph are the equivalence classes of vertices, and there is one arc F_x for each original vertex; F_x runs from the class containing x to the class containing the successors of x.

A minimal set of arc flows F_x that need to be measured in the reduced graph may be found by choosing any spanning subtree of the reduced graph; this will be a set of $k - 1$ arcs if there are k equivalence classes. The other $n - k + 1$ arcs correspond to frequency counts that need to be measured. A simple algorithm for finding spanning trees, and simultaneously deducing the relations expressing the flows in a spanning tree in terms of the other flows, appears for example in exercise 2.3.4.1–11 of [3].

In order to prove that $n-k+1$ is the minimum number of vertex flow measurements needed, it suffices to show that, whenever these $n-k+1$ flows F_x have been given arbitrary values, there will exist a consistent set of arc flows F_{ij} in the original flow chart. (We may ignore the fact that some of these arc flows might be negative; the point is that $n-k+1$ of the vertex flows are linearly independent. There exist some values of the $n-k+1$ selected vertex flows such that all the arc flows in the original flow chart are positive, otherwise we could simplify that flow chart. Hence the set of possible values for the $n-k+1$ selected vertex flows is a cone of dimension $n-k+1$, and we *must* make at least $n-k+1$ measurements.)

The proof will therefore be complete if we can take an arbitrary conservative flow in the reduced directed graph (a flow satisfying Kirchhoff's first law), and find a conservative flow in the original directed graph that reduces to it. For this purpose it suffices to undo each step of the reduction.

The reductions are of two kinds. One is a "trivial" reduction, where we combine two arcs F_{ij} and F_{ik} that happen to have the same final vertex since j and k have already been merged together. This is the situation that occurred just after Figure 3, when we combined F_{32} and F_{35}. (We "save" one measurement whenever such a reduction occurs in the transition from arc flows to vertex flows.) To undo such a reduction, we may assign an arbitrary value to F_{ij}, and let $F_{ik} = F_i' - F_{ij}$ where F_i' is the combined flow in the reduced graph.

The other reduction occurs when we combine two arcs F_{ij} and F_{ik} by merging the distinct nodes containing j and k. Figure 5 shows a typical situation before and after those nodes are merged.

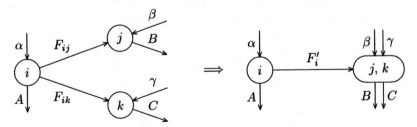

FIGURE 5. A typical merging step.

The flows in the reduced graph satisfy

$$\alpha = F_i' + A,$$
$$\beta + \gamma + F_i' = B + C.$$

By defining $F_{ij} = B - \beta$, $F_{ik} = C - \gamma$, we have $F_{ij} + F_{ik} = F_i'$ and there is conservative flow in the graph before reduction. A similar procedure works when there are additional incoming or outgoing arcs, or when $i = j$.

This completes the proof that $n - k + 1$ measurements are necessary. It might be worth remarking that some choices of $n - k + 1$ measuring points are better than others, since the overhead for measurement is proportional to the sum of the counts. Before the counts are taken we do not know for sure which will be the largest. After the counts have been made (thereby determining all the vertex flows) we can in retrospect find the $n - k + 1$ independent flows that would have been least costly to measure, by simply applying Prim's well-known algorithm [3, exercise 2.3.4.1–11] to find a spanning tree of the reduced graph having maximum total count. In general, a heuristic procedure can be followed to choose the best set of measurement points: If we guess that the frequencies will satisfy $F_1 \geq F_2 \geq \ldots \geq F_n$, we obtain the best measurement points by successively considering the arcs $F_1, F_2 \ldots$ in turn; F_i is selected for measurement if and only if it forms a cycle with a subset of the set of all preceding F_j that were not selected for measurement. For example, F_1 is selected if and only if it is a loop from some box to itself; if F_1 is not selected, F_2 is selected if and only if it is a loop or forms a cycle (possibly undirected) with F_1.

Connection with Nahapetian's Method

The reduction procedure described above is essentially equivalent to the measurement technique recently suggested by A. Nahapetian [6], but the connection is not easy to see since his formulation is quite different. Nahapetian defines an equivalence relation on the *arcs* of the flow chart, instead of on the vertices as we have done. Two arcs are equivalent by his definition, say $\alpha \sim \beta$, if α has the same initial vertex as β, or the same final vertex, or if α can be proved equivalent to β by a finite sequence of such steps. The vertices of his derived graph are the equivalence classes of arcs; and each arc of his derived graph, corresponding to vertex x in the flow chart, goes from the class of arcs entering x to the class of arcs leaving x.

In order to demonstrate the essential equivalence of the two methods we must establish a one-to-one correspondence between his arc equivalence classes and the vertex equivalence classes defined above. Let $[[\alpha]]$ be the arc equivalence class containing arc α, and let $[x]$ be the vertex equivalence class containing vertex x. Let $f([[\alpha]]) = [\text{fin } \alpha]$, and let $g([x])$ be $[[\alpha]]$, where α is some vertex with $x = \text{fin } \alpha$. (We write init α and fin α for the initial and final vertices of α.) To prove that f and g define a one-to-one correspondence, we shall prove that f and g are well defined, and that fg and gf are the identity mappings.

(1) f is well-defined; that is, if $\alpha \sim \beta$ then fin $\alpha \equiv$ fin β.

It suffices to verify this when init $\alpha = $ init β, and when fin $\alpha = $ fin β; both verifications are trivial.

(2) g is well-defined; that is, if $x \equiv y$ and $x = $ fin α and $y = $ fin β then $\alpha \sim \beta$.

It suffices to verify this when there are arcs α' and β' with init $\alpha' = $ init β' and $x = $ fin α', $y = $ fin β'. But then $\alpha \sim \alpha' \sim \beta' \sim \beta$.

(3) $f\big(g([x])\big) = [x]$, and $g\big(f([[\alpha]])\big) = [[\beta]]$ where fin $\alpha = $ fin β; hence f and g are inverse functions.

It follows now that Nahapetian's reduced directed graph is identical to the one described here. This removes the "mystery" of his method, since we can intuitively understand the reduced flow chart as a partitioning of the original steps of the algorithm.

Appendix

Details of an algorithm for determining the minimum measurement points corresponding to a given flow chart appear in the SIMULA 67 program that follows. The program has been written with brevity and clarity in mind, not efficiency.

The main body of the program below specifies a SIMULA class called *vertex*, whose objects represent the vertices of the original flow chart. The attributes of each vertex include, among other things, two procedures called *arcto*(*q*) and *insert*, which are intended to be used by a driver program in the following way.

Example driver program corresponding to Figure 1:
```
begin ref(vertex) array v[1 : 5];  integer i;
    for i := 1 step 1 until 5 do v[i] := new vertex;
```

Create the original flow chart:
$v[1].arcto(v[2]);$ $v[1].arcto(v[4]);$
$v[2].arcto(v[1]);$ $v[2].arcto(v[3]);$
$v[3].arcto(v[2]);$ $v[3].arcto(v[5]);$
$v[4].arcto(v[4]);$ $v[4].arcto(v[5]);$
$v[5].arcto(v[1]);$

Create the reduced flow chart:
$v[4].insert;$ $v[2].insert;$ $v[3].insert;$
$v[1].insert;$ $v[5].insert;$
end driver program

Thus, the driver program first calls $v.arcto(w)$ for all arcs from v to w in the original flow chart, in any order; this enables the SIMULA program to structure the data so that the equivalence classes of vertices (which form the boxes of the reduced flow chart) are determined. Then $v.insert$ is called for all vertices v of the original flow chart, in decreasing order of expected measurement cost; this enables the program to construct the reduced flowchart and to determine the minimal measurements that are necessary.

The net effect of the driver program is to cause the attributes *measure* and *flowlist* to be set up; these specify the minimal measurements in the following way:

$v.measure$ is a Boolean attribute that is set to **true** if the frequency count of vertex v should be measured, otherwise **false**;

$v.flowlist$ points to a list of *flowitem* objects that specify how to compute the frequency count of vertex v when $v.measure =$ **false**.

More precisely, a *flowitem* is defined by the following class declaration:

class *flowitem* $(v, d, suc);$
   ref (*vertex*) $v;$ **Boolean** $d;$ **ref** (*flowitem*) $suc;$
   begin comment Each object of this class represents an entry
      in the flow list of some vertex, namely
         if d **then** $v.count$ **else** $-v.count$
      and suc represents the next list element;

    integer procedure *sum*;
      comment Compute the sum of the counts represented by
        this *flowitem* and its successors;
      $sum :=$ (**if** d **then** $v.count$ **else** $-v.count$)
         $+$ (**if** $suc =$ **none then** 0 **else** $suc.sum$)
   end *flowitem*

If $v.count$ is set to the frequency count measurement for all v with $v.measure = $ **true**, then the frequency count measurements for any other vertex v may be computed by calling $v.flowlist.sum$.

The vertex class itself may now be declared as follows, with comments to indicate the uses of each variable and the way the program works:

class $vertex$;
    begin comment the vertices of the original flowchart;
        ref($vertex$) $parent$; **comment** If **this** $vertex$ is a "supervertex,"
                namely the representative of its equivalence class, then
                $parent \equiv $ **none**, otherwise $parent$ points to an equivalent
                vertex;
        ref($vertex$) **procedure** $super$; **comment** the supervertex equiva-
                lent to **this** vertex;
        $super :- $ **if** $parent \equiv $ **none then this** $vertex$ **else** $parent.super$;
        ref($vertex$) $follow$; **comment** a vertex to which **this** $vertex$ leads
                in the flow chart;
    procedure $arcto(w)$; **ref**($vertex$) w;
        comment Create an arc from **this** $vertex$ to w, in the original
            flow chart;
        if $follow \equiv $ **none then** $follow :- w$
        else begin Make w and $follow$ equivalent:
            $w :- w.super$;
            if $w \not\equiv follow.super$ **then** $w.parent :- follow.super$
        end;
    Boolean d; **ref**($vertex$) u, $cparent$;
        comment These three attributes are used only for supervertices.
            The connected components of the reduced flow chart created
            so far are represented as equivalence classes of supervertices,
            using $cparent$ in a way analogous to the $parent$ attribute
            above. However, when $cparent \not\equiv $ **none** it represents an
            actual arc of the spanning tree of the reduced flowchart,
            namely the arc from $u.super$ to $u.follow.super$. That arc
            runs from **this** $vertex$ to $cparent$ if $d = $ **true**, otherwise it
            runs from $cparent$ to **this** $vertex$;
    ref($vertex$) **procedure** $comp$; **comment** the representative of
            this supervertex's component in the reduced flowchart con-
            structed so far, analogous to $super$ above;
        $comp :- $ **if** $cparent \equiv $ **none then this** $vertex$
            else $cparent.comp$;

procedure *makecomp*; **comment** Transform the *d*, *u*, and *cparent* attributes of the supervertices so that this supervertex is the representative of its component;

if *cparent* ≢ **none then**
  begin *cparent.makecomp*;
    cparent.cparent :− **this** *vertex*;
    cparent.d := **not** *d*; *cparent.u* :− *u*;
    cparent :− **none**
  end *makecomp*;

integer *count*; **comment** the frequency count for **this** *vertex*;
Boolean *measure*; **comment** This *count* should be measured;
ref(*flowitem*) *flowlist*; **comment** if measure is **false**, the first entry on the corresponding flow list;

procedure *compute the count*;
  if not *measure* **then** *count* := *flowlist.sum*;

procedure *insert*; **comment** Create the arc corresponding to **this** *vertex*, in the reduced flow chart. Put the arc into the spanning tree if it reduces the number of components, otherwise augment the flow lists for the spanning tree arcs affected by this new independent flow;

begin ref(*vertex*) *v*, *w*;
  v :− *super*; *v.makecomp*;
  w :− *follow.super*;
  if *v* ≢ *w.comp* **then**
    begin Join the components:
      v.cparent := *w*;
      v.d := **true**; *v.u* := **this** *vertex*;
      measure := **false**
    end
  else begin Update the flow lists:
    measure := **true**;
    while *w* ≢ *v* **do**
      begin *w.u.flowlist* :−
        new *flowitem*(**this** *vertex*, *w.d*, *w.u.flowlist*);
        w :− *w.cparent*
      end
    end
  end *insert*
end *vertex* class declaration

This research was supported by Norges Almenvitenskapelige Forskningsråd and the United States Office of Naval Research.

References

[1] Yutze Chow and Etienne Cassignol, *Linear Signal-Flow Graphs and Applications* (New York: Wiley, 1962).

[2] Daniel Ingalls, "The execution time profile as a programming tool," in *Formal Semantics of Programming Languages*, edited by Randall Rustin, *Courant Computer Science Symposium* **2** (Englewood Cliffs, New Jersey: Prentice–Hall, 1970), 107–128.

[3] Donald E. Knuth, *The Art of Computer Programming*, Volumes 1–3 (Reading, Massachusetts: Addison–Wesley, 1968, 1969, 1973).

[4] Donald E. Knuth, "An empirical study of FORTRAN programs," *Software — Practice & Experience* **1** (1971), 105–133.

[5] S. J. Mason, "Feedback theory — some properties of signal-flow graphs," *Proceedings of the IRE* **4** (1953), 1144–1156.

[6] Armen Nahapetian, "Node flows in graphs with conservative flow," *Acta Informatica* **3** (1973), 37–41.

[7] Edwin H. Satterthwaite, "Debugging tools for high level languages," *Software — Practice & Experience* **2** (1972), 197–217.

Chapter 6

Estimating the Efficiency of Backtrack Programs

*[To Derrick H. Lehmer on his 70th birthday, 23 February 1975. Originally published in Mathematics of Computation **29** (1975), 121–136.]*

One of the chief difficulties associated with the so-called backtracking technique for combinatorial problems has been our inability to predict the efficiency of a given algorithm, or to compare the efficiencies of different approaches, without actually writing and running the programs. This paper presents a simple method that produces reasonable estimates for most applications, requiring only a modest amount of hand calculation. The method should prove to be of considerable utility in connection with D. H. Lehmer's branch-and-bound approach to combinatorial optimization.

The majority of all combinatorial computing applications can apparently be handled only by what amounts to an exhaustive search through all possibilities. Such searches can readily be performed by using a well-known "depth-first" procedure that R. J. Walker [21] has aptly called *backtracking*. (See Lehmer [16], Golomb and Baumert [6], and Wells [22] for general discussions of this technique, together with numerous interesting examples.)

Sometimes a backtrack program will run to completion in less than a second, while other applications of backtracking seem to go on forever. The author once waited all night for the output from such a program, only to discover that the answers would not be forthcoming for about 10^6 centuries. A "slight increase" in one of the parameters of a backtrack routine might slow down the total running time by a factor of a thousand; conversely, a "minor improvement" to the algorithm might cause a hundredfold improvement in speed; and a sophisticated "major improvement" might actually make the program ten times slower. These great discrepancies in execution time are characteristic of backtrack programs, yet we usually have no obvious way to predict what will happen until the algorithm has been coded and run on a machine.

Faced with these uncertainties, the author worked out a simple estimation procedure in 1962, designed to predict backtrack behavior in any given situation. This procedure was mentioned briefly in a survey article a few years later [8]; and during subsequent years, extensive computer experimentation has confirmed its utility. Several improvements on the original idea have also been developed during the last decade.

The estimation procedure we shall discuss is completely unsophisticated, and it probably has been used without fanfare by many people. Yet the idea works surprisingly well in practice, and some of its properties are not immediately obvious, hence the present paper might prove to be useful.

Section 1 presents a simple example problem, and Section 2 formulates backtracking in general, developing a convenient notational framework; this treatment is essentially self-contained, assuming no prior knowledge of the backtrack literature. Section 3 presents the estimation procedure in its simplest form, together with some theorems that describe the virtues of the method. Section 4 takes the opposite approach, by pointing out a number of flaws and things that can go wrong. Refinements of the original method, intended to counteract these difficulties, are presented in Section 5. Some computational experiments are recorded in Section 6, and Section 7 summarizes the practical experience obtained with the method to date.

1. Introduction to Backtrack

It is convenient to introduce the ideas of this paper by looking first at a small example. The problem we shall study is actually a rather frivolous puzzle, so it does not display the economic benefits of backtracking; but it does have the virtue of simplicity, since the complete solution can be displayed in a small diagram. Furthermore the puzzle itself seems to have been tantalizing people for at least sixty years (see [19]); it became extremely popular in the U.S.A. about 1967 under the name *Instant Insanity*.

Figure 1 shows four cubes whose faces are colored red (R), white (W), green (G), or blue (B); colors on the hidden faces are shown at the sides. The problem is to arrange the cubes in such a way that each of the four colors appears exactly once on the four back faces, once on the top, once in the front, and once on the bottom. Thus Figure 1 is not a solution, since there is no blue on the top nor white on the bottom; but a solution is obtained by rotating each cube 90°.

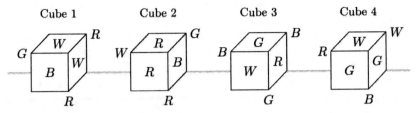

FIGURE 1. Instant Insanity cubes.

We can assume that these four cubes retain their relative left-to-right order in all solutions. Each of the six faces of a given cube can be on the bottom, and there are four essentially different positions having a given bottom face, so each cube can be placed in 24 different ways; therefore the "brute-force" approach to this problem is to try all of the $24^4 = 331776$ possible configurations. If done by hand, the brute force procedure might indeed lead to insanity, although not instantly.

It is not difficult to improve on the brute force approach by considering the effects of symmetry. Any solution clearly leads to seven other solutions, by simultaneously rotating the cubes about a horizontal axis parallel to the gray line in Figure 1, and/or by rotating each cube 180° about a vertical axis. Therefore we can assume without loss of generality that Cube 1 is in one of three positions, instead of considering all 24 possibilities. Furthermore it turns out that Cube 2 has only 16 essentially different placements, since it has two opposite red faces; see Figure 2, which shows that two of its 24 positionings have the same colors on the front, top, back, and bottom faces. The same observation applies to Cube 3. Hence the total number of essentially different ways to position the four cubes is only $3 \cdot 16 \cdot 16 \cdot 24 = 18432$; this is substantially less than 331776, but it might still be hazardous to one's mental health.

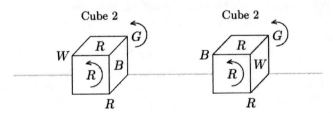

FIGURE 2. Rotation of this cube by 180° preserves the relevant colors.

A natural way to reduce the number of cases still further now suggests itself. Given one of the three placements for Cube 1, some of the 16 positionings of Cube 2 are obviously foolhardy since they cannot possibly lead to a solution. In Figure 1, for example, Cubes 1 and 2 both contain red on their bottom face, while a complete solution has no repeated colors on the bottom, nor on the front, top, or back. This placement of Cube 2 is incompatible with the given position of Cube 1, so we need not consider any of the $16 \cdot 24 = 384$ ways to place Cubes 3 and 4. Similarly, when Cubes 1 and 2 have been given a compatible placement, it makes sense to place Cube 3 so as to avoid duplicate colors on the relevant sides, before we even begin to consider Cube 4.

Such a sequential placement can be represented by a tree structure, as shown in Figure 3. The three nodes just below the root (top) of this tree stand for the three essentially different ways to place Cube 1. Below each such node are further nodes representing the possible placements of Cube 2 in a compatible position; and below the latter are the compatible placements of Cube 3 (if any), etc. Notice that there is only one solution to the puzzle, represented by the single node on Level 4.

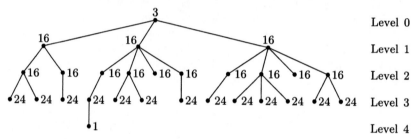

FIGURE 3. The Instant Insanity tree.

This procedure cuts the number of cases examined to $3 + 3 \cdot 16 + 10 \cdot 16 + 13 \cdot 24 + 1 = 524$; for example, each of the 10 nodes on Level 2 of the tree involves the consideration of 16 ways to place Cube 3. It is reasonable to assume that a sane person can safely remain *compos mentis* while examining 524 cases; thus, we may conclude that systematic enumeration can cut the work by several orders of magnitude even in simple problems like this one. (Actually a further refinement, which may be called the technique of "homomorphism and lifting," can be applied to the Instant Insanity problem, reducing the total number of cases examined to about 50, as shown originally in [1]; see also [7] for further discussion and for a half-dozen recent references. But such techniques are beyond the scope of the present paper.)

The tree of Figure 3 can be explored systematically, with comparatively little memory of what has gone before. The idea is to start at the root and continually to move downward when possible, taking the leftmost branch whenever a decision is necessary; but if it is impossible to continue downward, "backtrack" by considering the next alternative on the previous level. This is a special case of the classical Trémaux procedure for exploring a maze (see [17, pages 47–50] and [13, Chapter 3]).

2. The General Backtrack Procedure

Now that we understand the Instant Insanity example, let us consider backtracking in general. The problem we wish to solve can be expressed abstractly as the task of finding all sequences $(x_1, x_2, \ldots, x_n)$ that satisfy some property $P_n(x_1, x_2, \ldots, x_n)$. For example, in the case of Instant Insanity, we have $n = 4$; the symbol x_k denotes a placement of the kth cube; and $P_4(x_1, x_2, x_3, x_4)$ is the property that the four cubes exhibit all four colors on all four relevant sides.

The general backtrack approach consists of inventing intermediate properties $P_k(x_1, \ldots, x_k)$ such that

$$P_{k+1}(x_1, \ldots, x_k, x_{k+1}) \text{ implies } P_k(x_1, \ldots, x_k) \text{ for } 0 \leq k < n. \qquad (1)$$

In other words, if $(x_1, \ldots, x_k)$ *does not* satisfy property P_k, then no extended sequence $(x_1, \ldots, x_k, x_{k+1})$ can possibly satisfy P_{k+1}; hence by induction, no extended sequence $(x_1, \ldots, x_k, \ldots, x_n)$ can solve the original condition P_n. The backtrack procedure systematically enumerates all solutions $(x_1, \ldots, x_n)$ to the original problem by considering all partial solutions $(x_1, \ldots, x_k)$ that satisfy P_k, using the following general algorithm:

B1. [Initialize.] Set k to 0.

B2. [Compute the successors.]   (Now $P_k(x_1, \ldots, x_k)$ holds, and $0 \leq k < n$.) Set S_k to the set of all elements x_{k+1} such that $P_{k+1}(x_1, \ldots, x_k, x_{k+1})$ is true.

B3. [Have all successors been tried?] If S_k is empty, go to step B6.

B4. [Advance.] Choose any element of S_k, call it x_{k+1}, and delete it from S_k. Increase k by 1.

B5. [Solution found?] (Now $P_k(x_1, \ldots, x_k)$ holds, and $0 < k \leq n$.) If $k < n$, return to step B2. Otherwise output the solution $(x_1, \ldots, x_n)$ and go on to step B6.

B6. [Backtrack.] (All extensions of $(x_1, \ldots, x_k)$ have now been explored.) Decrease k by 1. If $k \geq 0$, return to step B3; otherwise the algorithm terminates.   □

Condition (1) does not uniquely define the intermediate properties P_k, so we often have considerable latitude when we choose them. For example, we could simply let P_k be true for all $(x_1, \ldots, x_k)$, when $k < n$; this is the weakest possible property satisfying (1), and it corresponds to the brute force approach, where some 24^4 possibilities would be examined in the cube problem. On the other hand the strongest property is obtained when $P_k(x_1, \ldots, x_k)$ is true if and only if there exist $x_{k+1}, \ldots, x_n$ satisfying $P_n(x_1, \ldots, x_k, x_{k+1}, \ldots, x_n)$. In our example this strongest property would reduce the search to the examination of a trivial twig of a tree, but the decisions at each node would require considerable calculation. In general, stronger properties limit the search but require more computation, so we want to find a suitable trade-off. The solution adopted in our example (namely to use symmetry considerations when placing Cubes 1, 2, and 3, and to let $P_k(x_1, \ldots, x_k)$ mean that no colors are duplicated on the four relevant sides) is fairly obvious, but in other problems the choice of P_k is not always so self-evident.

3. A Simple Estimate of the Running Time

For each $(x_1, \ldots, x_k)$ satisfying P_k with $0 < k < n$, the algorithm of Section 2 will execute steps B2, B4, B5, and B6 once, and step B3 twice. (To see this, note that it is true for steps B2, B5, and B6, and apply Kirchhoff's law as in [12].) Let us call the associated running time the cost $c(x_1, \ldots, x_k)$. When $k = n$, the corresponding cost amounts to one execution of steps B3, B4, B5, and B6. If we also let $c(\ )$ be the cost for $k = 0$ (that is, one execution of steps B1, B2, B3, and B6), the total running time of the algorithm comes to exactly

$$\sum_{k \geq 0} \sum_{P_k(x_1, \ldots, x_k)} c(x_1, \ldots, x_k). \tag{2}$$

This formula essentially distributes the total cost among the various nodes of the tree. Since the time to execute step B2 can vary from node to node, and since the time to execute step B5 depends on whether or not $k = n$, the running time is not simply proportional to the size of the tree except in simple cases.

Let T be the tree of all possibilities explored by the backtrack method; that is, let

$$T = \{(x_1, \ldots, x_k) \mid k \geq 0 \text{ and } P_k(x_1, \ldots, x_k) \text{ holds}\}. \tag{3}$$

Then we can rewrite (2) as

$$\text{cost}(T) = \sum_{t \in T} c(t). \tag{4}$$

Our goal is to find some way of estimating $\text{cost}(T)$, without knowing a great deal about the properties P_k, since the example of Section 1 indicates that these properties might be very complex.

A natural solution to this estimation problem is to try a Monte Carlo approach, based on a random exploration of the tree; for each partial solution $(x_1, \ldots, x_k)$ for $0 \leq k < n$, we can choose x_{k+1} at random from among the set S_k of all continuations, as in the following algorithm. (A related but more complicated procedure, which is intrinsically different because it is oriented to estimates for problems that have a certain geometric structure, has been published by Hammersley and Morton [10], and it has been the subject of numerous papers in the literature of mathematical physics; see [5].)

E1. [Initialize.] Set $k \leftarrow 0$, $D \leftarrow 1$, and $C \leftarrow c(\ )$. (Here C will be an estimate of (2), and D is an auxiliary variable used in the calculation of C, namely the product of all "degrees" encountered in the tree. An arrow '$\leftarrow$' denotes the assignment operation equivalent to ALGOL's ':='; and $c(\ )$ denotes the cost at the root of the tree, as in (2) when $k = 0$.)

E2. [Compute the successors.] Set S_k to the set of all x_{k+1} such that $P_{k+1}(x_1, \ldots, x_k, x_{k+1})$ is true, and let d_k be the number of elements of S_k. (If $k = n$, then S_k is empty and $d_k = 0$.)

E3. [Terminal position?] If $d_k = 0$, the algorithm terminates, with C an estimate of $\text{cost}(T)$.

E4. [Advance.] Choose an element $x_{k+1} \in S_k$ at random, each element being equally likely. (Thus, each choice occurs with probability $1/d_k$.) Set $D \leftarrow d_k D$, then set $C \leftarrow C + c(x_1, \ldots, x_{k+1})D$. Increase k by 1 and return to step E2.   ☐

This algorithm makes a random walk in the tree, without any backtracking, and computes the estimate

$$C = c(\ ) + d_0 c(x_1) + d_0 d_1 c(x_1, x_2) + d_0 d_1 d_2 c(x_1, x_2, x_3) + \cdots, \quad (5)$$

where d_k is a function of $(x_1, \ldots, x_k)$, namely the number of x_{k+1} satisfying $P_{k+1}(x_1, \ldots, x_k, x_{k+1})$. We may define $d_k = 0$ for all large k, thereby regarding (5) as an infinite series although only finitely many terms are nonzero.

The validity of estimate (5) can be proved as follows.

Theorem 1. *The expected value of C, as computed by Algorithm E above, is* $\mathrm{cost}(T)$ *as defined in* (4).

Proof. We shall consider two proofs, at least one of which should be convincing. First we can observe that for every $t = (x_1, \ldots, x_k) \in T$, the term

$$d_0 d_1 \ldots d_{k-1} c(x_1, \ldots, x_k) \tag{6}$$

occurs in (5) with probability $1/d_0 d_1 \ldots d_{k-1}$, since this is the chance that the algorithm will consider the partial solution $(x_1, \ldots, x_k)$. Hence the sum of all the terms (6) has the expected value (4).

The second proof is based on a recursive definition of $\mathrm{cost}(T)$, namely

$$\mathrm{cost}(T) = c(\,) + \mathrm{cost}(T_1) + \ldots + \mathrm{cost}(T_d), \tag{7}$$

where $d = d_0$ is the degree of the root of the tree and $T_1, \ldots, T_d$ are the respective subtrees of the root, namely

$$T_j = \{(x_1, \ldots, x_k) \in T \mid x_1 \text{ is the } j\text{th element of } S_0\}.$$

We also have $C = c(\,) + d_0 C'$, where $C' = c(x_1) + d_1 c(x_1, x_2) + d_1 d_2 c(x_1, x_2, x_3) + \ldots$ has the form of (5) and is an estimate of one of the T_j. Since each of the $d = d_0$ values of j is equally likely, the expected value of C is

$$\mathrm{E}\, C = c(\,) + d_0 \,\mathrm{E}\, C' = c(\,) + d_0 \big((\mathrm{E}\, C_1 + \ldots + \mathrm{E}\, C_d)/d\big),$$

where $\mathrm{E}\, C_j = \mathrm{cost}(T_j)$ by induction on the size of the tree. Hence $\mathrm{E}\, C = \mathrm{cost}(T)$. $\square$

This theorem demonstrates that C is indeed an appropriate statistic to compute, based on one random walk down the tree. As an example of the theorem, let us consider Figure 3 in Section 1, using the costs shown there (since they represent the time to perform step B2, which dominates the calculation). We have $\mathrm{cost}(T) = 524$, and if the estimation algorithm is applied to the tree it is not difficult to determine that the result will be $C = 243$, or 291, or 435, or 531, or 543, or 819, or 1107, with respective probabilities 1/6, 1/6, 1/6, 1/6, 1/12, 1/6, and 1/12. Thus, a fairly reasonable approximation will nearly always be obtained; and we know that the mean of repeated estimates will approach 524, by the law of large numbers.

Since the proof of Theorem 1 applies to all functions $c(t)$ defined over trees, we can apply it to other functions in order to obtain further information:

Corollary 1. *The expected value of D at the end of Algorithm E is the number of terminal nodes in the tree.*

Proof. Let $c(t) = 1$ if t is terminal, and $c(t) = 0$ otherwise; then $C = D$ at the end of the algorithm, hence $\mathrm{E}\,D = \mathrm{E}\,C = \sum c(t)$ is the number of terminal nodes by Theorem 1. $\square$

Corollary 2. *The expected value of the product $d_0 d_1 \ldots d_{k-1}$ for fixed k, when the d_j's are computed by Algorithm E, is the number of nodes on level k of the tree.*

Proof. Let $c(t) = 1$ for all nodes on level k, and $c(t) = 0$ otherwise; then $C = d_0 d_1 \ldots d_{k-1}$ at the end of the algorithm. (Note that $d_0 d_1 \ldots d_{k-1}$ is zero if the algorithm terminates before reaching level k.) $\square$

Corollary 2 gives some insight into the "meaning" of the individual terms of our estimate (5); the term $d_0 d_1 \ldots d_{k-1} c(x_1, \ldots, x_k)$ represents the number of nodes on level k times the cost associated with a typical one of these nodes.

4. Some Cautionary Remarks

The algorithm of Section 3 seems too simple to work, and there are many intuitive grounds for skepticism, since we are trying to predict the characteristics of an entire tree based on the knowledge of only one branch! The combinatorial realities of most backtrack applications make it clear that different partial solutions can have drastically different behavior patterns.

The mere knowledge that an experiment yields the right expected value is not much consolation in practice. For example, consider an experiment that produces a result of 1 with probability 0.999, while the result is 1,000,001 with probability 0.001; the expected value is 1001, but a limited sampling would almost always convince us that the true answer is 1.

There is reason to suspect that the estimation procedure of Section 3 will suffer from precisely this defect: It has the potential to produce huge values, but with very low probability, so that the expected value might be quite different from typical estimates.

Let N_k be the number of nodes on level k of the tree. In most backtrack applications, the vast majority of all nodes in the search tree are concentrated at only a few levels, so that in fact the *logarithm* of N_k (the number of digits in N_k) tends to follow a bell-shaped curve when plotted as a function of k:

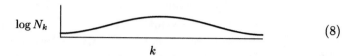

$$\text{(8)}$$

On the other hand our estimate of N_k in Corollary 2 is composed of a series of estimates $N_k' = d_0 d_1 \ldots d_{k-1}$ of a very special nature. The d's are integers, so the N_k' grow exponentially with k, until finally dropping to zero:

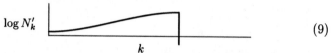

$$\text{(9)}$$

Although these two graphs have quite different characteristics, we are getting estimates that produce exponentials of (8) in the long run, as an average of exponentials of curves like (9).

Consider also Figure 3, where we have somewhat arbitrarily assigned a cost of 1 to the lone solution node on Level 4. Perhaps our output routine is so slow that the solution node should really have a cost of 10^6; this would now become the dominant portion of the total cost, but it would be considered only $1/12$ of the time, and it would then be multiplied by 12.

There is clearly a danger that our estimates will almost always be low, except for rare occasions when they will be much too high.

5. Refinements

Algorithm E can be modified in order to circumvent the difficulties sketched in Section 4. One idea is to introduce systematic bias into step E4, so that the choice of x_{k+1} is not completely random; then we might be able to investigate the more interesting or more difficult parts of the tree.

In other words, the algorithm can be generalized by using the following selection procedure in place of step E4.

E4'. [Generalized advance.] Determine, in any arbitrary fashion, a sequence of d_k nonnegative numbers $p_k(1),\ p_k(2),\ \ldots,\ p_k(d_k)$ whose sum is unity. Then choose a random integer J_k in the range $1 \le J_k \le d_k$ in such a way that J_k takes the value j with probability $p_k(j)$. Let x_{k+1} be the J_kth element of S_k, and set $D \leftarrow D/p_k(J_k), \quad C \leftarrow C + c(x_1, \ldots, x_{k+1})D$. Increase k by 1 and return to step E2. $\square$

(The original step E4 is the special case $p_k(j) = 1/d_k$ for all j.) Again we can prove that the expected value of C will be $\mathrm{cost}(T)$, no matter how strangely the probabilities $p_k(j)$ are biased in step E4'; in fact, both proofs of Theorem 1 are readily extended to yield this result. Notice, incidentally, that the calculation of D involves *a posteriori* probabilities, and D grows only slightly after a highly probable choice has been made. The technique embodied in step E4' is generally known as *importance sampling* [9, pages 57–59].

Some choices of the $p_k(j)$ are much better than others, of course, and the most interesting fact is that one of the possible choices is actually perfect:

Theorem 2. *If the probabilities $p_k(j)$ in step E4' are chosen appropriately, the estimate C will always be exactly equal to $\mathrm{cost}(T)$.*

Proof. For $1 \leq j \leq d_k$, let $p_k(j)$ be

$$p_k^*(j) = \frac{\mathrm{cost}(T(x_1, \ldots, x_k, x_{k+1}(j)))}{\mathrm{cost}(T(x_1, \ldots, x_k)) - c(x_1, \ldots, x_k)}, \qquad (10)$$

where $T(x_1, \ldots, x_k)$ is the set of all $t \in T$ having specified values $(x_1, \ldots, x_k)$ for the first k components, and where $x_{k+1}(j)$ is the jth element of S_k. Now we can prove that the relation

$$C + (\mathrm{cost}(T(x_1, \ldots, x_k)) - c(x_1, \ldots, x_k))D = \mathrm{cost}(T)$$

is invariant, in the sense that it always holds at the beginning and end of step E4'. Since $\mathrm{cost}(T(x_1, \ldots, x_k)) = c(x_1, \ldots, x_k)$ when $d_k = 0$, the algorithm terminates with $C = \mathrm{cost}(T)$.

Alternatively, using the notation in the second proof of Theorem 1, we have

$$C = c(\ ) + \frac{\mathrm{cost}(T) - c(\ )}{\mathrm{cost}(T_j)} C_j$$

for some j, and $C_j = \mathrm{cost}(T_j)$ by induction, hence $C = \mathrm{cost}(T)$.   □

Of course we generally need to know the cost of the tree before we know the exact values of these ideal probabilities $p_k^*(j)$, so we cannot achieve zero variance in practice. But the form of the $p_k^*(j)$ shows what kind of bias is likely to reduce the variance; any information or hunches that we have about relative subtree costs will be helpful. (In the case of Instant Insanity there is no simple *a priori* reason to prefer one cube position over another, so this idea does not apply. Perhaps Instant Insanity is a mind-boggling puzzle for precisely this reason, since intuition usually turns out to be much more valuable.)

Theorem 1 can be extended considerably; in fact we can derive a general formula for the variance. The probability generating function for C satisfies

$$C(z) = \mathrm{E}\, z^C = z^{c(\,)} \sum_{j=1}^{d} p_j C_j(z^{1/p_j}), \tag{11}$$

and from this equation it follows by differentiation that

$$\mathrm{var}(C) = C''(1) + C'(1) - C'(1)^2$$
$$= \sum_{j=1}^{d} \frac{\mathrm{var}(C_j)}{p_j} + \sum_{1 \le i < j \le d} p_i p_j \left(\frac{\mathrm{cost}(T_i)}{p_i} - \frac{\mathrm{cost}(T_j)}{p_j} \right)^2. \tag{12}$$

Iterating this recurrence shows that the variance can be expressed as

$$\sum_{t \in T} \frac{1}{p(t)} \sum_{1 \le i < j \le d(t)} p(t,i) p(t,j) \left(\frac{\mathrm{cost}(T(t,i))}{p(t,i)} - \frac{\mathrm{cost}(T(t,j))}{p(t,j)} \right)^2 \tag{13}$$

where $p(t)$ is the probability that node t is encountered, $d(t)$ is the degree of that node, $p(t,j)$ is the probability that we go from t to its jth successor, and $T(t,j)$ is the subtree rooted at that successor.

From this explicit formula we can get a bound on the variance, if the probabilities are reasonably good approximations to the relative subtree costs:

Theorem 3. *If the probabilities $p_k(j)$ in step E4' satisfy*

$$0 \le \frac{\mathrm{cost}(T(x_1, \ldots, x_k, x_{k+1}(j)))}{p_k(j)} \le \alpha \frac{\mathrm{cost}(T(x_1, \ldots, x_k, x_{k+1}(i)))}{p_k(i)}$$

for all i and j, where $\alpha \ge 1$ is a fixed constant, the variance of C in a tree of depth n is at most

$$\left(\left(\frac{\alpha^2 + 2\alpha + 1}{4\alpha} \right)^n - 1 \right) \mathrm{cost}(T)^2. \tag{14}$$

Proof. Let $q_j = \mathrm{cost}(T_j)/p_j$; then we have

$$\sum_{1 \le i < j \le d} p_i p_j (q_i - q_j)^2 = \sum_{j=1}^{d} \frac{\mathrm{cost}(T_j)^2}{p_j} - \left(\sum_{j=1}^{d} \mathrm{cost}(T_j) \right)^2.$$

The key to the proof is the inequality

$$\sum_{j=1}^{d} \frac{\mathrm{cost}(T_j)^2}{p_j} \le \frac{\alpha^2 + 2\alpha + 1}{4\alpha} \left(\sum_{j=1}^{d} \mathrm{cost}(T_j)\right)^2, \qquad (15)$$

which can be demonstrated as follows: If $q_d = \alpha_j q_j$, the left-hand side of (15) can be written

$$\left(\sum_{j=1}^{d} \alpha_j \, \mathrm{cost}(T_j)\right) \left(\sum_{j=1}^{d} \frac{\mathrm{cost}(T_j)}{\alpha_j}\right), \qquad (16)$$

because $p_1 + \cdots + p_d = 1$. We can assume without loss of generality that $\alpha = \alpha_1 \ge \cdots \ge \alpha_d = 1$. When $d = 2$, we have

$$(\alpha x + y)(x/\alpha + y) \le \beta(x + y)^2$$

for all x and y when $\beta = (\alpha^2 + 2\alpha + 1)/(4\alpha)$, and this constant β is best possible. And for $d > 2$, the maximum of (16) over the range $\alpha = \alpha_1 \ge \alpha_2 \ge \cdots \ge \alpha_d = 1$ occurs when $\alpha_2 = \alpha_1$ or $\alpha_2 = \alpha_3$; hence (15) follows by induction on d.

Finally, (14) follows from (15) by induction, since (12) now yields

$$\mathrm{var}(C) \le \sum_{j=1}^{d} \mathrm{var}(C_j)/p_j + (\beta - 1)\, \mathrm{cost}(T)^2$$

$$\le \sum_{j=1}^{d} (\beta^{n-1} - 1)\, \mathrm{cost}(T_j)^2 /p_j + (\beta - 1)\, \mathrm{cost}(T)^2$$

$$\le (\beta^n - \beta)\, \mathrm{cost}(T)^2 + (\beta - 1)\, \mathrm{cost}(T)^2. \qquad \square$$

Theorem 3 implies Theorem 2 when $\alpha = 1$. For $\alpha > 1$ the bound in (14) is not especially comforting, but it does indicate that a few runs of the algorithm will probably predict $\mathrm{cost}(T)$ with the right order of magnitude.

Another way to improve the estimates is to transform the tree into another one having the same total cost, and to apply the Monte Carlo procedure to the transformed tree. For example, the tree fragment

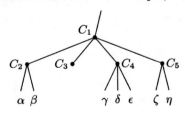

with costs $C_1, \ldots, C_5$ and subtrees $\alpha, \ldots, \eta$ can be replaced by

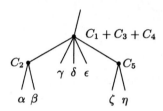

by identifying five nodes. Intermediate condensations such as

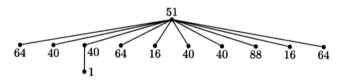

are also possible.

One application of this idea, if the estimates are being made by a computer program, is to eliminate all nodes on levels 1, 3, 5, 7, ... of the original tree, making the nodes formerly on levels $2k$ and $2k+1$ into a new level k. For example, Figure 4 shows the tree that results when this idea is applied to Figure 3. The estimates in the collapsed tree are $C = 211$, or 451, or 461, or 691, or 931, with respective probabilities .2, .3, .1, .3, .1, so we have a slightly better distribution than before.

FIGURE 4. Collapsed Instant Insanity tree.

Another use of this idea is to eliminate all terminal nodes having nonterminal siblings. Then we can ensure that the algorithm never moves directly to a configuration having $d_k = 0$ unless all possible moves are to such a terminal situation; in other words, "stupid" moves can be systematically avoided.

Still another improvement to the general estimation procedure can be achieved by "stratified sampling" [9, pages 55–57]. We can reduce the variance of a series of estimates by insisting for example that each experiment chooses a different value of x_1.

6. Computational Experience

The method of Section 3 has been tested on dozens of applications; and despite the dire predictions made in Section 4 it has consistently performed amazingly well, even on problems that were intended to serve as bad examples. In virtually every case the right order of magnitude for the tree size was found after ten trials. Three or four of the ten trials would typically be gross underestimates, but they were generally counterbalanced by overestimates, in the right proportion.

We shall describe only the largest experiment here, since the method is of most critical importance on a large tree. Figure 5 illustrates the problem that was considered, the enumeration of *uncrossed knight's tours*; these are nonintersecting paths of a knight on the chessboard, where the object is to find the longest possible tour of this kind. T. R. Dawson first proposed the problem in 1930 [2], and he gave the two 35-move solutions of Figure 5, stating that "il est probablement impossible de dénombrer la quantité de ces tours; ... vraisemblablement, on ne peut effectuer plus de 35 coups." Later [3, page 20][4, page 35] he stated without proof that 35 is maximum.

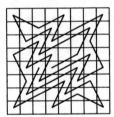 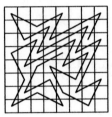

FIGURE 5. Uncrossed knight's tours.

The backtrack method provides a way to test his assertion; we may begin the tour in any of 10 essentially different squares, then continue by making knight's moves that do not cross previous ones, until reaching an impasse. But backtrack trees that extend across 30 levels or more can be extremely large; even if we assume an average of only 3 consistent choices at every stage, out of at most 7 possible knight moves to new squares, we are faced with a tree of about $3^{30} = 205,891,132,094,649$ nodes, and we would never finish. Actually $3^{20} = 3,486,784,401$ is nearer the upper limit of feasibility, since the task of testing whether or not one move crosses another is not especially simple. Thus it is certainly not clear *a priori* that an exhaustive backtrack search is economically feasible.

The simple procedure of Section 3 was therefore used to estimate the number of nodes in the tree, using $c(t) = 1$ for all t. Here are the estimated tree sizes found in the first ten independent experiments:

1571717091	209749511
315291281	58736818301
8231	311
1793651	259271
59761491	6071489081

The mean value is 6,696,688,822. The next sequence of ten experiments gave the estimates

567911	238413491
111	6697691
569585831	5848873631
111	161
411	140296511

for an average of only 680,443,586, although the four extremely low estimates make this value look highly suspicious. (The "stupid moves" that led to such low estimates could have been avoided by using the technique explained at the end of Section 5, but the simple original method was being followed faithfully here.) After 100 experiments had been conducted, the observed mean value of the estimates was 1,653,634,783.8, with an observed standard deviation of about 6.7×10^9.

The first few experiments were done by hand, but then a computer program was written and it performed 1000 experiments in about 30 seconds. The results of these experiments were extremely encouraging, because they were able to predict the size of the tree quite accurately as well as its "shape" (the number N_k of nodes per level), even though the considerations of Section 4 seem to imply that N_k cannot be estimated well. Table 1 shows how these estimates compare to the exact values, which were calculated later; there is surprisingly good agreement, although the experiment looked at fewer than 0.00001 of the nodes of the tree. Perhaps this was unusually good luck.

The uncrossed knight's tour problem reflects the typical growth of backtrack trees; the same problem on a 7×7 board generates a tree with 10,874,674 nodes and on a 6×6 board there are only 88,467. On a 9×9 board we need another method; the longest known tour has 47 moves [18]. The longest reentrant uncrossed knight's tour on an $n \times n$ board can be shown to have at least $n^2 - O(n)$ moves (see [11]).

k	Estimate, N'_k	True value, N_k
0	1.0	1
1	10.0	10
2	42.8	42
3	255.0	251
4	991.4	968
5	4352.2	4215
6	16014.4	15646
7	59948.8	56435
8	190528.7	182520
9	580450.8	574555
10	1652568.7	1606422
11	4424403.9	4376153
12	9897781.4	10396490
13	22047261.5	23978392
14	44392865.5	47667686
15	92464977.5	91377173
16	145815116.2	150084206
17	238608697.6	235901901
18	253061952.9	315123658
19	355460520.9	399772215
20	348542887.6	427209856
21	328849873.9	429189112
22	340682204.1	358868304
23	429508177.9	278831518
24	318416025.6	177916192
25	38610432.0	103894319
26	75769344.0	49302574
27	74317824.0	21049968
28	0.0	7153880
29	0.0	2129212
30	0.0	522186
31	0.0	109254
32	0.0	18862
33	0.0	2710
34	0.0	346
35	0.0	50
36	0.0	8
Total	3123375511.1	3137317290

TABLE 1. Estimates after 1000 random walks.

7. Use of the Method in Practice

There are two principal ways to apply this estimation method, namely by hand and by machine.

Hand calculation is especially recommended as the first step when embarking on any backtrack computations. For one thing, the algorithm is great fun to apply, especially when decimal dice [20] are used to guide the decisions. The reader is urged to try constructing a few random uncrossed knight's tours, recording the statistics d_k as the tours materialize; it is a captivating game that can lead to hours of enjoyment until the telephone rings.

Furthermore, the game is worthwhile, because it gives insight into the behavior of the algorithm, and such insight is of great use later when the algorithm is eventually programmed. Good ideas about data structures, and about various improvements to the backtracking strategy, usually suggest themselves. The assignment of nonuniform probabilities as suggested in Section 5 seems to improve the quality of the estimates, and adds interest to the game. Usually about three estimates are enough to give a feeling for the amount of work that will be involved in a full backtrack search.

For large-scale experiments, especially when the best procedure in some family of methods is being sought, involving parameters that must be selected, the estimates can be done rapidly by machine. Experience indicates that most of the refinements suggested in Section 5 are unnecessary; for example, the idea of collapsing the tree into half as many levels does not improve the quality of the estimates sufficiently to justify the greatly increased computation. Only the partial collapsing technique that avoids "stupid moves" is worth the effort, and even this makes the program so much more complex that it should probably be used only when provided as a system subroutine. (A collection of system routines or programming language features, with which the estimation algorithm and full backtracking can both be driven by the same source language program, proves to be quite useful.)

Perhaps the most important application of backtracking nowadays is to combinatorial optimization problems, as first suggested by D. H. Lehmer [15, pages 168–169]. In this case the method is commonly called a *branch-and-bound* technique (see [14]). The estimation procedure of Section 3 does not apply directly to branch-and-bound algorithms, but we can use it to estimate the amount of work needed to test any given bound for optimality. Thus we can get a good idea of the running time even in this case, provided that we can guess a reasonable bound. Again, hand calculations using a Monte Carlo approach are recommended as a first step in the approach to all branch-and-bound procedures, since the random experiments provide both insight and enjoyment.

Acknowledgments

I wish to thank Robert W. Floyd and George W. Soules for several stimulating conversations relating to this research. The knight's tour calculations were performed as "background computation" during a period of several weeks, on the Control Data 6600 computer at IDA-CRD in Princeton, New Jersey.

References

[1] F. de Carteblanche, "The coloured cubes problem," *Eureka* **9** (Cambridge, England: The Archimedeans, April 1947), 9–11.

[2] T. R. Dawson, "Echecs Feeriques," problem 186, *L'Echiquier* (2) **2** (1930), 1085–1086; solution in *L'Echiquier* (2) **3** (1931), 1150.

[3] T. R. Dawson, *Caissa's Wild Roses* (Surrey, England: C. M. Fox, 1935). Reprinted in *Five Classics of Fairy Chess* (New York: Dover, 1973).

[4] T. R. Dawson, "Chess facts and figures," in *Chess Pie III*, souvenir booklet of the International chess tournament (Nottingham, England: 1936), 34–36.

[5] Paul J. Gans, "Self-avoiding random walks. I. Simple properties of intermediate-walks," *Journal of Chemical Physics* **42** (1965), 4159–4163.

[6] Solomon W. Golomb and Leonard D. Baumert, "Backtrack programming," *Journal of the Association for Computing Machinery* **12** (1965), 516–524.

[7] N. T. Gridgeman, "The 23 colored cubes," *Mathematics Magazine* **44** (1971), 243–252.

[8] Marshall Hall, Jr., and D. E. Knuth, "Combinatorial analysis and computers," *American Mathematical Monthly* **72**, number 2, part II (1965), 21–28.

[9] J. M. Hammersley and D. C. Handscomb, *Monte Carlo Methods* (London: Methuen, 1965).

[10] J. M. Hammersley and K. W. Morton, "Poor man's Monte Carlo," *Journal of the Royal Statistical Society*, Series B, **16** (1954), 23–28; discussion on pages 61–75.

[11] Donald E. Knuth, "Uncrossed knight's tours" (letter to the editor), *Journal of Recreational Mathematics* **2** (1969), 155–157.

[12] Donald E. Knuth, *Fundamental Algorithms*, Volume 1 of *The Art of Computer Programming* (Reading, Massachusetts: Addison–Wesley, 1968).

[13] Dénes König, *Theorie der endlichen und unendlichen Graphen* (Leipzig: 1936). English translation, *Theory of Finite and Infinite Graphs* (Boston: Birkhäuser, 1990).

[14] E. L. Lawler and D. E. Wood, "Branch-and-bound methods: A survey," *Operations Research* **14** (1966), 699–719.

[15] Derrick H. Lehmer, "Combinatorial problems with digital computers," *Proceedings of the Fourth Canadian Mathematical Congress* (Toronto, Ontario: University of Toronto Press, 1959), 160–173. See also *Proceedings of Symposia in Applied Mathematics* **6** (Providence, Rhode Island: American Mathematical Society, 1956), 115, 124, 201.

[16] Derrick H. Lehmer, "The machine tools of combinatorics," Chapter 1 of *Applied Combinatorial Mathematics*, edited by Edwin F. Beckenbach (New York: Wiley, 1964), 5–31.

[17] Édouard Lucas, *Récréations Mathématiques* **1** (Paris: Gauthier-Villars, 1882).

[18] Michio Matsuda and S. Kobayashi, "Uncrossed knight's tours" (letter to the editor), *Journal of Recreational Mathematics* **2** (1969), 155–157.

[19] T. H. O'Bierne, *Puzzles and Paradoxes* (London: Oxford University Press, 1965).

[20] C. B. Tompkins, review of "Random-number generating dice" by the Japanese Standards Association, *Mathematics of Computation* **15** (1961), 94–95.

[21] R. J. Walker, "An enumerative technique for a class of combinatorial problems," *Proceedings of Symposia in Applied Mathematics* **10** (Providence, Rhode Island: American Mathematical Society, 1960), 91–94.

[22] Mark B. Wells, *Elements of Combinatorial Computing* (New York: Pergamon Press, 1971).

[23] L. D. Yarbrough, "Uncrossed knight's tours," *Journal of Recreational Mathematics* **1** (1968), 140–142.

Addendum

Pang C. Chen discovered an important extension of Algorithm E by introducing the notion of *strata* as a generalization of tree levels. When his estimation method was applied to the problem of uncrossed knight's tours, it reduced the variance corresponding to Table 1 by two orders of magnitude, without increasing the total amount of computation. ["Heuristic sampling: A method for predicting the performance of tree searching programs," *SIAM Journal on Computing* **21** (1992), 295–315. See also Pang-Chieh Chen, "Heuristic sampling on DAGs," *Algorithmica* **12** (1994), 458–475.]

Algorithm E has an amusing application to the purely mathematical problem of estimating the number $S_n(t)$ of integer sequences $(a_0, a_1, \ldots, a_n)$ such that $a_0 = 1$ and $1 \le a_{j+1} \le ta_j$ for $0 \le j < n$; here t is an integer ≥ 2. Corollary 2 implies that $S_n(t) = \mathrm{E}(d_0 d_1 \ldots d_{n-1})$ where $d_j = ta_j$, $a_{j+1} = \lceil U_j ta_j \rceil$, and the random variables U_0, U_1, $\ldots, U_{n-1}$ are independent uniform deviates. Removing the ceiling brackets gives the lower bound

$$S_n(t) \ge \mathrm{E}\,(t)(U_0 t^2) \ldots (U_0 \ldots U_{n-2} t^n)$$
$$= \mathrm{E}\,U_0^{n-1} U_1^{n-2} \ldots U_{n-2} t^{n(n+1)/2} = t^{n(n+1)/2}/n!.$$

And a closer analysis of the discretization error caused by removing the ceiling brackets shows that $\ln S_n(t) = \frac{n(n+1)}{2} \ln t - \ln n! + O(\log n)^2$. The sequence $S_n(2)$ was introduced by A. Cayley in *Philosophical Magazine* (4) **13** (1857), 245–248. An interesting way to compute the exact value of $S_n(t)$ and similar sequences in $O(n^6)$ steps has been discovered by Matthew Cook and Michael Kleber, "Tournament sequences and Meeussen sequences" [*Electronic Journal of Combinatorics* **7** (2000), #R44].

Chapter 7

Ordered Hash Tables

[Written with O. Amble. Originally published in The Computer Journal 17 (1974), 135–142.]

Some variants of the traditional hash method, making use of the numerical or alphabetical order of the keys, lead to faster searching at the expense of a little extra work when items are inserted. This paper presents the new algorithms and analyzes their average running time.

Traditional methods of search are usually based either on the numerical or alphabetical ordering of keys (for example, binary search), or on the keys' arithmetical properties (for example, hashing). By combining these two approaches we can obtain methods that are often superior to the traditional algorithms.

In this paper we shall discuss a new class of search procedures that use both the idea of ordering and the idea of "open" hash addressing. A mathematical analysis of the expected running time will also be given.

Definitions

Given a file or *table* of data containing N distinct *keys* $K_1, K_2, \ldots, K_N$, the search problem consists of taking a given *argument* K and determining whether or not $K = K_i$ for some i. In practice the key K_i is part of a larger record of information, R_i, which is being retrieved via its key. But for the purposes of our discussion we may concentrate solely on the keys themselves, since they are the only things that significantly enter into the search algorithms. If the search argument K is not in the table, we sometimes want to put it in; therefore we are generally interested in two algorithms, one for searching and one for insertion. A recent book [4] contains an extensive account of the algorithms that are commonly used for searching and insertion.

One of the important families of search algorithms is the so-called method of open addressing with double hashing, which works as follows.

The table is stored in a larger array of M positions, numbered 0 through $M-1$. If U is the universe of all possible keys that might ever be sought (for example, U might consist of all n-bit numbers or all n-character identifiers), we define two functions for each K in U, namely

$$h(K) = \text{the } hash\ address \text{ of } K,$$
$$i(K) = \text{the } hash\ increment \text{ of } K.$$

These functions are constrained so that $0 \le h(K) < M$, $1 \le i(K) < M$, and $i(K)$ is relatively prime to M, for all K. Thus if M is a power of 2, the increment $i(K)$ is allowed to be any odd positive number less than M; alternatively if M is prime, $i(K)$ is allowed to be *any* positive number less than M. For best results these functions are usually chosen to be efficiently computable, yet with the property that distinct keys will tend to have different hash addresses.

Some of the M positions of the hash table are unoccupied, while N of the positions contain keys. For convenience we shall assume that all keys have a strictly positive numeric value. The entries of the hash table will be denoted by T_0, T_1, ..., T_{M-1}, where $T_j = 0$ if that position is empty and $T_j > 0$ if T_j is the key stored in position j.

Algorithms

Using these definitions, it is possible to describe the conventional algorithm for open addressing with double hashing as follows.

Algorithm A. (Searching in a hash table.) Let K be the search argument.

A1. [Initialize.] Set $j \leftarrow h(K)$.

A2. [Equal?] If $T_j = K$, the algorithm terminates successfully.

A3. [Empty?] If $T_j = 0$, the algorithm terminates unsuccessfully.

A4. [Move on.] Set $j \leftarrow j - i(K)$. If now $j < 0$, set $j \leftarrow j + M$. Return to step A2.   ☐

The search is said to be *successful* or *unsuccessful* according as K has been found or not. After a successful search, it is possible to fetch the entire record having the given key.

A new record may be inserted into such a table by first searching for its key K; when the algorithm terminates unsuccessfully in step A3, the new record is then placed into the jth position of the table. Subsequent searches for this key will follow the same path to position j.

The fact that $i(K)$ is relatively prime to M ensures that no part of the table is examined twice, until all M locations have been probed.

Since we assume that there is at least one empty position, the search must terminate if K is not present.

This algorithm includes several noteworthy special cases. If $i(K)$ is identically 1 for all K, it is the well known method of *linear probing*. If $i(K) = 1$ and $h(K) = M - 1$ for all K, it reduces to the straightforward method of *sequential scanning*. If $i(K) = f(h(K))$ where f is a more-or-less random function, the algorithm is called double hashing with *secondary clustering*. On the other hand, if each of the possible values of the pair $(h(K), i(K))$ is equally likely, so that we have $h(K) = h(K')$ and $i(K) = i(K')$ with probability $1/(M\varphi(M))$ for every pair of keys K and K' in U, the method is called *independent double hashing*.

Algorithm A makes decisions only by testing for equality versus inequality. By using the numerical order of keys we obtain a new algorithm that is almost identical to the other:

Algorithm B. (Searching in an ordered hash table.)

B1. [Initialize.] Set $j \leftarrow h(K)$.

B2. [Equal?] If $T_j = K$, the algorithm terminates successfully.

B3. [Smaller?] If $T_j < K$, the algorithm terminates unsuccessfully.

B4. [Move on.] Set $j \leftarrow j - i(K)$. If now $j < 0$, set $j \leftarrow j + M$. Return to step B2. ☐

Only step B3 has changed, and the change is almost trivial. Unsuccessful searches will now be faster.

Of course we cannot use Algorithm B unless the positions of the hash table have been filled in a suitable way. If the keys have been inserted in decreasing order by the ordinary method (that is, if we start with an empty table, then insert the largest key, then the second-largest, and so on), it is easy to see that Algorithm B will work properly. This proves that there is always an arrangement of keys such that Algorithm B is valid.

In practice we need to be able to insert keys in arbitrary order, as they arrive "on line." The following method can be used:

Algorithm C. (Insertion into an ordered hash table.) Assume that $K \neq T_j$ for $0 \leq j < M$, and that at least two table positions are empty.

C1. [Initialize.] Set $j \leftarrow h(K)$.

C2. [Empty?] If $T_j = 0$, set $T_j \leftarrow K$ and terminate.

C3. [Smaller?] If $T_j < K$, interchange the values of $T_j \leftrightarrow K$.

C4. [Move on.] Set $j \leftarrow j - i(K)$. If now $j < 0$, set $j \leftarrow j + M$. Return to step C2. ☐

During this algorithm, the variable K takes on a decreasing sequence of values, and the increments in step C4 will vary (in general). This is a rather peculiar state of affairs, in spite of the innocuous appearance of Algorithm C, so it is helpful to look at an example.

Suppose that $M = 11$ and that there are $N = 8$ keys

$$145, \quad 293, \quad 397, \quad 458, \quad 553, \quad 626, \quad 841, \quad 931,$$

where the middle digit is the h-value and the rightmost digit is the i-value; thus, $h(293) = 9$ and $i(293) = 3$. Then the keys may be distributed in the T table as follows:

T_0	T_1	T_2	T_3	T_4	T_5	T_6	T_7	T_8	T_9	T_{10}
0	0	626	931	841	553	293	0	458	397	145

The reader may verify that Algorithm B will indeed retrieve each of these keys properly. Now if we wish to insert the new key 759, Algorithm C first replaces T_5 by 759 and sets $K \leftarrow 553$; after examining $T_2 = 626$, it sets $T_{10} \leftarrow 553$, $K \leftarrow 145$; and eventually $T_0 \leftarrow 145$. The table for all nine keys is therefore

T_0	T_1	T_2	T_3	T_4	T_5	T_6	T_7	T_8	T_9	T_{10}
145	0	626	931	841	759	293	0	458	397	553

To verify that Algorithm C is correct, consider the *path* corresponding to key K, namely the sequence of table position numbers

$$h(K), \quad h(K) - i(K), \quad h(K) - 2i(K), \quad \ldots, \quad h(K) - (M-1)i(K)$$

mod M. Since $i(K)$ is relatively prime to M, this sequence consists of the numbers $0, 1, \ldots, M-1$ in some order. Algorithm B works properly if and only if, for every key $K = T_j$ in the table, we do not have $K > T_{j'}$ for any j' that appears *earlier* than j in the path corresponding to K. (This is the essential invariant relation that is relevant to formal proofs of Algorithm B.) Since Algorithm C never decreases the value of any table position, it preserves this condition.

Analyses

Now let us attempt to determine how much faster (if at all) the new algorithms will go. The following uniqueness theorem is quite helpful in this regard.

Theorem. *A set of N keys $K_1, \ldots, K_N$ can be arranged in a table $T_0, T_1, \ldots, T_{M-1}$ of $M > N$ positions in one and only one way such that Algorithm B is valid.*

Proof. We have observed that at least one arrangement is possible. Suppose that there are at least two, and let K_j be the largest key that appears in different positions in two different arrangements. Thus, all keys larger than K_j occupy fixed positions in all possible arrangements. If we look at the path corresponding to K_j, as defined above, the positions of keys larger than K_j are predetermined; and all keys smaller than K_j must occur later than K_j. Therefore K_j must occupy the first vacant place in its path, after the larger keys, contradicting the assumption that K_j can appear in different places.   □

To know the behavior of these search algorithms, we want to know the corresponding average number of iterations or *probes* in the table, namely the average number of times steps A2, B2, or C2 are performed, respectively. Only the average number is generally considered in discussions of hashing, since the worst case is too horrible to contemplate.

The classical Algorithm A has been extensively investigated (see [4, Section 6.4] for a review of the literature), and the results can be summarized as follows. Let $\alpha = N/M$ be the load factor of the hash table. Let A_N be the average number of times step A2 is performed in a random successful search, and let A'_N be the corresponding number in a random unsuccessful search. By "random" and "average" we mean that the hash addresses of the keys are assumed to be independent and uniformly distributed in the range 0 through $M - 1$, and that each of the N keys of the table is equally likely in a successful search. Then the following approximate formulas have been derived, as M and N approach infinity:

Increment method	A_N	A'_N
linear probing	$\frac{1}{2}(1 + (1-\alpha)^{-1})$	$\frac{1}{2}(1 + (1-\alpha)^{-2})$
secondary clustering	$1 - \ln(1-\alpha) - \frac{1}{2}\alpha$	$(1-\alpha)^{-1} - \ln(1-\alpha) - \alpha$
independent double hashing	$-\alpha^{-1}\ln(1-\alpha)$	$(1-\alpha)^{-1}$

Since the number of probes needed to retrieve an item with Algorithm A is the same as the number needed to insert it, the average number of probes needed to find the kth item inserted is A'_{k-1}. It follows that

$$A_N = (A'_0 + A'_1 + \cdots + A'_{N-1})/N. \tag{1}$$

Now let us consider the performance of Algorithm B. We shall assume that there is no significant correlation between the hash addresses and the numerical ordering of the keys. Since the position of any fixed set of keys in the table is unique, we may as well assume that they have been inserted in decreasing order. Then the insertion algorithm is identical to that used with Algorithm A, and the average number of probes needed to find the kth largest item is A'_{k-1}. It follows that

$$B_N = (A'_0 + A'_1 + \cdots + A'_{N-1})/N = A_N. \tag{2}$$

In other words, Algorithm B is equivalent to Algorithm A with respect to successful searching, on the average.

In an unsuccessful search with Algorithm B, the number of probes is the same as would be required in a *successful* search if the keys were $\{K_1, K_2, \ldots, K_N, K\}$ instead of $\{K_1, K_2, \ldots, K_N\}$. Therefore

$$B'_N = B_{N+1} = A_{N+1}. \tag{3}$$

The formulas given for A_N and A'_N above show that this is indeed an improvement. For example, when $\alpha = 0.90$ (that is, when the table is 90% full), the quantities for unsuccessful search are

Increment method	A'_N	B'_N
linear probing	50.50	5.500
secondary clustering	11.40	2.853
independent double hashing	10.00	2.558

As $\alpha \to 1$, the ratio B'_N/A'_N approaches 0.

Finally let us investigate the new cost of insertion with Algorithm C. Let C_N be the average number of times step C2 is performed when inserting the Nth item. Each time we execute step C2, we increase by one the total number of probes needed to find one of the keys. Thus, if we sum over N insertions, we must have

$$C_1 + \cdots + C_N = NA_N.$$

This equation together with (1) implies that

$$C_N = A'_{N-1}. \tag{4}$$

In other words, the average number of probes needed to insert a new item is exactly the same as it was with Algorithm A.

It is worth noting that the probability distribution of C_N is not in general the same as that of A'_{N-1}, although the average value is the same. In fact, a single insertion with Algorithm C might take up to order N^2

iterations (although such an event is extremely rare). Consider again the case of three-digit keys whose middle digit is the h-value and whose rightmost digit is the i-value; and let $M = 10$. Then the insertion of 949 into the table

T_0	T_1	T_2	T_3	T_4	T_5	T_6	T_7	T_8	T_9
109	319	529	739	841	651	461	271	0	0

is amazingly slow, as the reader may verify. In general, the table might contain n keys in "organ-pipe order,"

$$0 = T_n < T_0 < T_{n-1} < T_1 < \cdots < T_{\lfloor n/2 \rfloor},$$

and we might have

$$i(T_j) = \begin{cases} M - 1, & \text{for } 0 \leq j < \lceil n/2 \rceil, \\ 1, & \text{for } \lceil n/2 \rceil \leq j < n; \end{cases}$$

then the insertion of a new largest key whose hash address is $\lfloor n/2 \rfloor$ will take maximum time, namely $(n + 1)n/2 + 1$ iterations of step C2.

We have now analyzed the average number of iterations in both Algorithms B and C. The analysis isn't complete, however, because we have not determined the average number of *interchanges* performed in step C3. This is an important consideration, since it is the number of times we need to compute an increment $i(K)$; with Algorithm A, the increment needs to be computed only once. Therefore let D_N be the average number of times the operation $T_j \leftrightarrow K$ is performed in step C3 while inserting the Nth item.

Unfortunately the analysis of D_N is complicated, and we must defer the calculations to Appendix 1. It turns out that D_N is approximately $(1 - \alpha)^{-1} + \alpha^{-1} \ln(1 - \alpha)$ for linear probing, and approximately equal to $A_N - 1$ for independent double hashing.

Further Development

The algorithms above can be extended in various ways, to gain further improvements. For example, it is easy to see that the ideas can immediately be generalized to the case of external searching, where each of the M table positions is a "bucket" containing at most b keys for some given capacity b.

Another type of extension will make unsuccessful searching still faster, at the expense of M more bits of memory. Let $B_0, B_1, \ldots, B_{M-1}$ be a vector of bits with all B_j initially 0. Suppose that we set

N/M (the load ratio)	25%	50%	75%	85%	90%	95%
Alg. A, linear probing	1.167	1.500	2.500	3.833	5.500	10.500
Alg. A, secondary clustering	1.163	1.443	2.011	2.472	2.853	3.521
Alg. A, independent double hashing	1.151	1.386	1.848	2.232	2.558	3.153
Alg. B, linear probing	1.167	1.500	2.500	3.833	5.500	10.500
Alg. B, secondary clustering	1.163	1.443	2.011	2.472	2.853	3.521
Alg. B, independent double hashing	1.151	1.386	1.848	2.232	2.558	3.153
Alg. B, linear, with pass bits	1.167	1.500	2.500	3.833	5.500	10.500
Alg. B, independent, with pass bits	1.151	1.386	1.848	2.232	2.558	3.153
Alg. B, linear, correlated, one ahead	1.871	1.797	2.245	3.306	4.825	9.667
Alg. X, bidirectional linear	1.1	1.3	1.7	2.3	2.9	4.2

TABLE 1. The average number of probes in a successful search.

$B_j \leftarrow 1$ in step C3 of the insertion algorithm, so that $B_j = 1$ if and only if some successful search "passes through" position j. Then if the search algorithm ever gets to step B3 and finds $B_j = 0$, the search must be unsuccessful.

This extra-bit approach applies to unordered hash tables as well as to ordered ones (see Furukawa [2]); and it is especially attractive in the ordered case because the extra testing can be done with almost no cost. We can combine the bit test with the ordinary test if we assume that each bit B_j appears at the left of T_j as a new significant bit. Then Algorithm B can be rewritten as follows.

B1. [Initialize.] Set $j \leftarrow h(K)$.

B2. [Smaller?] If $(B_j, T_j) < (1, K)$, the algorithm terminates successfully or unsuccessfully according as $T_j = K$ or not.

B3. [Equal?] If $(B_j, T_j) = (1, K)$, the algorithm terminates successfully.

B4. [Move on.] Set $j \leftarrow j - i(K)$. If now $j < 0$, set $j \leftarrow j + M$. Return to step B2. $\square$

Only steps B2 and B3 have changed, and the change is such that the computer time per iteration is the same as before; there is just a little more calculation at the end of a successful search, plus the cost of attaching a 1 at the left of the input argument K when the search begins.

The average number of probes per unsuccessful search with this modified algorithm appears to be difficult to analyze, but the empirical statistics in Tables 1 and 2 show that the idea can be worthwhile. Of course the number of probes per successful search is unaffected by the extra bits.

N/M (the load ratio)	25%	50%	75%	85%	90%	95%
Alg. A, linear probing	1.389	2.500	8.500	22.722	50.500	200.500
Alg. A, secondary clustering	1.371	2.193	4.636	7.715	11.402	22.045
Alg. A, independent double hashing	1.333	2.000	4.000	6.667	10.000	20.000
Alg. B, linear probing	1.167	1.500	2.500	3.833	5.500	10.500
Alg. B, secondary clustering	1.163	1.443	2.011	2.472	2.853	3.521
Alg. B, independent double hashing	1.151	1.386	1.848	2.232	2.558	3.153
Alg. B, linear, with pass bits	1.0	1.2	2.0	3.6	5.4	10.3
Alg. B, independent, with pass bits	1.0	1.1	1.3	1.6	1.7	2.2
Alg. B, linear, correlated, one ahead	2.0	2.2	2.9	4.0	5.8	11.0
Alg. X, bidirectional linear	1.3	1.5	2.1	2.6	3.1	4.4

TABLE 2. The average number of probes in an unsuccessful search.

So far none of the ideas mentioned have been of any use in the case of successful search. One possibility that suggests itself is to start searching one place ahead (that is, to start at position $h(K) - i(K)$), because this will save one probe if K is not at its hash address, and because we will be able to test whether K is in position $h(K)$ if the first search is unsuccessful. Since we have greatly improved the ability to detect unsuccessful searches, we can perhaps use some of this capability in connection with successful searches.

Unfortunately, a more careful analysis shows that such an idea is unsound; it actually *increases* the average number of probes for both successful and unsuccessful searching (see Appendix 2). There is, however, a case in which it does work, namely if we force $h(K)$ to be *correlated* with the magnitude of the table entry for K. Suppose we have a hash function such that

$$K \leq K' \quad \text{implies} \quad h(K) \leq h(K'),$$

and suppose further that we are using linear probing (namely that $i(K)$ is identically 1). Then it is not hard to see that the correlation causes the number of probes for successful search in an ordered hash table to have a much smaller variance; there will be fewer keys requiring very small or very large numbers of probes, although the average number will remain unchanged. Appendix 2 shows that this start-one-ahead approach will lead to fewer probes per successful search when the table is more than about 64.38% full. (The limiting value where the one-ahead method begins to excel is the root $\alpha \approx 0.6437977582$ of $2(1 - \alpha)(e^\alpha - 1) = \alpha$.)

An obvious problem arises, however, if we want the hash function to correlate with the keys in this way. Our options for the choice of hash function will be so drastically reduced that it will probably be impossible to find an efficiently computable $h(K)$ that works well with typical sets of keys. A solution to this dilemma is achieved if we store *transformed keys* in the T table, instead of the keys themselves. Thus, let $t(K)$ be any function that scrambles keys without loss of information:

$$t(K) = t(K') \quad \text{implies that} \quad K = K'.$$

Then we can store $t(K_1)$, $t(K_2)$, ... in the table, and search for $t(K)$ instead of K. We can now achieve the desired correlation between $h(K)$ and $t(K)$ by letting $h(K)$ be the leading bits of $t(K)$.

For example, if M is a prime number and if $h(K) = K \bmod M$, we can let $t(K)$ be a packed binary number whose leftmost bits are $h(K)$ and whose rightmost bits represent the quotient $\lfloor K/M \rfloor$. This transformed key $t(K)$ is one bit larger than the original key. Alternatively if $M = 2^m$ is a power of 2, we may let $t(K) = (aK) \bmod 2^w$, where w is the key length and a is any odd number; then $h(K)$ may be chosen as the leading m bits of $t(K)$.

The reader may justifiably feel at this point that the method is getting baroque. The last few paragraphs have discussed detailed refinements that are mildly interesting, but they can obviously never save more than one probe per search. Therefore the reader may wonder why we are going on and on, "beating a dead horse." The answer is that it was precisely the above train of thought, together with hand simulations on random numbers, that led the authors to consider another algorithm, which *does* offer a substantial improvement. We shall now discuss this improved algorithm, which uses the correlation between hash addresses and table entries in a somewhat different fashion.

Bidirectional Linear Probing

Let $t(K)$ be any one-to-one transformation of keys:

$$t(K) = t(K') \quad \text{implies} \quad K = K'.$$

Furthermore let $h(K)$ be a hash function such that

$$t(K) \leq t(K') \quad \text{implies} \quad h(K) \leq h(K').$$

We have already discussed practical ways of finding such functions; and it is natural to assume that a hash method using such transformations would keep the nonempty positions of the hash table in sorted order:

$$T_i \neq 0 \text{ and } T_j \neq 0 \text{ and } i < j \quad \text{implies} \quad T_i < T_j.$$

Consider now the following straightforward search procedure:

Algorithm X. (Bidirectional linear probing.)

X1. [Initialize.] Set $j \leftarrow h(K)$, and set $K \leftarrow t(K)$.

X2. [Compare.] If $T_j = K$, the algorithm terminates successfully. If $T_j = 0$, the algorithm terminates unsuccessfully. Otherwise go to step X3 if $T_j < K$, to step X5 if $T_j > K$.

X3. [Move up.] (At this point, $0 < T_j < K$.) Set $j \leftarrow j + 1$.

X4. [Compare.] If $T_j = K$, the algorithm terminates successfully. If $T_j = 0$ or $T_j > K$, the algorithm terminates unsuccessfully. Otherwise return to step X3.

X5. [Move down.] (At this point, $T_j > K$.) Set $j \leftarrow j - 1$.

X6. [Compare.] If $T_j = K$, the algorithm terminates successfully. If $T_j < K$, the algorithm terminates unsuccessfully. Otherwise return to step X5. ☐

This algorithm searches either up or down depending on the result of the first comparison. Its validity depends on having a table T_j whose nonempty entries are ordered as stated above, having the additional property that no empty space occurs between the location of any transformed key and its hash address. Furthermore there must be empty positions at the end of the table; we can take care of this by extending the boundaries so that $T_{-1} = T_M = 0$.

In this case there are, in general, many configurations of the T's that will guarantee correct retrieval. For example, suppose that $M = 10$ and consider the transformed keys 614, 621, 637, 641, 647, 698, 841, where $h(K)$ is the leading digit. (It is not typical to have so many keys with the same hash address, but our intent is to give a small example that exhibits some of the more interesting things that can happen.) If we use the ordinary method of linear probing (Algorithm B), the table is filled thus:

$j =$	0	1	2	3	4	5	6	7	8	9
$T_j =$	0	614	621	637	641	647	698	0	841	0
probes		6	5	4	3	2	1		1	

The bottom line shows how many table entries are examined when searching for T_j; for example, it takes four probes to find 637, since we start at T_6. Algorithm X allows us to rearrange the transformed keys so that many of them will be found sooner:

$j =$	0	1	2	3	4	5	6	7	8	9
$T_j =$	0	0	0	614	621	637	641	647	698	841
probes				4	3	2	1	2	3	2

The search for 841 goes upwards now, but we save two probes when searching for 614. The average number of probes per successful search has been reduced from

$$(6 + 5 + 4 + 3 + 2 + 1 + 1)/7 = 22/7$$

to

$$(4 + 3 + 2 + 1 + 2 + 3 + 2)/7 = 17/7.$$

Appendix 3 shows how to characterize the *optimum* arrangements for any given set of keys, namely those arrangements that minimize the average number of probes per successful search by Algorithm X. As a consequence of theory developed there, we may use the following algorithm to insert into a bidirectional hash table, maintaining optimum arrangements at all times.

Algorithm Y. (Optimum insertion for bidirectional linear probing.) In this algorithm we let $h'(T_j)$ stand for $h(t^{-1}(T_j))$; thus if $T_j = t(K_j)$ we have $h'(T_j) = h(K_j)$.

Y1. [Initialize.] Set $j \leftarrow h(K)$ and $K \leftarrow t(K)$.

Y2. [Empty?] If $T_j = 0$, set $T_j \leftarrow K$ and terminate the algorithm.

Y3. [Find bounds.] Set p to the largest index $< j$ such that $T_p = 0$. Set q to the smallest index $> j$ such that $T_q = 0$.

Y4. [Sort in.] Set $j \leftarrow q$. Then if $T_{j-1} > K$, repeatedly set $T_j \leftarrow T_{j-1}$ and $j \leftarrow j - 1$, until $T_{j-1} < K$. Finally set $T_j \leftarrow K$. (Thus K has been sorted into the proper place with respect to the other transformed keys.)

Y5. [Check displacements.] Set $d \leftarrow 0$. Then for $j \leftarrow p + 1, p + 2, \dots, q$ (in this order), repeatedly set

$$d \leftarrow d + 1, \qquad \text{if } h'(T_j) \geq j;$$
$$d \leftarrow d - 1, \qquad \text{if } h'(T_j) < j.$$

If at any time during this process d becomes negative go immediately to step Y6 without finishing the loop. But if d remains ≥ 0 throughout the entire loop, terminate the algorithm.

Y6. [Shift down.] Set $T_j \leftarrow T_{j+1}$ for $p \leq j < q$, and set $T_q \leftarrow 0$. ◻

Algorithm Y finds the smallest block of consecutive nonempty locations containing position $h(K)$, and inserts $t(K)$ into this block by shifting the transformed keys that are larger. Then step Y5 is used to decide whether it would have been better to shift the transformed keys that are smaller; if so, step Y6 moves the whole block down. (Empirical tests show that step Y6 is required only about $1/4$ as often as step Y5.)

It seems wise to avoid end effects by including a dozen or so extra table positions T_j for $j < 0$ and for $j \geq M$. (There are several ways to make the algorithm cyclically symmetric modulo M, but these are more complicated and time-consuming than simply to provide extra "breathing space" at both ends. The optimum arrangement rarely spills over very far; in our experiments with $M = 4096$ and tables 95% full, no more than five locations were needed at either end.)

The theory of linear probing shows that this insertion method isn't extremely slow; the average size $q - p$ of the block of keys considered when the $(N+1)$st key is being inserted will be $2A'_N - 2 \approx (1-\alpha)^{-2} - 1$ when $N/M = \alpha$. (See [4, exercise 6.4–47].) When this size is averaged over N insertions, it reduces to $2A_N - 2 \approx \alpha/(1 - \alpha)$. Thus, insertion by Algorithm Y is only four or five times slower than insertion by the classical linear probing algorithms. On the other hand, empirical results (see Tables 1 and 2) show that retrieval by Algorithm X is significantly better than classical linear probing.

Conclusions

Traditional hash methods are comparatively slow with respect to unsuccessful search. By extending them to make use of the inherent ordering of keys, we have shown that the time for unsuccessful search can be significantly reduced.

Two main algorithms have been presented in this paper. First we discussed Algorithm B, and the corresponding Algorithm C for insertion. This method reduces the time for unsuccessful search to the time for successful search, without significantly increasing the cost per insertion. Therefore it is attractive for applications in which unsuccessful searches are common. A refinement, adding "pass bits," makes unsuccessful search even faster. However, the method is never useful in typical compiler or assembler applications, where unsuccessful searches are almost always followed by insertions.

The second method we have discussed is Algorithm X, together with the corresponding Algorithm Y for insertion. Here both successful and unsuccessful search times are reduced, at the expense of greater insertion time and slightly more complex programs. (The method may be compared with a scheme recently published by Brent [1]; his method requires fewer probes than ours on successful searches, but it does not reduce the unsuccessful search time.)

Tables 1 and 2 present the behavioral characteristics of the algorithms discussed here, assuming random hash functions. Some of the results have been derived by theoretical analyses; these are shown to three decimal places. The other results, for which only one decimal place of accuracy appears, have not yet been verified theoretically. Every entry in these tables is the number of probes per search, namely the number of T_j entries examined. This information can be used to predict the behavior of each algorithm; but we should remember that the time per probe and the setup time will vary from one method to another. For example, linear probing and Algorithm X will have faster inner loops than independent double hashing, while the latter (especially with "pass bits") will involve fewer probes. Thus the number of probes is not an absolute measure of goodness; the entire algorithm must be considered when making comparisons.

The appendices that follow contain interesting mathematics that the authors hope some readers will enjoy.

Appendix 1. Analysis of Step C3

To analyze the quantity D_N defined in the text, let us assume that the keys are $K_1 < K_2 < \cdots < K_N$. Let D'_N be the average number of times, during N random insertions, that the variable K is set to the *smallest* key K_1 at some time during the insertion process. In other words, D'_N is the average number of times K_1 is moved. Then D'_{N-1} is the average number of times K_2 is moved, since the behavior of the algorithm on $\{K_2, \ldots, K_N\}$ is essentially independent of K_1. Similarly, D'_{N+1-i} is the average number of times K_i is moved. Therefore

$$D_1 + \cdots + D_N = (D'_1 - 1) + \cdots + (D'_N - 1)$$

for all N, and we have

$$D_N = D'_N - 1.$$

Consider now the case of independent double hashing. When M is large, this case is satisfactorily approximated by *uniform* hashing, where each key's path is a random permutation of $\{0, 1, \ldots, M - 1\}$, independent of all other keys. (See [5].) Under this assumption, which has been tacitly made in the text, the analysis of hashing algorithms usually becomes quite easy. However, the "organ pipe" example above indicates some of the complexities of Algorithm C, and a rather indirect approach to the analysis of D_N (or D'_N) seems to be necessary.

Let D_N'' be the probability that the smallest key K_1 is moved during the insertion of the Nth key. It follows that

$$D_N' = \frac{D_1'' + 2D_2'' + \cdots + ND_N''}{N},$$

since the probability that K_1 is moved on the jth insertion is D_j'' times j/N, the probability that K_1 appears among the first j keys inserted.

Consider the entire sequence of actions that occur when the keys $\{K_1, \ldots, K_N\}$ are inserted into the table in decreasing order. This sequence of actions states for example that, when K_j was inserted, a certain sequence of larger keys were encountered before an empty place was found. We shall call the elements of the latter sequence the *dominators* of K_j. Knowing all the sequences of dominators, in the decreasing-order case, we can deduce what actions will occur when the keys are inserted in any other specified order. Define the function p on the indices $\{2, \ldots, N\}$ such that, if K_j is the last of $\{K_2, \ldots, K_N\}$ to be inserted, then $K_{p(j)}$ will be the last of $\{K_2, \ldots, K_N\}$ to be moved. Now the very last insertion moves K_1 if and only if either (a) K_1 was the last element inserted, or (b) K_j was the last element inserted, for some $j \geq 2$, and $K_{p(j)}$ is one of the dominators of K_1.

For example, suppose $N = 3$, so that $K_3 > K_2 > K_1$. If K_3 is a dominator of K_2, we have $p(3) = p(2) = 2$, and K_1 is moved on the third insertion if and only if it is the last to be inserted or it is dominated by K_2. On the other hand if K_3 does not dominate K_2, then $p(3) = 3$ and $p(2) = 2$; hence K_1 is moved on the third insertion if and only if it is either the last to be inserted, or it is dominated by the last to be inserted.

For any fixed choice of dominator sequences on $\{K_2, \ldots, K_N\}$, and for fixed $j \geq 2$, the probability that $K_{p(j)}$ dominates K_1 is a function only of M and N, independent of j and the given actions, because of the assumptions of uniform hashing. This probability may be expressed as

$$\frac{1}{N-1} \sum_{r \geq 1} (r-1) P_r,$$

where P_r is the probability that K_1 has $r - 1$ dominators, since exactly

$$\binom{N-2}{r-2} \Big/ \binom{N-1}{r-1} = (r-1)/(N-1)$$

of the possible choices of $r - 1$ dominators include the given key $K_{p(j)}$. Since P_r is also the probability that r probes are needed to insert the

Nth item by Algorithm A, we have

$$\frac{1}{N-1}\sum_{r\geq 1}(r-1)P_r = \frac{1}{N-1}(A'_{N-1}-1).$$

The probability that K_j is inserted last is $1/N$; summing for $2 \leq j \leq N$, and adding $1/N$ for the case that K_1 comes last, gives

$$D''_N = \frac{N-1}{N}\left(\frac{1}{N-1}(A'_{N-1}-1)\right) + \frac{1}{N} = \frac{1}{N}A'_{N-1}.$$

The formulas above now yield the desired answer,

$$D_N = A_N - 1.$$

Such a simple result deserves a simpler proof; however, it is surprisingly easy to derive this formula by plausible but fallacious arguments, and the stated approach is the only reliable one for this analysis that is known to the authors.

We come finally to the case of linear probing. This is much more complicated, and the derivation will only be sketched here. Consider the M^n hash sequences $a_1 \ldots a_n$ to be equally likely, where the kth key inserted has $h(K) = a_k$. Then the probability that the $(n+1)$st key inserted moves K_1 and is not itself K_1 is

$$\frac{1}{N}\sum_{k=1}^{n} k \sum_{i=1}^{n} \frac{a(M,n,k,i)}{M^n}, \tag{$*$}$$

where $a(M,n,k,i)$ denotes the number of hash sequences $a_1 \ldots a_n$ that cause T_0 through T_{k-1} to be occupied, T_k to be empty, and $T_0 = K_1$ if the smallest key K_1 is the ith to be inserted. Let $g(M,n,k)$ be the number of hash sequences that cause T_0 through T_{k-1} to be occupied and $T_{M-1} = T_k = 0$, and let $f(M,n)$ be the number of hash sequences that cause $T_{M-1} = 0$. Then the formulas

$$f(m,n) = (m-n)m^{n-1},$$

$$g(m,n,k) = \binom{n}{k}f(k+1,k)f(m-k-1,n-k)$$

can be derived by simple arguments (see [4, equations 6.4–(37) and 6.4–(38)]). Also let b_n be the number of hash sequences $a_1 \ldots a_n$ that cause

$T_0, \ldots, T_{n-1}$ to be occupied in such a way that the pass bit B_j is set to 1 for $0 < j \le n - 1$. From the relation

$$f(n+1, n) = \sum_{k=0}^{n-1} \binom{n}{k} f(k+1, k) b_{n-k}$$

and Abel's binomial formula, we deduce that $b_n = (n-1)^{n-1}$. Now the value of $(*)$ may be expressed as

$$\frac{1}{N} \sum_{j=1}^{n} \binom{n}{j} jb_j \sum_{l \ge 0} (j+l) \frac{g(M - j + 1, n - j, l)}{M^n} \qquad (**)$$

because we obtain each sequence enumerated by $a(M, n, k, i)$ by piecing together, in $\binom{n}{j}$ ways, a sequence enumerated by b_j and a sequence enumerated by $g(M - j + 1, n - j, l)$, where $1 \le i \le j$ and $k = j + l$. The sum $(**)$ can be evaluated as described in [4, exercise 6.4–27]; the result is

$$\frac{1}{N} \left(\frac{n}{M} + 2 \frac{n(n-1)}{M^2} + 3 \frac{n(n-1)(n-2)}{M^3} + \cdots \right),$$

essentially an incomplete gamma function. Summing for $0 \le n < N$, and adding 1 for when K_1 is inserted, yields the desired result

$$D'_N = 1 + \frac{1}{2} \frac{N-1}{M} + \frac{2}{3} \frac{(N-1)(N-2)}{M^2} + \frac{3}{4} \frac{(N-1)(N-2)(N-3)}{M^3} + \cdots.$$

Appendix 2. Starting One Place Ahead

Consider the case of linear probing in an ordered hash table, when $h(K)$ is uncorrelated with the magnitude of K. Let P_r be the probability that exactly r probes are needed to find the $(n+1)$st largest key, for some fixed value of n. Then P_r is the probability that the positions occupied by the n largest keys include $h-1, h-2, \ldots, h-r+1$, but not position $h-r$, given any h; and P_{r+1} is the probability that $h, h-1, \ldots, h-r+1$ (but not $h - r$) are occupied. Hence $P_r - P_{r+1}$ is the probability that $h - 1, \ldots, h - r + 1$ are occupied, but neither h nor $h - r$, for any given h. It follows that the expected number of probes needed to locate the $(n+1)$st largest key K, if we begin searching at location $h(K) - 1$ instead of $h(K)$, is

$$\sum_{r \ge 2} (r-1) P_r + \sum_{r \ge 1} (r+1)(P_r - P_{r+1}) = P_1 + \sum_{r \ge 1} r P_r.$$

This always exceeds $\sum r P_r$, which is the corresponding average if we begin searching at the normal place $h(K)$.

Essentially the same argument applies to uniform hashing. So we may conclude that it is not a good idea to start probing at location $h(K) - i(K)$.

However, the situation is considerably different when $h(K)$ is correlated with K, so that $h(K) \leq h(K')$ whenever $K < K'$, since then T_{h-1} is almost always less than T_h. To analyze this situation, let us look first at the case that j never goes from 0 to $M - 1$ during a successful search. (In other words, the pass bit B_0 is 0.) Then the nonzero T_j's are sorted; hence if we start a search at $h(K) - 1$, we will lose only one probe when K is in its home position $h(K)$, while we save one probe whenever K is not. It follows that the one-ahead method is favorable, for successful searching, whenever the number of keys in home position is less than $\frac{1}{2} N$.

An assumption that greatly simplifies the analysis when $B_0 \neq 0$ is to restore cyclic symmetry, by assuming that keys behave as if they are larger than ordinary keys after they pass from position 0 to position $M - 1$. Under this assumption we shall prove below that the average number of keys in home position is exactly

$$(M - N)\left(\left(1 + \frac{1}{M}\right)^{N-1} - 1\right) + \left(1 + \frac{1}{M}\right)^{N-1}.$$

For $N/M = \alpha$ as $M \to \infty$, this number is approximately

$$(1 - \alpha) \frac{e^\alpha - 1}{\alpha} N;$$

curiously as $N \to M$ it drops to approximately e.

Without the symmetry assumption above, the number of keys in home position might be drastically different. For example, when $M = 10$ and $N = 8$, the hash sequence 9 8 7 6 5 1 1 1 leaves only one element in home position under cyclic symmetry, but there will be six keys in home position in the true ordered hash table. However, the average effect of this correction is bounded by the length of search A'_N for the smallest element, and for $N/M = \alpha < 1$ the correction is asymptotically negligible. Similarly we may ignore the fact that the search for a key in home position T_0 might be adversely affected by the presence of larger keys in T_{M-1}, T_{M-2}, etc.

To prove the formula for keys in home position under cyclic symmetry we can observe that the number of hash sequences $a_1 \ldots a_N$ that leave an element in home position $M - 1$ is exactly

$$f(M + 1, N) - f(M, N),$$

in the notation of Appendix 1. For if we add the $f(M, N)$ hash sequences that leave T_{M-1} empty, we obtain all the $f(M + 1, N)$ hash sequences that would leave T_M empty in a linearly probed hash table of size $M + 1$. Therefore the average total number of elements in home position, under cyclic symmetry, is

$$M\big(f(M + 1, N) - f(M, N)\big)/M^N.$$

The formula for f, given in Appendix 1, completes the proof.

It is interesting to study the cyclically symmetric algorithm further, namely to find the average number of elements displaced exactly d locations from their home position when $h(K)$ correlates with K. Let $h(M, n, k)$ be the number of hash sequences $a_1 \ldots a_n$ for which at most k elements pass from position 0 to $M - 1$ when they are inserted. Then, by considering the number of such sequences containing exactly j zeros, we obtain the recurrence

$$h(m, n, k) = \sum_j \binom{n}{j} h(m - 1, n - j, k + 1 - j)$$

for all $m, n, k \geq 0$. Furthermore we have the initial conditions

$$h(m, n, 0) = f(m + 1, n) = (m + 1 - n)(m + 1)^{n-1},$$

from which it is possible to deduce the general formula

$$h(m, n, k) = (m + 1 + k - n) \sum_{r=0}^{k} \binom{n}{r} (m + k + 1 - r)^{n-1-r} (r - k - 1)^r$$

for all $m, n, k \geq 0$. (Abel's binomial identity shows that this quantity equals m^n whenever $k \geq n - 1$.)

The hash sequence $a_1 \ldots a_N$ produces a key with home address 0 and displacement $d > 0$ if and only if it is a sequence with $\geq d$ keys passing from 0 to $M - 1$ but $\leq d$ passing from 1 to 0. The number of such hash sequences, when $d > 0$, is

$$h(M, N, d) - h(M, N, d - 1),$$

because $h(M, N, d)$ is the number of hash sequences with $\leq d$ keys passing from 1 to 0, while $h(M, N, d - 1)$ is the number with $< d$ passing from 0 to $M - 1$ and (consequently) $\leq d$ from 1 to 0. It follows that the average total number of keys with displacement $d > 0$ is

$$M(h(M, N, d) - h(M, N, d - 1))/M^N.$$

It would be interesting to obtain asymptotic data about this probability distribution. When $M = N$, the same formulas arise in connection with the classical Kolmogorov–Smirnov tests for random numbers: The quantity $h(n, n, k - 1)/n^n$ is the probability that the so-called statistic K_n^+ is $\leq k/\sqrt{n}$. According to a theorem of N. V. Smirnov in 1939, we have

$$\lim_{n \to \infty} \frac{h(n, n, s\sqrt{n})}{n^n} = 1 - e^{-2s^2};$$

see [3, Section 3.3.1C].

We can check some of these formulas by summing over all $d > 0$ to conclude that the total number of keys with home position 0 and positive displacement among all M^N hash sequences is $h(M, N, \infty) - h(M, N, 0) = M^N - f(M + 1, N)$. Adding the $f(M + 1, N) - f(M, N)$ that have displacement 0 now gives NM^{N-1}, as it should.

Appendix 3. Optimum Bidirectional Linear Probing

Given N keys $K_1 < \cdots < K_N$ and corresponding hash addresses $0 \leq h(K_1) \leq \cdots \leq h(K_N) < M$, we wish to place them into table positions so that K_j appears in $T_{p(j)}$ for $1 \leq j \leq N$, where $p(1) < \cdots < p(N)$. Writing $h_j = h(K_j)$, we also wish to find a placement that is *optimum*, in the sense that the sum

$$\sum_{j=1}^{N} |h_j - p(j)|$$

is minimized. We shall call this sum the *cost* of the placement. For convenience in exposition, we shall allow the positions $p(j)$ to be negative or greater than M, although the proofs could easily be extended to characterize the optimum arrangements subject to $p(1) \geq x$ and $p(N) \leq y$, for any desired bounds $x \leq 0$ and $y \geq M - 1$. Algorithm X requires a placement such that all positions between h_j and $p(j)$ are occupied, for each j; but we may ignore this condition, because all optimum placements automatically satisfy it.

Given any placement $p(1) < \cdots < p(N)$, we shall say that a *block* $[a..b]$ is a set of consecutive positions that are occupied by K_a through K_b; thus $p(j + 1) = p(j) + 1$ for $a \leq j < b$. An *up-block* is a block followed by an empty position, which would lead to smaller cost if it were shifted one place higher; in other words, it is a block $[a..b]$ such that the shifted placement p' costs less, where

$$p'(j) = \begin{cases} p(j) + 1 & \text{if } a \leq j \leq b; \\ p(j), & \text{otherwise.} \end{cases}$$

By the definition of cost, we find that $[a \mathinner{.\,.} b]$ is an up-block if and only if the following conditions hold:

a) either $b = N$ or $p(b+1) > p(b) + 1$; and

b) the number of indices j in the range $a \leq j \leq b$ for which $h_j > p(j)$ exceeds the number for which $h_j \leq p(j)$.

Thus it is easy to test a given placement for the presence of up-blocks. A *down-block* is defined similarly.

An optimum placement will, of course, contain neither up-blocks nor down-blocks. Conversely, this condition of local optimality is sufficient for global optimality:

Theorem. *Given N hash addresses $h_1 \leq \cdots \leq h_N$, a placement $p(1) < \cdots < p(N)$ is optimum if and only if it contains no up-blocks and no down-blocks.*

Proof. Let p be an arbitrary placement; we want to prove that p either contains an up-block, or a down-block, or is optimum. Let p' be an optimum placement. If $p(j) = p'(j)$ for all j, we are done. Otherwise suppose that $p(j_0) \neq p'(j_0)$. By symmetry we may assume that $p(j_0) < p'(j_0)$.

It would be nice if we could prove that $p(j_0)$ is part of an up-block, under these hypotheses. However, the following example shows that the argument cannot be quite so trivial:

$k =$	1	2	3	4	5	6	7	8
$h_k =$	4	4	4	4	4	6	6	6
$p(k) =$	0	1	2	3	4	6	7	8
$p'(k) =$	2	3	4	5	6	7	8	9

If $j_0 = 6$, we have $p(j_0) < p'(j_0)$, but $p(j_0)$ is actually part of a down-block.

We can circumvent such difficulties by arguing as follows. Let a' be minimal so that $[a' \mathinner{.\,.} j_0]$ is a block in placement p'. Then let b be maximal so that $[a' \mathinner{.\,.} b]$ is a block in placement p. Then let a be minimal so that $[a \mathinner{.\,.} b]$ is a block in placement p'. (In the example above, when $j_0 = 6$, we would have $a' = 1$ and $b = 5$ and $a = 1$.) In general we will always have $p(a') < p'(a')$ and $p(b) < p'(b)$; furthermore $[a \mathinner{.\,.} b]$ will always be a block in both placements. Thus, $p'(j) - p(j)$ has a constant value $t \geq 1$ for $a \leq j \leq b$. Moreover, position $p(b) + 1$ is empty in placement p, while $p'(a) - 1$ is empty in placement p'.

Let d_+ be the number of displacements $h_j - p(j)$ in block $[a \mathinner{.\,.} b]$ that are positive for placement p; also let d_- be the number of negative displacements in the block, and let d_k be the number of displacements that equal k. Define d'_+, d'_-, and d'_k similarly for placement p'. It follows that $d_k = d'_{k-t}$ for all k.

Now $[a .. b]$ is an up-block for p if and only if $d_+ > d_0 + d_-$, and it is a down-block for p' if and only if $d'_- > d'_0 + d'_+$. Our proof would be complete if $[a .. b]$ were an up-block for p, hence we may assume that

$$d_+ \leq d_0 + d_- .$$

The optimality of p' implies that

$$d'_- \leq d'_0 + d'_+ .$$

Now the latter inequality is equivalent to

$$d_- + \sum\{d_x \mid 0 \leq x < t\} \leq d_+ - \sum\{d_x \mid 0 < x < t\};$$

hence we have

$$d_+ \leq d_0 + d_- \leq d_+ - 2\sum\{d_x \mid 0 < x < t\}.$$

This can be true only if $d_+ = d_0 + d_-$ and $d'_- = d'_0 + d'_+$. If we shift block $[a .. b]$ one position down from where it was in p', we obtain a new placement p'' of cost equal to p', hence p'' is optimum. Furthermore p'' is *closer* to the given placement, in an obvious sense, so the proof will eventually terminate. □

It is interesting to note that this proof does not use the hypothesis $h_1 \leq \cdots \leq h_N$; it characterizes the optimum placements for *arbitrary* h_j, which need not even be integers. If $N = 2$, with $h_1 = 100$ and $h_2 = 1$, there are actually one hundred optimum placements, namely $p_k(j) = k + j$ for $-1 \leq k \leq 99$. The additional hypothesis $h_1 \leq \cdots \leq h_N$ leads to a slightly stronger theorem, showing that the optimum placements are more constrained: When $h_j \leq h_{j+1}$ we have

$$h_j - p(j) \leq h_{j+1} - p(j) = h_{j+1} - p(j+1) + 1,$$

for j and $j+1$ in the same block. The proof above can now be strengthened to show that if the h_j are integers, we have $d_1 > 0$ (and hence $t = 1$) whenever p has no up-blocks. Thus two optimum placements p and p' must have $|p(j) - p'(j)| \leq 1$ for all j, whenever the h_j form a nondecreasing sequence of integers.

Finally we are ready to verify Algorithm Y. Let α be a string of integers representing consecutive displacements $h_j - p(j)$ in a block of optimally placed elements. For example, α might be $10210\overline{1}\overline{2}\overline{2}0\overline{1}$, where $\overline{1}$ and $\overline{2}$ denote -1 and -2. We have observed that $\alpha_i \leq \alpha_{i+1} + 1$. A down-block is a prefix of α that contains more negative elements than nonnegative elements; an up-block is a suffix of α that contains more positive elements than nonpositive elements.

Let α^+ be the string obtained from α by adding 1 to each element, and let α^- be obtained similarly by subtracting 1. After inserting x into $\alpha\beta$ by Algorithm Y, we have either $\alpha x\beta^-$ or $\alpha^+x^+\beta$. The validity of that algorithm follows from two basic facts:

(1) *If $\alpha x\beta^-$ has a down-block then $\alpha^+x^+\beta$ has no up-block.* For the down-block must be $\alpha x\beta_1^-$, and the up-block must be $\alpha_1^+x^+\beta$, for some strings α_1 and β_1. Since α is not a down-block, $\alpha_1 x\beta_1^-$ is a down-block. Similarly $\alpha_1^+x^+\beta_1$ is an up-block. But that is absurd, since $\alpha_1^+x^+\beta_1 = (\alpha_1 x\beta_1^-)^+$.

(2) *The string $\alpha x\beta^-$ has no up-block.* For if β contains no positive elements, we must have $x \leq 0$. But if β does contain a positive element, it contains at least one $+1$; thus β^- contains more nonpositive elements than positive elements.

The preparation of this paper was supported in part by Norges Almenvitenskapelige Forskningsråd, and in part by the United States Office of Naval Research.

References

[1] Richard P. Brent, "Reducing the retrieval time of scatter storage techniques," *Communications of the ACM* **16** (1973), 105–109.

[2] Koichi Furukawa, "Hash addressing with conflict flag," *Information Processing in Japan* **13** (1973), 13–18.

[3] Donald E. Knuth, *Seminumerical Algorithms*, Volume 2 of *The Art of Computer Programming* (Reading, Massachusetts: Addison–Wesley, 1969).

[4] Donald E. Knuth, *Sorting and Searching*, Volume 3 of *The Art of Computer Programming* (Reading, Massachusetts: Addison–Wesley, 1973).

[5] George S. Lueker and Mariko Molodowitch, "More analysis of double hashing," *Combinatorica* **13** (1993), 83–96.

(References [2] and [5] were not cited in the original publication of this paper.)

Chapter 8

Activity in an Interleaved Memory

[Written with Gururaj S. Rao. Originally published in IEEE Transactions on Computers C-24 (1975), 943–944.]

A complicated expression for the average number of active modules, in a published model for interleaved memory, is shown to be a function well studied in other contexts.

In an n-way interleaved memory, the effective bandwidth depends on the average number of concurrently active modules. Hellerman [2, page 245] has proposed a theoretical model in order to estimate the effect of n-way interleaving for large n. We shall show in this correspondence that his model is equivalent to another that has occurred in studies of epidemics, and of random number generators, and in other statistical applications. We also present a simple "algebra" for dealing with sums of the type Hellerman encountered.

The theoretical model for interleaved memory assumes that a sequence of memory requests a_1, a_2, a_3, ... is made at high speed, where each a_i is a uniformly distributed random integer between 1 and n, independent of the other a_j. We find the smallest m such that $a_m = a_j$ for some $j < m$, and then the first $m - 1$ memory requests are serviced. The process continues on the next cycle by considering the sequence a_m, a_{m+1}, a_{m+2}, ... in the same way. Thus the model assumes the following. (1) The memory never idles from lack of work. (2) The time to inspect the requests can be overlapped with the accessing. (3) There is no queuing of requests on busy modules.

Hellerman proved that the average number of active modules is

$$\sum_{k=1}^{n} \frac{k^2 (n-1)!}{(n-k)! \, n^k}. \tag{1}$$

He tabulated this quantity for $1 \leq n \leq 45$ and suggested that $n^{0.56}$ would be a good approximation based on these data. We shall show that the preceding quantity equals $Q(n)$, a well-studied function whose value is

$$\left(\frac{\pi n}{2}\right)^{1/2} - \frac{1}{3} + \frac{1}{12}\left(\frac{\pi}{2n}\right)^{1/2} - \frac{4}{135}n^{-1} + O(n^{-3/2}). \qquad (2)$$

The sum in (1) takes the form

$$\frac{1^2}{n} + \frac{2^2}{n}\cdot\frac{n-1}{n} + \frac{3^2}{n}\cdot\frac{n-1}{n}\cdot\frac{n-2}{n} + \cdots + \frac{n^2}{n}\cdot\frac{n-1}{n}\cdot\frac{n-2}{n}\cdots\frac{1}{n} \qquad (3)$$

when written out term by term. In dealing with such sums it is convenient to define the notation

$$\langle a_0, a_1, a_2, \ldots \rangle = a_0 + a_1\frac{n-1}{n} + a_2\frac{n-1}{n}\frac{n-2}{n} + \cdots, \qquad (4)$$

regarding n as a fixed positive integer. We will use this notation for infinite sequences a_0, a_1, a_2, ...; but the quantity $\langle a_0, a_1, a_2, \ldots \rangle$ is actually independent of a_n, a_{n+1}, ..., since the terms on the right-hand side are eventually all multiplied by zero. Thus there is no problem of convergence, nor do we need to worry about the upper limit of summation.

The bracketed function in (4) is clearly linear in all components:

$$\langle a_0, a_1, a_2, \ldots \rangle + \langle b_0, b_1, b_2, \ldots \rangle = \langle a_0 + b_0, a_1 + b_1, a_2 + b_2, \ldots \rangle. \qquad (5)$$

Furthermore we have the identity

$$\langle a_0, a_1, a_2, \ldots \rangle = a_0 + \langle a_1, a_2, a_3, \ldots \rangle - \frac{1}{n}\langle 1a_1, 2a_2, 3a_3 \ldots \rangle, \qquad (6)$$

as is readily verified from the definition. Equation (6) is useful since it proves, for example, that $\langle 1, 2, 3, 4, \ldots \rangle = n$ if we set all the a_j to 1.

Hellerman's sum (3) is

$$\frac{1}{n}\langle 1^2, 2^2, 3^2, \ldots \rangle$$

and by setting $a_j = j$ for all j, we have

$$\frac{1}{n}\langle 1^2, 2^2, 3^2, \ldots \rangle = \langle 1, 2, 3, 4, \ldots \rangle - \langle 0, 1, 2, 3, \ldots \rangle = \langle 1, 1, 1, 1, \ldots \rangle$$

by (6) and (5). Therefore the average number of memory modules active per cycle is

$$\langle 1, 1, 1, 1, \ldots \rangle = 1 + \frac{n-1}{n} + \frac{n-1}{n}\frac{n-2}{n} + \cdots . \qquad (7)$$

This is precisely the function $Q(n)$ discussed in some detail in Section 1.2.11.3 of [3]. The asymptotic behavior of this function was investigated by Ramanujan in 1911 [5], who showed that

$$Q(n) = \frac{n!\, e^n}{2n^n} - \frac{1}{3} - \frac{4}{135}n^{-1} + \frac{8}{2835}n^{-2} + \frac{16}{8505}n^{-3} + O(n^{-4}). \quad (8)$$

The leading term of (8) can be approximated by using Stirling's formula.

The preceding memory-access model is equivalent to another model that has received considerable study, namely, the behavior of a *random mapping* from the set $\{1, 2, \ldots, n\}$ into itself, considering all n^n functions to be equally likely. If we start at any random point a_1 and then compute $a_2 = f(a_1)$, $a_3 = f(a_2)$, etc., until $a_m = f(a_{m-1})$ is first equal to a_j for some $j < m$, the sequences $a_1, a_2, \ldots, a_m$ have the same property as in the memory-accessing model, since the values $f(a_1)$, $f(a_2)$, $\ldots$, $f(a_{m-1})$ are independent of each other and of the choice of a_1. This problem was apparently first studied by Rapoport [6] and later by many other people (see, for example, [1]). The final value of $m - j$ is called the *period* of the random mapping starting at a_1 and the final value of $j - 1$ is called the length of the *tail*. It is not difficult to prove (see [4, exercise 3.1–12]) that the average tail length is $(Q(n) - 1)/2$ and the average period length is $(Q(n) + 1)/2$; hence we obtain another proof that $Q(n)$ is the average value of $m - 1$.

References

[1] Bernard Harris, "Probability distributions related to random mappings," *Annals of Mathematical Statistics* **31** (1960), 1045–1062.

[2] H. Hellerman, *Digital Computer System Principles*, second edition (New York: McGraw–Hill, 1973).

[3] Donald E. Knuth, *Fundamental Algorithms*, Volume 1 of *The Art of Computer Programming* (Reading, Massachusetts: Addison–Wesley, 1968).

[4] Donald E. Knuth, *Seminumerical Algorithms*, Volume 2 of *The Art of Computer Programming* (Reading, Massachusetts: Addison–Wesley, 1969).

[5] S. Ramanujan, "Questions for solution, number 294," *Journal of the Indian Mathematical Society* **3** (1911), 128; **4** (1912), 151–152. Reprinted in *Collected Papers of Srinivasa Ramanujan* (Cambridge: 1927), 323–324.

[6] Anatol Rapoport, "Cycle distributions in random nets," *Bulletin of Mathematical Biophysics* **10** (1948), 145–157.

This research was supported in part by the National Science Foundation, in part by the Office of Naval Research, and in part by National Scholarships for Study Abroad, Ministry of Education, Government of India.

Chapter 9

An Analysis of Alpha-Beta Pruning

[Written with Ronald W. Moore. Originally published in Artificial Intelligence **6** *(1975), 293–326.]*

The alpha-beta technique for searching game trees is analyzed in an attempt to provide some insight into its behavior. The first portion of this paper is an expository presentation of the method together with a proof of its correctness and a historical discussion. The alpha-beta procedure is shown to be optimal in a certain sense, and bounds are obtained for its running time with various kinds of random data.

> Put one pound of Alpha Beta Prunes
> in a jar or dish that has a cover.
> Pour one quart of boiling water over prunes.
> The longer prunes soak, the plumper they get.

—Alpha Beta Acme Markets, Inc., La Habra, California

0. Introduction

Computer programs for playing games like chess typically choose their moves by searching a large tree of potential continuations. A technique called "alpha-beta pruning" is generally used to speed up such search processes without loss of information. The purpose of this paper is to analyze the alpha-beta procedure in order to obtain some quantitative estimates of its performance characteristics.

Section 1 defines the basic concepts associated with game trees. Section 2 presents the alpha-beta method together with a related technique that is similar, but not as powerful, because it fails to make "deep cutoffs." The correctness of both methods is demonstrated, and Section 3 gives examples and further development of the algorithms. Several suggestions for applying the method in practice appear in Section 4, and the history of alpha-beta pruning is discussed in Section 5.

105

Section 6 begins the quantitative analysis, by deriving lower bounds on the amount of searching needed by alpha-beta and by *any* algorithm that solves the same general problem. Section 7 derives upper bounds, primarily by considering the case of random trees when no deep cutoffs are made. It is shown that the procedure is reasonably efficient even under these weak assumptions. Section 8 shows how to introduce some of the deep cutoffs into the analysis; and Section 9 shows that the efficiency improves when there are dependencies between successive moves.

This paper is essentially self-contained, except for a few mathematical results quoted in the later sections.

1. Games and Position Values

The two-person games we are dealing with can be characterized by a set of "positions," and by a set of rules for moving from one position to another, the players moving alternately. We assume that no infinite sequence of positions is allowed by the rules,[1] and that there are only finitely many legal moves from every position. It follows from the "infinity lemma" (see [11, Section 2.3.4.3]) that the tree of all possible games is finite.

If p is a position from which there are no legal moves, there is an integer-valued function $f(p)$ that represents the *value* of this position to the player whose turn it is to play from p; the value to the other player is assumed to be $-f(p)$.

If p is a position from which there are d legal moves $p_1, \ldots, p_d$, where $d > 1$, the problem is to choose the "best" move. We assume that the best move is one that achieves the greatest possible value when the game ends, if the opponent also chooses moves that are best. Let $F(p)$ be the greatest possible value achievable from position p against the optimal defensive strategy, from the standpoint of the player who is moving from that position. Since the value (to this player) after moving to position p_k will be $-F(p_k)$, we have

$$F(p) = \begin{cases} f(p), & \text{if } d = 0; \\ \max(-F(p_1), \ldots, -F(p_d)), & \text{if } d > 0. \end{cases} \quad (1)$$

---

[1] Strictly speaking, chess does not satisfy this condition, since its rules for repeated positions only give the players the option to *request* a draw, in certain circumstances; if neither player actually does ask for a draw, the game can go on forever. But this technicality is of no practical importance, since chess programs only look finitely many moves ahead. It is possible to deal with infinite games by assigning appropriate values to repeated positions, but such questions are beyond the scope of this paper.

This formula serves to define $F(p)$ for all positions p, by induction on the length of the longest game playable from p.

In most discussions of game-playing, a slightly different formalism is used; the two players are named Max and Min, where all values are given from Max's viewpoint. Thus, if p is a terminal position with Max to move, its value is $f(p)$ as before, but if p is a terminal position with Min to move its value is

$$g(p) = -f(p). \tag{2}$$

Max will try to maximize the final value, and Min will try to minimize it. There are now two functions corresponding to (1), namely

$$F(p) = \begin{cases} f(p), & \text{if } d = 0, \\ \max(G(p_1), \ldots, G(p_d)), & \text{if } d > 0, \end{cases} \tag{3}$$

which is the best value Max can guarantee starting at position p, and

$$G(p) = \begin{cases} g(p), & \text{if } d = 0, \\ \min(F(p_1), \ldots, F(p_d)), & \text{if } d > 0, \end{cases} \tag{4}$$

which is the best that Min can be sure of achieving. As before, we assume that $p_1, \ldots, p_d$ are the legal moves from position p. It is easy to prove by induction that the two definitions of F in (1) and (3) are identical, and that

$$G(p) = -F(p) \tag{5}$$

for all p. Thus the two approaches are equivalent.

Sometimes it is easier to reason about game-playing by using the "minimax" framework of (3) and (4) instead of the "negamax" approach of equation (1); the reason is that we are sometimes less confused if we consistently evaluate the game positions from one player's standpoint. On the other hand, formulation (1) is advantageous when we're trying to prove things about games, because we don't have to deal with two (or sometimes even four or eight) separate cases when we want to establish our results. Equation (1) is analogous to the "NOR" operation that arises in circuit design; two levels of NOR logic are equivalent to a level of ANDs followed by a level of ORs.

The function $F(p)$ is the maximum final value that can be achieved if both players play optimally; but we should remark that this reflects a rather conservative strategy that won't always be best against poor players or against the nonoptimal players we encounter in the real world. For example, suppose that there are two moves, to positions p_1 and p_2, where p_1 assures a draw (value 0) but cannot possibly win, while p_2 gives a chance of either victory or defeat depending on whether or not the opponent overlooks a rather subtle winning move. We may be better off gambling on the move to p_2, which is our only chance to win, unless we are convinced of our opponent's competence. Indeed, humans seem to beat chess-playing programs by adopting such a strategy.

2. Development of the Algorithm

The following algorithm (expressed in an ad hoc ALGOL-like language) clearly computes $F(p)$, by following definition (1):

```
integer procedure F(position p):
  begin integer m, k, t, d;
      Determine the successor positions p₁, ..., p_d;
      if d = 0 then F := f(p) else
      begin m := −∞;
          for k := 1 step 1 until d do
              begin t := −F(p_k);
                  if t > m then m := t;
              end;
          F := m;
      end;
  end.
```

Here ∞ denotes a value that is greater than or equal to $|f(p)|$ for all terminal positions of the game, hence $-\infty$ is less than or equal to $\pm F(p)$ for all p. This algorithm is a "brute force" search through all possible continuations (see Shannon [23]).

One way to improve on the brute-force approach is to use a "branch-and-bound" technique [14], ignoring moves that are incapable of being better than moves that are already known. For example, if $F(p_1) = -10$, then $F(p) \geq 10$, and we don't have to know the exact value of $F(p_2)$ if we can deduce that $F(p_2) \geq -10$ (namely that $-F(p_2) \leq 10$). Thus if p_{21} is a legal move from p_2 such that $F(p_{21}) \leq 10$, we need not bother to explore any other moves from p_2. In game-playing terminology, a move to p_2 can be "refuted" (relative to the alternative move p_1) if the opposing player can make a reply to p_2 that is at least as good as the best reply to p_1. Once a move has been refuted, we need not search for the best possible refutation.

This line of reasoning leads to a computational technique that avoids much of the computation done by F. We shall define $F1$ as a procedure on two parameters p and *bound*, and our goal is to achieve the following conditions:

$$F1\,(p, bound) = F(p), \qquad \text{if } F(p) < bound;$$
$$F1\,(p, bound) \geq bound, \qquad \text{if } F(p) \geq bound. \tag{6}$$

These relations do not fully define $F1$, but they are sufficiently powerful to calculate $F(p)$ for any starting position p because they imply that

$$F1\,(p, \infty) = F(p). \tag{7}$$

The following algorithm corresponds to this branch-and-bound idea.

> **integer procedure** $F1$ (**position** p, **integer** $bound$):
>   **begin integer** m, k, t, d;
>   Determine the successor positions $p_1, \ldots, p_d$;
>   **if** $d = 0$ **then** $F1 := f(p)$ **else**
>   **begin** $m := -\infty$;
>   **for** $k := 1$ **step** 1 **until** d **do**
>   **begin** $t := -F1\,(p_k, -m)$;
>   **if** $t > m$ **then** $m := t$;
>   **if** $m \geq bound$ **then go to** done;
>   **end**;
>   done: $F1 := m$;
>   **end**;
>   **end**.

We can prove that this procedure satisfies (6) by arguing as follows: At the beginning of the kth iteration of the **for** loop, we have the "invariant" condition

$$m = \max(-F(p_1), \ldots, -F(p_{k-1})) \tag{8}$$

just as in procedure F. (The max operation over an empty set is conventionally defined to be $-\infty$.) For if $-F(p_k)$ is $> m$, then we have $F1\,(p_k, -m) = F(p_k)$, by condition (6) and induction on the length of the game following p; therefore (8) will hold on the next iteration. And if $\max(-F(p_1), \ldots, -F(p_k)) \geq bound$ for any k, then $F(p) \geq bound$. It follows that condition (6) holds for all p.

The procedure can be improved further if we introduce both lower and upper bounds. This idea, which is called *alpha-beta* pruning, is a significant extension to the one-sided branch-and-bound method. (Unfortunately it doesn't apply to all branch-and-bound algorithms; it works only when a game tree is being explored.) We define a procedure $F2$

on three parameters p, *alpha*, and *beta*, for *alpha* < *beta*, satisfying the following conditions analogous to (6):

$$
\begin{aligned}
F2\,(p, alpha, beta) &\le alpha, &&\text{if } F(p) \le alpha; \\
F2\,(p, alpha, beta) &= F(p), &&\text{if } alpha < F(p) < beta; &&(9)\\
F2\,(p, alpha, beta) &\ge beta, &&\text{if } F(p) \ge beta.
\end{aligned}
$$

Again, these conditions do not fully specify $F2$, but they imply that

$$
F2\,(p, -\infty, \infty) = F(p). \tag{10}
$$

It turns out that this improved algorithm looks only a little different from the others, when it is expressed in a programming language:

```
integer procedure F2 (position p, integer alpha, integer beta):
    begin integer m, k, t, d;
        Determine the successor positions p₁, ..., p_d;
        if d = 0 then F2 := f(p) else
        begin m := alpha;
            for k := 1 step 1 until d do
                begin t := −F2 (p_k, −beta, −m);
                    if t > m then m := t;
                    if m ≥ beta then go to done;
                end;
        done: F2 := m;
        end;
    end.
```

To prove the validity of $F2$, we proceed as we did with $F1$. The invariant relation analogous to (8) is now

$$
m = \max(alpha, -F(p_1), \ldots, -F(p_{k-1})) \tag{11}
$$

and $m < beta$. If $-F(p_k) \ge beta$, then $-F2\,(p_k, -beta, -m)$ will also be $\ge beta$; and if $m < -F(p_k) < beta$, then $-F2\,(p_k, -beta, -m) = -F(p_k)$. So the proof goes through as before, establishing both (9) and (11) by induction.

Now that we have found two improvements of the minimax procedure, it is natural to ask whether still further improvement is possible. Is there an "alpha-beta-gamma" procedure $F3$, which makes use say of the second-largest value found so far, or some other gimmick? Section 6 below shows that the answer is no, or at least that there is a reasonable sense in which procedure $F2$ is optimum.

3. Examples and Refinements

As an example of these procedures, consider the tree in Figure 1, which represents a position that has three successors, each of which has three successors, etc., until we get to $3^4 = 81$ positions possible after four moves. These 81 positions have been assigned "random" f values according to the first 81 digits of π. Figure 1 shows the F values computed from the f's; thus, the root node at the top of the tree has an effective value of 2 after best play by both sides.

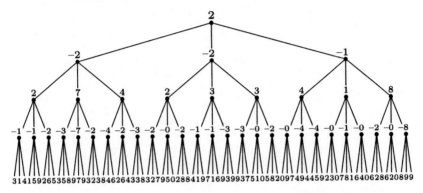

FIGURE 1. Complete evaluation of a game tree.

Figure 2 shows the same situation as it is evaluated by procedure $F1\,(p, \infty)$. Notice that only 36 of the 81 terminal positions are examined, and that one of the nodes at level 2 now has the "approximate" value 3 instead of its true value 7; but this approximation does not affect the value at the top, of course.

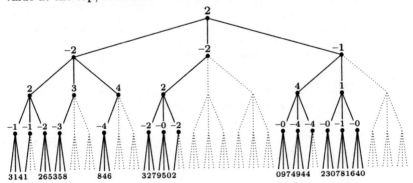

FIGURE 2. The game tree of Figure 1 evaluated with procedure $F1$ (branch-and-bound strategy).

Figure 3 shows the same situation as it is evaluated by the full alpha-beta pruning technique. Procedure $F2(p, -\infty, +\infty)$ will always examine the same nodes as $F1(p, \infty)$ until the fourth level of lookahead is reached, in any game tree; this is a consequence of the theory developed below. On levels 4, 5, ..., however, procedure $F2$ is occasionally able to make "deep cutoffs" that $F1$ is incapable of finding. A comparison of Figure 3 with Figure 2 shows that there are five deep cutoffs in this example.

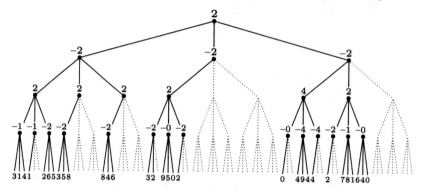

FIGURE 3. The game tree of Figure 1 evaluated with procedure $F2$ (alpha-beta strategy).

All of these illustrations present the results in terms of the "negamax" model of Section 1; readers who prefer to see them in "minimax" form can simply ignore all the minus signs in Figures 1–3. The procedures of Section 2 can readily be converted to the minimax conventions, for example by replacing $F2$ by the following two procedures:

```
integer procedure F2 (position p, integer alpha, integer beta):
  begin integer m, k, t, d;
    Determine the successor positions p₁, ..., p_d;
    if d = 0 then F2 := f(p) else
    begin m := alpha;
      for k := 1 step 1 until d do
        begin t := G2 (p_k, m, beta);
          if t > m then m := t;
          if m ≥ beta then go to done;
        end;
    done: F2 := m;
    end;
  end;
```

```
integer procedure G2(position p, integer alpha, integer beta):
  begin integer m, k, t, d;
    Determine the successor positions p₁, ..., p_d;
    if d = 0 then G2 := g(p) else
    begin m := beta;
      for k := 1 step 1 until d do
        begin t := F2(p_k, alpha, m);
          if t < m then m := t;
          if m ≤ alpha then go to done;
        end;
      done: G2 := m;
    end;
  end.
```

It is a simple but instructive exercise to prove that $G2(p, alpha, beta)$ always equals $-F2(p, -beta, -alpha)$.

The procedures above have made use of a magic routine that determines the successors $p_1, \ldots, p_d$ of a given position p. If we want to be more explicit about how positions are represented, we can conveniently use the format of linked records: When p is a reference to a record denoting a position, let $first(p)$ be a reference to the first successor of that position, or Λ (a null reference) if the position is terminal. Similarly if q references a successor p_k of p, let $next(q)$ be a reference to the next successor p_{k+1}, or Λ if $k = d$. Finally let $generate(p)$ be a procedure that creates the records for $p_1, \ldots, p_d$, sets their $next$ fields, and makes $first(p)$ point to p_1 (or to Λ if $d = 0$). Then the alpha-beta pruning method takes the following more explicit form.

```
integer procedure F2(ref(position) p,
                          integer alpha, integer beta):
  begin integer m, t; ref(position) q;
    generate(p);
    q := first(p);
    if q = Λ then F2 := f(p) else
    begin m := alpha;
      while q ≠ Λ and m < beta do
        begin t := -F2(q, -beta, -m);
          if t > m then m := t;
          q := next(q);
        end;
      F2 := m;
    end;
  end.
```

It is interesting to convert this recursive procedure to an iterative (nonrecursive) form by a sequence of mechanical transformations, and to apply simple optimizations that preserve program correctness (see [13]). The resulting procedure is surprisingly simple, but not as easy to prove correct as the recursive form:

```
integer procedure alphabeta (ref (position) p):
    begin integer l; comment the level of recursion;
        integer array a[−2 : L]; comment a stack for recursion,
            where a[l − 2], a[l − 1], a[l], a[l + 1] denote respectively
            alpha, −beta, m, −t in procedure F2;
        ref (position) array r[0 : L + 1]; comment another stack
            for recursion, where r[l] and r[l + 1] denote respectively
            p and q in procedure F2;
        l := 0;  a[−2] := a[−1] := −∞;  r[0] := p;
    F2: generate (r[l]);
        r[l + 1] := first (r[l]);
        if r[l + 1] = Λ then a[l] := f(r[l]) else
        begin a[l] := a[l − 2];
            loop: l := l + 1; go to F2;
            resume: if −a[l + 1] > a[l] then
                    begin a[l] := −a[l + 1];
                        if a[l + 1] ≤ a[l − 1] then go to done;
                    end;
                r[l + 1] := next (r[l + 1]);
                if r[l + 1] ≠ Λ then go to loop;
        end;
        done: l := l − 1; if l ≥ 0 then go to resume;
        alphabeta := a[0];
    end.
```

This procedure $alphabeta(p)$ will compute the same value as the procedure $F2(p, -\infty, +\infty)$; we must choose L large enough so that the level of recursion never exceeds L.

4. Applications

When a computer is playing a complex game, it will rarely be able to search all possibilities until truly terminal positions are reached; even the alpha-beta technique won't be fast enough to solve the game of chess! But we can still use the procedures above, if the routine that generates all moves is modified so that sufficiently deep positions are considered to be terminal. For example, if we wish to look six moves ahead (three for each player), we can pretend that the positions reached at level 6 have no successors. To compute f at such artificially-terminal positions, we must of course use our best guess about the true value, hoping that a sufficiently deep search will ameliorate the inaccuracy of our guess. (Most of the time will be spent in evaluating these guessed values for f, unless the determination of legal moves is especially difficult, so some quickly-computed estimate is needed.)

Instead of searching to a fixed depth, we might also decide to explore some lines further; for example, we could play out all sequences of captures. Robert W. Floyd suggested an interesting approach in 1965 [6], under which each move is assigned a "likelihood" according to the following general plan:[2] A forced move has likelihood 1, while implausible moves (like queen sacrifices in chess) get 0.01 or so. In chess a recapture has likelihood greater than 0.5; and the best strategic choice out of 20 or 30 possibilities gets a likelihood of about 0.1, while the worst choices get say 0.02. When the product of all likelihoods leading to a position becomes less than a given threshold (say 10^{-8}), we consider that position to be terminal and estimate its value without further searching. Under this scheme, the "most likely" branches of the tree get the most attention.

Whatever method is used to produce a tree of reasonable size, the alpha-beta procedure can be somewhat improved if we have an idea what the value of the initial position will be. Instead of calling $F2(p, -\infty, +\infty)$, we can try $F2(p, a, b)$ where we expect the value to be greater than a and less than b. For example, if $F2(p, 0, 4)$ is used instead of $F2(p, -10, +10)$ in Figure 3, the rightmost '−4' on level 3, and the '4' below it, do not need to be considered. If our expectation is fulfilled, we may have pruned off more of the tree; on the other hand if the value turns out to be low, say $F2(p, a, b) = v$ where $v \leq a$, we can use $F2(p, -\infty, v)$ to deduce the correct value. This idea has been used in some versions of Greenblatt's chess program [8].

5. History

Before we begin to make quantitative analyses of alpha-beta's effectiveness, let us look briefly at its historical development. The early history is somewhat obscure, because it is based on undocumented recollections and because some people have confused procedure *F1* with the stronger procedure *F2*; therefore the following account is based on the best information now available to the authors.

---

[2] Many chess-playing programs of the 1990s have adopted an almost identical scheme called the method of "fractional extensions."

John McCarthy [15] thought of the method during the Dartmouth Summer Research Conference on Artificial Intelligence in 1956, when Alex Bernstein described an early chess program [3] that didn't use any sort of alpha-beta. McCarthy "criticized it on the spot for this [reason], but Bernstein was not convinced. No formal specification of the algorithm was given at that time." It is plausible that McCarthy's remarks at that conference led to the use of alpha-beta pruning in game-playing programs of the late 1950s. Arthur Samuel has stated that the idea was present in his checker-playing programs, but he did not allude to it in his classic article [21] because he felt that the other aspects of his program were more significant.

The first published discussion of a method for game tree pruning appeared in Newell, Shaw, and Simon's description [16] of their early chess program. However, they illustrated only the "one-sided" technique used in procedure *F1* above, so it is not clear whether they made use of "deep cutoffs."

McCarthy coined the name "alpha-beta" when he first wrote a LISP program embodying the technique. His original approach was somewhat more elaborate than the method described above, since he assumed the existence of two functions "*optimistic value*(p)" and "*pessimistic value*(p)," which were to be upper and lower bounds on the value of a position. McCarthy's form of alpha-beta searching was equivalent to replacing the body of procedure *F2* above by

> **if** *optimistic value*(p) ≤ *alpha* **then** *F2* := *alpha*
> **else if** *pessimistic value*(p) ≥ *beta* **then** *F2* := *beta*
> **else begin** ⟨ the body of procedure *F2* ⟩ **end**.

Because of this elaboration, he thought of alpha-beta as a (possibly inaccurate) heuristic device, not realizing that it would also produce the same value as full minimaxing in the special case that *optimistic value*(p) = $+\infty$ and *pessimistic value*(p) = $-\infty$ for all p. He credits the latter discovery to Timothy Hart and Daniel Edwards, who wrote a memorandum [10] on the subject in 1961. Their unpublished memorandum gives examples of the general method, including deep cutoffs; but (as usual in 1961) no attempt was made to indicate why the method worked, much less to demonstrate its validity.

The first published account of alpha-beta pruning actually appeared in Russia, quite independently of the American work. A. L. Brudno, who was one of the developers of an early Russian chess-playing program, described an algorithm identical to alpha-beta pruning, together with a rather complicated proof, in 1963 (see [4]).

The full alpha-beta pruning technique finally appeared in "Western" computer-science literature in 1968, within an article on theorem-proving strategies by James Slagle and Philip Bursky [25], but their description was somewhat vague and they did not illustrate deep cutoffs. Thus we might say that the first real English descriptions of the method appeared in 1969, in articles by Slagle and Dixon [26] and by Samuel [22]; both of these articles clearly mention the possibility of deep cutoffs, and discuss the idea in some detail.

The alpha-beta technique seems to be quite difficult to communicate verbally, or in conventional mathematical language, and the authors of the papers cited above had to resort to rather complicated descriptions; furthermore, considerable thought seems to be required at first exposure to convince oneself that the method is correct, especially when it has been described in ordinary language and when "deep cutoffs" must be justified. Perhaps this is why many years went by before the technique was published. However, we have seen in Section 2 that the method is easily understood and proved correct when it has been expressed in algorithmic language; this makes a good illustration of a case where a "dynamic" approach to process description is conceptually superior to the "static" approach of conventional mathematics.

Excellent presentations of the method appear in the recent textbooks by Nilsson [18, Section 4] and Slagle [24, pages 16–24], but in prose style instead of the easier-to-understand algorithmic form. Alpha-beta pruning has become "well known"; yet to the authors' knowledge only two published descriptions have heretofore been expressed in an algorithmic language. In fact the first of these, by Wells [28, Section 4.3.3], isn't really the full alpha-beta procedure — it isn't even as strong as procedure *F1*. (Not only is his algorithm incapable of making deep cutoffs, it makes shallow cutoffs only on strict inequality.) The other published algorithm, by Dahl and Belsnes [5, Section 8.1], appears in a recent Norwegian-language textbook on data structures; however, the alpha-beta method is presented using label parameters, so the corresponding proof of correctness becomes somewhat difficult. Another recent textbook [17, Section 3.3.1] contains an informal description of what is called "alpha-beta pruning," but again it presents only the method of procedure *F1*. Apparently many people are unaware that the alpha-beta procedure is capable of making deep cutoffs.[3] For these reasons, the

---

[3] Indeed, one of the authors of the present paper (D.E.K.) did some of the research described in Section 7 approximately five years before he was aware that deep cutoffs were possible. It is easy to understand procedure *F1*, and

authors of the present paper do not feel it redundant to have presented a new exposition of the method in this paper, even though alpha-beta pruning has been in use for more than 15 years.

6. Analysis of the Best Case

Now let us turn to a quantitative study of the algorithm. How much of the tree needs to be examined?

For this purpose it is convenient to assign coordinate numbers to the nodes of the tree as in the "Dewey decimal system" [11, Section 2.3]: Every position on level l is assigned a sequence of positive integers $a_1 a_2 \ldots a_l$. The root node (the starting position) corresponds to the empty sequence, and the d successors of position $a_1 \ldots a_l$ are assigned the respective coordinates $a_1 \ldots a_l 1, \ldots, a_1 \ldots a_l d$. Thus, position 314 is reached after making the third possible move from the starting position, then the first move from that position, and then the fourth.

Let us call position $a_1 a_2 \ldots a_l$ *critical* if $a_k = 1$ for all even values of k or for all odd values of k. Thus, positions 21412, 131512, 11121113, and 11 are critical, and the root position is always critical; but 12112 is not, since it has non-1s in both even and odd positions. The relevance of this concept is due to the following theorem, which characterizes the action of alpha-beta pruning when we are lucky enough to look at the best move first from every position.

Theorem 1. *Consider a game tree for which the value of the root position is not $\pm\infty$, and for which the first successor of every position is optimum; that is,*

$$F(a_1 \ldots a_l) = \begin{cases} f(a_1 \ldots a_l), & \text{if } a_1 \ldots a_l \text{ is terminal}, \\ -F(a_1 \ldots a_l 1), & \text{otherwise}. \end{cases} \tag{12}$$

The alpha-beta procedure F2 examines precisely the critical positions of this game tree.

Proof. Let us say that a critical position $a_1 \ldots a_l$ is of type 1 if all the a_k are 1; it is of type 2 if a_j is its first entry > 1 and $l - j$ is even; otherwise (that is, when $l - j$ is odd, hence $a_l = 1$) it is of type 3. The following facts can easily be established by induction on the computation, namely by showing that they are invariant assertions:

(1) A type 1 position p is examined by calling $F2\,(p, -\infty, +\infty)$. If it is not terminal, its successor position p_1 is of type 1, and $F(p) =$

---

to associate it with the term "alpha-beta pruning" that your colleagues are talking about, without discovering $F2$.

$-F(p_1) \neq \pm\infty$. The other successor positions $p_2, \ldots, p_d$ are of type 2, and they are all examined by calling $F2(p_k, -\infty, F(p_1))$.

(2) A type 2 position p is examined by calling $F2(p, -\infty, beta)$, where $-\infty < beta \leq F(p)$. If it is not terminal, its successor position p_1 is of type 3, and $F(p) = -F(p_1)$; hence, by the mechanism of procedure $F2$ as defined in Section 2, the other successors $p_2, \ldots, p_d$ are not examined.

(3) A type 3 position p is examined by calling $F2(p, alpha, +\infty)$, where $+\infty > alpha \geq F(p)$. If it is not terminal, each of its successor positions p_k is of type 2 and examined by calling $F2(p_k, -\infty, -alpha)$.

Thus, by induction on l, every critical position is examined.   □

Corollary 1. *If every position on levels* 0, 1, $\ldots$, $l-1$ *of a game tree satisfying the conditions of Theorem 1 has exactly d successors, for some fixed constant d, then the alpha-beta procedure examines exactly*

$$d^{\lfloor l/2 \rfloor} + d^{\lceil l/2 \rceil} - 1 \tag{13}$$

positions on level l.

Proof. There are $d^{\lfloor l/2 \rfloor}$ sequences $a_1 \ldots a_l$ with $a_k = 1$ for all odd values of k and $1 \leq a_k \leq d$ for all k; there are $d^{\lceil l/2 \rceil}$ such sequences with $a_k = 1$ for all even values of k; and we subtract 1 for the sequence $1 \ldots 1$ that was counted twice.   □

This corollary was first derived by Michael Levin in 1961, but no proof was apparently ever written down at the time. In fact, the informal memo [10] by Hart and Edwards justifies the result by saying: "For a convincing personal proof using the new heuristic hand waving technique, see the author of this theorem." A proof was eventually published by Slagle and Dixon [26]. However, none of these authors pointed out that the value of the root position must not equal $\pm\infty$. Although the latter condition is a rare occurrence in nontrivial games, since it means that the root position is a forced win or loss, it is a necessary hypothesis for both the theorem and the corollary, since the number of positions examined on level l will be $d^{\lfloor l/2 \rfloor}$ when the root value is $+\infty$, and it will be $d^{\lceil l/2 \rceil}$ when the root value is $-\infty$. Roughly speaking, we gain a factor of 2 when the root value is $\pm\infty$.

The characterization of perfect alpha-beta pruning in terms of critical positions allows us to extend Corollary 1 to a much more general class of game trees, having any desired probability distribution of legal moves on each level.

Corollary 2. *Let a random game tree be generated in such a way that each position on level j has probability q_j of being nonterminal, and has an average of d_j successors. Then the expected number of positions on level l is $d_0 d_1 \ldots d_{l-1}$; and the expected number of positions on level l examined by the alpha-beta technique under the assumptions of Theorem 1 is*

$$
\begin{aligned}
d_0 q_1 \ldots d_{l-2} q_{l-1} + q_0 d_1 \ldots q_{l-2} d_{l-1} - q_0 q_1 \ldots q_{l-1}, & \quad l \text{ even;} \\
d_0 q_1 d_2 \ldots q_{l-2} d_{l-1} + q_0 d_1 q_2 \ldots d_{l-2} q_{l-1} - q_0 q_1 \ldots q_{l-1}, & \quad l \text{ odd.}
\end{aligned}
\tag{14}
$$

(More precisely, the assumptions underlying this random branching process are that level $j + 1$ of the tree is formed from level j as follows: Each position p on level j is assigned a probability distribution $\langle r_0(p), r_1(p), \ldots \rangle$, where $r_d(p)$ is the probability that p will have d successors; these distributions may be different for different positions p, but each must satisfy $r_0(p) = 1 - q_j$, and each must have the mean value $r_1(p) + 2r_2(p) + \cdots = d_j$. The number of successor positions for p is chosen at random from this distribution, independently of the number of successors of other positions on level j.) Notice that (14) reduces to (13) when $q_j = 1$ and $d_j = d$ for $0 \le j < l$.

Proof. If x is the expected number of positions of a certain type on level j, then $x d_j$ is the expected number of successors of these positions, and $x q_j$ is the expected number of "number 1" successors. It follows as in Corollary 1 that (14) is the expected number of critical positions on level l; for example, $q_0 q_1 \ldots q_{l-1}$ is the expected number of positions on level l whose identifying coordinates are all 1s.   □

Intuitively we might think that alpha-beta pruning would be most effective when the perfect-ordering assumption (12) holds, namely when the first successor of every position is the best possible move. But this is not always the case: Figure 4 shows two game trees that are identical except for the left-to-right ordering of successor positions; alpha-beta search will investigate more of the left-hand tree than the right-hand tree, although the left-hand tree has its positions perfectly ordered at every branch.

Thus the truly optimum order of game tree traversal isn't obvious. On the other hand there always does exist an order for processing the tree so that alpha-beta examines as few of the terminal positions as possible; no algorithm can do better. This can be demonstrated by strengthening the technique used to prove Theorem 1.

Theorem 2. *Alpha-beta pruning is optimum in the following sense: Given any game tree and any algorithm that computes the value of the*

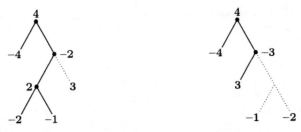

FIGURE 4. Perfect ordering is not always best.

root position, there is a way to permute the tree (by reordering successor positions if necessary) so that every terminal position examined by the alpha-beta method under this permutation is examined by the given algorithm. Furthermore if the value of the root is not $\pm\infty$, the alpha-beta procedure examines precisely the positions that are critical under this permutation.

(We assume that all terminal positions have independent values, or equivalently that the algorithm has no knowledge about dependencies between the values of terminal positions.) This result is due to G. M. Adelson-Velsky [1, Appendix 1]; a somewhat simpler proof will be presented here.

Proof. The following functions F_l and F_u define the best possible bounds on the value of any position p, based on the terminal positions examined by the given algorithm:

$$F_l(p) = \begin{cases} -\infty, & \text{if } p \text{ is terminal and not examined,} \\ f(p), & \text{if } p \text{ is terminal and examined,} \\ \max(-F_u(p_1), \ldots, -F_u(p_d)), & \text{otherwise;} \end{cases} \quad (15)$$

$$F_u(p) = \begin{cases} +\infty, & \text{if } p \text{ is terminal and not examined,} \\ f(p), & \text{if } p \text{ is terminal and examined,} \\ \max(-F_l(p_1), \ldots, -F_l(p_d)), & \text{otherwise.} \end{cases} \quad (16)$$

Notice that $F_l(p) \leq F_u(p)$ for all p. By independently varying the values at unexamined terminal positions in the subtree rooted at p, we can make $F(p)$ assume any given value between $F_l(p)$ and $F_u(p)$, but we can never go beyond these limits. When p is the root position we must therefore have $F_l(p) = F_u(p) = F(p)$.

Assume that the root value is not $\pm\infty$. We will show how to permute the tree so that every critical terminal position (according to the new numbering of positions) is examined by the given algorithm, and so that precisely the critical positions are examined by the alpha-beta procedure $F2$. The critical positions will be classified as type 1, 2, or 3 as in the proof of Theorem 1, the root being type 1. The following facts can be proved by induction:

(1) A type 1 position p has $F_l(p) = F_u(p) = F(p) \neq \pm\infty$, and it is examined during the alpha-beta procedure by calling $F2(p, -\infty, +\infty)$. If p is terminal, it must be examined by the given algorithm, since $F_l(p) \neq -\infty$. If p is not terminal, let j and k be such that $F_l(p) = -F_u(p_j)$ and $F_u(p) = -F_l(p_k)$. Then by (15) and (16) we have

$$F_l(p_k) \leq F_l(p_j) \leq F_u(p_j) = -F(p) = F_l(p_k),$$

hence $F_l(p_j) = F_l(p_k)$ and we may assume that $j = k$. By permuting the successor positions we may assume in fact that $j = k = 1$. Position p_1 (after permutation) is of type 1; the other successor positions $p_2, \ldots, p_d$ are of type 2, and they are all examined by calling $F2(p_i, -\infty, -F(p_1))$.

(2) A type 2 position p has $F_l(p) > -\infty$, and it is examined during the alpha-beta procedure by calling $F2(p, -\infty, beta)$, where $-\infty < beta \leq F_l(p)$. If p is terminal, it must be examined by the given algorithm. Otherwise let j be such that $F_l(p) = -F_u(p_j)$, and permute the successor positions if necessary so that $j = 1$. Position p_1 (after permutation) is of type 3 and is examined by calling $F2(p_1, -beta, +\infty)$. Since $F_u(p_1) = -F_l(p) \leq -beta$, this call returns a value $\leq -beta$; hence the other successors $p_2, \ldots, p_d$ (which are not critical positions) are not examined by the alpha-beta method, nor are their descendants.

(3) A type 3 position p has $F_u(p) < \infty$, and it is examined during the alpha-beta procedure by calling $F2(p, alpha, +\infty)$, where $F_u(p) \leq alpha < \infty$. If p is terminal, it must be examined by the given algorithm. Otherwise all its successor positions p_k are of type 2, and they are all examined by calling $F2(p_k, -\infty, -alpha)$. (There is no need to permute them; the ordering makes absolutely no difference here.)

A similar argument can be given when the root value is $+\infty$ (treating it as a type 2 position) or $-\infty$ (type 3). $\square$

A surprising corollary of this proof is that *the ordering of successors to type 3 positions in an optimally ordered tree has absolutely no effect on the behavior of alpha-beta pruning*. Type 1 positions constitute the so-called "principal variation," corresponding to the best strategy by both players. The alternative responses to moves on the principal variation are of type 2. Type 3 positions occur when the best move is made from a type 2 position, and the successors of type 3 positions are again of type 2. Hence about half of the critical positions of a perfectly ordered game tree are of type 3, and current game-playing algorithms are probably wasting nearly half of the time they now spend trying to put successor moves in order.

Let us say that a game tree is *uniform* of degree d and height h if every position on levels $0, 1, \ldots, h - 1$ has exactly d successors, and if every position on level h is terminal. For example, Figure 1 is a uniform tree of height 4 and degree 3, but the trees of Figure 4 are not uniform. Since all permutations of a uniform tree are uniform, Theorem 2 implies the following generalization of Corollary 1.

Corollary 3. *Any algorithm that evaluates a uniform game tree of height h and degree d must evaluate at least*

$$d^{\lceil h/2 \rceil} + d^{\lfloor h/2 \rfloor} - 1 \tag{17}$$

terminal positions. The alpha-beta procedure achieves this lower bound, if the best move is considered first at each position of types 1 and 2.   □

7. Uniform Trees Without Deep Cutoffs

Now that we have determined the best case of alpha-beta pruning, let's be more pessimistic and try to look at the worst that can happen. Given any finite tree, it is possible to find a sequence of values for the terminal positions so that the alpha-beta procedure will examine every node of the tree, without making any cutoffs unless the tree branches are permuted. (To see this, arrange the values so that whenever $F2\,(p, alpha, beta)$ is called, the condition $-alpha > F(p_1) > F(p_2) > \cdots > F(p_d) > -beta$ is satisfied.) On the other hand, there are game trees with distinct terminal values for which the alpha-beta procedure will always find some cutoffs no matter how the branches are permuted, as shown in Figure 5. (Procedure *F1* does not enjoy this property.)

Since game-playing programs usually use some sort of ordering strategy in connection with alpha-beta pruning, these facts about the worst case are of little or no practical significance. A more useful upper bound relevant to the behavior we may expect in practice can be based on the assumption of random data. Fuller, Gaschnig, and Gillogly have recently undertaken a study [7] of the average number of terminal positions examined when the alpha-beta procedure is applied to a uniform tree of degree d and height h, giving independent random values to the terminal positions on level h. They have obtained formulas by which this average number can be computed, in roughly d^h steps, and their theoretically predicted results were only slightly higher than empirically

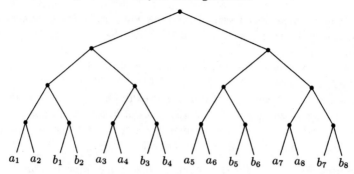

FIGURE 5. If $\max(a_1, \ldots, a_8) < \min(b_1, \ldots, b_8)$, the alpha-beta procedure will always find at least two cutoffs, no matter how we permute the branches of this game tree.

observed data obtained from a modified chess-playing program. Unfortunately, the formulas turn out to be extremely complicated, even for this reasonably simple theoretical model, and the asymptotic behavior for large d and/or h seems to defy analysis.

We are looking for upper bounds anyway, so it is natural to consider the behavior of the weaker procedure *F1*. This method is weaker since it doesn't find any "deep cutoffs"; but it is much better than complete minimaxing, and Figures 1–3 indicate that deep cutoffs probably have only a second-order effect on the efficiency. Furthermore, procedure *F1* has the great virtue that its analysis is much simpler than that of the full alpha-beta procedure *F2*.

On the other hand, the analysis of *F1* is by no means as easy as it looks, and the mathematics turns out to be extremely interesting. In fact, the authors' first analysis was found to be incorrect, although several competent people had checked it without seeing any mistakes. Since the error is quite instructive, we shall present our original (but fallacious) analysis here, challenging the reader to "find the bug"; then we shall study how to fix things up.

With this understanding, let us consider the following problem: A uniform game tree of degree d and height h is constructed with random values attached to its d^h terminal positions. What is the expected number of terminal positions examined when procedure *F1* is applied to this tree? The answer to this problem will be denoted by $T(d, h)$.

Since the search procedure depends only on the relative order of the terminal values, not on their magnitudes, and since there is zero probability that two different terminal positions get the same value, we may assume that the respective values assigned to the terminal positions are permutations of $\{1, 2, \ldots, d^h\}$, each permutation occurring with probability $1/(d^h)!$. From this observation it is clear that the d^l values of positions on each level l are also in random order, for $0 \le l \le h$. Although procedure $F1$ does not always compute the exact F values at every position, the decisions that it makes about cutoffs are easily seen to depend entirely on the F values (not on the approximate values $F1(p)$); see (8). We may conclude that the expected number of positions examined on level l is $T(d, l)$ for $0 \le l \le h$. This justifies restricting attention to a single level h when we count the number of positions examined.

In order to simplify the notation, let us consider first the case of ternary trees, $d = 3$; the general case will follow easily once this one is understood. Our first step is to classify the positions of the tree into types A, B, C as follows:

> The root position is type A.
>
> The first successor of every nonterminal position is type A.
>
> The second successor of every nonterminal position is type B.
>
> The third successor of every nonterminal position is type C.

Figure 6 shows the local "environment" of typical A, B, C positions as they appear below a nonterminal position p, which may be of any type. The F-values of these three positions are x_1, x_2, x_3, respectively, and their descendants have respective F-values $y_{11}, \ldots, y_{33}$. Our assumptions guarantee that $y_{11}, \ldots, y_{33}$ are in random order, no matter what level of the tree we are studying; hence the values

$$x_1 = \max(-y_{11}, -y_{12}, -y_{13}), \quad \ldots, \quad x_3 = \max(-y_{31}, -y_{32}, -y_{33})$$

are also in random order.

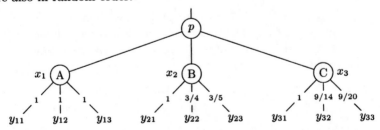

FIGURE 6. Part of a uniform ternary tree.

If position p is examined by calling $F1(p, bound)$, then position A will be examined by the subsequent call $F1(A, +\infty)$, by definition of $F1$.

(See Section 2.) Eventually the value x_1 will be returned; and if $-x_1 <$ *bound*, position B will be examined by calling $F1\,(\text{B}, x_1)$. Eventually the value x_2 will be returned; or, if $x_2 \geq x_1$, any value $x_2' \geq x_1$ may be returned. If $\max(-x_1, -x_2') < $ *bound*, position C will be examined by calling $F1\,(\text{C}, \min(x_1, x_2))$. Note that $-\max(-x_1, -x_2') = \min(x_1, x_2)$; the precise value of x_2' is not involved when C is called.

   This argument shows that all three successors of an A position are always examined (since the corresponding *bound* is $+\infty$). Each B position will examine its first successor, but (since its *bound* is $x_1 = -\min(y_{11}, y_{12}, y_{13})$) it will examine the second successor if and only if $-y_{21} < -\min(y_{11}, y_{12}, y_{13})$, that is, if and only if the values satisfy $\min(y_{11}, y_{12}, y_{13}) < y_{21}$. This happens with probability $\frac{3}{4}$, since the y's are randomly ordered and since the relation $\min(y_{11}, y_{12}, y_{13}) > y_{21}$ obviously holds with probability $\frac{1}{4}$. Similarly, the third successor of a B position is evaluated if and only if the values satisfy $\min(y_{11}, y_{12}, y_{13}) < \min(y_{21}, y_{22})$, and this has probability $\frac{3}{5}$. The probability that the second successor of a C position is evaluated is the probability that $\max(\min(y_{11}, y_{12}, y_{13}), \min(y_{21}, y_{22}, y_{23})) < y_{31}$, and this occurs $\frac{9}{14}$ of the time; the third successor is examined with probability $\frac{9}{20}$. (A general formula for these probabilities is derived below.)

   Let A_n, B_n, C_n be the expected number of positions examined n levels below an A, B, or C position that is examined by procedure $F1$ in a random game tree. Our discussion proves that

$$
\begin{aligned}
A_0 &= B_0 = C_0 = 1; \\
A_{n+1} &= A_n + B_n + C_n; \\
B_{n+1} &= A_n + \tfrac{3}{4}B_n + \tfrac{3}{5}C_n; \\
C_{n+1} &= A_n + \tfrac{9}{14}B_n + \tfrac{9}{20}C_n;
\end{aligned}
\tag{18}
$$

and $T(3, h) = A_h$ is the answer to our problem when $d = 3$.

   The solution to these simultaneous linear recurrences can be studied in many ways, and for our purposes the use of generating functions is most convenient. Let

$$
A(z) = \sum_{n \geq 0} A_n z^n, \qquad B(z) = \sum_{n \geq 0} B_n z^n, \qquad C(z) = \sum_{n \geq 0} C_n z^n,
$$

so that (18) is equivalent to

$$
\begin{aligned}
A(z) - 1 &= zA(z) + zB(z) + zC(z), \\
B(z) - 1 &= zA(z) + \tfrac{3}{4}zB(z) + \tfrac{3}{5}zC(z), \\
C(z) - 1 &= zA(z) + \tfrac{9}{14}zB(z) + \tfrac{9}{20}zC(z).
\end{aligned}
\tag{19}
$$

By Cramer's rule, $A(z) = U(z)/V(z)$, where

$$U(z) = \det \begin{pmatrix} -1 & z & z \\ -1 & \frac{3}{4}z - 1 & \frac{3}{5}z \\ -1 & \frac{9}{14}z & \frac{9}{20}z - 1 \end{pmatrix},$$

$$V(z) = \det \begin{pmatrix} z - 1 & z & z \\ z & \frac{3}{4}z - 1 & \frac{3}{5}z \\ z & \frac{9}{14}z & \frac{9}{20}z - 1 \end{pmatrix}$$

(20)

are polynomials in z. If the equation $z^3 V(1/z) = 0$ has distinct roots r_0, r_1, r_2, there will be a partial fraction expansion of the form

$$A(z) = \frac{c_0}{1 - r_0 z} + \frac{c_1}{1 - r_1 z} + \frac{c_2}{1 - r_2 z},$$

(21)

where

$$c_i = -r_i U(1/r_i)/V'(1/r_i).$$

(22)

Consequently $A(z) = \sum_{n \geq 0} (c_0(r_0 z)^n + c_1(r_1 z)^n + c_2(r_2 z)^n)$, and we have

$$A_n = c_0 r_0^n + c_1 r_1^n + c_2 r_2^n$$

by equating coefficients of z^n. If we number the roots so that $|r_0| > |r_1| \geq |r_2|$ (and the theorem of Perron [19] assures us that this can be done), we have asymptotically

$$A_n \sim c_0 r_0^n.$$

(23)

Numerical calculation gives $r_0 \approx 2.533911$, $c_0 \approx 1.162125$; thus, the alpha-beta procedure without deep cutoffs in a random ternary tree will examine about as many nodes as in a tree of the same height with average degree 2.534 instead of 3. (It is worthwhile to note that (23) predicts about 48 positions to be examined on the fourth level, while only 35 occurred in Figure 2; the reason for this discrepancy is chiefly that the one-digit values in Figure 2 are nonrandom because of frequent equalities.)

Elementary manipulation of determinants shows that the equation $z^3 V(1/z) = 0$ is the same as

$$\det \begin{pmatrix} 1 - z & 1 & 1 \\ 1 & \frac{3}{4} - z & \frac{3}{5} \\ 1 & \frac{9}{14} & \frac{9}{20} - z \end{pmatrix} = 0;$$

hence r_0 is the *largest eigenvalue* of the matrix

$$\begin{pmatrix} 1 & 1 & 1 \\ 1 & \frac{3}{4} & \frac{3}{5} \\ 1 & \frac{9}{14} & \frac{9}{20} \end{pmatrix}.$$

We might have deduced this directly from equation (18), if we had known enough matrix theory to calculate the constant c_1 by matrix-theoretic means instead of function-theoretic means.

This solves the case $d = 3$. For general d we find similarly that the expected number of terminal positions examined by the alpha-beta procedure without deep cutoffs, in a random uniform game tree of degree d and height h, is asymptotically

$$T(d, h) \sim c_0(d) r_0(d)^h \tag{24}$$

for fixed d as $h \to \infty$, where $r_0(d)$ is the largest eigenvalue of a certain $d \times d$ matrix

$$M_d = \begin{pmatrix} p_{11} & p_{12} & \cdots & p_{1d} \\ p_{21} & p_{22} & \cdots & p_{2d} \\ \vdots & \vdots & & \vdots \\ p_{d1} & p_{d2} & \cdots & p_{dd} \end{pmatrix} \tag{25}$$

and where $c_0(d)$ is an appropriate constant. The general matrix element p_{ij} in (25) is the probability that

$$\max_{1 \le k < i} (\min(Y_{k1}, \dots, Y_{kd})) < \min_{1 \le k < j} Y_{ik} \tag{26}$$

in a sequence of $(i - 1)d + (j - 1)$ independent identically distributed random variables $Y_{11}, \dots, Y_{i(j-1)}$.

When $i = 1$ or $j = 1$, the probability in (26) is 1, since the min over an empty set is $+\infty$ and the max is $-\infty$. When $i > 1$ and $j > 1$ we can evaluate the probability in several ways, of which the simplest seems to be combinatorial: For (26) to hold, the minimum of all the Y's must be $Y_{k't'}$, for some $k' < i$, and this occurs with probability $(i - 1)d / ((i - 1)d + j - 1)$; removing $Y_{k'1}, \dots, Y_{k'd}$ from consideration, the minimum of the remaining Y's must be $Y_{k''t''}$ for some $k'' < i$, and this occurs with probability $(i - 2)d / ((i - 2)d + j - 1)$; and so on. Therefore (26) occurs with probability

$$\begin{aligned} p_{ij} &= \frac{(i - 1)d}{(i - 1)d + j - 1} \cdot \frac{(i - 2)d}{(i - 2)d + j - 1} \cdot \cdots \cdot \frac{d}{d + j - 1} \\ &= 1 \Big/ \binom{i - 1 + (j - 1)/d}{i - 1}. \end{aligned} \tag{27}$$

This explicit formula allows us to calculate $r_0(d)$ numerically for small d without much difficulty, and to calculate $c_0(d)$ for small d with somewhat more difficulty using (22).

The form of (27) isn't very convenient for asymptotic calculations; fortunately there is a much simpler expression that yields an excellent approximation:

Lemma 1. *When $0 \le x \le 1$ and k is a positive integer,*

$$k^x \le \binom{k-1+x}{k-1} \le k^x/\Gamma(1+x). \tag{28}$$

(Numerically, $0.885603 < \Gamma(1+x) \le 1$ for $0 \le x \le 1$, with the minimum value occurring at $x \approx 0.461632$; hence the simple formula k^x is always within about 11% of the exact value of the binomial coefficient.)

Proof. When $0 \le x \le 1$ and $t > -1$ we have

$$(1+t)^x \le 1 + tx, \tag{29}$$

since the function $f(x) = (1+t)^x/(1+tx)$ satisfies $f(0) = f(1) = 1$, and since

$$f''(x) = \big((\ln(1+t) - t/(1+tx))^2 + t^2/(1+tx)^2\big) f(x) > 0.$$

Using (29) for $t = 1, \frac{1}{2}, \frac{1}{3}, \ldots$ yields

$$1 \le \frac{1+x}{2^x}$$

$$\le \frac{1+x}{2^x} \cdot \frac{1+\frac{1}{2}x}{(\frac{3}{2})^x} \le \cdots$$

$$\le \lim_{m\to\infty} \frac{(1+x)}{1} \frac{(2+x)}{2} \cdots \frac{(m+x)}{m} \frac{1}{(m+1)^x} = \frac{1}{\Gamma(1+x)}$$

and the kth term of this series of inequalities is $\binom{k-1+x}{k-1}/k^x$. $\quad\square$

For trees of height 2, deep cutoffs are impossible, and procedures *F1* and *F2* have an identical effect. How many of the d^2 positions at level 2 are examined? Our analysis gives an exact answer for this case, and Lemma 1 can be used to give a good approximate result that we may state as a theorem.

Theorem 3. *The expected number of terminal positions examined by the alpha-beta procedure on level 2 of a random uniform game tree of degree d is*

$$T(d, 2) = \sum_{1 \leq i,j \leq d} p_{ij}, \qquad (30)$$

where the p_{ij} are defined in (27). We have

$$C_1 \frac{d^2}{\log d} \leq T(d, 2) \leq C_2 \frac{d^2}{\log d} \qquad (31)$$

for certain positive constants C_1 and C_2.

Proof. Equation (30) follows from our previous remarks, and from Lemma 1 we know that

$$C\, S(d) \leq T(d, 2) \leq S(d),$$

where $C = 0.885603 \approx \inf_{0 \leq x \leq 1} \Gamma(1 + x)$ and

$$S(d) = \sum_{k=1}^{d} \sum_{j=1}^{d} k^{-(j-1)/d}$$

$$= d + \sum_{k=2}^{d} \left(\frac{1 - k^{-1}}{1 - k^{-1/d}} \right).$$

Now for $k = d^t$ we have $k^{-1/d} = \exp(-t \ln d / d) = 1 - t \ln d / d + O((\log d / d)^2)$; hence for $\sqrt{d} \leq k \leq d$, $(1 - k^{-1})/(1 - k^{-1/d})$ lies between $d/\ln d$ and $2d/\ln d$ times $1 + O(\log d / d)$. The bounds in (31) now follow easily.   □

When the values of $r_0(d)$ for $d \leq 30$ are plotted on log log paper, they seem to be approaching a straight line, suggesting that $r_0(d)$ is approximately of order $d^{0.75}$. In fact, a least-squares fit for $10 \leq d \leq 30$ yielded $d^{0.76}$ as an approximate order of growth; this can be compared to the lower bound $2d^{0.5}$ of an optimum alpha-beta search, or to the upper bound d of a full minimax search, or to the estimate $d^{0.72}$ obtained by Fuller, Gaschnig, and Gillogly [7] for random alpha-beta pruning when deep cutoffs are included. However, we shall see that the true order of growth of $r_0(d)$ as $d \to \infty$ is really $d/\log d$.

There is a moral to this story: If we didn't know the theoretical asymptotic growth, we would be quite content to think of it as $d^{0.76}$

when d is in a practical range. The formula $d/\log d$ seems much worse than $d^{0.76}$, until we realize the magnitude of $\log d$ in the range of interest. (A similar phenomenon occurs with respect to Shell's sorting method, see [12, pp. 93–95].) On the basis of this theory we may well regard the approximation $d^{0.72}$ in [7] with some suspicion.

But as mentioned above, there is a much more significant moral to this story. Formula (24) *is incorrect* because the proof overlooked what appears to be a rather subtle question of conditional probabilities. Did the reader spot a fallacy? The authors found it only by comparing their results to those of [7] in the case $h = 3$, $d = 2$, since procedures *F1* and *F2* are equivalent for heights ≤ 3. According to the analysis above, the alpha-beta procedure will examine an average of $6\frac{7}{9}$ nodes on level 3 of a random binary game tree, but according to [7] the number is $6\frac{89}{105}$. After the authors of [7] were politely informed that they must have erred, since we had proved that $6\frac{7}{9}$ was correct, they politely replied that simulation results (including a test on all 8! permutations) had confirmed that the correct answer is $6\frac{89}{105}$.

A careful scrutiny of the situation explains what is going on. Theorem 3 is correct, since it deals only with level 2, but trouble occurs at level 3. Our theory predicts a cutoff on the right subtree of every B node with probability $\frac{2}{3}$, so that the terminal values $(f_1, \ldots, f_8)$ in Figure 7 will be examined with respective probabilities $(1, 1, 1, \frac{2}{3}, 1, 1, \frac{2}{3}, \frac{4}{9})$. Actually f_8 is examined with probability $\frac{18}{35}$ instead of $\frac{4}{9}$; for f_8 is examined if and only if

$$f_7 > \min(f_5, f_6),$$
$$\min(f_5, f_6) < \max\big(\min(f_1, f_2), \min(f_3, f_4)\big). \tag{32}$$

Each of these two events has probability $\frac{2}{3}$, but they are not independent.

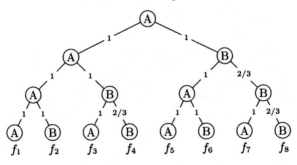

FIGURE 7. A tree that reveals the fallacious reasoning.

When the fallacy is stated in these terms, the error is quite plain, but the dependence was much harder to see in the diagrams we had been drawing for ourselves. For example, when we argued using Figure 6 that the second successor of a B position is examined with probability $\frac{3}{4}$, we neglected to consider that, when p is itself of type B or C, the B node in Figure 6 is entered only when $\min(y_{11}, y_{12}, y_{13})$ is less than the bound at p; so $\min(y_{11}, y_{12}, y_{13})$ is somewhat smaller than a random value would be. What we should have computed is the probability that $y_{21} > \min(y_{11}, y_{12}, y_{13})$ *given that* position B is not cut off. And unfortunately this can depend in a very complicated way on the ancestors of p.

To make matters worse, our error is in the wrong direction; the correction doesn't provide an upper bound for alpha-beta searching. It yields only a lower bound on an upper bound (which is nothing). In order to get information relevant to the behavior of procedure *F2* on random data, we need at least an upper bound on the behavior of procedure *F1*.

A correct analysis of the binary case $(d = 2)$ involves the solution of recurrences

$$A_{n+1} = A_n + B_n^{(0)},$$
$$B_{n+1}^{(k)} = A_n + p_k B_n^{(k+1)} \quad \text{for } k \geq 0, \tag{33}$$
$$A_0 = B_0^{(0)} = B_0^{(1)} = B_0^{(2)} = \cdots = 1,$$

where the p_k are appropriate probabilities. For example, $p_0 = \frac{2}{3}$; $p_0 p_1$ is the probability that (32) holds; and $p_0 p_1 p_2$ is the probability that fifteen independent random variables satisfy

$$f_{15} > f_{13} \wedge f_{14},$$
$$f_{13} \wedge f_{14} < (f_9 \wedge f_{10}) \vee (f_{11} \wedge f_{12}), \tag{34}$$
$$(f_9 \wedge f_{10}) \vee (f_{11} \wedge f_{12}) > ((f_1 \wedge f_2) \vee (f_3 \wedge f_4)) \wedge ((f_5 \wedge f_6) \vee (f_7 \wedge f_8)),$$

writing $\vee$ for max and $\wedge$ for min. These probabilities can be computed exactly by evaluating appropriate integrals, but the formulas are complicated and it is easier to look for upper bounds. We can at least show easily that the probability in (34) is $\leq \frac{4}{9}$, since the first and third conditions *are* independent, and they each hold with probability $\frac{2}{3}$. Thus we obtain an upper bound if we set $p_0 = p_2 = p_4 = \cdots = \frac{2}{3}$ and $p_1 = p_3 = p_5 = \cdots = 1$; this is equivalent to the recurrence

$$A_0 = B_0 = 1,$$
$$A_{n+1} = A_n + B_n, \tag{35}$$
$$B_{n+1} = A_n + \tfrac{2}{3} A_n.$$

Similarly in the case of degree 3, we obtain an upper bound on the average number of nodes examined without deep cutoffs by solving the recurrence

$$
\begin{aligned}
A_0 &= B_0 = C_0 = 1, \\
A_{n+1} &= A_n + B_n + C_n, \\
B_{n+1} &= A_n + \tfrac{3}{4}A_n + \tfrac{3}{5}A_n, \\
C_{n+1} &= A_n + \tfrac{9}{14}A_n + \tfrac{9}{20}A_n,
\end{aligned}
\tag{36}
$$

in place of (18). This is equivalent to

$$
A_{n+1} = A_n + (1 + \tfrac{3}{4} + \tfrac{3}{5} + 1 + \tfrac{9}{14} + \tfrac{9}{20})A_{n-1}
$$

and for general degree d we get the recurrence

$$
A_{n+1} = A_n + S_d A_{n-1},
\tag{37}
$$

where $A_0 = 1$, $A_1 = d$, and

$$
S_d = \sum_{i=2}^{d} \sum_{j=1}^{d} p_{ij}.
\tag{38}
$$

This gives a valid upper bound on the behavior of procedure *F1*, because it is equivalent to setting *bound* $\leftarrow +\infty$ at certain positions (and this operation never decreases the number of positions examined). Furthermore we can solve (37) explicitly, to obtain an asymptotic upper bound on $T(d, h)$ of the form $c_1(d)r_1(d)^h$, where the growth ratio is

$$
r_1(d) = \sqrt{S_d + \tfrac{1}{4}} + \tfrac{1}{2}.
\tag{39}
$$

Unfortunately it turns out that S_d is of order $d^2/\log d$, by Theorem 3; so (39) is of order $d/\sqrt{\log d}$, while an upper bound of order $d/\log d$ is desired.

Another way to get an upper bound relies on a more detailed analysis of the structural behavior of procedure *F1*, as in the following theorem.

Theorem 4. *The expected number of terminal positions examined by the alpha-beta procedure without deep cutoffs, in a random uniform game tree of degree d and height h, satisfies*

$$
T(d, h) < c^*(d)\, r^*(d)^h,
\tag{40}
$$

where $r^*(d)$ is the largest eigenvalue of the matrix

$$M_d^* = \begin{pmatrix} \sqrt{p_{11}} & \sqrt{p_{12}} & \cdots & \sqrt{p_{1d}} \\ \sqrt{p_{21}} & \sqrt{p_{22}} & \cdots & \sqrt{p_{2d}} \\ \vdots & \vdots & & \vdots \\ \sqrt{p_{d1}} & \sqrt{p_{d2}} & \cdots & \sqrt{p_{dd}} \end{pmatrix}, \tag{41}$$

and $c^*(d)$ is an appropriate constant.

(The p_{ij} in (41) are the same as in (25) and (38).)

Proof. Assign coordinates $a_1 \dots a_l$ to the positions of the tree as in Section 6. For $l \geq 1$, it is easy to prove by induction that position $a_1 \dots a_l$ has *bound* $= \min\{F(a_1 \dots a_{l-1}k) \mid 1 \leq k < a_l\}$ when it is examined by procedure *F1*; hence it is examined if and only if $a_1 \dots a_{l-1}$ is examined and either $l = 1$ or

$$- \min_{1 \leq k \leq a_l} F(a_1 \dots a_{l-1}k) < \min_{1 \leq k \leq a_{l-1}} F(a_1 \dots a_{l-2}k). \tag{42}$$

It follows that a terminal position $a_1 \dots a_h$ is examined by *F1* if and only if (42) holds for $2 \leq l \leq h$. Let us abbreviate (42) by P_l, so that $a_1 \dots a_h$ holds if and only if P_2 and $\dots$ and P_h. Condition P_l by itself holds with probability p_{ij} where $i = a_{l-1}$ and $j = a_l$, because of definition (26); hence if the P_l were independent we would have $a_1 \dots a_h$ examined with probability $p_{a_1 a_2} p_{a_2 a_3} \cdots p_{a_{h-1} a_h}$, and this is precisely equivalent to the analysis leading to (24). However, the P_l aren't independent, as we have observed in (32) and (34).

Condition P_l is a function of the terminal values

$$f(a_1 \dots a_{l-2} \, j \, k \, a_{l+1} \dots a_h),$$

where $j < a_{l-1}$ or $j = a_{l-1}$ and $k < a_l$. Hence P_l is *independent* of P_1, $P_2, \dots, P_{l-2}$. (This generalizes an observation we made about (34).) Let x be the probability that position $a_1 \dots a_h$ is examined, and assume for convenience in notation that h is odd. Then by the partial independence of the P_l's, we have

$$x < p_{a_1 a_2} p_{a_3 a_4} \cdots p_{a_{h-2} a_{h-1}},$$
$$x < p_{a_2 a_3} p_{a_4 a_5} \cdots p_{a_{h-1} a_h};$$

hence

$$x < \sqrt{p_{a_1 a_2} p_{a_2 a_3} \cdots p_{a_{h-1} a_h}}$$

and the theorem follows by choosing $c^*(d)$ large enough. $\quad\square$

Now we are ready to establish the correct asymptotic growth rate of the branching factor for procedure *F1*.

Theorem 5. *The expected number $T(d, h)$ of terminal positions examined by the alpha-beta procedure without deep cutoffs, in a random uniform game tree of degree d and height h, has a branching factor*

$$\lim_{h \to \infty} T(d, h)^{1/h} = r(d) \tag{43}$$

that satisfies

$$C_3 \frac{d}{\log d} \leq r(d) \leq C_4 \frac{d}{\log d} \tag{44}$$

for certain positive constants C_3 and C_4.

Proof. We have

$$T(d, h_1 + h_2) \leq T(d, h_1) T(d, h_2), \tag{45}$$

since the right-hand side of (45) is the number of positions that would be examined by *F1* if *bound* were set to $+\infty$ for all positions at height h_1. Furthermore the arguments above prove that

$$\liminf_{h \to \infty} T(d, h) \geq r_0(d), \qquad \limsup_{h \to \infty} T(d, h) \leq r^*(d).$$

By a standard argument about subadditive functions (see, for example, [20, Problem 1.98]) it follows that the limit (43) exists.

To prove the lower bound in (44) we shall show that $r_0(d) \geq C_3 \, d/\log d$. The largest eigenvalue of a matrix with positive entries p_{ij} is known to be $\geq \min_i(\sum_j p_{ij})$, according to the theory of Perron [19]; see [27, Section 2.1] for a modern account of this theory.[4] Therefore by Lemma 1,

$$r_0(d) \geq C \min_{1 \leq k \leq d} \left(\sum_{1 \leq j \leq d} k^{-(j-1)/d} \right)$$

$$= C \min_{2 \leq k \leq d} \left(\frac{1 - k^{-1}}{1 - k^{-1/d}} \right) = C \frac{1 - d^{-1}}{1 - d^{-1/d}} > C \frac{d-1}{\ln d},$$

where $C = 0.885603 \approx \inf_{0 \leq x \leq 1} \Gamma(1+x)$, since $d^{-1/d} = \exp(-\ln d / d) > 1 - \ln d / d$.

---

[4] We are indebted to Dr. J. H. Wilkinson for suggesting this proof of the lower bound.

To get the upper bound in (44), we shall prove that $r^*(d) < C_4\, d/\log d$, using a rather curious matrix norm. If s and t are positive real numbers with

$$\frac{1}{s} + \frac{1}{t} = 1, \tag{46}$$

then all eigenvalues λ of a matrix A with entries a_{ij} satisfy

$$|\lambda| \le \left(\sum_i \left(\sum_j |a_{ij}^t|\right)^{s/t}\right)^{1/s}. \tag{47}$$

To prove this, let $Ax = \lambda x$, where x is a nonzero vector; by Hölder's inequality [9, Section 2.7],

$$|\lambda|\left(\sum_i |x_i^s|\right)^{1/s} = \left(\sum_i \left|\sum_j a_{ij}x_j\right|^s\right)^{1/s}$$

$$\le \left(\sum_i \left(\sum_j |a_{ij}^t|\right)^{s/t}\left(\sum_j |x_j^s|\right)\right)^{1/s}$$

$$= \left(\sum_i \left(\sum_j |a_{ij}^t|\right)^{s/t}\right)^{1/s}\left(\sum_i |x_i^s|\right)^{1/s}$$

and (47) follows.

If we let $s = t = 2$, inequality (47) yields $r^*(d) = O(d/\sqrt{\log d}\,)$, while if s or $t \to \infty$ the upper bound is merely $O(d)$. Therefore some care is necessary in selecting the best s and t; for our purposes we choose $s = f(d)$ and $t = f(d)/(f(d) - 1)$, where $f(d) = \frac{1}{2}\ln d /\ln\ln d$. Then

$$r^*(d) \le \left(\sum_{k=1}^d \left(\sum_{j=1}^d k^{-t(j-1)/2d}\right)^{s/t}\right)^{1/s}$$
$$< \left(\sqrt{d}\, d^{s/t} + (d - \sqrt{d})\left(\sum_{j\ge 1}(\sqrt{d}\,)^{-t(j-1)/2d}\right)^{s/t}\right)^{1/s}. \tag{48}$$

The inner sum is $g(d) = 1/(1 - d^{-t/4d}) = (4d/\ln d)(1 + O(\ln\ln d / \ln d))$, so

$$d\, g(d)^{s/t} = d^{f(d)-1/2}\exp(\tfrac{1}{2}\ln 4\ln d / \ln\ln d + \ln\ln d + O(1)).$$

Hence the right-hand side of (48) is

$$\exp\bigl(\ln d - \ln\ln d + \ln 4 + O((\ln\ln d)^2 / \ln d)\bigr);$$

d	$r_0(d)$	$r_1(d)$	$r^*(d)$		d	$r_0(d)$	$r_1(d)$	$r^*(d)$
2	1.847	1.884	1.912		17	8.976	11.378	11.470
3	2.534	2.666	2.722		18	9.358	11.938	12.021
4	3.142	3.397	3.473		19	9.734	12.494	12.567
5	3.701	4.095	4.186		20	10.106	13.045	13.108
6	4.226	4.767	4.871		21	10.473	13.593	13.644
7	4.724	5.421	5.532		22	10.836	14.137	14.176
8	5.203	6.059	6.176		23	11.194	14.678	14.704
9	5.664	6.684	6.805		24	11.550	15.215	15.228
10	6.112	7.298	7.420		25	11.901	15.750	15.748
11	6.547	7.902	8.024		26	12.250	16.282	16.265
12	6.972	8.498	8.618		27	12.595	16.811	16.778
13	7.388	9.086	9.203		28	12.937	17.337	17.288
14	7.795	9.668	9.781		29	13.277	17.861	17.796
15	8.195	10.243	10.350		30	13.614	18.383	18.300
16	8.589	10.813	10.913		31	13.948	18.903	18.802

TABLE 1. Bounds for the branching factor in a random tree of degree d when no deep cutoffs are performed.

we have proved that

$$r^*(d) \leq (4d/\ln d)(1 + O((\ln \ln d)^2/\ln d)) \qquad \text{as } d \to \infty. \quad \square$$

Table 1 shows the various bounds we have obtained on $r(d)$, namely the lower bound $r_0(d)$ and the upper bounds $r_1(d)$ and $r^*(d)$. We have proved that $r_0(d)$ and $r^*(d)$ grow as $d/\log d$, and that $r_1(d)$ grows as $d/\sqrt{\log d}$; but the table shows that $r_1(d)$ is actually a better bound than $r^*(d)$ for $d \leq 24$.

8. Discussion of the Model

The theoretical model we have studied gives us an upper bound on the actual behavior obtained in practice. It is an upper bound for four separate reasons:

(a) the deep cutoffs are not considered;
(b) the ordering of successor positions is random;
(c) the terminal positions are assumed to have distinct values;
(d) the terminal values are assumed to be independent of each other.

Each of these conditions makes our model pessimistic; for example, we are usually able in practice to make plausible guesses that some moves will be better than others. Furthermore, the large number of equal terminal values in typical games helps to provide additional cutoffs. The effect of assumption (d) is less clear, and it will be studied in Section 9.

In spite of all these pessimistic assumptions, the results of our calculations show that alpha-beta pruning will be reasonably efficient.

Let us now try to estimate the effect of deep cutoffs versus no deep cutoffs. One way to study this is in terms of the best case: Under ideal ordering of successor positions, what is the analog for procedure *F1* of the theory developed in Section 6? It is not difficult to see that the positions $a_1 \ldots a_l$ examined by *F1* in the best case are precisely those with no two non-1s in a row, namely those for which $a_k > 1$ implies $a_{k+1} = 1$.

In the ternary case under best ordering, we obtain the recurrence

$$\begin{aligned}
A_0 &= B_0 = C_0 = 1, \\
A_{n+1} &= A_n + B_n + C_n, \\
B_{n+1} &= A_n, \\
C_{n+1} &= A_n,
\end{aligned} \qquad (49)$$

hence $A_{n+1} = A_n + 2A_{n-1}$. For general d the corresponding recurrence is

$$A_0 = 1, \qquad A_1 = d, \qquad A_{n+2} = A_{n+1} + (d-1)A_n. \qquad (50)$$

The solution to this recurrence is

$$A_n = \frac{1}{\sqrt{4d-3}}\left(\left(\sqrt{d-\tfrac{3}{4}}+\tfrac{1}{2}\right)^{n+2} - \left(-\sqrt{d-\tfrac{3}{4}}+\tfrac{1}{2}\right)^{n+2}\right); \qquad (51)$$

so the growth rate or effective branching factor is $\sqrt{d-\tfrac{3}{4}}+\tfrac{1}{2}$, not much higher than the value $\sqrt{d}$ obtained for the full method including deep cutoffs. This result tends to support the contention that deep cutoffs have only a second-order effect, although we must admit that poor ordering of successor moves will make deep cutoffs increasingly valuable.

9. Dependent Terminal Values

Our model gives independent values to all the terminal positions, but such independence doesn't happen very often in real games. For example, if $f(p)$ is based on the piece count in a chess game, all the positions following a blunder will tend to have low scores for the player who loses material.

In this section we shall try to account for such dependencies by considering a *total dependency* model, which has the following property for all nonterminal positions p: For each i and j, all of the terminal successors of p_i either have greater value than all terminal successors of p_j, or they all have lesser value. This model is equivalent to assigning a permutation of $\{0, 1, \ldots, d-1\}$ to the moves at every position, and then using the concatenation of all move numbers leading to a terminal position as that position's value, considered as a radix-d number. For example, Figure 8 shows a uniform ternary game tree of height 3 constructed in this way.

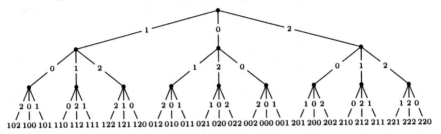

FIGURE 8. A tree with "totally dependent" values.

Another way to look at this model is to imagine assigning the values $0, 1, \ldots, d^h - 1$ in d-ary notation to the terminal positions, and then to apply a random permutation to the branches emanating from every nonterminal position. It follows that the F value at the root is always $-(0c0c\ldots c0)_d$ if h is odd, $+(c0c0\ldots c0)_d$ if h is even, where $c = d - 1$.

Theorem 6. *The expected number of terminal positions examined by the alpha-beta procedure, in a random totally dependent uniform game tree of degree d and height h, is*

$$\frac{d - H_d}{d - H_d^2}\left(d^{\lceil h/2 \rceil} + H_d d^{\lfloor h/2 \rfloor} - H_d^{h+1} - H_d^h\right) + H_d^h, \tag{52}$$

where H_d is the harmonic number $1 + \frac{1}{2} + \cdots + \frac{1}{d}$.

Proof. As in our other proofs, we divide the positions of the tree into a finite number of classes or types for which recurrence relations can be given. In this case we use three types, somewhat as in our proof of Theorems 1 and 2.

A type 1 position p is examined by calling $F2\,(p, alpha, beta)$ where all terminal descendants q of p have $alpha < \pm f(q) < beta$; here the $+$ or $-$ sign is used according as p is an even or an odd number of levels from the bottom of the tree. If p is nonterminal, its successors are assigned a definite ranking; let us say that p_k is *relevant* if $F(p_k) < F(p_j)$ for all $1 \leq j < k$. Then all of the relevant successors of p are examined by calling $F2(p_k, -beta, -m)$ where $F(p_k)$ lies between $-beta$ and $-m$, hence the relevant p_k are again of type 1. The irrelevant p_k are examined by calling $F2(p_k, -beta, -m)$ where $F(p_k) > -m$, and we shall call them type 2.

A type 2 position p is examined by calling $F2(p, alpha, beta)$ where all terminal descendants q of p have $\pm f(q) > beta$. If p is nonterminal, its first successor p_1 is classified as type 3, and it is examined by calling $F2(p_1, -beta, -alpha)$. This procedure call eventually returns a value $\leq -beta$, causing an immediate cutoff.

A type 3 position p is examined by calling $F2(p, alpha, beta)$ where all terminal descendants q of p have $\pm f(q) < alpha$. If p is nonterminal, all its successors are classified type 2, and they are examined by calling $F2(p_k, -beta, -alpha)$; they all return values $\geq -alpha$.

Let A_n, B_n, C_n be the expected number of terminal positions examined in a random totally dependent uniform tree of degree d and height h, when the root is of type 1, 2, or 3 respectively. Our argument shows that the following recurrence relations hold:

$$A_0 = B_0 = C_0 = 1;$$
$$A_{n+1} = A_n + (\tfrac{1}{2}A_n + \tfrac{1}{2}B_n) + (\tfrac{1}{3}A_n + \tfrac{2}{3}B_n) + \cdots$$
$$+ ((1/d)A_n + ((d-1)/d)B_n)$$
$$= H_d A_n + (d - H_d)B_n; \tag{53}$$
$$B_{n+1} = C_n;$$
$$C_{n+1} = dB_n.$$

Consequently $B_n = d^{\lfloor n/2 \rfloor}$, and A_h has the value stated in (52). □

Corollary 4. *When $d \geq 3$, the average number of positions examined by alpha-beta search under the assumption of totally dependent terminal values is bounded by a constant[5] times the optimum number of positions specified in Corollary 3.*

Proof. The growth of (52) as $h \to \infty$ is order $d^{h/2}$. The stated constant is approximately

$$(d - H_d)(1 + H_d)/(2(d - H_d^2)).$$

(When $d = 2$ the growth rate of (52) is order $(\tfrac{3}{2})^h$ instead of $(\sqrt{2})^h$.)

---

[5] This "constant" depends on the degree d, but not on the height h.

Incidentally, we can also analyze procedure *F1* under the same assumptions; the restriction of deep cutoffs leads to the recurrence

$$A_0 = 1, \qquad A_1 = 1, \qquad A_{n+2} = H_d A_{n+1} + (d - H_d) A_n, \qquad (54)$$

and the corresponding growth rate is of order $(\sqrt{d - H_d + \frac{1}{4} H_d^2} + \frac{1}{2} H_d)^h$; again the branching factor is roughly $\sqrt{d}$ for large d.   □

The authors of [7] have suggested another model to account for dependencies between positions: Each branch of the uniform game tree is assigned a random number between 0 and 1, and the value of each terminal position is taken to be the sum of all values on the branches leading to that position. If we apply the naïve approach of Section 7 to the analysis of this model without deep cutoffs, the probability needed in place of equation (26) is the probability that

$$\max_{1 \le k < i} (X_k + \min(Y_{k1}, \ldots, Y_{kd})) < X_i + \min_{1 \le k < j} Y_{ik} \qquad (55)$$

where as before the Y's are independent and identically distributed random variables, and where $X_1, \ldots, X_i$ are independent uniform random deviates. Balkema [2] has shown that (55) never occurs with greater probability than the value p_{ij} derived in Section 7, regardless of the distribution of the Y's (as long as that distribution is continuous). Therefore we have good grounds to believe that dependencies between position values tend to make alpha-beta pruning more efficient than it would be if all terminal positions had independent values.

Acknowledgments

We wish to thank J. R. Slagle, whose lecture at Caltech in 1967 originally stimulated some of the research reported here, and we also wish to thank Forest Baskett, Robert W. Floyd, John Gaschnig, James Gillogly, John McCarthy, and James H. Wilkinson for discussions that contributed significantly to our work.

This research was supported in part by the National Science Foundation and in part by the Office of Naval Research. Computer time for our numerical experiments was supported in part by the Advanced Research Projects Agency (ARPA) and in part by IBM Corporation.

References

[1] G. M. Adel'son-Vel'skiĭ, V. L. Arlazarov, A. R. Bitman, A. A. Zhivotovskiĭ, and A. V. Uskov, "О программировании игры вычислительной машины в шахматы," *Uspekhi Matematicheskikh*

Nauk **25**, 2 (1970), 221–260. English translation, "Programming a computer to play chess," *Russian Mathematical Surveys* **25**, 2 (1970), 221–262.

[2] G. Balkema, Personal communication (19 July 1974).

[3] A. Bernstein, M. de V. Roberts, T. Arbuckle, and M. A. Belsky, "A chess playing program for the IBM 704," *Proceedings of the Western Joint Computer Conference* **13** (1958), 157–159; discussion on pages 171–172.

[4] A. L. Brudno, "Грани и оценки для сокращения перебора вариантов," *Problemy Kibernetiki* **10** (1963), 141–150.

[5] Ole-Johan Dahl and Dag Belsnes, *Algoritmer og Datastrakturer* (Lund, Sweden: Studentlitteratur, 1973).

[6] R. W. Floyd, Personal communication (18 January 1965).

[7] S. H. Fuller, J. G. Gaschnig, and J. J. Gillogly, "Analysis of the alpha-beta pruning algorithm," Technical Report, Department of Computer Science (Pittsburgh, Pennsylvania: Carnegie–Mellon University, July 1973), ii + 51 pages.

[8] Richard D. Greenblatt, Donald E. Eastlake, III, and Stephen D. Crocker, "The Greenblatt chess program," *Proceedings of the AFIPS Fall Joint Computer Conference* **31** (1967), 801–810.

[9] G. H. Hardy, J. E. Littlewood, and G. Pólya, *Inequalities* (Cambridge: Cambridge University Press, 1934).

[10] Timothy P. Hart and Daniel J. Edwards, "The tree prune (TP) algorithm," M.I.T. Artificial Intelligence Project Memo #30 (Cambridge, Massachusetts: Research Laboratory of Electronics and Computation Center, Massachusetts Institute of Technology, 4 December 1961), 6 pages. Revised form, "The α-β heuristic," by Daniel J. Edwards and Timothy P. Hart (28 October 1963), 4 pages.

[11] Donald E. Knuth, *Fundamental Algorithms*, Volume 1 of *The Art of Computer Programming* (Reading, Massachusetts: Addison–Wesley, 1968).

[12] Donald E. Knuth, *Sorting and Searching*, Volume 3 of *The Art of Computer Programming* (Reading, Massachusetts: Addison–Wesley, 1973).

[13] Donald E. Knuth, "Structured programming with **go to** statements," *Computing Surveys* **6** (1974), 261–301. Reprinted with revisions as Chapter 2 of *Literate Programming*, CSLI Lecture

Notes 27 (Stanford, California: Center for the Study of Language and Information, 1992), 17–89.

[14] E. L. Lawler and D. E. Wood, "Branch-and-bound methods: A survey," *Operations Research* **14** (1966), 699–719.

[15] John McCarthy, Personal communication (1 December 1973).

[16] Allen Newell, J. C. Shaw, and H. A. Simon, "Chess-playing programs and the problem of complexity," *IBM Journal of Research and Development* **2** (1958), 320–355. Reprinted with minor corrections in *Computers and Thought*, edited by E. A. Feigenbaum and J. Feldman (New York: McGraw–Hill, 1963), 109–133.

[17] Jurg Nievergelt, J. Craig Farrar, and Edward M. Reingold, *Computer Approaches to Mathematical Problems* (Englewood Cliffs, New Jersey: Prentice–Hall, 1974).

[18] Nils J. Nilsson, *Problem-Solving Methods in Artificial Intelligence* (New York: McGraw–Hill, 1971).

[19] Oskar Perron, "Zur Theorie der Matrices," *Mathematische Annalen* **64** (1907), 248–263.

[20] G. Pólya and G. Szegö, *Aufgaben und Lehrsätze aus der Analysis* **1** (Berlin: Springer, 1925).

[21] A. L. Samuel, "Some studies in machine learning using the game of checkers," *IBM Journal of Research and Development* **3** (1959), 210–229. Reprinted with minor additions and corrections in *Computers and Thought*, edited by E. A. Feigenbaum and J. Feldman (New York: McGraw–Hill, 1963), 71–105.

[22] A. L. Samuel, "Some studies in machine learning using the game of checkers. II — Recent progress," *IBM Journal of Research and Development* **11** (1967), 601–617.

[23] Claude E. Shannon, "Programming a computer for playing chess," *The Philosophical Magazine* (7) **51** (1950), 256–275. Reprinted in *Computer Chess Compendium*, edited by D. N. L. Levy (Springer, 1989), 2–13.

[24] James R. Slagle, *Artificial Intelligence: The Heuristic Programming Approach* (New York: McGraw–Hill, 1971).

[25] James R. Slagle and Philip Bursky, "Experiments with a multipurpose, theorem-proving heuristic program," *Journal of the Association for Computing Machinery* **15** (1968), 85–99.

[26] James R. Slagle and John K. Dixon, "Experiments with some programs that search game trees," *Journal of the Association for Computing Machinery* **16** (1969), 189–207.

[27] Richard S. Varga, *Matrix Iterative Analysis* (Englewood Cliffs, New Jersey: Prentice–Hall, 1962).

[28] Mark B. Wells, *Elements of Combinatorial Computing* (New York: Pergamon, 1971).

Addendum

Equation (42) implicitly establishes a nice characterization of the nodes visited by procedure *F1*, which can be made explicit as follows. Let us say that node q is *prior* to node p if q is either a left sibling of p or prior to p's parent. (No node is prior to the root.) Then p is pruned away by *F1* if and only if there are nodes q and r prior to p such that $F(q) + F(r) \leq 0$, with q and r on adjacent levels of the tree. Similarly, p is pruned away by *F2* if and only if there are nodes q and r prior to p such that $F(q) + F(r) \leq 0$, with an odd number of levels between q and r in the tree. (The latter condition is equivalent to Theorem 1 of [7].) If independent random values are assigned to terminal nodes of a game tree, the values of $F(q)$ for all nodes q prior to any given node p are independent.

Several years after the paper above was published, Judea Pearl established the exact value of the asymptotic branching factor $\rho(d) = \lim_{h \to \infty} \tau(d, h)^{1/h}$, where $\tau(d, h)$ is the expected number of terminal positions of a random uniform game tree of degree d and height h that are examined by procedure *F2*, including deep cutoffs ["The solution for the branching factor of the alpha-beta pruning algorithm and its optimality," *Communications of the ACM* **25** (1982), 559–564]. It is the unique positive value that satisfies $\rho^d = (\rho + 1)^{d-1}$. For example, $\rho(2) = \phi \approx 1.61803$; $\rho(3) \approx 2.1479$; $\rho(4) \approx 2.6297$; $\rho(10) \approx 5.0635$; $\rho(100) \approx 28.926$; $\rho(1000) \approx 189.91$; $\rho(10000) \approx 1382.21$; $\rho(100000) \approx 10770$. If x is the solution to $x \ln x = d$, we have $\rho(d) = x - (\ln x + 2)/(2 \ln x + 2) + O(1/x)$. Pearl's analysis was based on an ingenious way to study the probability distribution of the values $F(p)$ at the roots of such game trees; chapters 8 and 9 of his book *Heuristics* (Reading, Massachusetts: Addison–Wesley, 1984) connect this analysis to other methods of search and consider also trees that have nonuniform branching degrees. Curiously, his methods do not apply directly to the study of the growth factor $r(d)$ when deep cutoffs are not allowed. Thus we have a paradoxical situation in which the expected behavior of procedure *F2* on random data has been well analyzed, but the behavior of the supposedly simpler procedure *F1* remains an open question even when $d = 2$.

Another interesting case of alpha-beta searching arises when we consider a *randomized* version of procedure *F1* or *F2*, applying a random permutation to the successors of every branch node p. How many terminal nodes are visited, on the average, when such a procedure is applied to an arbitrary (but fixed) uniform game tree of degree d and height h? The worst case, with respect to procedure *F1*, arises in a tree like the one illustrated for the special case $d = 3$ and $h = 4$ in Figure 9: At most one successor of each branch node can lead to early termination of *F1*, and the other successors make the least possible improvements to the *bound*. (A similar tree with $1 + h(d - 1)$ distinct values can be constructed for the general case; when h is even, we put the middle value at the root, then introduce $d - 1$ new values on each new level.)

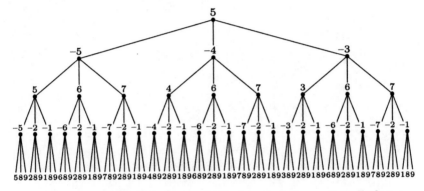

FIGURE 9. A tree for which the randomized version of procedure *F1* has the most difficulty finding cutoffs. (As in Figure 8, we imagine that all permutations of each branch are equally likely.)

When the randomized variant of *F1* is applied to such a tree, two kinds of nodes arise: Type A, where *bound* is never attained, and type B, where *bound* is exceeded by exactly one successor. Node p_k is of type A if and only if $-F(p_k)$ exceeds $\max\big(-F(p_1),\ldots,-F(p_{k-1})\big)$; node p_k is pruned if and only if node p is type B and $\max\big(-F(p_1),\ldots,-F(p_d)\big) = -F(p_j)$ for some $j < k$. It follows that the expected number of terminal nodes examined is A_d, where $A_0 = B_0 = 1$ and

$$A_{n+1} = H_d A_n + (d - H_d) B_n ; \tag{56}$$

$$B_{n+1} = H_d A_n + (\tfrac{1}{2}(d + 1) - H_d) B_n . \tag{57}$$

Thus $A_1 = d$ and $A_{n+1} = \frac{d+1}{2}A_n + \frac{d-1}{2}H_d A_{n-1}$; the asymptotic growth ratio is

$$\frac{1}{4}\left(d+1+\sqrt{(d+1)^2 + 8(d-1)H_d}\right) = \frac{1}{2}d + H_d + \frac{1}{2} + O\left(\frac{(\log d)^2}{d}\right). \tag{58}$$

[See Yanjun Zhang, "On the optimality of randomized α-β search," *SIAM Journal on Computing* **24** (1995), 138–147.]

When procedure *F2* is applied to a tree like that of Figure 9, eight kinds of nodes arise, and the recurrences analogous to (56) and (57) turn out to be

$$A_{n+1}^+ = dC_n^-, \tag{59}$$

$$A_{n+1} = dC_n, \tag{60}$$

$$B_{n+1}^{-+} = B_n^{-+} + (H_d - 1)B_n^- + (d - H_d)C_n^-, \tag{61}$$

$$B_{n+1}^- = B_n^+ + (H_d - 1)B_n + (d - H_d)C_n, \tag{62}$$

$$B_{n+1}^+ = B_n^- + (d - 1)C_n^-, \tag{63}$$

$$B_{n+1} = B_n + (d - 1)C_n, \tag{64}$$

$$C_{n+1}^- = A_n + B_n^+ + (H_d - 2)B_n + (\tfrac{1}{2}(d + 1) - H_d)C_n$$
$$+ \tfrac{1}{d}(B_n - B_n^+ + A_n^+ - A_n), \tag{65}$$

$$C_{n+1} = A_n + \tfrac{1}{2}(d - 1)C_n. \tag{66}$$

Here A, B, and C refer to cases where a node's final value will be respectively less than *alpha*, between *alpha* and *beta*, or greater than *beta*; superscripts indicate cases where $alpha = -\infty$ and/or $beta = +\infty$. The generating function $\sum_{n \geq 0} B_n^{-+} z^n$ turns out to be a rational function with denominator $(1 - z)(1 - dz^2)\left(1 - \frac{1}{2}(d - 1)z - dz^2\right)$; therefore the growth ratio is

$$\frac{1}{4}\left(d - 1 + \sqrt{(d - 1)^2 + 16d}\right) = \frac{1}{2}d + \frac{3}{2} + O\left(\frac{1}{d}\right). \tag{67}$$

However, there seems to be no obvious way to prove that trees like Figure 9 are necessarily the worst case for procedure *F2*, since a "greedy" approach to constructing a difficult game tree might not apply with respect to deep cutoffs. The true worst-case behavior of randomized alpha-beta pruning is therefore not yet known. Incidentally, Michael Saks and Avi Wigderson have proved that no randomized algorithm of any kind can achieve a branching factor less than (67) when searching a uniform game tree of degree d ["Probabilistic Boolean decision trees and the complexity of evaluating game trees," *IEEE Symposium on Foundations of Computer Science* **27** (1986), 29–38].

Don Beal and Martin C. Smith recently conducted an amusing experiment on random *nonuniform* game trees. They programmed a computer to play chess with 5 levels of lookahead, giving totally random values $f(p)$ to all nodes at depth 5. When this program was matched with another one that simply used random evaluations at depth 1 (unless checkmate was imminent), the level-5-lookahead version won 200 games out of 200! [See "Random evaluations in chess," *ICCA Journal* **17** (Maastricht, The Netherlands: International Computer Chess Association, 1994), 3–9.]

For more recent developments in the art of high-speed game tree evaluation, see Ernst A. Heinz, *Scalable Search in Computer Chess* (Wiesbaden: Vieweg Verlag, 2000).

Chapter 10

Notes on Generalized Dedekind Sums

[Originally published in Acta Arithmetica **33** *(1977), 297–325.]*

When Richard Dedekind prepared a commentary on one of Bernhard Riemann's fragmentary manuscripts, for publication in Riemann's collected works [5], he introduced a number-theoretic function that has recently arisen in several different contexts. Let

$$\delta(x) = \begin{cases} 1, & \text{if } x \text{ is an integer,} \\ 0, & \text{otherwise;} \end{cases} \tag{0.1}$$

$$((x)) = x - \lfloor x \rfloor - \tfrac{1}{2} + \tfrac{1}{2}\delta(x) = x - \lceil x \rceil + \tfrac{1}{2} - \tfrac{1}{2}\delta(x). \tag{0.2}$$

(Here $\lfloor x \rfloor$ denotes the greatest integer $\leq x$ and $\lceil x \rceil$ denotes the least integer $\geq x$.) Then Dedekind's sum was the special case $c = 0$ of the *generalized Dedekind sum*

$$\sigma(h, k, c) = 12 \sum_{j=0}^{k-1} \left(\left(\frac{j}{k}\right)\right)\left(\left(\frac{hj + c}{k}\right)\right), \tag{0.3}$$

defined for all positive integers h, k and all real values c.

Our primary purpose in this paper is to examine this sum closely, and in particular to show that $k\sigma(h, k, c)$ is always an integer that can be calculated by an efficient all-integer algorithm. In view of the applications of generalized Dedekind sums, we shall also be interested in estimating and/or computing the minimum and maximum values of $\sigma(h, k, c)$ when h and k are fixed and c varies.

A secondary purpose of this paper is to illustrate the fruitful interplay between computer science and mathematics. On the one hand, we shall see that symbolic formula manipulation by computer is an aid to the development of number theory. The quest for efficient means of calculation is also shown to lead to nontrivial results of a purely mathematical nature that would probably not have been discovered otherwise. Furthermore, the mathematical results derived here have immediate application to the problem of generating random numbers on a computer, as discussed in [8] and [11].

In recent years important new results about generalized Dedekind sums have been derived by U. Dieter and J. Ahrens [7], and this has substantially improved the analysis of random numbers generated by a linear congruential recurrence relation. In their forthcoming book [8], they make use of the even more generalized Dedekind sum

$$s(a, c \mid x, y) = \sum_{0 \le j < |c|} \left(\!\!\left(\frac{j+y}{c}\right)\!\!\right) \left(\!\!\left(\frac{a(j+y)}{c} + x\right)\!\!\right), \qquad (0.4)$$

where a, c are arbitrary integers and x, y are arbitrary reals. (See Rademacher and Grosswald [13] for a comprehensive survey of Dedekind sums and their generalizations.) It is not difficult to verify that

$$s(a, c \mid x, y) = s(a, -c \mid -x, y) = s(a, c \mid x - \lfloor x \rfloor, y - \lfloor y \rfloor) \qquad (0.5)$$

and that

$$s(a, c \mid x, y) = \frac{1}{12}\sigma(a, c, ay{+}cx) + \frac{yd}{c}\left(\!\!\left(\frac{ay{+}cx}{d}\right)\!\!\right) - \frac{1}{2}\left(\!\!\left(\frac{ay{+}cx}{c}\right)\!\!\right) \qquad (0.6)$$

when $c > 0$, $0 < y < 1$, and $d = \gcd(a, c)$; hence it suffices for our purposes to work with the simpler function $\sigma(h, k, c)$.

Equations (0.5) and (0.6) follow readily from the well-known identities

$$((-x)) = -((x)), \qquad (0.7)$$

$$((x + n)) = ((x)), \qquad \text{integer } n, \qquad (0.8)$$

$$\sum_{k=0}^{n-1} \left(\!\!\left(x + \frac{k}{n}\right)\!\!\right) = ((nx)), \qquad \text{integer } n > 0, \qquad (0.9)$$

which are used freely below without explicit mention.

1. Preliminary Transformations

For the most part we shall study $\sigma(h, k, c)$ only when h is relatively prime to k and when c is an integer. This limitation will be sufficient to establish the general behavior, because we have

Lemma 1. *Let h and k be relatively prime, and let $hh' \equiv 1$ (modulo k). Then the following identities hold for all real c:*

$$\sigma(dh, dk, dc) = \sigma(h, k, c), \qquad \text{integer } d > 0; \qquad (1.1)$$

$$\sigma(h, k, c) = \sigma(h, k, \lfloor c \rfloor) + 6((h' \lfloor c \rfloor / k)). \qquad (1.2)$$

Proof. For (1.1), we have

$$\sum_{j=0}^{dk-1} \left(\left(\frac{j}{dk}\right)\right) \left(\left(\frac{hj+c}{k}\right)\right) = \sum_{i=0}^{d-1} \sum_{j=0}^{k-1} \left(\left(\frac{ik+j}{dk}\right)\right) \left(\left(\frac{hj+c}{k}\right)\right)$$

$$= \sum_{j=0}^{k-1} \left(\left(\frac{j}{k}\right)\right) \left(\left(\frac{hj+c}{k}\right)\right).$$

For (1.2), let c be an integer and $0 < \theta < 1$. Then

$$\sum_{j=0}^{k-1} \left(\left(\frac{j}{k}\right)\right) \left(\left(\frac{hj+c+\theta}{k}\right)\right) = \sum_{j=0}^{k-1} \left(\left(\frac{j}{k}\right)\right) \left(\left(\left(\frac{hj+c}{k}\right)\right) + \frac{\theta}{k} - \frac{1}{2}\delta\left(\frac{hj+c}{k}\right)\right)$$

$$= \sum_{j=0}^{k-1} \left(\left(\frac{j}{k}\right)\right) \left(\left(\frac{hj+c}{k}\right)\right) + 0 + \frac{1}{2}\left(\left(\frac{h'c}{k}\right)\right).$$

Note that this result is independent of θ.   □

Four other simple transformations will be useful:

Lemma 2. *If $0 < h < k$ and n is any nonnegative integer,*

$$\sigma(nk + h, k, c) = \sigma(h, k, c); \qquad (1.3)$$

$$\sigma(k - h, k, c) = -\sigma(h, k, c); \qquad (1.4)$$

$$\sigma(h, k, c + nk) = \sigma(h, k, c); \qquad (1.5)$$

$$\sigma(h, k, -c) = \sigma(h, k, c). \qquad (1.6)$$

Proof. Equations (1.3) and (1.5) are obvious; equation (1.4) follows if j is replaced by $k - j$; and equation (1.6) follows from (1.4) since $\sigma(k - h, k, c)$ obviously equals $-\sigma(h, k, -c)$.   □

The key tool in algorithms for efficient evaluation of $\sigma(h, k, c)$ is the so-called *reciprocity law* for generalized Dedekind sums, first proved in general by U. Dieter [6].

Lemma 3. *Let h and k be relatively prime and let $0 \le c < k, 0 < h \le k$. Then*

$$\sigma(h, k, c) + \sigma(k, h, c) = f(h, k, c) \tag{1.7}$$

where

$$f(h, k, c) = \frac{h}{k} + \frac{k}{h} + \frac{1 + 6\lfloor c \rfloor \lceil c \rceil}{hk} - 6\left\lfloor \frac{c}{h} \right\rfloor - 3e(h, c); \tag{1.8}$$

$$e(h, c) = \begin{cases} 1, & \text{if } c = 0 \text{ or } c \not\equiv 0 \pmod{h}, \\ 0, & \text{if } c > 0 \text{ and } c \equiv 0 \pmod{h}. \end{cases} \tag{1.9}$$

Proof. We shall defer the proof for $c = 0$ until Section 5. Assume that c is an integer, $0 < c < k$, and let h', k' be integers satisfying

$$hh' + kk' = 1. \tag{1.10}$$

Since

$$\left(\!\!\left(\frac{hj+c+1}{k}\right)\!\!\right) = \left(\!\!\left(\frac{hj+c}{k}\right)\!\!\right) + \frac{1}{k} - \frac{1}{2}\delta\left(\frac{hj+c}{k}\right) - \frac{1}{2}\delta\left(\frac{hj+c+1}{k}\right), \tag{1.11}$$

an argument like the one we used in Lemma 1 to derive (1.2) proves that

$$\sigma(h, k, c+1) = \sigma(h, k, c) + 6\left(\!\!\left(\frac{h'c}{k}\right)\!\!\right) + 6\left(\!\!\left(\frac{h'(c+1)}{k}\right)\!\!\right). \tag{1.12}$$

It follows by induction on c that

$$\sigma(h, k, c) = \sigma(h, k, 0) + 12\sum_{j=1}^{c-1}\left(\!\!\left(\frac{h'j}{k}\right)\!\!\right) + 6\left(\!\!\left(\frac{h'c}{k}\right)\!\!\right). \tag{1.13}$$

We also have, for $0 < j < k$,

$$\left(\!\!\left(\frac{h'j}{k}\right)\!\!\right) = \left(\!\!\left(\frac{j}{hk} - \frac{k'j}{h}\right)\!\!\right) = -\left(\!\!\left(\frac{k'j}{h} - \frac{j}{hk}\right)\!\!\right)$$
$$= -\left(\!\!\left(\frac{k'j}{h}\right)\!\!\right) + \frac{j}{hk} - \frac{1}{2}\delta\left(\frac{k'j}{h}\right). \tag{1.14}$$

Hence, adding (1.13) to itself with h and k interchanged,

$$\sigma(h, k, c) + \sigma(k, h, c) = \sigma(h, k, 0) + \sigma(k, h, 0)$$
$$+ 12\sum_{j=1}^{c-1}\left(\frac{j}{hk} - \frac{1}{2}\delta\left(\frac{k'j}{h}\right)\right) + 6\frac{c}{hk} - 3\delta\left(\frac{k'c}{h}\right)$$
$$= \sigma(h, k, 0) + \sigma(k, h, 0) + 6\frac{c^2}{hk} - 6\left\lfloor\frac{c}{h}\right\rfloor + 3\delta\left(\frac{c}{h}\right)$$
$$= \sigma(h, k, 0) + \sigma(k, h, 0) + f(h, k, c) - f(h, k, 0).$$

When $0 < \theta < 1$, equations (1.2) and (1.14) imply that

$$\sigma(h, k, c + \theta) + \sigma(k, h, c + \theta) = \sigma(h, k, c) + \sigma(h, k, c) + \frac{6c}{hk} - 3\delta\left(\frac{c}{h}\right).$$

Therefore (1.8) has been established for arbitrary values of c.   □

2. A Euclidean Algorithm

The results reviewed in Section 1 lead immediately to an efficient scheme for evaluating $\sigma(h, k, c)$. Let h and k be relatively prime, with $0 < h < k$, and let c be an integer with $0 \le c < k$. By Lemmas 2 and 3,

$$\begin{aligned}
\sigma(h, k, c) &= f(h, k, c) - \sigma(k, h, c) \\
&= f(h, k, c) - \sigma(k \bmod h, h, c \bmod h);
\end{aligned} \tag{2.1}$$

hence the evaluation problem for (h, k) reduces to the same problem for $(k \bmod h, h)$. (We write "$x \bmod y$" for the remainder of x divided by y, namely $x - y\lfloor x/y \rfloor$.) The same recurrence underlies Euclid's algorithm for determining the greatest common divisor of h and k.

Certain simplifications will become apparent when we write the process out in detail. Let us set

$$\begin{aligned}
m_0 = k, \quad m_1 &= h, \quad c_0 = c, \\
a_j = \lfloor m_j/m_{j+1} \rfloor, \quad b_j &= \lfloor c_j/m_{j+1} \rfloor, \\
m_{j+2} = m_j \bmod m_{j+1}, \quad c_{j+1} &= c_j \bmod m_{j+1},
\end{aligned} \tag{2.2}$$

for $0 \le j < t$, where t is the least integer such that

$$m_{t+1} = 0. \tag{2.3}$$

For example, if $t = 4$ we have the tableau

$$\begin{aligned}
m_0 &= a_0 m_1 + m_2, & c_0 &= b_0 m_1 + c_1, \\
m_1 &= a_1 m_2 + m_3, & c_1 &= b_1 m_2 + c_2, \\
m_2 &= a_2 m_3 + m_4, & c_2 &= b_2 m_3 + c_3, \\
m_3 &= a_3 m_4, & c_3 &= b_3 m_4 + c_4.
\end{aligned}$$

Since h and k are relatively prime it follows that

$$m_t = 1, \qquad\qquad c_t = 0. \tag{2.4}$$

Furthermore the partial quotients $a_0, \ldots, a_{t-1}$ are positive integers, and (2.2) implies that

$$0 < m_{j+1} < m_j, \quad 0 \le c_j < m_j, \quad 0 \le b_j \le a_j, \quad \text{for} \quad 0 \le j < t. \quad (2.5)$$

Equation (2.1) says that

$$\sigma(m_{j+1}, m_j, c_j) = f(m_{j+1}, m_j, c_j) - \sigma(m_{j+2}, m_{j+1}, c_{j+1}), \quad 0 \le j < t,$$

and $\sigma(m_{t+1}, m_t, c_t) = \sigma(0, 1, 0) = 0$; hence by iterating this recurrence we have

$$\sigma(h, k, c) = \sum_{j=0}^{t-1} (-1)^j \left(\frac{m_{j+1}}{m_j} + \frac{m_j}{m_{j+1}} + \frac{1 + 6c_j^2}{m_j m_{j+1}} - 6b_j - 3e(m_{j+1}, c_j) \right).$$

$$(2.6)$$

This equation can be simplified in several ways. In the first place, $m_j/m_{j+1} = a_j + m_{j+2}/m_{j+1}$, so the first two terms in the summand reduce to a_j plus a telescoping series. In the second place, the term $e(m_{j+1}, c_j)$ is easy to deal with: If z is the least subscript such that $c_z = 0$, we have

$$\sum_{j=0}^{t-1} (-1)^j e(m_{j+1}, c_j) = (t \bmod 2) + (-1)^z - \delta_{z0}. \quad (2.7)$$

In the third place, it is well known from the theory of continued fractions that the sum $\sum_{j=0}^{t-1} (-1)^j / m_j m_{j+1}$ is a fraction whose denominator is $m_0 = k$. Therefore equation (1.11) implies by induction on c that $k\sigma(h, k, c)$ is an integer. In other words, the sum

$$\sum_{j=0}^{t-1} (-1)^j \frac{c_j^2}{m_j m_{j+1}}, \quad (2.8)$$

which is a certain rational function in the indeterminates $a_0, \ldots, a_{t-1}$, $b_0, \ldots, b_{t-1}$, always evaluates to a rational number, and the denominator of this rational number is a divisor of m_0.

From these considerations we can be pretty sure that the rational function (2.8) can be simplified in general, and the author therefore used the MACSYMA symbol manipulation system [12] for $t = 5$ to guess the general form to which (2.8) simplifies. (MACSYMA is a large collection of computer programs, written to perform symbolic mathematical calculations as well as numerical operations on numbers of arbitrary precision. In particular, MACSYMA is able to simplify rational functions in any number of indeterminates. The total elapsed time between the moment that the author thought of simplifying (2.8) and the time when his computer terminal typed out the simplified numerator and denominator was less than ten minutes; this can be considered an excellent demonstration of the use of symbolic mathematical systems in the discovery of new mathematics. In principle, of course, Euler would have been able to discover the same identity in the 18th century, if he had set himself the problem; but such a task would almost certainly have taken him much longer, and perhaps the lengthy formula manipulation would have been quite frustrating.) The resulting formula is stated in the following lemma.

Lemma 4. *Let*

$$p_0 = 1, \quad p_1 = a_0, \quad \text{and} \quad p_j = a_{j-1}p_{j-1} + p_{j-2} \quad \text{for } 2 \le j \le t. \quad (2.9)$$

Then the definitions (2.2) imply that

$$\sum_{j=0}^{t-1} (-1)^j \frac{c_j^2}{m_j m_{j+1}} = \frac{1}{m_0} \sum_{j=0}^{t-1} (-1)^j b_j (c_j + c_{j+1}) p_j. \quad (2.10)$$

Proof. Littlewood [4, page 34] has said that any identity, once written down, is trivial; however, we would like to understand what lies behind equation (2.10), so we don't simply wish to prove it by induction.

According to a well-known identity of Euler, rediscovered by Sylvester and easily proved by induction on j, we have

$$m_0 = p_j m_j + p_{j-1} m_{j+1} \quad \text{for} \quad 0 < j < t. \quad (2.11)$$

As an alternative to induction, *this* identity can be "understood" by using Euler's characterization of the continuant polynomials p_j (see, for example, exercise 4.5.3–32 of [11]). Equation (2.11) leads immediately to the formula

$$\sum_{j=0}^{r-1} \frac{(-1)^j}{m_j m_{j+1}} = (-1)^r \frac{p_r}{m_0 m_{r+1}}. \quad (2.12)$$

Now by an appropriate interchange of summation,

$$m_0 \sum_{j=0}^{t-1} \frac{(-1)^j}{m_j m_{j+1}} \left(\sum_{j \le r < t} b_r m_{r+1} \right)^2$$

$$= m_0 \sum_{r=0}^{t-1} \sum_{s=0}^{t-1} b_r b_s m_{r+1} m_{s+1} \sum_{j=0}^{\min(r,s)} \frac{(-1)^j}{m_j m_{j+1}}$$

$$= \sum_{r=0}^{t-1} \sum_{s=0}^{t-1} b_r b_s m_{r+1} m_{s+1} (-1)^{\min(r,s)} \frac{p_{\min(r,s)}}{m_{\min(r,s)+1}}$$

$$= \sum_{0 \le r \le s < t} b_r b_s (-1)^r p_r m_{s+1} + \sum_{0 \le r < s < t} b_r b_s (-1)^s p_s m_{r+1}$$

$$= \sum_{r=0}^{t-1} (-1)^r b_r p_r c_r + \sum_{s=0}^{t-1} (-1)^s b_s p_s c_{s+1}. \quad \square$$

Using the proof technique of Lemma 4 it is possible to derive the considerably more general identity

$$\sum_{j=0}^{t-1} (-1)^j \frac{f(c_j)}{m_j m_{j+1}} = \sum_{j=0}^{t-1} (-1)^j b_j \left(\frac{f(c_j) - f(c_{j+1}) + f(0)\delta_{j(t-1)}}{c_j - c_{j+1}} \right) p_j$$

(2.13)

where f is any polynomial (and hence, any function analytic at zero); this is an observation one does not expect MACSYMA to make. One of the advantages of computer-aided mathematics is that it spurs us on, as we strive to maintain our superiority over the machine.

Combining Lemma 4 with equation (2.6), and setting $r = t - 1$ in (2.12), yields

$$\sigma(h, k, c) = \frac{1}{k} \left(h - (-1)^t p_{t-1} + 6 \sum_{j=0}^{t-1} (-1)^j b_j (c_j + c_{j+1}) p_j \right)$$

$$+ \sum_{j=0}^{t-1} (-1)^j \left(a_j - 6b_j - 3e(m_{j+1}, c_j) \right). \quad (2.14)$$

Therefore the following algorithm is suggested:

Algorithm 1. Let h and k be relatively prime, $0 < h < k$, and let c be an integer with $0 \le c < k$. This algorithm will output the value of $\sigma(h, k, c)$. (For brevity and precision, it has been stated in ALGOL notation, which is explained below for readers not familiar with computer programming languages.)

```
0.   procedure sigma(integer value h, k, c);
1.      begin integer a, b, p, pp, r, s, sigma1, sigma2;
2.          sigma1 := 0;  sigma2 := h;
3.          p := 1;  pp := 0;  s := 1;
4.          while h > 0 do
5.              begin comment At this point we have
6.                      k = m_j,  h = m_{j+1},  c = c_j,  p = p_j,
7.                      pp = p_{j-1}, and s = (-1)^j for some j < t;
8.                  a := ⌊k/h⌋;  b := ⌊c/h⌋;  r := c mod h;
9.                  comment Now a = a_j,  b = b_j,  r = c_{j+1};
10.                 if r = 0 and c ≠ 0 then sigma1 := sigma1 + 3 × s;
11.                 if h = 1 then sigma2 := sigma2 + p × s;
12.                 sigma1 := sigma1 + (a - 6 × b) × s;
13.                 sigma2 := sigma2 + 6 × b × p × (c + r) × s;
14.                 c := r;  s := -s;
15.                 r := k mod h;  k := h;  h := r;
16.                 r := a × p + pp;  pp := p;  p := r;
17.              end;
18.          comment Now s = (-1)^t and p is the original value of k;
19.          if s < 0 then sigma1 := sigma1 - 3;
20.          output(sigma1 + sigma2/p);
21.      end.
```

(Algorithms in ALGOL notation are expressed as a sequence of instructions separated by semicolons. A sequence of instructions surrounded by **begin** and **end** acts as a single instruction, just as parentheses are used to group algebraic expressions; the instructions are performed one by one in the stated sequence. Line 0 of the program states that the following instructions constitute a procedure for evaluating $\sigma(h, k, c)$, given the integer values h, k, and c; line 1 means that the symbols a, b, p, pp, r, s, $sigma1$, and $sigma2$ are used as auxiliary integer-valued variables in the program. If v is a variable and E is an expression, the instruction '$v := E$' means that the value of v is replaced by the present value of E. Thus, '$sigma2 := h$' in line 2 means that variable $sigma2$ should be set to the (initially given) value of h, and '$s := -s$' in line 14 means that the value of the variable s should be negated when we reach that point of the program. The instruction '**if** R **then** I', where R is a relation and I is an instruction, means "if R

is presently true, do instruction I, otherwise do nothing." The instruction 'while R do I', where R is a relation and I is an instruction, is equivalent to 'if R then begin I; while R do I end'; in other words, the instruction I is performed zero or more times until R becomes false. Thus lines 5–17 are performed repeatedly until h is not positive. Relationships stated between 'comment' and the following semicolon are not part of the program, but they may be used to prove the correctness of the program; we assert that the stated relationships between the current values of the variables will hold whenever this point in the program is reached. The idea of the program is to set *sigma1* equal to the second sum in (2.14) and to set *sigma2* equal to the coefficient of $1/k$; comments appearing within the program provide the basis for a rigorous proof of this fact.)

Lines 10 and 19 of Algorithm 1 have the effect of subtracting 3 times (2.7) from *sigma1*. A simpler alternative would be to delete line 19 and to use the definition of $e(m_{j+1}, c_j)$ directly in line 10:

$$\text{if } r \neq 0 \text{ or } c = 0 \text{ then } \textit{sigma1} := \textit{sigma1} - 3 \times s;$$

this change requires only slightly more computation and makes the algorithm slightly easier to prove. Therefore the original sequence of instructions would be frowned upon by contemporary aesthetes of programming style. The author apologizes for his bias towards using mathematics to avoid computation.

To evaluate $\sigma(h, k, c + \theta)$ for $0 < \theta < 1$, it suffices to replace '$c + r$' by '$c + r + 1$' in line 13, and to delete line 10.

The algorithm works entirely with integers, although the integers can become large when k is large. If necessary, multiples of k can be subtracted from *sigma2* and the quotient added to *sigma1*. We have

$$b_j p_j (c_j + c_{j+1}) < a_j p_j (m_j + m_{j+1})$$
$$= a_j m_0 + m_{j+1}(a_j p_j - p_{j-1}) < (a_j + 1) m_0$$

by (2.11). Therefore the size of numbers in line 13 is reasonably well controlled.   □

3. Extreme Values of Dedekind Sums

Let h and k be relatively prime, $0 < h < k$. We shall now develop an algorithm to calculate an integer c that maximizes $\sigma(h, k, c)$, for fixed h and k. Such an algorithm can also be used to find the c that minimizes $\sigma(h, k, c)$, since c minimizes $\sigma(h, k, c)$ if and only if it maximizes $\sigma(k - h, k, c)$, by (1.4).

The alternating character of our formulas in Section 2, namely the presence of the factor $(-1)^j$, makes it very difficult to see how to maximize $\sigma(h, k, c)$; indeed, the form of the answer we shall obtain shows that the correct value of c would be very difficult to discover by working directly with the Euclidean construction of Section 2. For our present purposes it is much more convenient to work with a "subtractive" process, using $\lceil x \rceil$ in place of $\lfloor x \rfloor$ in the previous formulas.

Let us set

$$M_0 = k, \quad M_1 = h, \quad C_0 = c,$$
$$A_j = \lceil M_j/M_{j+1} \rceil, \quad B_j = \lceil C_j/M_{j+1} \rceil, \tag{3.1}$$
$$M_{j+2} = (-M_j) \bmod M_{j+1}, \quad C_{j+1} = (-C_j) \bmod M_{j+1},$$

for $0 \le j < T$, where T is the least integer such that

$$M_{T+1} = 0. \tag{3.2}$$

(Compare with (2.2) and (2.3).) For example, if $T = 4$ we have the tableau

$$\begin{aligned}
M_0 &= A_0 M_1 - M_2, & C_0 &= B_0 M_1 - C_1, \\
M_1 &= A_1 M_2 - M_3, & C_1 &= B_1 M_2 - C_2, \\
M_2 &= A_2 M_3 - M_4, & C_2 &= B_2 M_3 - C_3, \\
M_3 &= A_3 M_4, & C_3 &= B_3 M_4 - C_4.
\end{aligned}$$

As in the additive process we have

$$M_T = 1, \qquad\qquad C_T = 0. \tag{3.3}$$

The analog of (2.5) is

$$0 < M_{j+1} < M_j, \quad 0 \le C_j < M_j, \quad 0 \le B_j \le A_j, \quad \text{for } 0 \le j < T, \tag{3.4}$$

and we also have $A_0, \ldots, A_{T-1} \ge 2$. The important advantage of the subtractive process is that we now have an additive recurrence,

$$\begin{aligned}
\sigma(M_{j+1}, M_j, C_j) &= f(M_{j+1}, M_j, C_j) - \sigma(M_j, M_{j+1}, C_j) \\
&= f(M_{j+1}, M_j, C_j) + \sigma(M_{j+2}, M_{j+1}, C_{j+1}), \quad 0 \le j < T,
\end{aligned}$$

by equations (1.3), (1.4), and (1.6); hence the $(-1)^j$ factor does not appear in

$$\sigma(h, k, c) = \sum_{j=0}^{T-1} \left(\frac{M_{j+1}}{M_j} + \frac{M_j}{M_{j+1}} + \frac{1 + 6C_j^2}{M_j M_{j+1}} - 6B_j + 3E(M_{j+1}, C_j) \right), \tag{3.5}$$

where

$$E(M,C) = \begin{cases} -1, & \text{if } C = 0; \\ 0, & \text{if } C \neq 0 \text{ and } C \bmod M = 0; \\ +1, & \text{if } C \bmod M \neq 0. \end{cases} \quad (3.6)$$

Our interest in (3.5) rests solely in the terms that depend on c; we obtain the maximum of $\sigma(h,k,c)$ if and only if we maximize

$$\sum_{j=0}^{T-1} \left(\frac{C_j^2}{M_j M_{j+1}} - B_j + \frac{1}{2} E(M_{j+1}, C_j) \right) \quad (3.7)$$

over all the appropriate choices of B_0, B_1, ..., B_{T-1}.

Theorem 1. *Let h and k be relatively prime integers, with $0 < h < k$. The maximum value of $\sigma(h,k,c)$, over all integers c in the range $0 < c < k$, occurs when $B_j = 1$ for $0 \leq j < T$ in the subtractive process (3.1), (3.2).*

Proof. Let

$$P_0 = 1, \quad P_1 = A_0, \quad P_j = A_{j-1} P_{j-1} - P_{j-2} \quad (3.8)$$

be the subtractive analog of (2.9). Then it is easy to verify that the analogs of (2.11) and (2.12) are

$$M_0 = P_j M_j - P_{j-1} M_{j+1}, \quad 0 < j \leq T; \quad (3.9)$$

$$\sum_{j=0}^{r} \frac{1}{M_j M_{j+1}} = \frac{P_r}{M_0 M_{r+1}}. \quad (3.10)$$

Since each $A_j \geq 2$, we have $P_j \geq 2P_{j-1} - P_{j-2}$; in other words, the P's are convex,

$$P_j - P_{j-1} \geq P_{j-1} - P_{j-2}. \quad (3.11)$$

It follows that

$$P_j \geq 2P_{j-1} - 2P_{j-2} + 2P_{j-3} - \cdots, \quad (3.12)$$

where we may assume that $P_{-1} = P_{-2} = \cdots = 0$. Equality holds in (3.12) if and only if j is odd and $A_{j-1} = A_{j-3} = \cdots = 2$. A similar inequality applies to the M's, namely

$$M_j \geq 2M_{j+1} - 2M_{j+2} + 2M_{j+3} - \cdots. \quad (3.13)$$

Now let c be a value that maximizes $\sigma(h, k, c)$. We may assume that $c \le \frac{1}{2}k$, by (1.6); and under this assumption we shall prove that $B_0 = B_1 = \cdots = B_{T-1} = 1$ yields the maximum.

For convenience in notation, suppose we have proved that $B_0 = B_1 = B_2 = 1$ and we wish to show that $B_3 = 1$; essentially the same argument will work for all B_j. If $C_3 \ne 0$, the first three terms of (3.7) are

$$\varphi(C_3) = \frac{(M_1-M_2+M_3-C_3)^2}{M_0 M_1} + \frac{(M_2-M_3+C_3)^2}{M_1 M_2} + \frac{(M_3-C_3)^2}{M_2 M_3} - \frac{3}{2}$$

$$= \frac{C_3^2 P_2}{M_0 M_3} - 2C_3 \left(\frac{M_1 - M_2 + M_3}{M_0 M_1} + \frac{-M_2 + M_3}{M_1 M_2} + \frac{M_3}{M_2 M_3} \right) + W$$

$$= \frac{1}{M_0} \left(\frac{C_3^2 P_2}{M_3} - 2C_3(P_2 - P_1 + P_0) \right) + W, \tag{3.14}$$

where W is independent of C_3. Since $P_2/(M_3 M_0) > 0$, the minimum of this quadratic $\varphi(C_3)$ occurs when the derivative is zero, namely when

$$C_3/M_3 = (P_2 - P_1 + P_0)/P_2;$$

and we have $(P_2 - P_1 + P_0)/P_2 \ge 1/2$, by (3.12).

We may now conclude that $C_3 \ge \frac{1}{2}M_3$, by using the following argument. Suppose $C_3 > \frac{1}{2}M_3$, and let c' be the value defined by

$$c' = C_0' = M_1 - C_1', \quad C_1' = M_2 - C_2', \quad C_2' = M_3 - C_3', \quad C_3' = M_3 - C_3.$$

Since the minimum of $\varphi(C_3)$ occurs at a point $\ge \frac{1}{2}M_3$, we must have $\varphi(C_3') \ge \varphi(C_3)$. Furthermore $\sigma(M_4, M_3, C_3) = \sigma(M_4, M_3, M_3 - C_3)$ by (1.6), so we have $\sigma(h, k, c') \ge \sigma(h, k, c)$. The optimality of c implies that $\sigma(h, k, c') = \sigma(h, k, c)$; hence $\varphi(C_3') = \varphi(C_3)$; hence $(P_0 - P_1 + P_2)/P_2 = 1/2$. But that is impossible.

A slightly different argument is used to show that $C_4 \le \frac{1}{2}M_4$, since we might have $(P_3-P_2+P_1-P_0)/P_3 = 1/2$ when $A_2 = A_0 = 2$. However, the relations $C_4 > \frac{1}{2}M_4$ and $A_2 = 2$ imply that $C_2 > M_3 - M_4 + \frac{1}{2}M_4 = \frac{1}{2}M_2$, a contradiction.

The fourth term of (3.7) is

$$\psi(B_3) = \frac{(B_3 M_4 - C_4)^2}{M_3 M_4} - B_3 + \frac{1}{2}E(M_4, C_3),$$

and this quadratic $\psi(B_3)$ has its minimum when

$$\frac{2(B_3 M_4 - C_4)}{M_3} - 1 = 0,$$

namely when $C_3 = \frac{1}{2}M_3$. Therefore if $B_3 > 1$, decreasing B_3 (while holding C_4 fixed) causes both $\psi(B_3)$ and $\varphi(C_3)$ to increase. It follows that $B_3 = 1$ when $C_3 \neq 0$.

All of our arguments so far have been made under the assumption that the C_j were nonzero. We have proved that there is a subscript $z \geq 1$ such that $B_j = 1$ for $0 \leq j < z$, and $B_j = 0$ for $z \leq j < T$. It remains to choose the best value of z. Formula (3.7) reduces to

$$\sum_{j=0}^{z-1} \frac{\left(\sum_{r=j+1}^{z}(-1)^r M_r\right)^2}{M_j M_{j+1}} - \frac{T+1}{2}. \tag{3.15}$$

For example, the value of (3.7) when $z = 4$ is

$$\frac{(M_1 - M_2 + M_3 - M_4)^2}{M_0 M_1} + \frac{(M_2 - M_3 + M_4)^2}{M_1 M_2} + \frac{(M_3 - M_4)^2}{M_2 M_3}$$
$$+ \frac{M_4^2}{M_3 M_4} - \frac{T+1}{2}.$$

Let

$$\varphi_4(X) = \frac{(M_1 - M_2 + M_3 - X)^2}{M_0 M_1} + \frac{(M_2 - M_3 + X)^2}{M_1 M_2} + \frac{(M_3 - X)^2}{M_2 M_3} + \frac{X^2}{M_3 M_4}.$$

Then

$$\varphi_4(M_4) - \varphi_3(M_3) = \varphi_4(M_4) - \varphi_4(0)$$
$$= \frac{1}{M_0}\left(M_4^2 \frac{P_3}{M_4} - 2M_4(P_2 - P_1 + P_0)\right)$$
$$= \frac{M_4}{M_0}(P_3 - 2P_2 + 2P_1 - 2P_0) \geq 0.$$

Similar arguments apply for all z. Hence

$$\varphi_1(M_1) \leq \varphi_2(M_2) \leq \cdots \leq \varphi_T(M_T). \quad \square$$

Theorem 1 only claims to find the maximum over the restricted range $0 < c < k$; it is possible that an even larger value will occur when $c = 0$. In fact, this happens if and only if

$$\varphi_T(M_T) < \tfrac{1}{2} \tag{3.16}$$

in the notation of the proof. If $A_j = 2$ for any j, we have

$$\varphi_T(M_T) \geq \varphi_j(M_j) \geq M_j^2/(M_{j-1}M_j) = M_j/(2M_j - M_{j+1}) \geq \tfrac{1}{2},$$

so $\sigma(h,k,0)$ will not be maximum. But on the other hand if $A_j = x$ for all j, we have $\varphi_T(M_T) \sim T/x$ as $x \to \infty$, hence the maximum will occur at $c = 0$ for sufficiently large x.

The proof of Theorem 1 demonstrates that there is exactly one integer value of $0 < c \leq \tfrac{1}{2}k$ where the maximum occurs. (For if $\varphi_T(M_T) = \varphi_{T-1}(M_{T-1})$, we have T even and $A_{T-2} = A_{T-4} = \cdots = A_0 = 2$. But then $B_{T-1} = 0$ implies that $C_{T-2} = M_{T-1} > \tfrac{1}{2}M_{T-2}$.)

It is possible to generalize the proof of Theorem 1 in order to find the maximum of $\sigma(h,k,c)$ over all real c; it turns out that the maximum, over all real c including $c = 0$, occurs when

$$c = M_1 - M_2 + \cdots + (-1)^T M_{T-1} + \frac{1}{2}(-1)^{T+1}. \qquad (3.17)$$

Let us now connect up the additive and subtractive processes. In order to simplify the formulas that occur, we shall assume that t is always even in the additive Euclidean algorithm. (If t is odd,

replace	by	
$m_{t-1} = a_{t-1}m_t$	$m_{t-1} = (a_{t-1} - 1)m_t + m_{t+1}$	
$m_t = 1$	$m_t = (1)m_{t+1}$	(3.18)
$m_{t+1} = 0$	$m_{t+1} = 1$	
	$m_{t+2} = 0$	

and increase t by 1.) This yields an even number of partial quotients $a_0, a_1, \ldots, a_{t-1}$, which we shall call the *canonical sequence* for (h,k). The formulas that we have derived for the evaluation of $\sigma(h,k,c)$ still hold for the canonical sequence, since Lemma 3 includes the case $h = k = 1$.

The subtractive quotients $A_0, \ldots, A_{T-1}$ can be expressed readily in terms of the canonical sequence, as

$$a_0 + 1, (a_1 - 1) \times 2, a_2 + 2, (a_3 - 1) \times 2, \ldots, a_{t-2} + 2, (a_{t-1} - 1) \times 2, \quad (3.19)$$

where $(a_j - 1) \times 2$ stands for a sequence of $a_j - 1$ elements each equal to 2. Thus in particular

$$T = \sum_{j=0}^{t/2-1} a_{2j+1}. \qquad (3.20)$$

For example, if $h = 3141592621$ and $k = 2^{35} = 34359738368$, the additive partial quotients are

$$10, 1, 14, 1, 7, 1, 1, 1, 3, 3, 3, 5, 2, 1, 8, 7, 1, 4, 1, 2, 4, 2,$$

and the subtractive ones are

$$11, 16, 9, 3, 5, 2, 2, 5, 2, 2, 2, 2, 4, 10, 2, 2, 2, 2, 2, 2, 3, 2, 2, 2, 3, 2, 6, 2.$$

The canonical sequence for the pair of numbers whose subtractive quotients are $A_0, A_1, \ldots, A_{T-1}$, when all $A_j \geq 3$, is

$$A_0 - 1, 1, A_1 - 2, 1, \ldots, A_{T-1} - 2, 1.$$

If $h = k - 1$ the additive quotients are 1, $k - 1$ and the subtractive ones are $(k-1) \times 2$. Thus the subtractive process can be exponentially slower than the additive one, although it can also be twice as fast in favorable cases.

The subtractive convergents $M_0, M_1, \ldots, M_T$ are easily expressed as

$$m_0, \ \langle jm_2 + m_3 \rangle_{a_1}^1, \ \langle jm_4 + m_5 \rangle_{a_3}^1, \ldots, \ \langle jm_t + m_{t+1} \rangle_{a_{t-1}}^1, \qquad (3.21)$$

where $\langle f(j) \rangle_a^1$ stands for $f(a), f(a-1), \ldots, f(1)$.

It is now possible to express the number c of Theorem 1 in terms of the canonical partial quotients, so that we obtain an efficient algorithm for the evaluation of c. The first $a = a_1$ steps of the subtractive process give

$$\begin{aligned}
C_0 &= M_1 - C_1, &\text{that is,}& &C_0 &= am_2 + m_3 - C_1, \\
C_1 &= M_2 - C_2, & & &C_1 &= (a-1)m_2 + m_3 - C_2, \\
&\ \vdots & & & &\ \vdots \\
C_{a-1} &= M_a - C_a, & & &C_{a-1} &= m_2 + m_3 - C_a,
\end{aligned}$$

and it follows that

$$C_0 = \begin{cases} (a/2)m_2 + C_a, & a \text{ even}; \\ ((a+1)/2)m_2 + m_3 - C_a, & a \text{ odd}. \end{cases} \qquad (3.22)$$

Similarly, if $b = a_3$ we have

$$C_a = \begin{cases} (b/2)m_4 + C_{a+b}, & b \text{ even}; \\ ((b+1)/2)m_4 + m_5 - C_{a+b}, & b \text{ odd}. \end{cases}$$

And so on.

Notice that

$$C_0 - \tfrac{1}{2}m_1 = C_0 - \tfrac{1}{2}am_2 - \tfrac{1}{2}m_3 = \begin{cases} C_a - \tfrac{1}{2}m_3, & a \text{ even;} \\ \tfrac{1}{2}m_2 - (C_a - \tfrac{1}{2}m_3), & a \text{ odd.} \end{cases}$$

Hence we have the following rather curious rule for evaluating the number c of Theorem 1: Look at the odd numbered elements $a_1, a_3, \ldots, a_{t-1}$ of the canonical sequence for (h, k) and strike out all the *even* quotients in this list. If the remaining partial quotients are $a_{2j(0)+1}, a_{2j(1)+1}, \cdots,$ $a_{2j(u-1)+1}$ for $0 \le j(0) < \cdots < j(u-1) < t/2$ and $u \ge 0$, the value of c is

$$\tfrac{1}{2}\left(m_1 + m_{2j(0)+2} - m_{2j(1)+2} + \cdots + (-1)^{u-1}m_{2j(u-1)+2}\right). \qquad (3.23)$$

The following algorithm evaluates this formula.

Algorithm 2. Let h and k be relatively prime, $0 < h < k$. This algorithm will output the unique integer value of $c \le \tfrac{1}{2}k$ that maximizes $\sigma(h, k, c)$ for $0 < c < k$.

```
0.    procedure maxc(integer value h, k);
1.        begin integer a, r, s, sigma;
2.            s := 1;  sigma := h;
3.        while h > 0 do
4.            begin comment At this point we have k = m_2j
5.                and h = m_{2j+1} for some 0 ≤ j < ⌊t/2⌋, and s is
6.                the sign of the next term to be added in (3.23);
7.                r := k mod h;  k := h;  h := r;
8.                if h = 0 then
9.                    begin comment t = 2j + 1, convert to 2j + 2;
10.                        sigma := sigma + s;
11.                    end
12.                else begin a := ⌊k/h⌋;  comment a = a_{2j+1};
13.                        if a mod 2 = 1 then
14.                            begin sigma := sigma + s × h;  s := -s;
15.                            end;
16.                        r := k mod h;  k := h;  h := r;
17.                    end;
18.            end;
19.        output(sigma/2);
20.    end.
```

We have $0 < sigma \le k$ throughout the algorithm.   □

4. Estimates for Dedekind Sums

Our goal in this section is to obtain tight bounds on $|\sigma(h, k, c)|$ in terms of the canonical sequence of partial quotients $a_1, a_2, \ldots, a_{t-1}$ for (h, k), where t is even (see (3.18)). Throughout this section h and k are relatively prime, $0 < h < k$, and c is an integer.

We have proved in (2.14) that

$$\sigma(h, k, 0) = \frac{h - p_{t-1}}{k} + \sum_{j=0}^{t-1} (-1)^j a_j. \tag{4.1}$$

It is well known from the theory of continued fractions that

$$p_{t-1} h \equiv -1 \pmod{k}. \tag{4.2}$$

(See, for example, equation 4.5.3–(8) of [11].) Hence if h' is the inverse of h modulo k, so that

$$hh' \equiv 1 \pmod{k} \quad \text{and} \quad 0 < h' < k, \tag{4.3}$$

we have $p_{t-1} = k - h'$, and (4.1) takes the more symmetrical form

$$\sigma(h, k, 0) = \frac{h + h'}{k} - 1 + \sum_{j=0}^{t-1} (-1)^j a_j. \tag{4.4}$$

(Note that since $k = p_t = a_{t-1} p_{t-1} + p_{t-2}$, we have $h' \leq \frac{1}{2} k$ if and only if $a_{t-1} = 1$ in the canonical sequence.)

In order to estimate $\sigma(h, k, c)$ for $c \neq 0$ we shall first determine the sequences $b_1, b_2, \ldots, b_{t-1}$ and $c_1, c_2, \ldots, c_{t-1}$ defined in connection with Algorithm 1, for the special value c of Theorem 1 and equation (3.23). It is not difficult to prove that

$$b_{2j} = 0, \qquad c_{2j} = c_{2j+1}; \tag{4.5}$$

$$b_{2j+1} = \frac{1}{2} a_{2j+1}, \quad \text{if} \quad a_{2j+1} \text{ is even}; \tag{4.6}$$

$$b_{2j(r)+1} = \frac{1}{2} \left(a_{2j(r)+1} + (-1)^r \right), \quad \text{for} \quad 0 \leq r < u; \tag{4.7}$$

$$c_{2j+1} = \frac{1}{2} \left(m_{2j+1} + \sum_{\substack{0 \leq r < u \\ j(r) \geq j}} (-1)^r m_{2j(r)+2} \right); \tag{4.8}$$

for these values satisfy $c_j = b_j m_{j+1} + c_{j+1}$, $0 \le c_{j+1} < m_{j+1}$, *with one exception*. The exception occurs when $a_{t-1} = 1$ and u is odd; for then $2j(u-1) + 1 = t - 1$, and $c_{t-2} = \frac{1}{2}(m_{t-1} + m_t) = 1$, and b_{t-2} should be 1, and c_{t-1} should be 0. We shall use equations (4.5)–(4.8) even in this exceptional case, and take care of the exception later.

The proof we shall discuss can be expressed very compactly in terms of $\sum$ notation, etc., but such a derivation would be quite hard to understand without some indication of how it could have been discovered. Indeed, equations (4.5)–(4.8) are not very easy to conceptualize until an example has been written down. Therefore, it will be helpful to consider an example in which $t = 10$; a_1, a_5, and a_9 are odd; a_3 and a_7 are even. We have the following tableau:

$$m_0 = a_0 m_1 + m_2, \qquad m_1 = a_1 m_2 + m_3,$$
$$c_0 = c_1 = \tfrac{1}{2}(a_1 + 1)m_2 + c_2 = \tfrac{1}{2}(m_1 + m_2 - m_6 + m_{10});$$
$$m_2 = a_2 m_3 + m_4, \qquad m_3 = a_3 m_4 + m_5,$$
$$c_2 = c_3 = \tfrac{1}{2}a_3 m_4 + c_4 = \tfrac{1}{2}(m_3 - m_6 + m_{10});$$
$$m_4 = a_4 m_5 + m_6, \qquad m_5 = a_5 m_6 + m_7,$$
$$c_4 = c_5 = \tfrac{1}{2}(a_5 - 1)m_6 + c_6 = \tfrac{1}{2}(m_5 - m_6 + m_{10});$$
$$m_6 = a_6 m_7 + m_8, \qquad m_7 = a_7 m_8 + m_9,$$
$$c_6 = c_7 = \tfrac{1}{2}a_7 m_8 + c_8 = \tfrac{1}{2}(m_7 + m_{10});$$
$$m_8 = a_8 m_9 + m_{10}, \qquad m_9 = a_9 m_{10} + m_{11},$$
$$c_8 = c_9 = \tfrac{1}{2}(a_9 + 1)m_{10} + c_{10} = \tfrac{1}{2}(m_9 + m_{10});$$
$$m_{10} = 1, \qquad m_{11} = 0, \qquad c_{10} = 0.$$

According to (2.14) the major unknown term in the evaluation of $\sigma(h, k, c)$ is

$$\sum_{j=0}^{t-1} (-1)^j b_j (c_j + c_{j+1}) p_j,$$

and since $b_{2j} = 0$ we can express $-4 \sum (-1)^j b_j (c_j + c_{j+1}) p_j$ as follows:

$$
\begin{aligned}
& (a_1 + 1)p_1(m_1 + m_2 + m_3 - 2m_6 + 2m_{10}) \\
+ \; & a_3 p_3(m_3 + m_5 - 2m_6 + 2m_{10}) \\
+ \; & (a_5 - 1)p_5(m_5 - m_6 + m_7 + 2m_{10}) \\
+ \; & a_7 p_7(m_7 + m_9 + 2m_{10}) \\
+ \; & (a_9 + 1)p_9(m_9 + m_{10})
\end{aligned}
$$

We can rearrange these terms into $S+T$, where S is the portion that will be present whenever $t = 10$, regardless of the evenness or oddness of a_1, a_3, ..., a_9, namely

$$S = a_1 p_1(m_1 + m_3) + a_3 p_3(m_3 + m_5) + \cdots + a_9 p_9 m_9.$$

Fortunately this sum turns out to be simply

$$S = (a_1 + a_3 + a_5 + a_7 + a_9)m_0 - m_1, \tag{4.9}$$

as we will see in Lemma 5 below.

The remaining sum T can be written

$$
\begin{aligned}
T = \quad & p_1(m_1 + m_3 + m_2 - 2m_6 + 2m_{10}) + a_1 p_1(\ m_2 - 2m_6 + 2m_{10}) \\
& \qquad\qquad\qquad\qquad\qquad\qquad\quad + a_3 p_3(\qquad\quad -2m_6 + 2m_{10}) \\
& - p_5(m_5 + m_7 \qquad\quad - m_6 + 2m_{10}) + a_5 p_5(\qquad\quad -m_6 + 2m_{10}) \\
& \qquad\qquad\qquad\qquad\qquad\qquad\quad + a_7 p_7(\qquad\qquad\qquad +2m_{10}) \\
& + p_9(m_9 \qquad\qquad\quad + m_{10}) + a_9 p_9(\qquad\qquad\qquad\quad m_{10}) \\
= \quad & p_1(2m_3 + m_2 \qquad - 2m_6 + 2m_{10}) + a_1 p_1(2m_2 - 2m_6 + 2m_{10}) \\
& \qquad\qquad\qquad\qquad\qquad\qquad\quad + a_3 p_3(\qquad\quad -2m_6 + 2m_{10}) \\
& - p_5(2m_7 \qquad\qquad - m_6 + 2m_{10}) + a_5 p_5(\qquad\quad -2m_6 + 2m_{10}) \\
& \qquad\qquad\qquad\qquad\qquad\qquad\quad + a_7 p_7(\qquad\qquad\qquad 2m_{10}) \\
& + p_9(2m_{11} \qquad\qquad + m_{10}) + a_9 p_9(\qquad\qquad\qquad 2m_{10})
\end{aligned}
$$

Now $a_j p_j = p_{j+1} - p_{j-1}$, so we get some helpful telescoping:

$$
\begin{aligned}
T = \ & 2m_2(p_2 - p_0) - 2m_6(p_6 - p_0) + 2m_{10}(p_{10} - p_0) \\
& + 2m_3 p_1 - 2m_7 p_5 + 2m_{11} p_9 \\
& + m_2 p_1 + m_6(p_5 - 2p_1) + m_{10}(p_9 - 2p_5 + 2p_1).
\end{aligned}
$$

Furthermore, $m_0 = m_2 p_2 + m_3 p_1 = m_6 p_6 + m_7 p_5 = m_{10} p_{10} + m_{11} p_9$ by (2.11), so

$$T = 2m_0 + m_2(p_1 - 2) + m_6(p_5 - 2p_1 + 2) + m_{10}(p_9 - 2p_5 + 2p_1 - 2). \tag{4.10}$$

The coefficients of m_6 and m_{10} are nonnegative, since we have $p_1 = 1$ and $p_j \geq 2p_{j-2}$ for $2 \leq j < t$; hence

$$T \geq 2m_0 + m_2(a_0 - 2). \tag{4.11}$$

Finally $m_j p_{j-1} = m_j(p_j - p_{j-2})/a_{j-1} \leq m_j p_j / a_{j-1} \leq m_0 / a_{j-1}$, so

$$T \leq m_0(2 + 1/a_1 + 1/a_5 + 1/a_9). \tag{4.12}$$

(Notice that if $a_0 = a_2 = a_4 = a_6 = a_8 = x$, then

$$T/m_0 \to 2 + 1/a_1 + 1/a_5 + 1/a_9 \quad \text{as} \quad x \to \infty;$$

thus the upper bound in (4.12) is sharp.)

Let us now prove that the analog of (4.9) holds in general.

Lemma 5. *If* $m_j = a_j m_{j+1} + m_{j+2}$ *and* $p_{j+1} = a_j p_j + p_{j-1}$ *for* $0 \leq j < t$, *where* $p_0 = 1$, $p_{-1} = 0$, $m_t = 1$, $m_{t+1} = 0$, *and* t *is even, then*

$$m_1 + \sum_{\substack{0 \leq j < t \\ j \text{ odd}}} a_j p_j (m_j + m_{j+2}) = m_0 \sum_{\substack{0 \leq j < t \\ j \text{ odd}}} a_j; \qquad (4.13)$$

$$\sum_{\substack{0 \leq j < t \\ j \text{ even}}} a_j p_j (m_j + m_{j+2}) = p_{t-1} + m_0 \sum_{\substack{0 \leq j < t \\ j \text{ even}}} a_j. \qquad (4.14)$$

Proof. Since $p_j m_j + p_{j-1} m_{j+1} = m_0$, we have

$$
\begin{aligned}
a_j p_j (m_j + m_{j+2}) &= a_j m_0 - a_j p_{j-1} m_{j+1} + a_j p_j m_{j+2} \\
&= a_j m_0 - p_{j-1}(m_j - m_{j+2}) + (p_{j+1} - p_{j-1}) m_{j+2} \\
&= a_j m_0 - p_{j-1} m_j + p_{j+1} m_{j+2}
\end{aligned}
$$

for $0 \leq j < t$. Hence the sums on the left of (4.13) and (4.14) are immediately evaluated.   □

We are now ready to prove our main result.

Theorem 2. *Let* h *and* k *be relatively prime,* $0 < h < k$, *and let* c *be an integer. Let* $a_0, a_1, \ldots, a_{t-1}$ *be the canonical sequence of partial quotients for* (h, k), *with* t *even (see (3.18)). Also let*

$$S_e = \sum_{\substack{0 \leq j < t \\ j \text{ even}}} a_j, \qquad S_o = \sum_{\substack{0 \leq j < t \\ j \text{ odd}}} a_j. \qquad (4.15)$$

Then

$$\sigma(h, k, c) \leq S_e + \frac{1}{2} S_o - \frac{1}{2}. \qquad (4.16)$$

Moreover, there exists a value of c *for which*

$$\sigma(h, k, c) \geq S_e + \frac{1}{2} S_o - 4 - \frac{3}{2} \sum_{\substack{0 \leq j < t \\ j \text{ odd} \\ a_j \text{ odd}}} \frac{1}{a_j}. \qquad (4.17)$$

Proof. By (2.6) we have

$$\sigma(h, k, c) = \sigma(h, k, 0) - 3(-1)^z + 6 \sum_{j=0}^{t-1} (-1)^j \left(\frac{c_j^2}{m_j m_{j+1}} - b_j \right)$$

for $0 < c < k$, where z is the least subscript such that $c_z = 0$. The value (3.23) of c that maximizes $\sigma(h, k, c)$ always has z even except when $a_{t-1} = 1$ and u is odd (see the discussion following (4.8)). It follows that the formula

$$\max_{0<c<k} \sigma(h, k, c) = \sigma(h, k, 0) - 3 + 6 \sum_{j=0}^{t-1} (-1)^j \left(\frac{c_j^2}{m_j m_{j+1}} - b_j \right) \quad (4.18)$$

holds *without* exception when the b_j and c_j are defined by (4.5)–(4.8). Now

$$-6 \sum_{j=0}^{t-1} (-1)^j b_j = 3 \sum_{j=0}^{t/2-1} a_{2j+1} + 3 \sum_{r=0}^{u-1} (-1)^r$$

$$= 3 S_o + 3 (u \bmod 2). \quad (4.19)$$

The argument leading up to (4.10) proves in general that

$$6 \sum_{j=0}^{t-1} \frac{(-1)^j c_j^2}{m_j m_{j+1}} = \frac{6}{m_0} \sum_{j=0}^{t-1} (-1)^j b_j (c_j + c_{j+1}) p_j$$

$$= \frac{3}{2} \left(\frac{m_1}{m_0} - S_o - R \right) - 3 (u \bmod 2), \quad (4.20)$$

where

$$R = \sum_{r=0}^{u-1} \frac{m_{2j(r)+2}}{m_0} \left(p_{2j(r)+1} + 2 \sum_{s=0}^{r-1} (-1)^{r-s} p_{2j(s)+1} - 2(-1)^r \right). \quad (4.21)$$

As in (4.11) and (4.12) we conclude that

$$\frac{h}{k} - 1 \le \frac{m_2 (a_0 - 2)}{m_0} \le R \le \sum_{r=0}^{u-1} \frac{1}{a_{2j(r)+1}} \le u. \quad (4.22)$$

Notice that $R = 0$ when $u = 0$; thus we have an *exact* result when the odd-numbered partial quotients $a_1, a_3, \ldots, a_{t-1}$ are all even. Combining (4.4) with (4.18), (4.19), and (4.20) now yields

$$\max_{0<c<k} \sigma(h, k, c) = S_e + \frac{1}{2} S_o + \frac{3}{2} \frac{h}{k} + \frac{h + h'}{k} - \frac{3}{2} R - 4. \quad (4.23)$$

Since (4.16) is easily verified when $c = 0$, the proof of (4.16) and (4.17) is immediate. $\square$

It is amusing to note that when $a_{2j} = x$ and $a_{2j+1} = 2y$ for all j, we have $h' = k - xh/2y$, and there is a simple explicit formula

$$\max_{0<c<k} \sigma(h, k, c) = \tfrac{1}{2} (x + y) t + \tfrac{1}{2} (5 - x/y) h/k - 3.$$

Theorem 2 can also be used to obtain bounds on the minimum value of $\sigma(h, k, c)$:

Theorem 3. *Under the assumptions of Theorem 2,*

$$\sigma(h, k, c) \geq -\frac{1}{2}S_e - S_o + \frac{1}{2}. \tag{4.24}$$

Moreover, there exists a value of c for which

$$\sigma(h, k, c) \leq -\frac{1}{2}S_e - S_o + 4 + \frac{3}{2}\sum_{\substack{0 \leq j < t \\ j \text{ even} \\ a_j \text{ odd}}}\frac{1}{a_j}. \tag{4.25}$$

Proof. Since $k - h' = p_{t-1}$, the canonical sequence for $(k - h', k)$ is

$$a_{t-1}, a_{t-2}, \ldots, a_0. \tag{4.26}$$

Notice that even and odd positions are interchanged here (as are the p's and the m's). Now

$$
\begin{aligned}
\sigma(k - h', k, h'c) &= -12\sum_{j=0}^{k-1}\left(\!\left(\frac{j}{k}\right)\!\right)\left(\!\left(\frac{h'j - h'c}{k}\right)\!\right) \\
&= -12\sum_{j=0}^{k-1}\left(\!\left(\frac{j+c}{k}\right)\!\right)\left(\!\left(\frac{h'j}{k}\right)\!\right) \\
&= -12\sum_{j=0}^{k-1}\left(\!\left(\frac{hj + c}{k}\right)\!\right)\left(\!\left(\frac{h'hj}{k}\right)\!\right) \\
&= -\sigma(h, k, c); \tag{4.27}
\end{aligned}
$$

hence maximizing $\sigma(k - h', k, c)$ is equivalent to minimizing $\sigma(h, k, c)$ and changing the sign. □

Corollary. *Under the hypotheses of Theorem 2,*

$$|\sigma(h, k, c)| \leq \sum_{j=0}^{t-1}a_j - \frac{t+2}{4}. \tag{4.28}$$

Proof. In fact, by combining (4.16) and (4.24) we have

$$|\sigma(h, k, c)| \leq S_e + S_o - \tfrac{1}{2} - \tfrac{1}{2}\min(S_e, S_o). □$$

A combination of (4.17) and (4.25) yields

$$\max_{c} \sigma(h, k, c) - \min_{c} \sigma(h, k, c) \geq \frac{3}{2} \sum_{j=0}^{t-1} \left(a_j - \frac{a_j \bmod 2}{a_j} \right) - 8. \quad (4.29)$$

This bound is weakest (indeed, trivial) when we have the Fibonacci case $a_0 = a_1 = \cdots = a_{t-1} = 1$, $h = F_t$, $k = F_{t+1}$, where

$$F_0 = 0, \quad F_1 = 1, \quad F_{j+2} = F_{j+1} + F_j; \quad (4.30)$$

so it will be of interest to examine the maximum and minimum in this case. Both max and min have the same magnitude whenever the partial quotients of the canonical sequence satisfy $(a_0, a_1, \ldots, a_{t-1}) = (a_{t-1}, a_{t-2}, \ldots, a_0)$, by the proof of Theorem 3, because of the fact that $\sigma(h, k, c) = -\sigma(h, k, hc)$ when $h + h' = k$. Hence it suffices to consider $\max \sigma(F_t, F_{t+1}, c)$. Equation (4.23) tells us that

$$\max_{0 < c < F_{t+1}} \sigma(F_t, F_{t+1}, c) = \frac{3}{4}t + \frac{3}{2}\frac{h}{k} - \frac{3}{2}R - 3, \quad (4.31)$$

where we have, for example,

$$R = \frac{1}{F_9} \left(F_7(F_2 - 2) + F_5(F_4 - 2F_2 + 2) + F_3(F_6 - 2F_4 + 2F_2 - 2) \right.$$

$$\left. + F_1(F_8 - 2F_6 + 2F_4 - 2F_2 + 2) \right)$$

when $t = 8$. Let $L_n = F_{n+1} + F_{n-1}$. Using the easily verified identities

$$F_{2r} - 2F_{2r-2} + \cdots + (-1)^{r-1}2F_2 + (-1)^r 2 = \frac{L_{2r} + (-1)^r 8}{5}, \quad (4.32)$$

$$F_{2n-1}L_2 + F_{2n-3}L_4 + \cdots + F_1 L_{2n} = nF_{2n+1} + F_{2n}, \quad (4.33)$$

we find

$$R = \frac{1}{5F_9} \left(F_7(L_2 - 8) + F_5(L_4 + 8) + F_3(L_6 - 8) + F_1(L_8 + 8) \right)$$

$$= \frac{1}{5F_9} \left(4F_9 + F_8 - 8(F_8 - 2F_6 + 2F_4 - 2F_2) \right)$$

$$= \frac{1}{5F_9} \left(4F_9 + F_8 - 8\left(\frac{1}{5}(L_8 + 8) - 2 \right) \right),$$

and in general we obtain the exact formula

$$R = \frac{1}{5F_{t+1}} \left(\frac{t}{2}F_{t+1} + F_t - 8\left(\frac{1}{5}(L_t + (-1)^{t/2}8) - (-1)^{t/2}2 \right) \right)$$

$$= \frac{1}{10}t - \frac{16}{25} + \frac{13}{25}\frac{h}{k} + \frac{16}{25}\frac{(-1)^{t/2}}{k} \quad (4.34)$$

when $h = F_t$ and $k = F_{t+1}$, and t is even.

Instead of using a strict Euclidean algorithm to compute $\sigma(h, k, c)$, we could also use the so-called *least remainder algorithm*, which replaces h by $k - h$, if necessary, to ensure that $h \leq \frac{1}{2}k$ at each step. The least remainder algorithm is a combination of the additive and subtractive processes, and it can be obtained from the additive process as follows: When $a_j = 1$ and $a_{j-1} > 1$,

$$
\begin{array}{ll}
\text{replace} & \text{by} \\[1em]
m_{j-1} = a_{j-1}m_j + m_{j-1} & m_{j-1} = (a_{j-1} - 1)m_j + m_{j+2} \\
m_j = m_{j+1} + m_{j+2} & m_j = (a_{j+1} + 1)m_{j+2} + m_{j+3} \\
m_{j+1} = a_{j+1}m_{j+2} + m_{j+3} &
\end{array}
\qquad (4.35)
$$

This saves one iteration for each partial quotient 1 that is immediately preceded by an even number of partial quotients equal to 1, and it is known [11, exercise 4.5.3–29 in early editions, later exercise 4.5.3–30] that the number of iterations decreases by about $2 - \lg(1 + \sqrt{5}) \approx 31\%$ on the average. The transformation increases $\sum a_j$ by 1, so it increases the bound (4.28). Other changes from an additive to a subtractive procedure also increase the bound, except when $a_{t-1} > 1$ is replaced by $(a_{t-1} - 1, 1)$.

Such considerations lead us to the following result:

Corollary. *The bound*

$$
|\sigma(h, k, c)| \leq \sum_{j=0}^{t-1} a_j - \frac{t}{4}
\qquad (4.36)
$$

holds for all sequences of positive integers $a_0, a_1, \ldots, a_{t-1}$ *such that* $m_0 = k$, $m_1 = h$, $m_j = a_j m_{j+1} \pm m_{j+2}$, $m_t = 1$, *and* $m_{t+1} = 0$; *in particular, it holds for the least remainder algorithm.*

Proof. Let θ be any number between 0 and $1/3$; we will prove that the minimum value of $\sum a_j - \theta t$, over all sequences $a_0, \ldots, a_{t-1}$ as described in the corollary, occurs when the a_j are defined by the additive Euclidean algorithm modified so that $a_{t-1} = 1$.

It is not quite easy to prove this statement rigorously, since there is no obvious quantity that can be used as the basis of a valid proof by induction. In fact, the result would be false for $\theta > 1/3$, although this is not immediately evident. For example let $h = 2$, $k = 7$; the modified Euclidean algorithm has $(a_0, \ldots, a_{t-1}) = (3, 1, 1)$ and the sum is $5 - 3\theta$, but the sequence $(a_0, \ldots, a_{t-1}) = (1, 1, 1, 1, 1, 1)$ has a sum of $6 - 6\theta$.

Our approach will be to consider an infinite directed graph on the vertices (h, k), for all pairs (h, k) of nonnegative, relatively prime integers. The arcs of this directed graph will go from (h, k) to $(|k - ah|, h)$ for all positive integers a, and every such arc will be assigned a "distance" $a - \theta$. In order to prove that the modified Euclidean algorithm gives the "shortest path" from (h, k) to $(0, 1)$ for all h and k, it suffices to prove that $f(h, k) \leq a - \theta + f(|k - ah|, h)$ for all $a \geq 1$, when $f(h, k)$ is the distance to $(0, 1)$ in the modified Euclidean algorithm.

Let $f(0, 1) = 0$, $f(1, 1) = 1 - \theta$, $f(1, k) = k - 2\theta$ for $k \geq 2$, $f(h, k) = 1 - \theta + f(h - k, k)$ for $h > k$, and $f(h, k) = \lfloor k/h \rfloor - \theta + f(k \bmod h, h)$ for $1 < h < k$. It follows that

$$f(h, k) = f(k, h) + \begin{cases} 1, & \text{if } h > k > \frac{1}{2}h, \\ 1 - \theta, & \text{if } \frac{1}{2}h = k, \\ 1 - 2\theta, & \text{if } \frac{1}{2}h > k, \end{cases}$$

and

$$f(h, ah - k) = a - 2 + f(h, k), \quad \text{if} \quad h > k \quad \text{and} \quad a \geq 2.$$

We must prove that $f(h, k) \leq a - \theta + f(|k - ah|, h)$ for all $a \geq 1$. This inequality is readily verified for $h = 1$. When $1 < h < k$, let $b = \lfloor k/h \rfloor$, so that equality holds for $a = b$. If $1 \leq a < b$, we have $f(|k - ah|, h) \geq 1 - 2\theta + f(h, k - ah) = 1 - 2\theta + f(h, k) - a \geq f(h, k) - a + \theta$ since $\theta \leq 1/3$; if $a = b + 1$, we have $f(|k - ah|, h) = f(h - (k \bmod h), h) = f(h, k \bmod h) - 1 + \theta \geq 1 - 2\theta + f(k \bmod h, k) - 1 + \theta = f(h, k) - a + 1 > f(h, k) - a + \theta$; and if $a > b + 1$, we have

$$\begin{aligned} f(|k - ah|, h) &= f\big((a - b)h - (k \bmod h), h\big) \\ &\geq 1 - 2\theta + f\big(h, (a - b)h - (k \bmod h)\big) \\ &= 1 - 2\theta + (a - b - 2) + f(h, k \bmod h) \\ &\geq 1 - 2\theta + (a - b - 2) + 1 - 2\theta + f(k \bmod h, h) \\ &= a - 2b - 3\theta + f(h, k) > -a + \theta + f(h, k). \end{aligned}$$

Finally if $h > k$ and $a \geq 2$ we have

$$\begin{aligned} f(|k - ah|, h) &= f(ah - k, h) \\ &\geq 1 - 2\theta + f(h, ah - k) \\ &= a - 1 - 2\theta + f(h, k) > f(h, k) - a + \theta. \quad \square \end{aligned}$$

The inequality (4.36) is a slight improvement on the results of U. Dieter and J. Ahrens ([8, Theorem 4.8]) who showed that

$$|\sigma(h, k, c)| \leq \sum_{j=0}^{t-1} a_j + 3t + 5.$$

For applications to random number generation, we would like to know that $\sigma(h, k, c)$ is not too large. A. Khintchine has shown [9] that for all $\epsilon > 0$ the measure of the set of real numbers with

$$\left| \frac{a_0 + \cdots + a_{n-1}}{n \log_2 n} - 1 \right| > \epsilon \tag{4.37}$$

approaches zero as $n \to \infty$. Hence by applying Lemma 4.5.3M of [11] we can show that (for sufficiently large fixed n and all large k) the number of values of h whose first n partial quotients satisfy (4.37) is less than ϵk. This is not as strong a result as one would like, but it does suggest that the average sum of partial quotients ought to satisfy

$$\frac{1}{k} \sum_{h=1}^{k} \sum_{j=0}^{t-1} a_j \leq C (\log k)(\log \log k) \tag{4.38}$$

for some appropriate constant C. (It is well known that $t \leq \log_\phi k$, where $\phi = (1 + \sqrt{5})/2$; see [11, Corollary 4.5.3L].)

Yao and Knuth [14] have recently established the somewhat surprising fact that (4.38) is false; in fact,

$$\frac{1}{k} \sum_{h=1}^{k} \sum_{j=0}^{t-1} a_j = \frac{6(\ln k)^2}{\pi^2} + O\big((\log k)(\log \log k)^2\big) \tag{4.39}$$

as $k \to \infty$. Apparently the "middle" partial quotients tend to be larger than the first ones.

The results in [14] imply that the average of S_o is asymptotically $3(\ln k)^2/\pi^2$; thus the value of our bound on $|\sigma(h, k, c)|$ is $\sim \frac{9}{2}(\ln k)^2/\pi^2$ for fixed k, when averaged over $1 \leq h \leq k$. It follows that at most $O\big((\log k)^{-\epsilon}\big)$ choices of h will have $|\sigma(h, k, c)| > (\log k)^{2+\epsilon}$. This supports the empirically observed phenomenon that "random" choices of h almost always lead to satisfactory random number generators.

5. A General Reciprocity Law

It remains for us to prove Lemma 3 in the case $c = 0$. Let us consider first an extremely general identity:

Lemma 6. *Let $f(x)$ and $g(x)$ be any real-valued functions defined over the nonnegative integers. Let m and n be positive integers, and let α be any positive real number. Then*

$$\sum_{0 \le j < \alpha n} \big(f(j+1) - f(j)\big)g(\lfloor mj/n \rfloor + 1) + \sum_{0 \le r < \alpha m} f(\lceil rn/m \rceil)\big(g(r+1) - g(r)\big)$$

$$= f(\lceil \alpha n \rceil)g(\lceil \alpha m \rceil) - f(0)g(0). \qquad (5.1)$$

Proof. Consider the change of variable $r = \lfloor mj/n \rfloor$, a condition that holds if and only if

$$\left\lceil \frac{rn}{m} \right\rceil \le j < \left\lceil \frac{(r+1)n}{m} \right\rceil.$$

This range of values of j is used for those r with

$$\frac{(r+1)n}{m} < \alpha n;$$

the next value of r satisfies

$$\frac{rn}{m} \le j < \alpha n \le \frac{(r+1)n}{m},$$

that is, $r = \lceil \alpha m \rceil - 1$. Hence

$$\sum_{0 \le j < \alpha n} \big(f(j+1) - f(j)\big)g(\lfloor mj/n \rfloor + 1)$$

$$= \sum_{0 \le r < \alpha m - 1} g(r+1)\big(f(\lceil (r+1)n/m \rceil) - f(\lceil rn/m \rceil)\big) +$$

$$+ g(\lceil \alpha m \rceil)\big(f(\lceil \alpha n \rceil) - f(\lceil (\lceil \alpha m \rceil - 1)n/m \rceil)\big).$$

Rearranging the latter sum by grouping terms with the same value of $f(\lceil rn/m \rceil)$ yields the result. ☐

(Stieltjes integration by parts can be used to give another proof of (5.1) and formulas of even greater generality.)

Corollary. *For all nonnegative integers* m, n, p, q *and real* α *we have*

$$\sum_{0 \le j < \alpha m} \binom{j}{p}\binom{\lceil jn/m \rceil}{q+1} + \sum_{0 \le j < \alpha n} \binom{\lfloor mj/n \rfloor + 1}{p+1}\binom{j}{q}$$
$$= \binom{\lceil \alpha m \rceil}{p+1}\binom{\lceil \alpha n \rceil}{q+1}. \qquad (5.2)$$

Proof. Set $f(x) = \binom{x}{q+1}$ and $g(x) = \binom{x}{p+1}$ in (5.1). □

The general reciprocity law of this corollary, with $\alpha = 1/2$ and $p = q = 0$, lies at the heart of Eisenstein's proof of the law of quadratic reciprocity for prime numbers (see [10, exercise 1.2.4–47] and [2]). We shall now show that another special case immediately yields the reciprocity law for Dedekind sums $\sigma(h, k, 0)$.

Let $\alpha = 1$, $p = 1$, $q = 0$, $m = h$, and $n = k$ in (5.2); also express $\lfloor\ \rfloor$ and $\lceil\ \rceil$ in terms of $((\ ))$. Assuming that h and k are relatively prime, we have

$$kh(h-1) = \sum_{j=1}^{k-1} \left(\frac{hj}{k} - \left(\left(\frac{hj}{k}\right)\right) + \frac{1}{2}\right)\left(\frac{hj}{k} - \left(\left(\frac{hj}{k}\right)\right) - \frac{1}{2}\right)$$

$$+ 2\sum_{j=1}^{h-1}\left(\frac{kj}{h} - \left(\left(\frac{kj}{h}\right)\right) + \frac{1}{2}\right)j$$

$$= \sum_{j=1}^{k-1}\left(\left(\frac{hj}{k}\right)^2 + \left(\left(\frac{hj}{k}\right)\right)^2 - \left(\left(\frac{hj}{k}\right)\right)\left(2h\left(\left(\frac{j}{k}\right)\right)+h\right) - \frac{1}{4}\right)$$

$$+ \sum_{j=1}^{h-1}\left(\frac{2kj^2}{h} - \left(\left(\frac{kj}{h}\right)\right)\left(2h\left(\left(\frac{j}{h}\right)\right)+h\right)+j\right)$$

$$= \sum_{j=1}^{k-1}\left(\left(\frac{hj}{k}\right)^2 + \left(\frac{j}{k}-\frac{1}{2}\right)^2 - 2h\left(\left(\frac{hj}{k}\right)\right)\left(\left(\frac{j}{k}\right)\right) - \frac{1}{4}\right)$$

$$+ \sum_{j=1}^{h-1}\left(\frac{2kj^2}{h} - 2h\left(\left(\frac{kj}{h}\right)\right)\left(\left(\frac{j}{h}\right)\right) + j\right).$$

Everything can now be summed, and we obtain the desired law,

$$kh^2 - kh + \frac{h^2}{6k} + \frac{k}{6} + \frac{1}{6k} - \frac{h}{2} - \frac{h}{6}\left(\sigma(h,k,0) + \sigma(k,h,0)\right)$$
$$= kh(h-1).$$

It is important to note that the existence of a reciprocity formula connecting $f(h, k)$ with $g(k, h)$ does not necessarily imply that we have an efficient "Euclidean" algorithm for the evaluation of f and g; it is also necessary to have relations between $f(h \bmod k, k)$, $g(k \bmod h, h)$ and $f(h, k)$, $g(k, h)$.

For example, let us try to develop a reciprocity formula for cubic analogs of Dedekind sums, by taking $p = 2$ in (5.2). A derivation like that above yields

$$\sum_{j=0}^{k-1}\left(h^2\left(\!\left(\tfrac{j}{k}\right)\!\right)^2\left(\!\left(\tfrac{hj}{k}\right)\!\right) - h\left(\!\left(\tfrac{j}{k}\right)\!\right)\left(\!\left(\tfrac{hj}{k}\right)\!\right)^2\right)$$

$$+ \sum_{j=0}^{h-1} h^2\left(\!\left(\tfrac{j}{h}\right)\!\right)^2\left(\!\left(\tfrac{kj}{h}\right)\!\right) = \varphi(h, k), \qquad (5.3)$$

where $\varphi(h, k)$ can be explicitly evaluated in terms of h, k, and ordinary Dedekind sums. However, this is a rather pointless identity, because the substitutions $j \to k - j$ and $j \to h - j$ show that both sides of (5.3) are zero! Turning to $p = 3$, we find

$$\frac{k^3}{6}\sigma_{31}(k, h) - \frac{k^2}{4}\sigma_{22}(k, h) + \frac{k}{6}\sigma_{13}(k, h) + \frac{k^3}{6}\sigma_{31}(h, k) = \psi_1(h, k), \quad (5.4)$$

where

$$\sigma_{mn}(h, k) = \sum_{j=0}^{k-1}\left(\!\left(\tfrac{j}{k}\right)\!\right)^m\left(\!\left(\tfrac{hj}{k}\right)\!\right)^n. \qquad (5.5)$$

This equation by itself does not imply an efficient evaluation procedure; but if we set $q = 1$, $p = 2$ we get an independent reciprocity formula,

$$\frac{hk^2}{2}\sigma_{31}(k, h) - \frac{hk}{2}\sigma_{22}(k, h) + \frac{h}{6}\sigma_{13}(k, h) + \frac{hk^2}{2}\sigma_{31}(h, k) - \frac{k^2}{4}\sigma_{22}(h, k)$$

$$= \psi_2(h, k). \quad (5.6)$$

Equations (5.4) and (5.6) combine to give an efficient procedure:

Theorem 4. *There is an algorithm that computes* $\sigma_{13}(h, k)$, $\sigma_{22}(h, k)$, *and* $\sigma_{31}(h, k)$ *in* $O(\log k)$ *arithmetic operations.*

Proof. By definition, $\sigma_{mn}(h, k) = \sigma_{mn}(h \bmod k, k)$. Equations (5.4) and (5.5) tell us that

$$\tfrac{1}{6}k^3\sigma_{31}(h, k) = \psi_1(h, k) - \tfrac{1}{6}k^3\sigma_{31}(k, h) + \tfrac{1}{4}k^2\sigma_{22}(k, h) - \tfrac{1}{6}k\sigma_{13}(k, h),$$

$$\tfrac{1}{4}k^2\sigma_{22}(h, k) = -\psi_2(h, k) + \tfrac{1}{2}hk^2\sigma_{31}(h, k) + \tfrac{1}{2}hk^2\sigma_{31}(k, h)$$
$$- \tfrac{1}{2}hk\sigma_{22}(k, h) + \tfrac{1}{6}h\sigma_{13}(k, h),$$

$$\tfrac{1}{6}k\sigma_{13}(h, k) = \psi_2(k, h) + \tfrac{1}{2}hk\sigma_{22}(h, k) - \tfrac{1}{2}h^2k\sigma_{31}(h, k)$$
$$- \tfrac{1}{2}h^2k\sigma_{31}(k, h) + \tfrac{1}{4}h^2\sigma_{22}(k, h).$$

Therefore a Euclidean algorithm applies.   □

A similar argument shows that we can evaluate any $\sigma_{mn}(h, k)$ in $O\big((m + n)^3 \log k\big)$ operations.

Reciprocity laws for sums of polynomials such as (5.6), but in a completely different notation, have previously been obtained by T. M. Apostol [1] and L. Carlitz [3].

In order to carry the application to random-number generators further, it will be necessary to deal with sums of a still more general type, such as

$$\sum_{j=0}^{k-1} \left(\!\left(\frac{j}{k}\right)\!\right)\left(\!\left(\frac{h_1 j + c_1}{k}\right)\!\right)\left(\!\left(\frac{h_2 j + c_2}{k}\right)\!\right).$$

Reciprocity laws for such sums (even if we had them only in the three special cases $h_2 = 1$, $h_2 = h_1$, and $h_2 = h_1^2$) would be useful for further development of the theory.

Acknowledgment

The MACSYMA system was very useful not only for discovering Algorithm 1, but also for much of the formula manipulation and experimental computations as the theorems were developed. MACSYMA's exact rational arithmetic and its ability to compute functions symbolically proved to be of considerable utility.

This research was supported in part by the National Science Foundation and the Office of Naval Research. Some computer experiments reported herein were done via the ARPA network with the MACSYMA system, a project supported by the Advanced Research Projects Agency.

References

[1] T. M. Apostol, "Theorems on generalized Dedekind sums," *Pacific Journal of Mathematics* **2** (1952), 1–9.

[2] Bruce C. Berndt, "A generalization of a theorem of Gauss on sums involving [x]," *American Mathematical Monthly* **82** (1975), 44–51.

[3] L. Carlitz, "A reciprocity and four-term relation for generalized Dedekind sums," *Indagationes Mathematicæ* **36** (1974), 413–422.

[4] J. W. S. Cassels, *An Introduction to the Geometry of Numbers* (Berlin: Springer, 1959).

[5] R. Dedekind, "Erläuterungen zu den Fragmenten XXVIII," in *Bernhard Riemann's gesammelte Mathematische Werke und Wissenschaftlicher Nachlass*, edited by Heinrich Weber, 2nd edition, (Leipzig: Teubner, 1892), 466–478.

[6] Ulrich Dieter, "Das Verhalten der Kleinschen Funktionen $\log \sigma_{g,h}(\omega_1, \omega_2)$ gegenüber Modultransformationen und verallgemeinerte Dedekindsche Summen," *Journal für die reine und angewandte Mathematik* **201** (1959), 37–70.

[7] U. Dieter and J. Ahrens, "An exact determination of serial correlations of pseudo-random numbers," *Numerische Mathematik* **17** (1971), 101–123.

[8] U. Dieter and J. Ahrens, *Uniform Random Numbers* (Graz, Austria: Institut für Mathematische Statistik, Technische Hochschule Graz, 1974). [A planned book that was never completed.]

[9] A. Ya. Khintchine, "Metrische Kettenbruchprobleme," *Compositio Mathematica* **1** (1935), 361–382.

[10] Donald E. Knuth, *Fundamental Algorithms*, Volume 1 of *The Art of Computer Programming* (Reading, Massachusetts: Addison–Wesley, 1968).

[11] Donald E. Knuth, *Seminumerical Algorithms*, Volume 2 of *The Art of Computer Programming* (Reading, Massachusetts: Addison–Wesley, 1969).

[12] The Mathlab Group, *MACSYMA Reference Manual*, version six (Cambridge, Massachusetts: Massachusetts Institute of Technology, Project MAC, 1974).

[13] Hans Rademacher and Emil Grosswald, *Dedekind Sums*, Carus Mathematical Monograph Number 16 (Mathematical Association of America, 1972).

[14] Andrew C. Yao and Donald E. Knuth, "Analysis of the subtractive algorithm for greatest common divisors," *Proceedings of the National Academy of Sciences of the United States of America* **72** (1975), 4720–4722. [Reprinted with additional material as Chapter 13 of the present volume.]

Chapter 11

The Distribution of Continued Fraction Approximations

*[Originally published in Journal of Number Theory **19** (1984), 443–448.]*

The continued fraction convergents to a random real number are shown to approximate that number with a limiting probability distribution that had been conjectured by H. W. Lenstra, Jr.

One of the best methods known for factoring large numbers is based on the continued fraction approximations to a quadratic irrationality $\sqrt{d}$. The details of this factoring procedure are not of concern here, but the general idea is to work with the quantities

$$x_n = (u_n + \sqrt{d})/v_n$$

that arise in the continued fraction for $\sqrt{d}$; if v_n consists entirely of small prime factors, we can obtain information that is helpful in discovering factors of d. Therefore it is of interest to know something about the expected size of the numbers v_n. It is well known that $0 < v_n < 2\sqrt{d}$, but the distribution is not uniform in that range.

In this paper we study this problem in the more general setting of continued fractions, based on an idea communicated to the author by H. W. Lenstra, Jr.: If p_n/q_n is the nth convergent to a random real number x, we shall study the distribution of the quantity

$$\theta_n(x) = q_n|p_n - q_n x|,$$

which is well known to lie between 0 and 1. It turns out that when n is large the density function for $\theta_n(x)$ is approximately equal to

$$l(\theta) = \min(1, \theta^{-1} - 1)/\ln 2,$$

in agreement with a conjecture that Lenstra had made when he posed the problem.

To see why $\theta_n(x)$ is related to the size of v_n in the factoring procedure, we can use the fact that $v_{n+1} = |p_n^2 - dq_n^2|$; see, for example, [5, exercise 4.5.3–12(c)]. Therefore

$$v_{n+1} = q_n|p_n - \sqrt{d}q_n| \left(\frac{p_n}{q_n} + \sqrt{d}\right)$$

$$= q_n|p_n - \sqrt{d}q_n| \left(2\sqrt{d} + O\left(\frac{1}{q_n^2}\right)\right)$$

$$= 2\sqrt{d}\,q_n|p_n - \sqrt{d}q_n| + O(q_n^{-2})$$

and we have plausible grounds for assuming that $v_{n+1}/(2\sqrt{d})$ has the density $l(\theta)$.

Of course, the stated result does not constitute a rigorous proof that the numbers v_n will have any particular distribution, since the set of quadratic irrationalities has measure zero. The analysis of quadratic irrationalities appears to be quite formidable, and there may never be a way to obtain precise estimates about the behavior of continued fraction factoring. At the present time we must apparently be content with heuristic arguments that are valid only when we take the average over all real numbers.

1. Preliminaries

If x is any irrational number between 0 and 1, we define its continued fraction $x = /\!/a_1, a_2, \ldots /\!/$ by the formulas

$$x_0 = x;$$

$$1/x_n = a_{n+1} + x_{n+1} \qquad \text{where} \quad a_{n+1} = \lfloor 1/x_n \rfloor.$$

Thus $0 < x_n < 1$ for all n, and the "partial quotients" a_n are positive integers. The nth "convergent" is

$$p_n/q_n = /\!/a_1, \ldots, a_n/\!/,$$

where the continued fraction $/\!/a_1, \ldots, a_n/\!/$ is defined to be 0 if $n = 0$, otherwise it is defined recursively by the formula

$$/\!/a_1, \ldots, a_n/\!/ = \frac{1}{a_1 + /\!/a_2, \ldots, a_n/\!/}.$$

The well known *continuant polynomials* $K_n(z_1, \ldots, z_n)$ are defined by the relations $K_0 = 1$, $K_1(z_1) = z_1$,

$$K_{n+2}(z_1, \ldots, z_{n+2}) = K_{n+1}(z_1, \ldots, z_{n+1})z_{n+2} + K_n(z_1, \ldots, z_n),$$

and we have

$$p_n = K_{n-1}(a_2, \ldots, a_n),$$
$$q_n = K_n(a_1, \ldots, a_n).$$

The quantity of interest to us can be expressed as

$$\theta_n(x) = q_n|p_n - q_n x| = \frac{1}{x_n^{-1} + q_{n-1}/q_n} \, ;$$

this formula follows from the well-known identity

$$p_{n-1}q_n - p_n q_{n-1} = (-1)^n$$

together with the relation

$$x = //a_1, \ldots, a_{n-1}, a_n + x_n// = \frac{p_n + p_{n-1}x_n}{q_n + q_{n-1}x_n}.$$

Since $0 \leq \theta_n(x) < 1$, it is clear that p_n/q_n is an excellent approximation to x.

Let $f_n(y)$ be the density function for x_n. Thus $f_n(y)\,dy$ is the probability that x_n lies between y and $y + dy$, so it is the sum of the quantity

$$\left| \frac{p_n + p_{n-1}(y + dy)}{q_n + q_{n-1}(y + dy)} - \frac{p_n + p_{n-1}y}{q_n + q_{n-1}y} \right| = \frac{dy + O(dy^2)}{(q_n + q_{n-1}y)^2}$$

over all n-tuples $(a_1, \ldots, a_n)$ of positive integers, if we assume that $x = x_0$ is uniformly distributed. Paul Lévy [6] proved that $f_n(y)$ converges rapidly to

$$\frac{1}{(1 + y)\ln 2}$$

as $n \to \infty$; sharp estimates of the asymptotic behavior of $f_n(y)$ have been obtained more recently by Eduard Wirsing [7] and K. I. Babenko [1]. Consequently we have

$$\sum_{(a_1, \ldots, a_n)} \frac{1}{(q_n + q_{n-1}y)^2} = \frac{c}{1 + y} + O(\lambda^n),$$

where $c = 1/\ln 2$, $\lambda \approx 0.30366$, and the sum is over all n-tuples $(a_1, a_2, \ldots, a_n)$ of partial quotients.

2. A Metric Lemma

The main result we shall need is the formula

$$\sum_{q_{n-1} < zq_n} \frac{1}{q_n^2} = cz + O(\psi^n),$$

where $c = 1/\ln 2$, $\psi = (\sqrt{5} - 1)/2 \approx 0.61803$, and the sum is over all n-tuples $(a_1, a_2, \ldots, a_n)$ of partial quotients such that the corresponding convergent denominators satisfy $q_{n-1} < zq_n$, where $0 \le z \le 1$.

To prove this lemma, let m be less than n, and consider the sum of q_n^{-2} over all $(a_1, \ldots, a_n)$ such that q_{n-1}/q_n lies between $//b_m, \ldots, b_1//$ and $//b_m, \ldots, b_1, 1//$, for some given integers $(b_1, \ldots, b_m)$. Since

$$q_{n-1}/q_n = //a_n, \ldots, a_1//,$$

this is equal to the sum of q_n^{-2} over all $(a_1, \ldots, a_n)$ such that $a_n = b_m$, $a_{n-1} = b_{m-1}, \ldots, a_{n-m+1} = b_1$. Furthermore we have $q_n = q_{n-m}\bar{q}_m + q_{n-m-1}\bar{p}_m$, where $\bar{p}_m/\bar{q}_m = //b_1, \ldots, b_m//$, because of Euler's formula

$$K_n(a_1, \ldots, a_n) = K_{n-m}(a_1, \ldots, a_{n-m})K_m(a_{n-m+1}, \ldots, a_n)$$
$$+ K_{n-m-1}(a_1, \ldots, a_{n-m-1})K_{m-1}(a_{n-m+2}, \ldots, a_n).$$

Therefore the sum of q_n^{-2} in the stated range is

$$\sum_{(a_1, \ldots, a_{n-m})} \frac{1}{(q_{n-m}\bar{q}_m + q_{n-m-1}\bar{p}_m)^2} = \frac{c}{\bar{q}_m(\bar{q}_m + \bar{p}_m)} + O\left(\frac{\lambda^{n-m}}{\bar{q}_m^2}\right).$$

But

$$\frac{1}{\bar{q}_m(\bar{q}_m + \bar{p}_m)} = \left| //b_m, \ldots, b_1// - //b_m, \ldots, b_1, 1// \right|$$

is just the size of the interval containing the values of q_{n-1}/q_n over which we were summing. This is what we want, since our goal is to establish that the sum for q_{n-1}/q_n lying in any interval is approximately c times the size of that interval.

To complete the proof, we observe that the sum for $0 \le q_{n-1}/q_n < z$ is the sum over all intervals strictly less than z that are defined by $(b_1, \ldots, b_m)$ as in the preceding paragraph, plus a correction term depending on the interval containing z. The latter correction is bounded by the size of the interval, which is $O(1/\bar{q}_m^2)$. The sum of the error term $O(\lambda^{n-m}/\bar{q}_m^2)$, taken over all $(b_1, \ldots, b_m)$, is $O(\lambda^{n-m})$. Therefore the entire sum is $cz + O(1/\bar{q}_m^2) + O(\lambda^{n-m})$; and the error is $O(\psi^n)$ if we choose $m = \lfloor n/2 \rfloor$, since $\bar{q}_m \ge \psi^{1-m}$ and $\lambda < \psi^2$.   □

3. A Metric Theorem

Let $l_n(\theta)\,d\theta$ be the probability that the quantity $\theta_n(x)$ defined in Section 1 lies between θ and $\theta + d\theta$. We shall prove that

$$l_n(\theta) = c\min(1, \theta^{-1} - 1) + O(\psi^n).$$

This is almost an immediate consequence of the lemma proved above, once we set the problem up correctly. If p_n and q_n are given, the probability that x lies between $p_n/q_n + (-1)^n\theta/q_n^2$ and $p_n/q_n + (-1)^n(\theta + d\theta)/q_n^2$ is, of course, $d\theta/q_n^2$. A sequence $(a_1, \ldots, a_n)$ of partial quotients leads to values of p_n and q_n that can occur with $\theta(x) = \theta$ if and only if the number x_n defined in the formula $\theta = 1/(x_n^{-1} + q_{n-1}/q_n)$ lies between 0 and 1, that is, if and only if $q_{n-1}/q_n \le \theta^{-1} - 1$. Therefore $l_n(\theta)$ is the step function $\sum 1/q_n^2$ summed over all $(a_1, \ldots, a_n)$ such that $q_{n-1}/q_n \le \theta^{-1} - 1$. If $\theta \le \frac{1}{2}$, this is the sum over all $(a_1, \ldots, a_n)$, so it equals $f_n(0) = c + O(\lambda^n)$. If $\theta > \frac{1}{2}$, our lemma proves that the sum is $c(\theta^{-1} - 1) + O(\psi^n)$.   □

4. Concluding Remarks

It is interesting to consider the initial distribution $f_0(x) = c/(1 + x)$ as an alternative to the uniform distribution. Then $f_n(x) = f_0(x)$ for all x, and we can show that $l_n(\theta) = l(\theta) + O(\psi^{2n})$, using the relation

$$\sum_{q_{n-1} < yq_n} \frac{1}{q_n(p_n + q_n)} = y + O(\psi^{2n}).$$

This estimate is sharp, since an error of order ψ^{2n} occurs when y is near ψ.

Harry Kesten [4] has studied a related problem: Let

$$\Theta_N(x) = N \cdot \min_{1 \le p, q \le N} |p - qx|$$

be a measure of the error in approximations to x by fractions whose numerator and denominator are at most N. It is well known that

$$\Theta_N(x) = N|p_n - q_n x|,$$

where $q_n \le N < q_{n+1}$ in the sequence of complete quotients $(q_1, q_2, \ldots)$ in the continued fraction for x; hence $\Theta_N(x) = (N/q_n)\theta_n(x)$, where q_n is a function of N and x. We have proved that $\theta_n(x)$ approaches a limiting distribution independent of x, as $n \to \infty$; but it does not follow that Θ_N has the same limiting distribution multiplied by the "average" value of N/q_n. Indeed, the inequality

$$\Theta_N(x) < q_{n+1}/(q_n x_n^{-1} + q_{n-1}) < 1$$

proves that when $\theta_n(x)$ is near 1, the quantity N/q_n cannot be very large. Kesten adapted an interesting elementary construction of Friedman and Niven [3] to prove that the density function of Θ_N approaches the limiting value $L(\theta)$ as $N \to \infty$, where

$$L(\theta) = \begin{cases} \dfrac{12}{\pi^2}, & \text{if } 0 \leq \theta \leq \frac{1}{2}; \\ \dfrac{12}{\pi^2}\left(\dfrac{1-\theta}{\theta}\ln\dfrac{\theta e}{1-\theta}\right), & \text{if } \frac{1}{2} \leq \theta \leq 1. \end{cases}$$

It is interesting to note that both $l(\theta)$ and $L(\theta)$ are uniform when $\theta \leq \frac{1}{2}$.

When Lenstra posed the problem of analyzing $\theta_n(x)$, he was actually interested in the infinite sequence of values $\big(\theta_1(x), \theta_2(x), \theta_3(x), \dots\big)$ corresponding to a single x, rather than the distribution of $\theta_n(x)$ for fixed n as x varies. This more difficult problem is close to what actually arises in the application to factorization, because a single value of x is used for each d. Lenstra's conjecture has recently been resolved in a strong form by W. Bosma, H. Jager, and F. Wiedijk [2], who proved (among other things) that

$$\lim_{N \to \infty} \frac{1}{N}\,(\text{number of } n \leq N \text{ with } \theta_n(x) \leq \theta) = \int_0^\theta l(t)\,dt$$

for almost all x.

Acknowledgments

The author is grateful to the editor and the referees, who pointed out the relevance of reference [4].

This research was supported in part by the National Science Foundation and the Office of Naval Research.

References

[1] K. I. Babenko, "Об одной задаче Гаусса," *Doklady Akademii Nauk SSSR* **238** (1978), 1021–1024. English translation, "On a

problem of Gauss," *Soviet Mathematics — Doklady* **19** (1978), 136–140.

[2] W. Bosma, H. Jager, and F. Wiedijk, "Some metrical observations on the approximation by continued fractions," *Indagationes Mathematicæ* **45** (1983), 281–299.

[3] Bernard Friedman and Ivan Niven, "The average first recurrence time," *Transactions of the American Mathematical Society* **92** (1959), 25–34.

[4] Harry Kesten, "Some probabilistic theorems on Diophantine approximations," *Transactions of the American Mathematical Society* **103** (1962), 189–217.

[5] Donald E. Knuth, *Seminumerical Algorithms*, Volume 2 of *The Art of Computer Programming* (Reading, Massachusetts: Addison–Wesley, 1969).

[6] Paul Lévy, "Sur les lois de probabilité dont dépendent les quotients complets et incomplets d'une fraction continue," *Bulletin de la Société mathématique de France* **57** (1929), 178–194.

[7] Eduard Wirsing, "On the theorem of Gauss–Kusmin–Lévy and a Frobenius-type theorem for function spaces," *Acta Arithmetica* **24** (1974), 507–528.

Addendum

Subsequent work by Hendrik Jager ["Continued fractions and ergodic theory," in *Transcendental Numbers and Related Topics* (Kyoto: Research Institute of Mathematical Sciences, 1986), 55–59] showed that the result can be obtained as a corollary of a two-dimensional distribution theorem. An alternative way to prove Lenstra's conjecture was discovered by D. Barbolosi, "Une application du théorème ergodique sous-additif à la théorie métrique des fractions continues," *Journal of Number Theory* **66** (1997), 172–182. The error term in the theorem of Section 3 was improved to $O(\lambda^n)$ by C. Faivre, "The rate of convergence of approximations of a continued fraction," *Journal of Number Theory* **68** (1998), 21–28.

Chapter 12

Evaluation of Porter's Constant

[Originally published in Computers and Mathematics with Applications 2 (1976), 137–139.]

A 40-digit value is computed for the constant that J. W. Porter has recently derived in connection with the analysis of Euclid's algorithm. A closed form for this constant, due to J. W. Wrench, Jr., is also presented.

1. Introduction and Summary

Let τ_n be the average number of iterations used by Euclid's algorithm to compute $\gcd(m, n)$, when n is fixed and m is randomly chosen from the set of all integers relatively prime to n. Empirical calculations by Knuth [2, Section 4.5.3] indicated that

$$\tau_n \approx 0.843 \ln n + 1.47, \tag{1}$$

and Heilbronn [1] proved that

$$\tau_n = \frac{12 \ln 2}{\pi^2} \ln n + O(\log \log n)^4. \tag{2}$$

The error estimate was improved to $O(\log \log n)^2$ by Tonkov [6], and recent work by Porter [3] has finally established (1) in the sharp form

$$\tau_n = \frac{12 \ln 2}{\pi^2} \ln n + (4P + 2.5) + O(n^{-\frac{1}{6}+\epsilon}), \tag{3}$$

for all $\epsilon > 0$. Here P is the constant defined by

$$P = \frac{6}{\pi^2} \left(B + \frac{3}{16} + \left(\gamma + \frac{5}{16} \right) \ln 2 - \frac{7}{8} (\ln 2)^2 + 2I - \frac{6}{\pi^2} \zeta'(2) \ln 2 \right), \tag{4}$$

189

where

$$B = \sum_{k \geq 1} \frac{1}{k}(H_{2k-1} - H_k - \ln 2), \tag{5}$$

$$I = \int_0^{1/\sqrt{8}} \frac{t^2 \ln t}{(t^2 + 1)^{\frac{1}{2}}} \, dt, \tag{6}$$

and H_k denotes the sum $1 + \frac{1}{2} + \cdots + \frac{1}{k}$. Porter established by hand that $P > -0.3$.

In this paper we apply standard techniques to evaluate these constants to 40 decimal digits, in particular obtaining the values

$12\pi^{-2} \ln 2 = 0.84276\ 59132\ 72194\ 51690\ 72631\ 93963\ 96411\ 55945+$

$4P + 2.5 = 1.46707\ 80794\ 33975\ 47289\ 77984\ 84707\ 22995\ 34499+$

$-P = 0.25823\ 04801\ 41506\ 13177\ 55503\ 78823\ 19251\ 16375+$

$-B = 1.16448\ 10529\ 30025\ 01180\ 53126\ 40319\ 36021\ 74884-$

$-I = 0.01958\ 27168\ 97011\ 53218\ 32291\ 14034\ 54827\ 84625+$

As a by-product of these calculations, we also obtain several 40-digit values of $\zeta'(k)$ (see below).

2. Calculation Procedure

The integral I is readily evaluated by expanding into power series,

$$I = \int_0^{1/\sqrt{8}} \sum_{k \geq 0} \binom{-\frac{1}{2}}{k} t^{2+2k} \ln t \, dt$$

$$= \sum_{k \geq 0} (-1)^{k+1} \binom{2k}{k} \frac{2^{-5k-4.5}}{(2k+3)^2}(1 + (3k+4.5)\ln 2). \tag{7}$$

To evaluate B, let $B' = B + \frac{1}{2}\zeta(2)$, so that $B' = \sum_{k \geq 1} A_k/k$ where

$$A_n = H_{2n} - H_n - \ln 2$$

$$= -\frac{1}{4n} + \sum_{k=1}^{r} \frac{B_{2k}}{2k} \frac{(1 - 2^{-2k})}{n^{2k}} + O(n^{-2r-2}) \tag{8}$$

by Euler's summation formula. Letting $\zeta_m(s) = \sum_{k \geq m} k^{-s} = O(m^{1-s})$, we have

$$B' = \sum_{k=1}^{m-1} \frac{1}{k} A_k - \frac{1}{4}\zeta_m(2) + \sum_{k=1}^{r} \frac{B_{2k}}{2k}(1 - 2^{-2k})\zeta_m(2k+1) + O(m^{-2r-2}), \tag{9}$$

for all fixed r. The necessary values of $\zeta_m(s)$ can themselves be obtained from Euler's summation formula,

$$\zeta_m(s) = \frac{m^{1-s}}{s-1} + \frac{m^{-s}}{2} + \sum_{k=1}^{r} \binom{s+2k-2}{s-1} \frac{B_{2k}}{2k} m^{-s-2k+1} + O(m^{-s-2r-1}).$$

(10)

For suitably large m, (9) and (10) will converge to the desired accuracy. An excellent check on the results (and the algorithms) is obtained by choosing two different values of m.

Finally we need to compute $\zeta'(2)$. Once again Euler's summation formula gives a satisfactory approach, since it implies that

$$-\zeta'_m(s) = \frac{m^{1-s}\ln m}{s-1} + \frac{m^{1-s}}{(s-1)^2} + \frac{\ln m}{2m^s}$$

$$+ \sum_{k=1}^{r} \binom{s+2k-2}{s-1} \frac{B_{2k}}{2k} m^{-s-2k+1}(\ln m + H_{s-1} - H_{s+2k-2})$$

$$+ O(m^{-s-2r-1}\log m).$$

(11)

3. Derivatives of the Zeta Function

A general program for $\zeta'(s)$ is almost as easy to write as a program for the special case $s = 2$, so the following values were also determined.

$$-\zeta'(2) = 0.93754\ 82543\ 15843\ 75370\ 25740\ 94567\ 86497\ 78979-$$
$$-\zeta'(3) = 0.19812\ 62428\ 85636\ 85333\ 06818\ 21503\ 28579\ 68755+$$
$$-\zeta'(4) = 0.06891\ 12658\ 96125\ 37984\ 88293\ 65587\ 44082\ 71500+$$
$$-\zeta'(5) = 0.02857\ 37805\ 09462\ 95008\ 03898\ 17083\ 80121\ 26482+$$

(The most precise previous calculation of $\zeta'(s)$ was apparently done by Rosser and Schoenfeld [4, Table 4], who gave 17-digit values for $2 \leq s < 30$. Their results are in agreement with the calculations above. See also [5], where it is observed that K. F. Gauss once calculated the first ten digits of $\zeta'(2)$.)

4. A Closed Form

John W. Wrench, Jr. [7] has pointed out that the constants B and I, and hence P, can be expressed in closed form, namely

$$B = (\ln 2)^2 - \frac{\pi^2}{6},$$

(12)

$$I = \frac{1}{96}\left(2\pi^2 + 30(\ln 2)^2 - 39\ln 2 - 9\right), \tag{13}$$

$$P = -\frac{3}{4} + \frac{6}{\pi^2}\left(\frac{3}{4}(\ln 2)^2 + \left(\gamma - \frac{1}{2}\right)\ln 2 - \frac{6}{\pi^2}\zeta'(2)\ln 2\right). \tag{14}$$

These formulas lead to independent confirmation of the 40-digit values above. (In his derivation, Wrench made use of the intermediate results

$$B' = -\sum_{k\geq 1}\frac{1}{k}\int_0^1 \frac{t^{2k}}{1+t}\,dt = \int_0^1 \frac{\ln(1-t^2)}{1+t}\,dt; \tag{15}$$

$$\int_0^a \frac{t^2\ln t}{(t^2+1)^{\frac{1}{2}}}\,dt = \frac{a}{2}A\ln a - \frac{a}{4}A - \frac{1}{4}\ln(A+a) - \frac{1}{4}\mathrm{Li}_2((A-a)^2)$$
$$- \frac{1}{4}\left(\ln\frac{A+a}{2}\right)^2 + \frac{\pi^2}{24} + \frac{1}{4}(\ln 2)^2, \tag{16}$$

where $A = (a^2+1)^{\frac{1}{2}}$ and

$$\mathrm{Li}_2(x) = \int_0^x \ln\left(\frac{1}{1-t}\right)\frac{dt}{t} = \sum_{k\geq 1}\frac{x^k}{k^2} \tag{17}$$

is the dilogarithm function.)

This research was supported in part by the National Science Foundation and the Office of Naval Research. The computations and formula manipulation were done with the MACSYMA system supported by the Advanced Research Projects Agency (ARPA).

References

[1] Hans Heilbronn, "On the average length of a class of finite continued fractions," in *Number Theory and Analysis* (Papers in honor of Edmund Landau), edited by Paul Turán (Plenum, 1969), 87–96. Reprinted in Heilbronn's *Collected Papers* (1988), 518–525.

[2] Donald E. Knuth, *Seminumerical Algorithms*, Volume 2 of *The Art of Computer Programming* (Reading, Massachusetts: Addison–Wesley, 1969).

[3] J. W. Porter, "On a theorem of Heilbronn," *Mathematika* **22** (1975), 20–28.

[4] J. Barkley Rosser and Lowell Schoenfeld, "Approximate formulas for some functions of prime numbers," *Illinois Journal of Mathematics* **6** (1962), 64–94.

[5] D. Shanks, Review of [4], *Mathematics of Computation* **17** (1963), 307–308.

[6] Tonko Tonkov, "On the average length of finite continued fractions," *Acta Arithmetica* **26** (1974), 47–57.

[7] John W. Wrench, Jr., Personal communications (24 March 1976 and 3 May 1976).

Addendum

A long-forgotten paper by Gustav Lochs ["Statistik der Teilnenner der zu den echten Brüchen gehörigen regelmäßigen Kettenbrüche," *Monatshefte für Mathematik* **65** (1961), 27–52] deserves to be mentioned here, because his work preceded that of Porter by nearly 15 years and involved essentially the same constant. Lochs computed an asymptotic formula for a quantity he called $h(N)$, which is equal to

$$\sum_{n=1}^{N} n(T_n - 1), \qquad T_n = \frac{1}{n}\sum_{d\backslash n} d\tau_d \tag{18}$$

in the notation of [2]. His formula was, in essence,

$$h(N) = \frac{6\ln 2}{\pi^2} N^2 \ln N - LN + O(N^{3/2}), \tag{19}$$

where

$$L = \frac{1}{2} + \frac{3}{\pi^2}\left(\left(\ln 2 + 3 - 4\gamma + \frac{12}{\pi^2}\zeta'(2)\right)\ln 2 - \frac{\pi^2}{12} - A\right), \tag{20}$$

$$A = 8\sum_{m=1}^{\infty}\sum_{n=1}^{\infty}\frac{r_n(m)}{3^{2n+1}}, \tag{21}$$

$$r_n(m) = \frac{1}{m^{2n+2}}\sum_{k=1}^{m}(2k-m)^{2n} - \frac{1}{(2n+1)m}$$

$$= \frac{1}{2n+1}\sum_{k=1}^{n}\binom{2n+1}{2k}\frac{2^{2k}B_{2k}}{m^{2k+1}}. \tag{22}$$

Numerical evaluation gives

$$L = 0.21732\,42870\,38481\,33931\,06086\,86618\,44603\,45935- \tag{23}$$

(although Lochs believed in 1961 that the value was ≈ 0.21807).

If we insert (3) into (18) we find that L and P must be related by the formula

$$4P + \frac{5}{2} - \frac{1}{2} - \frac{12\ln 2}{\pi^2}\left(\frac{1}{2} - \frac{6}{\pi^2}\zeta'(2)\right) = -2L + \frac{1}{2} \tag{24}$$

[see G. H. Norton, "On the asymptotic analysis of the Euclidean algorithm," *Journal of Symbolic Computation* **10** (1990), 53–58]. By (14) and (20), this relation is equivalent to

$$A = 4(\ln 2)^2 - \frac{\pi^2}{6}; \tag{25}$$

and sure enough, numerical evaluation confirms this formula, at least to 40 decimal places.

Perhaps we should therefore refer henceforth to the *Lochs–Porter constant*, instead of simply saying "Porter's constant."

Chapter 13

Analysis of the Subtractive Algorithm for Greatest Common Divisors

*[Written with Andrew C. Yao. Dedicated to the memory of Hans A. Heilbronn (1908–1975). Amplification of a paper originally published in Proceedings of the National Academy of Sciences of the United States of America **72** (1975), 4720–4722.]*

The sum of all partial quotients in the regular continued fraction expansions of m/n, for $1 \leq m \leq n$, is shown to be $6\pi^{-2}n(\ln n)^2 + O(n \log n (\log \log n)^2)$. This result is applied to the analysis of what is perhaps the oldest nontrivial algorithm for number-theoretic computations.

An ancient Greek method [1] for finding the greatest common divisor of two positive integers by mutual subtraction (ἀνταναίρεσις) can be described as follows: "Replace the larger number by the difference of the two numbers until both are equal; then the answer is this common value." For example, the computation of $\gcd(18, 42)$ requires four subtraction steps $\{18, 42\} \to \{18, 24\} \to \{18, 6\} \to \{12, 6\} \to \{6, 6\}$; the answer is 6.

Let $S(n)$ denote the average number of steps to compute $\gcd(m, n)$ by this method, when m is uniformly distributed in the range $1 \leq m \leq n$. We shall prove the following result:

Theorem. $S(n) = 6\pi^{-2}(\ln n)^2 + O(\log n (\log \log n)^2)$.

1. Preliminaries

Let $\lfloor x \rfloor$ denote the largest integer less than or equal to x, and let $x \bmod y = x - y\lfloor x/y \rfloor$ be the remainder of x after division by y. We represent the continued fraction $1/(x_1 + 1/(x_2 + \cdots + 1/x_r)\cdots)$ by $//x_1, x_2, \ldots, x_r//$.

If $1 \leq m \leq n$, it is well known that there is a unique sequence of positive integers $q_1, \ldots, q_r$ such that $m/n = //q_1, \ldots, q_r, 1//$, where $r = r(m, n) \geq 0$. The number of subtraction steps needed to compute $\gcd(m, n)$ is precisely $q_1 + \cdots + q_r$; for this is evident when m divides n, and otherwise $q_1 = \lfloor n/m \rfloor$ subtraction steps replace $\{m, n\}$ by $\{m, n \bmod m\}$, where $(n \bmod m)/m = //q_2, \ldots, q_m, 1//$. Therefore $S(n)$ may be interpreted as one less than the average total sum of partial quotients in the continued fraction representation of fractions with denominator n.

Let us say that (x, x', y, y') is an *H-representation* of n if

$$n = xx' + yy', \quad x > y > 0, \quad \gcd(x, y) = 1, \quad \text{and } x' \geq y' > 0. \quad (1.1)$$

We begin our analysis with the following sharpened form of a fundamental observation due to H. A. Heilbronn [2]:

Lemma 1. *There is a one-to-one correspondence between H-representations of n and the set of ordered pairs*

$$\{(m, j) \mid 0 < m < n/2 \text{ and } 1 \leq j \leq r(m, n)\}.$$

Furthermore if (x, x', y, y') corresponds to (m, j), the jth partial quotient q_j in the continued fraction $m/n = //q_1, q_2, \ldots, q_r, 1//$ is $\lfloor x/y \rfloor$.

Proof. Given $0 < m < n/2$, let $d = \gcd(m, n)$, $r = r(m, n)$, and $m/n = //q_1, q_2, \ldots, q_r, 1//$. Let the reversed fraction $//1, q_r, \ldots, q_2, q_1//$ be m'/n; then $n/2 < m' < n$, and the correspondence $m \leftrightarrow m'$ between integers in the intervals $(0 .. n/2)$ and $(n/2 .. n)$ is one-to-one.

Now let the pair (m, r) correspond to the H-representation $(m'/d, d, (n-m')/d, d)$; and if (m, j) corresponds to (x_j, x'_j, y_j, y'_j) for some $j > 1$, let $(m, j-1)$ correspond to $(y_j, q_j x'_j + y'_j, x_j - q_j y_j, x'_j)$. It follows readily that $\lfloor x_j/y_j \rfloor = q_j$ for $1 \leq j \leq r$ and that $y_1 = 1$, since this construction parallels the continued fraction process for m'/n.

To complete the proof, we start with a given H-representation (x, x', y, y') and show that it corresponds to a unique (m, j). This is obvious if $x' = y'$, since the construction clearly treats every such H-representation exactly once. If $x' > y'$ let $x' = qy' + x''$ where $0 < x'' \leq y'$ and $q \geq 1$. By induction on x', the H-representation $(y + qx, y', x, x'')$ corresponds uniquely to some (m, j), where $j > 1$ since $x > 1$; hence (x, x', y, y') corresponds uniquely to $(m, j-1)$. $\quad \square$

Corollary. $nS(n) = 2\sum\lfloor x/y\rfloor + 1 - (n \bmod 2)$, where the sum is over all H-representations of n.

Proof. By the lemma, $\sum\lfloor x/y\rfloor$ is the total number of subtractions to compute $\gcd(m,n)$ for $1 \le m < n/2$. It is also the total number for $n/2 < m < n$, since $\{m,n\}$ and $\{n-m,n\}$ both reduce to $\{m,n-m\}$ after one step. Finally we add the cases $m = n$ (0 steps) and $m = n/2$ (1 step if n is even).   □

2. Reduction of the Problem

Let $\sum'\lfloor x/y\rfloor$ denote the sum over all H-representations with $x'y < n/2$. Notice that

$$x/y < n/(x'y) = x/y + y'/x' \le x/y + 1; \qquad (2.1)$$

hence the excluded H-representations with $x'y \ge n/2$ have $\lfloor x/y\rfloor = 1$. Since $r(m,n) = O(\log n)$, Lemma 1 implies that

$$\sum\lfloor x/y\rfloor = \sum'\lfloor x/y\rfloor + O(n\log n). \qquad (2.2)$$

Lemma 2. Given $x' > 0$, $y > 0$, and $x'y < n/2$, there exist H-representations (x, x', y, y') of n if and only if

$$\gcd(y,n) = \gcd(y,x'). \qquad (2.3)$$

Furthermore, when (2.3) holds there are exactly $\gcd(y,n)\prod(1 - p^{-1})$ such H-representations, where the product is over all primes p that divide $\gcd(y,n)$ but not $y/\gcd(y,n)$.

Proof. The necessity of (2.3) is obvious, since $\gcd(x,y) = 1$. Let $d = \gcd(y,n) = \gcd(y,x') = ax' + by$. The set of all solutions (x,y') to $n = xx' + yy'$ is given by $((an + qy)/d, (bn - qx')/d)$, for integer q. Exactly d values of q will satisfy $0 < bn - qx' \le dx'$, that is, $y' \le x'$; and when $y' \le x'$ we have $x = (n - yy')/x' \ge n/x' - y > y$.

It remains to count how many of these d solutions have $\gcd(x,y) = 1$. If p is a prime divisor of y/d, then p does not divide an/d, hence p does not divide x. On the other hand, let $p_1, \ldots, p_r$ be the primes that divide d but not y/d; then $p_1 \ldots p_r$ consecutive values of q will make $(an + qy)/d$ run through a complete residue class modulo $p_1 \ldots p_r$, hence $(p_1 - 1)\ldots(p_r - 1)$ of these values will be relatively prime to y.   □

Let $P(n)$ denote $\varphi(n)/n = \prod(1 - p^{-1})$, where the product is over all prime divisors of n, and let $P(n \setminus m)$ denote the similar product over all primes that divide n but not m. From (2.1) and Lemma 2 we have

$$\sum' \left\lfloor \frac{x}{y} \right\rfloor = \sum_{d \setminus n} d \sum_{\substack{y \geq 1 \\ \gcd(y,n)=d}} P\left(d \setminus \frac{y}{d}\right) \sum_{\substack{1 \leq x' < n/(2y) \\ \gcd(x',y)=d}} \left(\frac{n}{x'y} + O(1)\right).$$

Replacing n, y, x' respectively by md, jd, kd and applying (2.2) yields

$$\sum \left\lfloor \frac{x}{y} \right\rfloor = \sum_{m \setminus n} \sum_{\substack{j \geq 1 \\ \gcd(j,m)=1}} P\left(\frac{n}{m} \setminus j\right) \sum_{\substack{1 \leq k < m^2/(2nj) \\ \gcd(k,j)=1}} \frac{m}{jk} + O(n \log n), \quad (2.4)$$

since the total number of H-representations is $O(n \log n)$.

3. Asymptotic Formulas

Lemma 3.

$$\sum_{\substack{p \setminus n \\ p \text{ prime}}} \frac{\log p}{p} = O(\log \log n). \tag{3.1}$$

Proof. Let n be divisible by k primes, and let c_1 and c_2 be constants such that the jth prime lies between $c_1 j \log j$ and $c_2 j \log j$. Then

$$\sum_{\substack{p \setminus n \\ p \text{ prime}}} \frac{\log p}{p} \leq \sum_{j=1}^{k} \frac{\log p_j}{p_j} = O\left(\sum_{j=1}^{k} \frac{\log j}{j \log j}\right) = O(\log k). \quad \square$$

Consequently

$$\sum_{d \setminus n} \frac{\mu(d)}{d} \log\left(\frac{1}{d}\right) = \sum_{\substack{p \setminus n \\ p \text{ prime}}} \frac{\log p}{p} P(n \setminus p) = O(\log \log n). \tag{3.2}$$

Lemma 4.

$$\sum_{d \setminus n} \frac{\log d}{d} = O(\log \log n)^2. \tag{3.3}$$

Proof. The left-hand side is

$$\sum_{p^j \backslash\backslash n} (\log p) \left(\frac{1}{p} + \frac{2}{p^2} + \cdots + \frac{j}{p^j} \right) \sigma_{-1}\left(\frac{n}{p^j} \right) < \sum_{\substack{p\backslash n \\ p\,\text{prime}}} \frac{4 \log p}{p} \sigma_{-1}(n),$$

where the notation $p^j \backslash\backslash n$ means that n is divisible by p^j but not by p^{j+1}, and where $\sigma_{-1}(n) = \sum_{d\backslash n} d^{-1} = \left(\sum_{d\backslash n} d \right)/n$. It is well known [3, §22.9] that $\sigma_{-1}(n) = O(\log \log n)$. □

Lemma 5.

$$\sum_{d\backslash n} \frac{\mu(d)}{d} (\log d)^2 = O(\log \log n)^2. \tag{3.4}$$

Proof. The sum is $- \sum_{\substack{p\backslash n \\ p\,\text{prime}}} \frac{(\log p)^2}{p} P(n \backslash p) + O\left(\sum_{\substack{p\backslash n \\ p\,\text{prime}}} \frac{\log p}{p} \right)^2$, and

$\sum_{p\backslash n,\, p\,\text{prime}} (\log p)^2/p = O(\log \log n)^2$ by the argument of Lemma 3. □

We shall now evaluate (2.4) step by step, beginning with the sum on k.

Lemma 6.

$$\sum_{\substack{k<x \\ \gcd(k,j)=1}} \frac{1}{k} = P(j) \ln x + O(\log \log j). \tag{3.5}$$

Proof. The sum is $\sum_{d\backslash j} \mu(d) \sum_{kd<x} \frac{1}{kd} = \sum_{d\backslash j} \frac{\mu(d)}{d} \left(\ln \frac{x}{d} + O(1) \right)$. □

Let $\mu_m(n) = (-1)^r$ if n is the product of $r \geq 0$ distinct primes, none of which divide m, otherwise $\mu_m(n) = 0$.

Lemma 7.

$$\sum_{\substack{j<x \\ \gcd(j,m)=1}} \frac{P(j\backslash d)}{j} = P(m) \ln x \sum_{\substack{r<x \\ \gcd(r,m)=1}} \frac{\mu_d(r)}{r^2} + O(\log \log m). \tag{3.6}$$

Proof. The sum is

$$\sum_{\substack{j<x \\ \gcd(j,m)=1}} \frac{1}{j} \sum_{r\backslash j} \frac{\mu_d(r)}{r} = \sum_{\substack{r<x \\ \gcd(r,m)=1}} \frac{\mu_d(r)}{r} \sum_{\substack{j<x/r \\ \gcd(j,m)=1}} \frac{1}{jr} \,;$$

apply (3.5). □

Lemma 8.

$$\sum_{\substack{j<x \\ \gcd(j,m)=1}} \frac{P(j \backslash d) \ln j}{j} = \frac{1}{2} P(m)(\ln x)^2 \sum_{\substack{r<x \\ \gcd(r,m)=1}} \frac{\mu_d(r)}{r^2}$$

$$+ O(\log \log m)^2 + O(\log x \log \log m). \quad (3.7)$$

Proof. Arguing as in Lemma 6, we have

$$\sum_{\substack{k<x \\ \gcd(k,j)=1}} \frac{\ln k}{k} = \sum_{d \backslash j} \mu(d) \sum_{kd<x} \frac{\ln kd}{kd}$$

$$= \sum_{\substack{d<x \\ d \backslash j}} \frac{\mu(d)}{d} \left(\frac{1}{2} \left(\ln \frac{x}{d} \right)^2 + \left(\ln \frac{x}{d} \right) (\ln d) + O(\log d) \right)$$

$$= \sum_{\substack{d<x \\ d \backslash j}} \frac{\mu(d)}{d} \left(\frac{(\ln x)^2 - (\ln d)^2}{2} + O(\log d) \right)$$

$$= \frac{P(j)(\ln x)^2}{2} + O(\log \log j)^2 + O(\log x \log \log j)$$

by Lemma 5. Now we can argue as in Lemma 7.   □

4. Concluding Steps

Putting the results of Section 3 into (2.4), letting N stand for $m^2/2n$, and using the fact that $P(a \backslash b)P(b) = P(ab) = P(b \backslash a)P(a)$, we have

$$\sum \left\lfloor \frac{x}{y} \right\rfloor = \sum_{m \backslash n} m \sum_{\substack{j<N \\ \gcd(j,m)=1}} \frac{P(n/m)P(j \backslash (n/m))}{j} \ln \left(\frac{N}{j} \right)$$

$$+ O(n\sigma_{-1}(n) \log n \log \log n)$$

$$= \sum_{m \backslash n} mP(n/m) \left(\frac{1}{2} P(m)(\ln N)^2 \sum_{\substack{r<N \\ \gcd(r,m)=1}} \frac{\mu_{n/m}(r)}{r^2} \right)$$

$$+ O(n \log n (\log \log n)^2)$$

$$= \frac{1}{2} \sum_{m \backslash n} mP(n/m)P(m) \left(\ln \frac{n}{2} - 2 \ln \frac{n}{m} \right)^2 \sum_{r<N} \frac{\mu_n(r)}{r^2}$$

$$+ O(n \log n (\log \log n)^2).$$

Since

$$\sum_{m\backslash n} m \log \frac{n}{m} = n \sum_{d\backslash n} \frac{\log d}{d} = O(n (\log \log n)^2)$$

by (3.3), and

$$\sum_{m\backslash n} m \left(\log \frac{n}{m}\right)^2 = n \sum_{d\backslash n} \frac{(\log d)^2}{d} = O(n \log n) \sum_{d\backslash n} \frac{\log d}{d}$$

$$= O(n \log n (\log \log n)^2),$$

we can simplify this to

$$\frac{1}{2} \sum_{m\backslash n} m P(n/m) P(m) (\ln n)^2 \sum_{r<N} \frac{\mu_n(r)}{r^2} + O(n \log n (\log \log n)^2).$$

And we can extend the sum on r to ∞, since

$$\sum_{m\backslash n} m \sum_{r\geq N} \frac{1}{r^2} \leq \sum_{\substack{m\backslash n \\ m\leq\sqrt{n}}} m \sum_{r\geq 1} \frac{1}{r^2} + \sum_{\substack{m\backslash n \\ m>\sqrt{n}}} m\, O\left(\frac{n}{m^2}\right)$$

$$= O\left(\sqrt{n} \sum_{m\backslash n} 1\right) = O(n^{\frac{1}{2}+\epsilon})$$

for all $\epsilon > 0$ by [3, §18.1]. Now

$$\sum_{r\geq 1} \frac{\mu_n(r)}{r^2} = \prod_{\substack{p\nmid n \\ p \text{ prime}}} \left(1 - \frac{1}{p^2}\right) = \frac{6}{\pi^2} \prod_{\substack{p\backslash n \\ p \text{ prime}}} \left(1 - \frac{1}{p^2}\right)^{-1}.$$

It remains to evaluate $\sum_{m\backslash n} m P(n/m) P(m)$, and since this is a multiplicative function we need only do the evaluation when $n = p^k$ and $k > 0$. In that case we obtain

$$\sum_{j=0}^{k} p^j \left(1 - \frac{1}{p}\right)^2 + (p^0 + p^k)\left(\left(1 - \frac{1}{p}\right) - \left(1 - \frac{1}{p}\right)^2\right) = p^k \left(1 - \frac{1}{p^2}\right),$$

hence

$$\sum_{m\backslash n} m P(n/m) P(m) = n \prod_{\substack{p\backslash n \\ p \text{ prime}}} \left(1 - \frac{1}{p^2}\right). \qquad (4.1)$$

Putting everything together yields

$$\sum \left\lfloor \frac{x}{y} \right\rfloor = \frac{3}{\pi^2} n (\ln n)^2 + O(n \log n \, (\log \log n)^2),$$

and this proves the theorem in view of the corollary to Lemma 1.   □

The theorem shows that the sum of all partial quotients for m/n is $O((\log n)^{2+\epsilon})$ for all but $o(n)$ values of $m \le n$, as $n \to \infty$, and this establishes a conjecture made in [4]. The application in [4] involves the sums of even-numbered and odd-numbered partial quotients separately. If $S_o(n)$ denotes the average of $q_1 + q_3 + q_5 + \cdots$ and $S_e(n)$ the average of $q_2 + q_4 + q_6 + \cdots$, it is easy to see from the relation between m/n and $(n - m)/n$ that $n(S_o(n) - S_e(n)) = n - 1$. Hence $S_o(n) \sim S_e(n) \sim 3\pi^{-2}(\ln n)^2$.

In a sense our theorem is surprising, since Khintchine [5] proved that the sum of the first k partial quotients of a real number x is asymptotically $k \log_2 k$ except for x in a set of measure zero. Thus we originally expected $S(n)$ to be of order $(\log n)(\log \log n)$ instead of $(\log n)^2$.

This research was supported in part by the National Science Foundation, the Office of Naval Research, and IBM Corporation.

References

[1] O. Becker, "Eudoxus Studien, I," *Quellen und Studien zur Geschichte der Mathematik, Astronomie und Physik* (B) **2** (1933), 311–333.

[2] Hans Heilbronn, "On the average length of a class of finite continued fractions," in *Number Theory and Analysis* (Papers in honor of Edmund Landau), edited by Paul Turán (Plenum, 1969), 87–96. Reprinted in Heilbronn's *Collected Papers* (1988), 518–525.

[3] G. H. Hardy and E. M. Wright, *An Introduction to the Theory of Numbers*, 4th edition (Oxford: Clarendon Press, 1960).

[4] D. E. Knuth, "Notes on Generalized Dedekind Sums," *Acta Arithmetica* **33** (1977), 297–325. [Reprinted as Chapter 10 of the present volume.]

[5] A. Ya. Khintchine, "Metrische Kettenbruchprobleme," *Compositio Mathematica* **1** (1935), 361–382.

Addendum

The value of $S(n)$ is, of course, influenced by the number of divisors of n, since the continued fraction for m/n is the same as the continued fraction for $(m/d)/(n/d)$ when $d = \gcd(m, n)$. We have, for example,

$n =$	10000000	10000001	10000002	10000003	10000004
$\sigma_{-1}(n) =$	2.49	1.09	2.04	1.08	2.11
$nS(n) =$	1625742939	1781148640	1669237795	1785226894	1646972073

But when we restrict consideration to prime numbers, the behavior of $S(p)$ turns out to be quite smooth:

$p =$	10000019	10000079	10000103	10000121	10000139
$pS(p) =$	1817768500	1817781215	1817788192	1817789062	1817794776

Similarly, if we restrict consideration to the average number $\widehat{S}(n)$ of subtraction steps when $1 \le m \le n$ and m is required to be relatively prime to n, the behavior is only slightly erratic:

$n =$	10000000	10000001	10000002	10000003	10000004
$\widehat{S}(n) =$	183.92	182.476	183.49	182.444	184.012

The condition $\gcd(m, n) = d$ corresponds to $\gcd(x', y') = d$ in Lemma 1.

A detailed study of the case $\gcd(m, n) = 1$ was carried out by A. A. Panov ["О средних по елементам одново класса конечных непрерывных дробей," *Uspekhi Matematicheskikh Nauk* **35**, 4 (1980), 201–202; "О среднем для суммы елементов по одному классу конечных непрерывных дробей," *Matematicheskie Zametki* **32** (1982), 593–600; English translations, "Averages over elements of a certain class of finite continued fractions," *Russian Mathematical Surveys* **35**, 4 (1980), 182–183; "Mean for the sum of elements over a class of finite continued fractions," *Mathematical Notes of the Academy of Sciences of the USSR* **32** (1982), 781–785], who proved that

$$\widehat{S}(n) = 6\pi^{-2}(\ln n)^2 + a \ln n + b + c(n) + O(n^{-\frac{1}{8}+\epsilon}),$$

where

$$\frac{e^{\gamma z}}{\zeta(2z+2)\Gamma(z+2)} = \frac{6}{\pi^2} + az + bz^2 + O(z^3)$$

and

$$c(n) = \frac{12}{\pi^2} \prod_{j=1}^{t} \frac{p_j(\ln p_j)^2}{(p_j - 1)^2}\left(1 - \frac{1}{p_j^{e_j}}\right) = O(\log n)$$

when n has the prime factorization $p_1^{e_1} \ldots p_t^{e_t}$.

Using the values

$$-\zeta'(2) = 0.93754\,82543\,15843\,75370\,25740\,94567\,86497\,78979-$$
$$\zeta''(2) = 1.98928\,02342\,98901\,02342\,08586\,87421\,51638\,14945-$$

we can evaluate Panov's constants to high precision:

$$a = 1.57374\,49203\,32491\,07890\,70569\,28048\,44170\,10544+;$$
$$-b = 1.52438\,38319\,22824\,99882\,07213\,30417\,42471\,09766+.$$

Panov also stated without proof that the average value of $q_1^k+\cdots+q_r^k$ is asymptotically $2n^{k-1}\zeta(k)^2/\zeta(2k)$, when n is prime and k is a given integer ≥ 2. This formula reduces to $5n$ when $k = 2$.

Computer calculations when the denominator n equals any of the first ten prime numbers $> 10^7$ confirm that the average value of $q_1^2 + \cdots + q_r^2$ over all possible numerators is indeed nearly $5n$, as is the average value of $(q_1+\cdots+q_r)^2$; thus the standard deviation is $\approx \sqrt{5n}$. Moreover, in all ten cases the minimum number of subtractions over the range $1 \leq m < n$ turns out to be exactly $35 = \lceil\log_\phi n\rceil + 1$, and the median number proves to be exactly 71. The maximum is, of course, $n-1$. The large variance, due to occasional large quotients, explains why the mean value is of order $(\log n)^2$ instead of order $(\log n)(\log\log n)$.

Gerald Myerson ["On semi-regular finite continued fractions," *Archiv der Mathematik* 48 (1987), 420–425] discovered that the quantity $S(n)$ arises also in another context: Suppose we form the continued fractions

$$m/n = 1/(Q_1-1/(Q_2-\cdots-1/Q_R)\cdots) = /\!/Q_1,-Q_2,\ldots,(-1)^{R-1}Q_R/\!/$$

instead of using regular continued fractions. In this case $Q_1 = \lceil n/m \rceil$ instead of $\lfloor n/m \rfloor$; and if $1 \leq m < n$ we have $Q_j \geq 2$ for $1 \leq j \leq R = R(m,n)$. Then the average value of R for $1 \leq m \leq n$ turns out to be exactly $\frac{1}{2}\left(S(n)+1+\frac{1}{n}\right)$. Moreover, the average value of $Q_1 + \cdots + Q_R$ is exactly $\frac{1}{2}\left(3S(n)+1+\frac{1}{n}\right)$. These surprisingly simple formulas follow from the easily proved facts that, if the regular continued fraction for m/n is $/\!/q_1,\ldots,q_r,1/\!/$, the sum $R(m,n)+R(n-m,n)$ is $q_1+\cdots+q_r+1$ while the sum of the Q's for m/n and $(n-m)/n$ is $3q_1 + \cdots + 3q_r + 1$, except when m/n equals $1/2$ or $1/1$.

Chapter 14

Length of Strings for a Merge Sort

[Originally published in Communications of the ACM **6** (1963), 685–688. "The author's first published analysis of an algorithm."]

Detailed statistics are given on the length of maximal sorted strings that result from the first (internal sort) phase of a merge sort onto tapes. It is shown that the strings produced by an alternating method (which produces ascending and descending strings alternately) tend to be only three-fourths as long as those in a method that produces only ascending strings, contrary to statements that have appeared previously in the literature. A slight modification of the read-backward polyphase merge algorithm is therefore suggested.

Introduction

The first pass of a tape sorting algorithm commonly takes the records that are to be sorted and distributes them onto magnetic tapes. Since the time spent by the merging process that follows is largely determined by the number of sorted substrings present after this distribution phase, it becomes advantageous to sort groups of records in the computer's internal memory during this pass, in an attempt to make the sorted substrings as long as possible.

The well-known *replacement selection* technique yields strings that are actually longer than the number of records that can be held in the computer memory. Several things have been claimed about the length of these strings in papers published on the subject, but those statements were usually made without proof. It is the purpose of this note to give detailed information about the lengths, since these lengths are an important consideration when estimating the running time required by a merge sort.

The replacement sorting technique may be described in the following way. Let m be the number of records to be sorted that can be held in the internal memory of the computer. We imagine that these memory areas are "registers," and that each of the m "registers" can be in the state "on" or "off." The algorithm is:

R1. Fill the m registers with records from the input to be sorted.

R2. Put all registers into the "on" state.

R3. Select the register that has the smallest key, of all the registers that are "on."

R4. Transfer the contents of the selected register to the output.

R5. Replace the contents of the selected register by the next input record. If the new record has a key higher than the key just transmitted, return to step R3; if the keys are equal, go to step R4; finally if the new record has a lower key, proceed to step R6.

R6. Turn the selected register "off." If all registers are now off, we are at an impasse; a sentinel record is written on the output, and we return to step R2 to begin another sorted substring. Otherwise return to step R3. □

This algorithm, as stated, never terminates; several straightforward methods can easily be devised to complete the procedure when the input is exhausted. It is usually a bit tricky to get the very last string out. The last string tends to be rather short, with length less than $\frac{1}{2}m$ on the average.

For convenience, however, we shall assume that there are an infinite number of records to be sorted. This will give formulas that need only a slight correction when the number of input records is reasonably large, say $10m$ or more. The average lengths derived will actually be very slightly smaller than the true values, for if n is any integer no matter how large, there is a finite probability that a sorted substring of length n may be taken from an infinite sequence. These extremely unlikely events are averaged into our formulas, but the correction is negligible because they have such small probability.

We will assume that all of the input records have distinct keys. Any equalities that occur will make the strings slightly longer.

The most important assumption made is that the input records are in random order. Another way to state this is that we suppose all permutations of the input keys to be equally probable. If the input is partially sorted, it will tend to produce longer strings (although if replacement selection is applied again to its own output, no change will occur).

The Effect of Changing m

Under these assumptions, let us scrutinize the algorithm carefully. As it proceeds, each of the m registers runs through a subsequence of the input. For example, suppose $m = 3$ and the input keys are 5, 2, 9, 7, 0, 8, 1, 6, 3, 4, ... The stages in the execution are

	"registers"		output
5	2	9	
5	7	9	2
0	7	9	5
0	8	9	7
0	1	9	8
0	1	6	9
3	1	6	0
3	4	6	1
	. . .		. . .

The sequences in the registers are

$$5, 0, 3, \ldots; \qquad 2, 7, 8, 1, 4, \ldots; \qquad 9, 6, \ldots$$

respectively. It is important to observe that *the original permutation can be uniquely constructed from these sequences*, merely by running through the algorithm in reverse. The set of sequences is therefore in one-to-one correspondence with the set of permutations. Moreover, the individual sequence for each register is enough to completely specify whether that register is "on" or "off." These sequences are independent of each other, by the nature of the algorithm, and each register does nothing more than act out the algorithm above for the simple case $m = 1$. Formally, if $P(n, m, k)$ denotes the probability that the nth string in an m-register algorithm has length k, we see that

$$P(n, m, k) = \sum_{j=1}^{k-1} P(n, m-1, j) P(n, 1, k-j). \tag{1}$$

This independence allows us to dispose with the general case and to consider only $m = 1$; and this simplification is extraordinarily useful, since the algorithm with $m = 1$ does not change the order of the input, and we merely need to study the "runs" in a random permutation.

Generating Functions

Exact estimates of the timing for nearly all sorting methods can be obtained rather easily by introducing *generating functions*

$$g(z) = P(0) + P(1)z + P(2)z^2 + \cdots = \sum_{k=0}^{\infty} P(k)z^k,$$

where $P(k)$ is the probability that some random variable equals k. If the generating function is given, all of the probabilities are uniquely determined, and this provides essentially the complete knowledge of the situation.

Obviously $g(1) = 1$, since it is the sum of all the probabilities. The expected value is given by a simple differentiation:

$$\text{mean}(g) = \sum_{k=0}^{\infty} kP(k) = g'(1). \tag{2}$$

All of the other moments can be obtained easily by further differentiation; for example, the variance is

$$\text{var}(g) = \sum_{k=0}^{\infty} k^2 P(k) - \text{mean}(g)^2 = g''(1) + g'(1) - g'(1)^2. \tag{3}$$

If $g(z)$ and $h(z)$ are both generating functions, elementary calculations give us simple relations for the product gh:

$$\begin{aligned} \text{mean}(gh) &= \text{mean}(g) + \text{mean}(h), \\ \text{var}(gh) &= \text{var}(g) + \text{var}(h). \end{aligned} \tag{4}$$

(Such an additive relationship will hold for all of the semi-invariants; this may be proved easily by observing that the characteristic function corresponding to a generating function is simply $\phi(t) = g(e^{it})$.)

For the purposes of this note, we will use the generating function

$$g(n, m) = P(n, m, 0) + P(n, m, 1)z + P(n, m, 2)z^2 + \cdots, \tag{5}$$

where $P(n, m, k)$ is as defined above. The independence relation (1) now tells us that

$$g(n, m) = g(n, 1)^m \tag{6}$$

and hence, by (4), we have the

Theorem. *The mean and variance of the string lengths produced by the replacement selection algorithm are proportional to m. The standard deviation is proportional to $\sqrt{m}$.*

Length of the First Three Strings

The first string is very easy to analyze. We see immediately that $P(1, 1, k)$ is just $1/(k + 1)!$ times the number of permutations on $k + 1$ elements such that

$$a_1 < a_2 < \cdots < a_k > a_{k+1}. \tag{7}$$

There are k such permutations, since there are k choices for a_{k+1} and then the remainder of the permutation is completely specified.

Hence $P(1, 1, k) = k/(k + 1)!$, and we get the generating function

$$g(1, m) = \left(\frac{e^z(z - 1) + 1}{z} \right)^m. \tag{8}$$

Turning to the second string, we have for $k \geq 1$

$$P(2, 1, k) = \sum_{r=1}^{\infty} \frac{A(k, r)}{(r + k + 1)!}, \tag{9}$$

where $A(k, r)$ is the number of permutations on $r + k + 1$ elements that have the pattern

$$a_1 < a_2 < \cdots < a_r > a_{r+1} < \cdots < a_{r+k} > a_{r+k+1}. \tag{10}$$

Questions of this kind are discussed in [3, Chapters 4 and 5]. An elementary combinatorial argument shows that

$$A(k, r) = \binom{r + k + 1}{r} k - r - k, \tag{11}$$

and by inserting this formula in (9) we find

$$P(2, 1, k) = (k(e - 1) - 1)/(k + 1)!. \tag{12}$$

The corresponding generating function is therefore

$$g(2, m) = (eg(1, 1) + 1 - e^z)^m. \tag{13}$$

The third string can be handled in a similar manner, setting

$$P(3, 1, k) = \sum_{r=2}^{\infty} \frac{B(k, r)}{(r + k + 1)!}, \tag{14}$$

where $B(k, r)$ is the number of permutations of $r + k + 1$ elements with

$$a_1 < \cdots < a_s > a_{s+1} < \cdots < a_r$$
$$> a_{r+1} < \cdots < a_{r+k} > a_{r+k+1}, \tag{15}$$

for $1 \le s < r$. The difficulties are increasing, but we can show that

$$B(k, r) = \binom{r + k + 1}{r} k (2^r - r - 1)$$
$$- \sum_{s=1}^{r} \left(\binom{r + k + 1}{r - s} (k + s) - r - k \right) \tag{16}$$

and this yields (after still more work)

$$P(3, 1, k) = \sum_{r=0}^{\infty} \frac{1}{(r + k - 1)!} + \frac{(e^2 - 2e)k - e}{(k + 1)!} - \frac{k + 1}{k!}. \tag{17}$$

The corresponding generating function can be derived from (17):

$$g(3, m) = ((1 - e)(1 - g(2, 1)) + 1 - e^z + (e - e^z)/(1 - z))^m. \tag{18}$$

Limiting Case

We could proceed to calculate the generating functions for the fourth, fifth, and further strings, but that is left as an exercise for the reader. Actually there is not much variation, and it is more fruitful to consider the limiting distribution. This can be done easily by calculating the average length of a run in a permutation of s elements. Run-length probabilities are fairly well known, since they are used in the tests for "runs up" and "runs down" that are commonly applied to pseudorandom number generators. The probability that a given run is of length r, for $1 \le r < s$, is exactly

$$2 \left(\frac{1}{(r + 2)!} - \frac{2}{(r + 1)!} + \frac{1}{r!} \right) - \frac{2}{s + 1} \left(\frac{1}{(r + 1)!} - \frac{2}{r!} + \frac{1}{(r - 1)!} \right). \tag{19}$$

This formula may be obtained by counting all the runs of length r among the $s!$ permutations, and dividing by $(s+1)!/2$, the total number of runs.

As s approaches infinity, the second term of (19) may be neglected, and we obtain

$$P(\infty, 1, k) = 2\big(1/(k + 2)! - 2/(k + 1)! + 1/k!\big). \tag{20}$$

The corresponding generating function is

$$g(\infty, m) = \big(2(1 - 1/z)g(1, 1) + 1\big)^m. \tag{21}$$

Alternating Directions

When preparing for a "read-backward polyphase merge" [2], the replacement selection algorithm is modified so that each time we reach step R2 we reverse the direction so that the 1st, 3rd, 5th, ... strings are in *ascending* order, while the 2nd, 4th, 6th, ... are in *descending* order.

Let $h(n, m)$ and $Q(n, m, k)$ correspond to $g(n, m)$ and $P(n, m, k)$ in the discussion above. Clearly the length of the *first* string is unaffected. But when we attack the *second* string, we find for $k \geq 1$,

$$Q(2, 1, k) = \sum_{r=1}^{\infty} \frac{C(r, k)}{(r + k + 1)!}, \tag{22}$$

where $C(r, k)$ is the number of permutations with

$$a_1 < \cdots < a_r > a_{r+1} > \cdots > a_{r+k} < a_{r+k+1}. \tag{23}$$

Here either a_r or a_{r+k+1} must be the largest element, hence

$$C(r, k) = \binom{r + k}{r - 1} k + \binom{r + k - 1}{r - 1}. \tag{24}$$

Some rather involved summations of infinite series can now be carried out, giving

$$Q(2, 1, k) = 2R_{k+1}/k! - e/(k + 1)!, \tag{25}$$

where

$$R_t = \sum_{s=0}^{\infty} \frac{1}{(s + t)s!}, \tag{26}$$

and we find

$$R_{t+1} = (-1)^t t! \left(e \left(1 - 1 + \frac{1}{2!} - \cdots \pm \frac{1}{t!} \right) - 1 \right), \tag{27}$$

leading at last to the generating function

$$h(2, m) = \left(\frac{2}{1 + z} (e^{1+z} + z) - \frac{e}{z} (e^z - 1 + z) \right)^m. \tag{28}$$

The *limiting* distribution for the alternating method is somewhat simpler. In a long permutation (discarding the first string) we find that the *ascending* runs of length r for the alternating algorithm are precisely the ascending runs of length $r + 1$ in the straight algorithm. The *descending* runs of length r are in the same place as the descending runs of length $r+1$ in a pure descending algorithm. Therefore, for $k \geq 1$, we find

$$
\begin{aligned}
Q(\infty, 1, k) &= P(\infty, 1, k+1)/(1 - P(\infty, 1, 1)) \\
&= \tfrac{3}{2} P(\infty, 1, k+1)
\end{aligned}
\tag{29}
$$

since $P(\infty, 1, 1) = \tfrac{1}{3}$. The generating function is therefore

$$
h(\infty, m) = \left(\tfrac{3}{2} (g(\infty, 1)/z - \tfrac{1}{3}) \right)^m .
\tag{30}
$$

Summary of Results

The generating functions (8), (13), (18), (21), (28), (30) derived above can be used to calculate, in particular, the mean and variance, using equations (2) and (3). (The functions as written sometimes have a denominator of $1 - z$, so they are not defined for $z = 1$; but they are actually all entire functions so it is a simple matter to calculate the limits as $z \to 1$ using L'Hospital's rule.)

We find the following *expected length of strings*:

first string	$(e - 1)m$	$\approx 1.718\,m$
second string	$(e^2 - 2e)m$	$\approx 1.952\,m$
third string	$(e^3 - 3e^2 + \tfrac{3}{2}e)m$	$\approx 1.996\,m$
limiting case	$2m$	$= 2.000\,m$

It is clear from this data that the length rapidly approaches $2m$ after the first string. The expected length of these strings has already been derived by B. J. Gassner [1], who gave the following formula for the average length of the jth string:

$$
jm \sum_{r=1}^{j} \frac{(-1)^{j-r} e^r r^{j-r-1}}{(j-r)!}, \quad j > 1.
$$

The reader may be surprised at first that the behavior of subsequent strings is different from the behavior of the first string. A simple interpretation accounts for this fact: The numbers in the "off" registers, as we prepare to begin the second string, tend to be lower than normal, since they were the "step-downs" that caused the register to go "off."

This is a desirable effect, since the second string will have lower values to begin with and thus a better chance to reach a longer string. The third string enjoys an even better beginning.

The *variances* of these expected values are as follows:

first string	$(-e^2 + 3e)m$	$\approx 0.766\,m$
second string	$(-e^4 + 4e^3 - 3e^2 - e)m$	$\approx 0.859\,m$
third string	$(-e^6 + 6e^5 - 12e^4 + 10e^3 - \frac{17}{4}e^2 - \frac{1}{6}e)m$	$\approx 0.871\,m$
limiting case	$(4e - 10)m$	$\approx 0.873\,m$

The square roots of these values (namely the standard deviations) are small compared to the mean, at least with reasonable sizes of m.

The expected lengths with alternating directions are:

first string	$(e - 1)m$	$\approx 1.718\,m$
second string	$(\frac{1}{2}e^2 - e + \frac{1}{2})m$	$\approx 1.476\,m$
limiting case	$\frac{3}{2}m$	$= 1.500\,m$

with the following variances:

first string	$(3e - e^2)m$	$\approx 0.766\,m$
second string	$(-e^4 + e^3 - \frac{3}{2}e^2 + 2e - \frac{1}{4})m$	$\approx 0.539\,m$
limiting case	$(6e - \frac{63}{4})m$	$\approx 0.560\,m$

The smaller average length in this case is exactly what we would expect, since the distribution at the beginning of the second string, biased towards low elements as mentioned above, works *against* a descending string, and the distribution at the beginning of the third string works against the chances of a long ascending string, etc. Therefore we obtain strings of length only 1.5m, rather than $2m - 1$ as was claimed in [2].

It is possible to avoid this difficulty somewhat, by designing an algorithm that produces as many strings in a single direction as possible before switching directions; this will tend to give strings of length $2m$, except some of length 1.5m when changing directions. If T is the total number of merge tapes, the shorter strings would then occur approximately $1/(T-1)$ of the time; thus the expected length when using such an algorithm would be nearly $\left(2 - 1/(2(T-1))\right)m$.

References

[1] Betty Jane Gassner, "Sorting by replacement selecting," *Communications of the ACM* **10** (1967), 89–93.

[2] R. L. Gilstad, "Read-backward polyphase sorting," *Communications of the ACM* **6** (1963), 220–223.

[3] P. A. MacMahon, *Combinatory Analysis* **1** (Cambridge: The University Press, 1915).

Addendum

Sequences of ordered records in a merge sort were conventionally called "strings" when this paper was written in 1963, but they are now more often called "runs." Further details about the subject of this paper, developed after 1963, can be found in exercises 5.1.3–11 and 5.4.1–24 of *The Art of Computer Programming*, Volume 3.

The heuristic analysis in the final paragraph of the paper is incorrect. For example, after a long sequence of ascending runs has been produced, the approximate average length of the first subsequent descending run will be not $1.5m$ but $(2e-4)m \approx 1.437m$. A second descending run will then have approximate length $(2e^2-4e-2)m \approx 1.905m$, etc. If runs are produced in a pattern A, A, D, D, A, A, D, D, ..., always switching to the opposite direction after two consecutive runs have been generated in one direction, the average run lengths tend to be alternately

$$\frac{2t}{1+t}m \approx 1.442m \qquad \text{and} \qquad \frac{12-2t}{1+t}m \approx 1.907m,$$

where $t = 3\sqrt{2}\tanh(1/\sqrt{2})$. (These results follow from the methods of exercise 5.4.1–24.)

Chapter 15

The Average Height of
Planted Plane Trees

[Written with N. G. de Bruijn and S. O. Rice. Originally published in Graph Theory and Computing, edited by R. C. Read (Academic Press, 1972), 15–22.]

A *planted plane tree*, sometimes called an ordered tree, is a rooted tree that has been embedded in the plane; thus the relative order of subtrees at each branch is part of its structure. In this paper we shall say simply *tree* instead of *planted plane tree*, following the custom of computer scientists.

The *height* of a tree is the number of nodes on a maximal simple path starting at the root. For example, there are exactly five trees with five nodes and height 4, namely

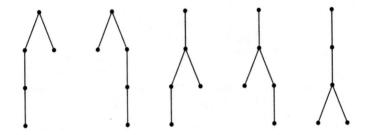

A tree's height is of interest in computing because it represents the maximum size of a stack used in algorithms that traverse the tree [3, Section 2.3.1]. Our goal in this paper is to study the average height of a tree with n nodes, assuming that all n-node trees are equally likely. The corresponding problem for *oriented trees* (that is, rooted but unordered trees) has been solved by Rényi and Szekeres [6]. Our principal results are stated in equations (32) and (34).

215

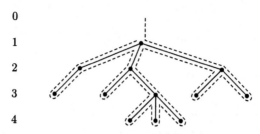

FIGURE 1. A tree as a random walk.

Trees appear in many disguises, and in particular there is a natural correspondence between trees of height less than or equal to h and discrete random walks in a straight line, with absorbing barriers at 0 and $h + 1$. If we wander around a tree with n nodes, as shown by the dotted lines in Figure 1, the vertical component of successive positions describes a path of length $2n - 1$ from 1 to 0. For example, the path in Figure 1 is

$$1, 2, 3, 2, 1, 2, 3, 2, 3, 4, 3, 4, 3, 4, 3, 2, 1, 2, 3, 2, 3, 2, 1, 0;$$

it is one way that a gambler can lose \$1 before winning \$5. This construction, suggested by Harris [2] in 1952, is clearly reversible.

The height of trees plays a similar role in the classical ballot problem. How many ways are there to arrange n ballots for candidate A and n for candidate B in a sequence so that the number of votes for A never lags behind the number for B as the ballots are counted, but A is never more than h votes ahead? The answer is the number of trees with $n + 1$ nodes and height less than or equal to $h + 1$, again by the construction indicated in Figure 1. The ballot sequence corresponding to that tree is AABBAABAABABABBBAABABB.

We shall begin our study of the asymptotic properties of height by reviewing some known results. Let A_{nh} be the number of trees with n nodes and height less than or equal to h, and let

$$A_h(z) = \sum_n A_{nh} z^n \tag{1}$$

be the corresponding generating function. We obtain all trees with height less than or equal to $h + 1$ by taking a root node and attaching zero or more subtrees each of which has height less than or equal to h. Therefore,

$$\begin{aligned} A_{h+1}(z) &= z(1 + A_h(z) + A_h(z)^2 + A_h(z)^3 + \cdots) \\ &= z/(1 - A_h(z)), \qquad \text{for all } h \geq 0. \end{aligned} \tag{2}$$

$n = 1$	2	3	4	5	6	7	8	9	10	11	12
$h = 1$	1	0	0	0	0	0	0	0	0	0	0	0
2	1	1	1	1	1	1	1	1	1	1	1	1
3	1	1	2	4	8	16	32	64	128	256	512	1024
4	1	1	2	5	13	34	89	233	610	1597	4181	10946
5	1	1	2	5	14	41	122	365	1094	3281	9842	29525
6	1	1	2	5	14	42	131	417	1341	4334	14041	45542

TABLE 1. Trees with n nodes and height $\leq h$.

Clearly $A_0(z) = 0$. Relation (2) yields a simple recurrence for the numbers A_{nh}, namely

$$A_{n,h+1} = A_{n-1,h+1} A_{1,h} + A_{n-2,h+1} A_{2,h} + \cdots + A_{1,h+1} A_{n-1,h} \quad (3)$$

for $n \geq 2$ and $h \geq 0$; thus we can easily calculate the first few values, as shown in Table 1. Since no tree with n nodes can have a height greater than n, we have

$$A_{nh} = A_{nn} = \binom{2n-2}{n-1}\frac{1}{n}, \qquad \text{for all } h \geq n; \quad (4)$$

this is the well-known formula for the total number of trees with n nodes [3, Section 2.3.4.4].

Iteration of (2) yields a continued fraction representation of $A_h(z)$. For example,

$$A_4(z) = \cfrac{z}{1 - \cfrac{z}{1 - \cfrac{z}{1 - z}}}. \quad (5)$$

This form suggests expressing the generating function as a quotient of polynomials

$$A_h(z) = zp_h(z)/p_{h+1}(z), \quad (6)$$

where

$$p_0(z) = 0, \qquad p_1(z) = 1, \qquad p_{h+1}(z) = p_h(z) - zp_{h-1}(z). \quad (7)$$

The solution to recurrence (7) is

$$p_h(z) = (1 - 4z)^{-\frac{1}{2}} \left(\left(\frac{1 + (1 - 4z)^{\frac{1}{2}}}{2} \right)^h - \left(\frac{1 - (1 - 4z)^{\frac{1}{2}}}{2} \right)^h \right), \quad (8)$$

and the form of this solution suggests setting $z = 1/(4\cos^2\theta)$. We obtain

$$p_h\big((4\cos^2\theta)^{-1}\big) = \sin h\theta \big/ \big((2\cos\theta)^{h-1}\sin\theta\big). \tag{9}$$

Incidentally it is easy to verify that $p_h(-1)$ is the Fibonacci number F_h, and that

$$p_h(z) = \sum_{0 \le k < h} \binom{h-1-k}{k}(-z)^k, \qquad h \ge 1. \tag{10}$$

This leads to another recurrence for the numbers A_{nh}.

Since $p_h(z)^2 - p_{h+1}(z)\,p_{h-1}(z) = z^{h-1}$, there is a simple generating function for the number of trees with n nodes and height exactly h,

$$A_h(z) - A_{h-1}(z) = z^h / p_{h+1}(z)\,p_h(z). \tag{11}$$

This formula was recently derived by Kreweras [4, page 37].

The polynomial p_h has degree $\lfloor (h-1)/2 \rfloor$, and by (9) the roots of $p_h(z) = 0$ are $(4\cos^2(j\pi/h))^{-1}$, for $1 \le j < h/2$. Hence we obtain a partial fraction expansion of the generating function

$$A_h(z) = \sum_{1 \le j \le h/2} \frac{\tan^2\theta_{jh}}{(h+1)(1 - (4\cos^2\theta_{jh})z)} + a_h + b_h z, \tag{12}$$

where $\theta_{jh} = j\pi/(h+1)$ and

$$a_{2m} = -m, \qquad\qquad b_{2m} = 0,$$
$$a_{2m+1} = \frac{-m(2m+1)}{6(m+1)}, \qquad b_{2m+1} = \frac{1}{m+1}. \tag{13}$$

This representation leads immediately to the explicit formula

$$A_{nh} = \frac{4^n}{h+1} \sum_{1 \le j \le h/2} \sin^2\!\left(\frac{j\pi}{h+1}\right) \cos^{2n-2}\!\left(\frac{j\pi}{h+1}\right), \qquad n \ge 2. \tag{14}$$

It is quite remarkable that this formula gives a constant value for fixed n and all $h \ge n$. It is perhaps even more remarkable that Lagrange [5, §62] derived a formula in 1775 that essentially includes this one as a special case. Feller [1, §XIV.5] observes that the formula has been rediscovered many times, although it appears in many texts on probability in connection with the equivalent gambler's ruin problem. As a special case of (14) we have the asymptotic formula

$$A_{nh} \sim \frac{4^n}{h+1} \tan^2\left(\frac{\pi}{h+1}\right) \cos^{2n}\left(\frac{\pi}{h+1}\right), \quad \text{fixed } h, \ n \to \infty. \quad (15)$$

Another interesting expression for A_{nh} can be derived by applying complex variable theory. We have

$$A_{nh} = \frac{1}{2\pi i} \oint \frac{dz}{z^{n+1}} A_h(z)$$
$$= \frac{1}{2\pi i} \oint \frac{dz}{z^n}(1+u)\frac{1-u^h}{1-u^{h+1}}, \quad (16)$$

where

$$u = \frac{1-(1-4z)^{\frac{1}{2}}}{1+(1-4z)^{\frac{1}{2}}}, \quad (17)$$

by (6) and (8). Since

$$z = u/(1+u)^2 \quad (18)$$

we have $u \approx z$ when $|z| \ll 1$. Hence we may change variables in (16) to obtain

$$A_{nh} = \frac{1}{2\pi i} \oint \frac{du}{u^n}(1-u)(1+u)^{2n-2}\frac{1-u^h}{1-u^{h+1}}. \quad (19)$$

In other words A_{nh} is the coefficient of u^{n-1} in the expression $(1-u)(1+u)^{2n-2}(1-u^h)/(1-u^{h+1})$. Some simplification now occurs when we consider the number of trees with height *greater* than h,

$$B_{nh} = A_{nn} - A_{nh}$$
$$= \frac{1}{2\pi i} \oint \frac{du}{u^{n+1}}(1-u)^2(1+u)^{2n-2}\frac{u^{h+1}}{1-u^{h+1}}. \quad (20)$$

It follows that

$$B_{n+1,h-1} = \sum_{k\geq 1}\left(\binom{2n}{n+1-kh} - 2\binom{2n}{n-kh} + \binom{2n}{n-1-kh}\right). \quad (21)$$

The *average height* of a tree with n nodes is S_n/A_{nn}, where S_n is the finite sum

$$
\begin{aligned}
S_n &= \sum_{h \geq 1} h(A_{nh} - A_{n,h-1}) \\
&= \sum_{h \geq 1} h(B_{n,h-1} - B_{nh}) \\
&= \sum_{h \geq 0} B_{nh} \\
&= \frac{1}{2\pi i} \oint \frac{du}{u^{n+1}} (1-u)^2 (1+u)^{2n-2} \sum_{h \geq 1} \frac{u^h}{1-u^h} \\
&= \frac{1}{2\pi i} \oint \frac{du}{u^{n+1}} (1-u)^2 (1+u)^{2n-2} \sum_{h \geq 1} d(k) u^k. \qquad (22)
\end{aligned}
$$

As usual, $d(k)$ denotes the number of positive divisors of k. Therefore,

$$
S_{n+1} = \sum_{k \geq 1} d(k) \left(\binom{2n}{n+1-k} - 2\binom{2n}{n-k} + \binom{2n}{n-1-k} \right). \qquad (23)
$$

We shall now proceed to obtain an asymptotic series for the sum

$$
f_a(n) = \sum_{k \geq 1} d(k) \binom{2n}{n+a-k} \Big/ \binom{2n}{n}, \qquad \text{fixed } a, \quad n \to \infty; \qquad (24)
$$

this will lead to an asymptotic series for S_n.

Let $x = (k-a)/n$. By Stirling's approximation we have

$$
\binom{2n}{n+a-k} \Big/ \binom{2n}{n} = \exp\left(-2n \left(\frac{x^2}{1 \cdot 2} + \frac{x^4}{3 \cdot 4} + \cdots \right) \right.
$$
$$
+ \left(\frac{x^2}{2} + \frac{x^4}{4} + \cdots \right)
$$
$$
\left. - \frac{x^2 + x^4 + \cdots}{6n} + O(x^2 n^{-3}) \right) \qquad (25)
$$

when $-\frac{1}{2} < x < \frac{1}{2}$; and

$$
\binom{2n}{n+a-k} \Big/ \binom{2n}{n} = O(\exp(-n^{2\epsilon}))
$$

when $k \geq n^{\frac{1}{2}+\epsilon} + a$, for all fixed $\epsilon > 0$. Therefore the sum of all terms in (24) for $k \geq n^{\frac{1}{2}+\epsilon} + a$ is negligible, being $O(n^{-m})$ for all $m > 0$, and we may take $x = O(n^{-\frac{1}{2}+\epsilon})$ in (25).

We now turn to the asymptotic behavior of the function

$$g_b(n) = \sum_{k \geq 1} k^b d(k) \exp(-k^2/n), \qquad \text{fixed } b, \quad n \to \infty. \qquad (26)$$

Again the terms for $k \geq n^{\frac{1}{2}+\epsilon}$ are negligible, so we can use (25) to express f in terms of g:

$$f_a(n) = g_0(n) + \frac{2a}{n} g_1(n) - \frac{a^2}{n} g_0(n) + \frac{4a^2 + 1}{2n^2} g_2(n) - \frac{1}{6n^3} g_4(n)$$
$$- \frac{2a^3 + a}{n^2} g_1(n) + \frac{4a^3 + 5a}{3n^3} g_3(n) - \frac{a}{3n^4} g_5(n)$$
$$+ O(n^{-2+\epsilon} g_0(n)). \qquad (27)$$

In principle such an expansion could be carried out as far as we like. Hence, the problem of obtaining an asymptotic expansion for $f_a(n)$ reduces to the analogous problem for $g_b(n)$.

The behavior of $g_b(n)$ can be derived by starting with the well-known formula

$$e^{-x} = \frac{1}{2\pi i} \int_{c-i\infty}^{c+i\infty} \Gamma(z) x^{-z} dz, \qquad c > 0, \quad x > 1, \qquad (28)$$

obtained, for example, by Fourier inversion of $\Gamma(c + 2\pi i t)$. Then since $\zeta(z)^2 = \sum_{k \geq 1} d(k)/k^z$, we find

$$g_b(n) = \sum_{k \geq 1} \frac{1}{2\pi i} \int_{c-i\infty}^{c+i\infty} n^z \Gamma(z) k^{b-2z} d(k) \, dz$$
$$= \frac{1}{2\pi i} \int_{c-i\infty}^{c+i\infty} n^z \Gamma(z) \zeta(2z - b)^2 \, dz, \qquad (29)$$

where now $c > \frac{1}{2}(b+1)$. Let q be a fixed positive number. When the real part of s exceeds $-q$, we have $\zeta(s) = O(|s|^{q+\frac{1}{2}})$ as $s \to \infty$. Since $n^z \Gamma(z)$ gets small on vertical lines we can shift the line of integration to the left as far as we please, as long as we take the residues into account. There is a double pole at $z = \frac{1}{2}(b+1)$, and possibly some simple poles at $z = 0, -1, -2, \ldots$. Letting $w = z - \frac{1}{2}(b+1)$, we have

$$n^z \Gamma(z) \zeta(2z - b)^2 = n^{(b+1)/2} \Gamma\left(\frac{b+1}{2}\right) (1 + w \ln n + O(w^2))$$
$$\times \left(1 + w\psi\left(\frac{b+1}{2}\right) + O(w^2)\right)\left(\frac{1}{2w} + \frac{\gamma}{w} + O(1)\right),$$

where $\psi(z) = \Gamma'(z)/\Gamma(z)$; hence the residue at the double pole is

$$n^{\frac{1}{2}(b+1)}\Gamma(\tfrac{1}{2}(b+1))(\tfrac{1}{4}\ln n + \tfrac{1}{4}\psi(\tfrac{1}{2}(b+1)) + \gamma). \tag{30}$$

The residue at $z = -k$ is

$$n^{-k}(-1)^k\zeta(-2k-b)^2/k! = n^{-k}(-1)^k B_{2k+b+1}^2/\big((2k+b+1)^2 k!\big), \tag{31}$$

which is almost always zero when b is even. The sum of (30) and (31) for all $k \geq 0$ gives an asymptotic series for $g_b(n)$. Hence we have, for all $m > 0$,

$$g_0(n) = \tfrac{1}{4}(\pi n)^{\frac{1}{2}}\ln n + (\tfrac{3}{4}\gamma - \tfrac{1}{2}\ln 2)(\pi n)^{\frac{1}{2}} + \tfrac{1}{4} + O(n^{-m});$$

$$g_1(n) = \tfrac{1}{4}n\ln n + \tfrac{3}{4}\gamma n + \tfrac{1}{144} - \tfrac{1}{14400}n^{-1} + O(n^{-2}); \tag{32}$$

$$g_2(n) = \tfrac{1}{8}n(\pi n)^{\frac{1}{2}}\ln n + (\tfrac{1}{4} + \tfrac{3}{8}\gamma - \tfrac{1}{4}\ln 2)n(\pi n)^{\frac{1}{2}} + O(n^{-m});$$

etc. These formulas have been verified by computer calculation. For example, when $n = 10$ we have $g_0(n) \approx 3.9604175$ and $\tfrac{1}{4}(\pi n)^{\frac{1}{2}}\ln n + (\tfrac{3}{4}\gamma - \tfrac{1}{2}\ln 2)(\pi n)^{\frac{1}{2}} + \tfrac{1}{4} \approx 3.9604169$.

Returning to our original problem about trees, we have

$$\frac{S_{n+1}}{(n+1)A_{n+1,n+1}} = f_1(n) - 2f_0(n) + f_{-1}(n)$$

$$= \frac{-2g_0(n)}{n} + \frac{4g_2(n)}{n^2} + O(n^{-\frac{3}{2}}\log n) \tag{33}$$

by (4), (23), (24), and (27); and this is equal to $(\pi/n)^{-\frac{1}{2}} - \tfrac{1}{2}n^{-1} + O(n^{-\frac{3}{2}}\log n)$. We have proved the following result.

Theorem. *The average height of a planted plane tree with n nodes, considering all such trees to be equally likely, is*

$$(\pi n)^{\frac{1}{2}} - \tfrac{1}{2} + O(n^{-\frac{1}{2}}\log n). \qquad \square \tag{34}$$

The same method can be used to obtain as many further terms of the expansion as desired. The factor $\log n$ in the error term turns out to be unnecessary.

We wish to thank Dr. John Riordan for pointing out references [2] and [4]. This research was supported in part by the National Science Foundation and the Office of Naval Research.

References

[1] William Feller, *An Introduction to Probability Theory and Its Applications*, Volume 1, second edition (New York: Wiley, 1957).

[2] T. E. Harris, "First passage and recurrence distributions," *Transactions of the American Mathematical Society* **73** (1952), 471–486.

[3] Donald E. Knuth, *Fundamental Algorithms*, Volume 1 of *The Art of Computer Programming* (Reading, Massachusetts: Addison–Wesley, 1968).

[4] G. Kreweras, "Sur les eventails de segments," *Cahiers du Bureau Universitaire de Recherche Operationelle* **15** (1970), 1–41.

[5] de la Grange [J. L. Lagrange], "Recherches sur les suites récurrentes dont les termes varient de plusieurs manières différentes, ou sur l'intégration des équations linéaires aux différences finies & partielles; & sur l'usage de ces équations dans la théorie des hazards," *Nouveaux Mémoires de l'Académie royale des Sciences et Belles-Lettres*, Berlin (1775), 183–272. Reprinted in Œuvres de Lagrange **4** (Paris: 1869), 149–251.

[6] A. Rényi and G. Szekeres, "On the height of trees," *Journal of the Australian Mathematical Society* **7** (1967), 497–507.

[7] J. Riordan, "The enumeration of trees by height and diameter," *IBM Journal of Research and Development* **4** (1960), 473–478.

[8] John Riordan, "Ballots and trees," *Journal of Combinatorial Theory* **6** (1969), 408–411.

Addendum

The quantities $g_b(n)$ for odd b do not arise in formula (33) because they occur only with odd powers of a in (27). This observation holds in general when we seek further terms in the expansion of (34); we find, for example,

$$\frac{S_n}{A_{nn}} = (\pi n)^{\frac{1}{2}} - \frac{1}{2} - \frac{25}{24}\left(\frac{\pi}{n}\right)^{\frac{1}{2}} + \frac{1}{2n} + \frac{101}{5760}\left(\frac{\pi}{n^3}\right)^{\frac{1}{2}} + O(n^{-\frac{5}{2}}).$$

Chapter 16

The Toilet Paper Problem

[Originally published in the American Mathematical Monthly **91** *(1984), 465–470.]*

1. Introduction

The toilet paper dispensers in a certain building are designed to hold two rolls of tissues, and a person can use either roll.

There are two kinds of people who use the rest rooms in the building: *big-choosers* and *little-choosers*. A big-chooser always takes a piece of toilet paper from the roll that is currently larger; a little-chooser always does the opposite. However, when the two rolls are the same size, or when only one roll is nonempty, everybody chooses the nearest nonempty roll. When both rolls are empty, everybody has a problem.

Let us assume that people enter the toilet stalls independently at random, with probability p that they are big-choosers and probability $q = 1 - p$ that they are little-choosers. If the janitor supplies a particular stall with two fresh rolls of toilet paper, both of length n, let $M_n(p)$ be the average number of portions left on one roll when the other roll first empties. (We assume that everyone uses the same amount of paper, and that the lengths are expressed in terms of this unit.) For example, it is easy to establish that $M_1(p) = 1$, $M_2(p) = 2-p$, $M_3(p) = 3-2p-p^2+p^3$; $M_n(0) = n$; $M_n(1) = 1$.

The purpose of this paper is to study the asymptotic value of $M_n(p)$ for fixed p as n approaches ∞. We will see that the generating function $\sum_n M_n(p)\, z^n$ has a surprisingly simple form, from which the asymptotic behavior can readily be deduced. Along the way we will encounter several other interesting facts.

225

2. Recurrence Relations

Let us begin by generalizing the problem slightly, using the notation $M_{mn}(p)$ to stand for the mean number of portions left when one roll empties if we start with m on one roll and n on the other. Thus

$$M_n(p) = M_{nn}(p)\,;$$
$$M_{m0}(p) = m\,;$$
$$M_{nn}(p) = M_{n(n-1)}(p)\,, \qquad \text{if} \quad n > 0\,;$$
$$M_{mn}(p) = p\,M_{(m-1)n}(p) + q\,M_{m(n-1)}(p)\,, \qquad \text{if} \quad m > n > 0\,.$$

The value of $M_n(p)$ can be computed for all n from these recurrence relations, since no pairs (m, n) with $m < n$ will arise.

It is convenient to visualize the recurrence by drawing certain arcs between adjacent lattice points in the plane, where the arc from (m, n) to $(m-1, n)$ has weight p and from (m, n) to $(m, n-1)$ has weight q, for all $0 < n < m$; the arc from (n, n) to $(n, n-1)$ has weight 1 for all $n > 0$; and there are no other arcs. Then $M_{mn}(p)$ is the sum, over all $k \geq 1$, of k times the sum of the weights of all paths from (m, n) to $(k, 0)$, where the weight of a path is the product of the individual arc weights.

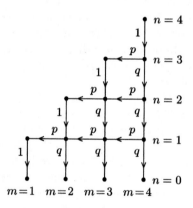

A path that starts at the diagonal point (n, n) must go first to $(n, n-1)$; then it either returns to the diagonal at $(n-1, n-1)$ or goes to $(n, n-2)$, etc. Let c_k be the number of paths from (n, n) to $(n-k, n-k)$ whose intermediate points do not touch the diagonal, and let d_{nk} be the number of paths from $(n, n-1)$ to $(k, 1)$, whose points do not ever touch the diagonal. A path that starts at (n, n) either returns to the diagonal for the first time at some point $(n-k, n-k)$, or never returns to the diagonal at all; consequently

$$M_n(p) = c_1 p\, M_{n-1}(p) + c_2 p^2 q\, M_{n-2}(p) + \cdots$$
$$+ c_{n-1} p^{n-1} q^{n-2}\, M_1(p) + L_n(p)$$
$$= \sum_{0<k<n} c_k p^k q^{k-1}\, M_{n-k}(p) + L_n(p);$$
$$L_n(p) = \sum_{2\le k\le n} k\, d_{nk} p^{n-k} q^{n-1}, \qquad \text{for } n \ge 2; \qquad L_1(p) = 1.$$

(Each path from (n, n) to $(n - k, n - k)$ has weight $p^k q^{k-1}$ if no intermediate diagonal points are involved, since the step to $(n, n - 1)$ has weight 1 and then there are k steps of weight p and $k - 1$ of weight q, in some order. Similarly, each diagonal-avoiding path from $(n, n - 1)$ to $(k, 1)$ has weight $p^{n-k} q^{n-2}$.)

The coefficients c_k are the well-known Catalan numbers, and the coefficients d_{nk} are the well-known numbers that arise in the classical ballot problem; see, for example, [2, §III.1] and [3, exercise 2.2.1–4]. We can discover the required values by observing that d_{nk} is the number of decreasing paths from $(n, n-1)$ to $(k, 1)$ minus the number of decreasing paths from $(n, n - 1)$ to $(1, k)$, where a "decreasing path" is any path that decreases either the left component or the right component by unity at each step. This follows because there is a one-to-one correspondence between all decreasing paths from $(n, n - 1)$ to $(k, 1)$ that do touch the diagonal and all decreasing paths from $(n, n - 1)$ to $(1, k)$; the idea [1] is to reflect the path about the diagonal, starting after the place where it first touches a diagonal point. Since the number of decreasing paths from (a, b) to (c, d) is $\binom{a+b-c-d}{a-c} = \binom{a+b-c-d}{b-d}$ for all $a \ge c$ and $b \ge d$, we have

$$d_{nk} = \binom{2n - k - 2}{n - 2} - \binom{2n - k - 2}{n - 1} = \binom{2n - k - 2}{n - 2} \frac{k - 1}{n - 1}.$$

Furthermore $c_{n-1} = d_{n2}$, hence

$$c_n = \binom{2n - 2}{n - 1} \frac{1}{n}.$$

3. Special Power Series

The generating function for Catalan numbers,

$$C(z) = c_1 z + c_2 z^2 + \cdots = \sum_{n \geq 1} \binom{2n-2}{n-1} \frac{1}{n} z^n = \frac{1 - \sqrt{1-4z}}{2},$$

can be derived in many ways. For our purposes it seems best to make use of the general identity

$$\sum_{k \geq 0} \binom{2k+w}{k} z^k = \frac{1}{\sqrt{1-4z}} \left(\frac{1 - \sqrt{1-4z}}{2z} \right)^w. \qquad (*)$$

This well-known identity, which holds for all complex numbers w, can be proved easily by contour integration: The coefficient of z^k in the Maclaurin expansion of the right-hand side is

$$\frac{1}{2\pi i} \oint \frac{1}{\sqrt{1-4z}} \left(\frac{1 - \sqrt{1-4z}}{2z} \right)^w \frac{dz}{z^{k+1}} = \frac{1}{2\pi i} \oint \frac{dt}{(1-t)^{w+k+1} t^{k+1}}$$

if we make the substitutions $t = \frac{1}{2}(1 - \sqrt{1-4z})$, $z = t - t^2$, $dz = (1 - 2t)\, dt$. The latter integral is the residue of the integrand, namely the coefficient of t^k in $(1-t)^{-w-k-1}$, namely $\binom{-w-k-1}{k}(-1)^k = \binom{2k+w}{k}$. (A more elementary proof can be found in [3, exercise 1.2.6–26].)

The derivative of $C(z)/z$ with respect to z is

$$C(z)^2/(z^2\sqrt{1-4z});$$

hence we can replace w by $w+1$ in $(*)$ and integrate, obtaining the companion formula

$$\sum_{k \geq 0} \frac{w}{k+w} \binom{2k+w-1}{k} z^k = \left(\frac{1 - \sqrt{1-4z}}{2z} \right)^w.$$

Again, this result is valid for all complex w, if we evaluate the coefficient by continuity when $k + w = 0$. The case $w = 1$ of this formula reduces to the generating function for Catalan numbers stated earlier.

These power series converge for $|z| < 1/4$, because the right-hand side is singular only when z is infinite or $\sqrt{1-4z}$ is singular. A curious thing happens when $z = pq$, $p \geq 0$, $q \geq 0$, and $p+q = 1$: In this case we have $1 - 4z = (p-q)^2$, hence $\sqrt{1-4z} = |p-q| = \max(p,q) - \min(p,q)$, and we obtain the interesting formula

$$C(pq) = \sum_{n \geq 1} \binom{2n-2}{n-1} \frac{1}{n} p^n q^n = \min(p,q).$$

The product pq is always less than $1/4$ unless $p = q = 1/2$; the formula holds also in the latter case, by Abel's limit theorem.

4. Generating Functions

Let us now set

$$M(z) = \sum_{n \geq 1} M_n(p) z^n \,; \qquad L(z) = \sum_{n \geq 1} L_n(p) z^n \,.$$

The recurrence relation for $M_n(p)$ in Section 2 is equivalent to

$$M(z) - L(z) = q^{-1} C(pqz) M(z) \,,$$

and we also have

$$L(z) = z + \sum_{2 \leq k \leq n} \frac{q^{n-1}}{n-1} k(k-1) p^{n-k} \binom{2n-k-2}{n-2} z^n$$

$$= \sum_{j,k \geq 0} \frac{q^{j+k-1}}{j+k-1} k(k-1) p^j \binom{2j+k-2}{j} z^{j+k}$$

$$= \sum_{k \geq 0} q^{k-1} k\, z^k \sum_{j \geq 0} \frac{k-1}{j+k-1} \binom{2j+k-2}{j} (pqz)^j \,.$$

By the identity in Section 3, the latter sum is

$$= \sum_{k \geq 0} q^{k-1} k\, z^k \left(\frac{1 - \sqrt{1 - 4pqz}}{2pqz} \right)^{k-1}$$

$$= z \sum_{k \geq 0} k\, p^{1-k} C(pqz)^{k-1} = \frac{p^2 z}{\big(p - C(pqz)\big)^2} \,.$$

We can now eliminate $L(z)$ and solve for $M(z)$, obtaining a "closed form" for the desired generating function:

$$M(z) = z \left(\frac{p}{p - C(pqz)} \right)^2 \left(\frac{q}{q - C(pqz)} \right) \,.$$

Such a simple form for $M(z)$ is unexpected; but in fact, we can do even more! We have

$$\big(p - C(pqz)\big)\big(q - C(pqz)\big) = pq - C(pqz) + C(pqz)^2 = pq(1-z) \,,$$

because $C(z) - C(z)^2 = z$. Hence the denominator of $M(z)$ can be vastly simplified:

$$M(z) = \frac{z}{(1-z)^2} \left(\frac{q - C(pqz)}{q} \right) \,.$$

This is the product $(z + 2z^2 + 3z^3 + \cdots)(1 - c_1 pz - c_2 p^2 qz^2 - \cdots)$, so the coefficient of z^n can be written

$$M_n(p) = n - (n-1)c_1 p - (n-2)c_2 p^2 q - \cdots - 1 c_{n-1} p^{n-1} q^{n-2}.$$

When a formula turns out to be so simple, it must have a simple explanation. But the author hasn't been able to think of any direct proof. For some reason, $M_n(p)$ is not only the expected size of the remaining roll when one roll empties, it is also the expected value of the "first return to the diagonal," in the following sense: Suppose the two toilet paper rolls start in the full state (n, n), and they are used by big-choosers and little-choosers until the empty state $(0, 0)$ is reached; and suppose that the rolls first become equal in size again at state $(n-k, n-k)$. Then the average value of k is $M_n(p)$. (This follows from our formula for $M_n(p)$, because $c_k p^k q^{k-1}$ is the probability of first return to $(n-k, n-k)$ for each $k < n$, and $1 - c_1 p - \cdots - c_{n-1} p^{n-1} q^{n-2}$ is the probability that the diagonal is not encountered until state $(0, 0)$ is reached.)

Is there an easy way to prove that the same expected value occurs in both problems? The distributions are different, but the mean values are the same.

5. The Limiting Behavior

Now that $M(z)$ has been put into a fairly simple form, we are ready to deduce the asymptotic value of $M_n(p)$ for fixed p as $n \to \infty$.

Let's assume first that $p \neq q$. Then $4pq < 1$, and the function $C(pqz) = \frac{1}{2}\left(1 - \sqrt{1 - 4pqz}\right)$ is analytic for $|z| < 1/(4pq)$; so $C(pqz)$ is analytic in a neighborhood of $z = 1$. In fact, a simple computation proves that its Taylor series at the point $z = 1$ involves the Catalan numbers once again:

$$C(pqz) = \min(p, q) + \left(\max(p, q) - \min(p, q)\right) C\left(\frac{pq(z-1)}{(p-q)^2}\right).$$

(This formula generalizes our observation that $C(pq) = \min(p, q)$.)

If $q < p$, our formula for $M(z)$ reduces to

$$M(z) = \frac{z}{(1-z)^2}\, \frac{q-p}{q}\, C\left(\frac{pq(z-1)}{(p-q)^2}\right)$$

$$= \frac{z}{1-z}\, \frac{p}{p-q} - z\left(c_2 \frac{p^2 q}{(p-q)^3} + c_3 \frac{p^3 q^2}{(p-q)^5}(z-1) + \cdots\right)$$

$$= \frac{z}{1-z}\, \frac{p}{p-q} + f(z),$$

where $f(z)$ is analytic in the region $|z| < 1/(4pq)$. This determines the value of $M_n(p)$ quite accurately:

Theorem 1. *Let r be any value greater than $4pq$. Then*

$$M_n(p) = \begin{cases} p/(p-q) + O(r^n), & \text{if } q < p; \\ ((q-p)/q)n + p/(q-p) + O(r^n), & \text{if } q > p. \end{cases}$$

(The constants implied by O in these formulas depend on p and r, but not on n.)

Proof. If $q < p$, the value of $M_n(p)$ is the coefficient of z^n in $M(z)$, which is $p/(p-q)$ plus the coefficient of z^n in $f(z)$. But $f(z)$ converges absolutely when $z = 1/r$, hence its nth coefficient is $O(r^n)$.

If $q > p$, the stated result follows from the formula for $q < p$, using the identity

$$q\, M_n(p) + pn = p\, M_n(q) + qn$$

which is an immediate consequence of the formula for $M_n(p)$ in Section 4.   □

For example, if $p = 2/3$ and $q = 1/3$, so that big-choosers outnumber little-choosers by 2 to 1, the average size of the remaining roll will be very close to 2, when n is large; but when $p = 1/3$ and $q = 2/3$ the average will be approximately $\frac{1}{2}n + 1$. (In fact, $M_{100}(2/3) \approx 1.9999998$ and $M_{100}(1/3) \approx 50.99999991$.)

Such rapid convergence to the limit is a surprise, but the general behavior predicted by Theorem 1 agrees with our intuition: If little-choosers predominate, the size of the larger roll will tend to be proportional to n, when the smaller roll is used up. But if big-choosers are in the majority, the larger roll will tend to be reduced to a bounded size, independent of the initial size n.

6. The Transition Point

But what about the boundary case, $p = q$? Does it lead to lengths of order n, or order 1, or something in between?

This is actually the simplest case to analyze, because everybody is a random-chooser when $p = q = 1/2$; the problem then reduces to a fairly simple "random walk." In fact, we are essentially dealing here with "Banach's match box problem" as discussed by Feller [2, §IX.3(f)]. According to our general formula, the generating function in this case is simply

$$M(z) = \frac{z}{(1-z)^{3/2}},$$

so there is a solution in closed form:

$$M_n\left(\frac{1}{2}\right) = \binom{-3/2}{n-1}(-1)^{n-1} = \frac{2n}{4^n}\binom{2n}{n}.$$

By Stirling's approximation we have

Theorem 2. $M_n(p) = 2\sqrt{\dfrac{n}{\pi}} - \dfrac{1}{4}\sqrt{\dfrac{1}{\pi n}} + O(n^{-3/2})$, when $p = q$. ☐

The function $M_n(p)$ is a polynomial in p of degree $2n-3$, for $n \geq 2$, and it decreases monotonically from n down to 1 as p increases from 0 to 1. The remarkable thing about this decrease is that it changes in character rather suddenly when p passes $1/2$. Here, for example, is the graph of $M_{100}(p)$:

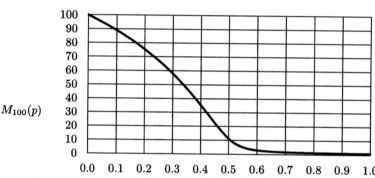

We can't use the formulas of Theorem 1 when p is too close to $1/2$, even if n is extremely large. For example, if we set $n = 10^{10}$ and $p = 1/2 \pm 10^{-20}$, the approximations in Theorem 1 give the ridiculous estimates $M_n(p) \approx \frac{1}{4} \times 10^{20}$. Indeed, we know that $M_n(1/2)$ is of order $\sqrt{n}$, so the approximations can be valid only when $|p - \frac{1}{2}|$ is of order $1/\sqrt{n}$ at least.

The slope of $M_n(p)$ at $p = 1/2$ can be calculated by differentiating $M(z)$ with respect to p and extracting the coefficient of z^n. The derivative is

$$-\frac{z}{(1-z)^2}\frac{d}{dp}\left(\frac{C(p(1-p)z)}{1-p}\right)$$

$$= -\frac{z}{(1-z)^2}\left(\frac{(1-2p)zC'(p(1-p)z)}{1-p} + \frac{C(p(1-p)z)}{(1-p)^2}\right)$$

and at $p = 1/2$ this equals $-2z(1-z)^{-2} + 2z(1-z)^{-3/2}$. Hence

$$M_n'(1/2) = -2n + 2M_n(1/2);$$

this slope is consistent with $M_n(p)$ dropping from n to a small value as p goes from 0 to $1/2$.

Acknowledgments

I wish to thank the architect of the computer science building at Stanford University for implicitly suggesting this problem, and Richard Beigel for the insight that led to the closed form of $L(z)$. Andrei Broder offered helpful comments and computed the graph of $M_{100}(p)$. My research was supported in part by the National Science Foundation.

References

[1] Désiré André, "Solution directe du problème résolu par M. Bertrand," *Comptes Rendus hebdomadaires des séances de l'Académie des Sciences* **105** (Paris: 1887), 436–437.

[2] William Feller, *An Introduction to Probability Theory and Its Applications*, Volume 1, second edition (New York: Wiley, 1957).

[3] Donald E. Knuth, *Fundamental Algorithms*, Volume 1 of *The Art of Computer Programming* (Reading, Massachusetts: Addison–Wesley, 1968).

[4] Wallace Reyburn, *Flushed with Pride* (London: Macdonald & Jane's, 1973).

Addendum

David Stirzaker ["A generalization of the matchbox problem," *The Mathematical Scientist* **13** (1988), 104–114] has suggested the more sanitary name *transparent matchbox problem* for the question treated above. He used martingales and renewal theory to study not only the average number $M_n(p)$ of portions that remain but also the corresponding probability distribution. Let $P_{nk}(p)$ be the probability that exactly k portions remain when we begin in state (n, n); then equation (22) of his paper can be put into the remarkably simple form

$$\sum_{k,n} P_{nk}(p)w^k z^n = \frac{pqwz}{\big(p - C(pqz)w\big)\big(q - C(pqz)\big)},$$

as observed by Wolfgang Stadje ["Asymptotic probabilities in a sequential urn scheme related to the matchbox problem," *Advances in Applied*

Probability **30** (1998), 831–849]. We obtain the formula derived earlier for $M(z) = \sum_n M_n(p)z^n$ from this more general expression if we differentiate with respect to w and then set $w = 1$. Moreover, the general expression has a nice combinatorial interpretation: One factor

$$\frac{qz}{q-C} = z\left(1 + \frac{C}{q} + \frac{C^2}{q^2} + \cdots\right), \qquad C = C(pqz),$$

is the generating function for paths from (n, n) to $(1, 1)$, because $z(C/q)^m$ is the generating function for such paths that return to the diagonal m times. And the other factor

$$\frac{pw}{p-Cw} = w\left(1 + \frac{Cw}{p} + \frac{C^2w^2}{p^2} + \cdots\right), \qquad C = C(pqz),$$

is z^{-1} times the generating function for paths from (n, n) that never return to the diagonal, because $zw^k(C/p)^{k-1}$ corresponds to such paths that end at $(k, 0)$.

Chapter 17

An Analysis of Optimum Caching

[Originally published in Journal of Algorithms **6** *(1985), 181–199.]*

A cache memory that is maintained clairvoyantly, that is, with perfect knowledge of the future, can be surprisingly effective even when it is applied to completely random data. This paper shows that a cache of size h, applied optimally to a uniformly random sequence on an alphabet of size d, is able to avoid faults with probability of order $\sqrt{h/d}$. The analysis of this question involves several subproblems that are of interest in themselves.

1. Introduction

The technique of "cache memory," which was originally used for register allocation in the design of high-speed computers and later applied to page allocation in virtual-memory machines, is now being used in many different kinds of software. The purpose of the present paper is to explore some of the theoretical questions associated with this technique.

The basic idea of caching is to maintain high-speed access to h items from a larger collection of d items that cannot all be accessed so quickly. We can formulate the essential properties in the following abstract way: A sequence $(a_1, a_2, a_3, \dots)$ is given in which each element a_i is a "d-git," that is, a radix-d digit, an integer in the range $0 \leq a_i < d$; this sequence represents the items that need to be accessed at time 1, 2, 3, ... A multiset C_0 of size h is also given; this represents the initial state of the cache. For all integers $t \geq 1$, the cache C_t at time t is defined by the formula

$$C_t = C_{t-1} - \{b_t\} + \{a_t\},$$

where b_t is an element of C_{t-1}; in other words, C_t is obtained by deleting b_t from C_{t-1}, and then inserting a_t. Hence C_t always has size h, and a_t is always in C_t. The particular choice of b_t depends on what caching strategy is being used.

If $b_t \neq a_t$, so that the cache actually changes at time t, we say that a "fault" has occurred. Changes to the cache can be expensive, so the goal of a caching strategy is to minimize the number of faults by judiciously choosing the element b_t that is replaced at time t.

An optimum caching strategy can be obtained by the following intuitively plausible rules: "If $a_t \in C_{t-1}$, let $b_t = a_t$. Otherwise if C_{t-1} contains at least one element that does not occur in the remaining sequence $(a_t, a_{t+1}, \dots)$, let b_t be such an element. Otherwise let b_t be the element of C_{t-1} whose first occurrence in $(a_t, a_{t+1}, \dots)$ is as remote as possible." The optimality of this strategy was first stated by Belady [1], and first proved by Mattson, Gecsei, Slutz, and Traiger [9]; the same result had been discovered independently by R. Shapiro of Computer Associates in Massachusetts, and perhaps by others, during the early 1960s. (See Fuchs and Knuth [3] for some slightly more general results.)

Suppose the sequence $(a_1, a_2, \dots)$ is random, so that each a_t has a given d-git as its value with probability $1/d$, independently of the other elements of the sequence. Let f_t be the probability that a fault occurs at time t, when the optimum strategy is used. Then f_t is a random variable, determined by the alphabet size d, the time t, the cache size h, and the initial contents C_0.

Section 2 of this paper proves that f_t approaches a limiting value $f(h, d)$ independent of C_0 as $t \to \infty$, and Section 3 derives an explicit formula for the case $h = 2$. Larger values of h lead to more complicated situations, so it appears unlikely that any simple formula for $f(h, d)$ exists when $d \gg h \geq 3$. However, it is possible to obtain bounds on $f(h, d)$ that are not too far apart; a lower bound is derived in Section 4, and an upper bound in Sections 5–7. Section 6 is devoted to "Q-algebra," a type of discrete mathematics that is needed for these upper bound calculations; similar formulas have arisen in connection with several other algorithms, so Q-algebra seems worthy of attention in its own right.

Section 8 discusses a nonuniform model of stochastic sequences $(a_1, a_2, \dots)$, intended to capture the degree of locality observed in typical applications. It is shown, somewhat paradoxically, that a random sequence based on the past is equivalent to a random sequence based on the future. The analysis of optimum caching for such sequences is proposed as a topic for further research.

2. Beginning the Analysis

Let $(a_1, a_2, \dots)$ be a sequence of d-gits in which every d-git occurs infinitely often. For each d-git x and time $t \geq 1$, let $\pi_t(x)$ be the number of distinct d-gits that occur before the first appearance of x in the sequence $(a_t, a_{t+1}, \ldots)$. Then $(\pi_t(0), \pi_t(1), \ldots, \pi_t(d-1))$ is a permutation of $\{0, 1, \ldots, d-1\}$. Let $(\rho_t(0), \rho_t(1), \ldots, \rho_t(d-1))$ be the inverse permutation; thus, $\rho_t(0)$ is the first d-git to appear in $(a_t, a_{t+1}, \ldots)$, namely a_t itself, and $\rho_t(1)$ is the second, etc. If m_t distinct d-gits occur between a_t and the first appearance of a_t in $(a_{t+1}, a_{t+2}, \ldots)$, we have

$$(\rho_{t+1}(0), \rho_{t+1}(1), \ldots, \rho_{t+1}(d-1))$$
$$= (\rho_t(1), \ldots, \rho_t(m_t), \rho_t(0), \rho_t(m_t+1), \ldots, \rho_t(d-1)).$$

Thus if $\sigma(m)$ denotes the cyclic permutation $(0\,1\,\ldots\,m)$ and if $\sigma^-(m)$ is the inverse permutation $(m\,\ldots\,1\,0)$, we have

$$\rho_{t+1} = \sigma(m_t)\rho_t, \quad \pi_{t+1} = \pi_t \sigma^-(m_t);$$

consequently

$$\pi_t = \pi_1 \sigma^-(m_1) \sigma^-(m_2) \ldots \sigma^-(m_{t-1}).$$

For example, if $d = 4$ and $(a_1, a_2, \ldots) = (2, 1, 1, 3, 3, 2, 3, 1, 1, 1, 0, \ldots)$, we have

$$(\pi_1(0), \pi_1(1), \pi_1(2), \pi_1(3)) = (3, 1, 0, 2),$$
$$(\rho_1(0), \rho_1(1), \rho_1(2), \rho_1(3)) = (2, 1, 3, 0),$$
$$(\pi_2(0), \pi_2(1), \pi_2(2), \pi_2(3)) = (3, 0, 2, 1),$$
$$(\rho_2(0), \rho_2(1), \rho_2(2), \rho_2(3)) = (1, 3, 2, 0),$$

and $m_1 = 2$. In cycle form the permutations are

$$\pi_1 = (0\ 3\ 2), \qquad\qquad \rho_1 = (0\ 2\ 3);$$
$$\pi_2 = (0\ 3\ 1) = \pi_1 \cdot (2\ 1\ 0), \qquad \rho_2 = (0\ 3\ 2) = (0\ 1\ 2) \cdot \rho_1.$$

We must have $m_t = d-1$ for infinitely many t, otherwise $\rho_t(d-1)$ would be constant for all large t and this d-git would never appear again.

Conversely, we can reconstruct the sequence $(a_1, a_2, \ldots)$ from the permutation π_1 and the sequence $(m_1, m_2, \ldots)$; and if $m_t = d-1$ for infinitely many t, the corresponding sequence $(a_1, a_2, \ldots)$ will include every d-git infinitely often. For if $0 \le x < d$ we have $\pi_{t+1}(x) \le \pi_t(x)$ unless $\pi_t(x) = 0$, and $\pi_{t+1}(x) = \pi_t(x) - 1$ when $m_t = d-1$ and $\pi_t(x) > 0$; hence $\pi_t(x)$ will be zero infinitely often. But $\pi_t(x) = 0$ if and only if $x = a_t$, so the proof is complete. Thus we have a one-to-one correspondence between the sequences $(a_1, a_2, \ldots)$ and the pairs $(\pi_1, (m_1, m_2, \ldots))$.

When $(a_1, a_2, \dots)$ is a random sequence, it is clear that π_1 is a random permutation and that $(m_1, m_2, \dots)$ is a random sequence. Hence we can study the behavior of optimum caching on a random sequence $(a_1, a_2, \dots)$ by studying its behavior on a random π_1 and a random $(m_1, m_2, \dots)$. This transformation is useful because π_1 and $(m_1, m_2, \dots)$ contain all the "lookahead" information necessary to control optimum caching in a simple way: A fault occurs at time t if and only if no element x of C_{t-1} has $\pi_t(x) = 0$; furthermore, if a fault occurs, b_t is the element of C_{t-1} having maximum $\pi_t(x)$.

Let us now transform the sets C_t in the analogous way, by defining

$$\Gamma_t = \{\pi_t(x) \mid x \in C_t\}.$$

The optimum caching algorithm acts as follows at time t:

(1) If $0 \notin \Gamma_{t-1}$, a fault occurs: Let $\Gamma_t^* = \Gamma_{t-1} - \{\max(\Gamma_{t-1})\} + \{0\}$. Otherwise, no fault occurs; let $\Gamma_t^* = \Gamma_{t-1}$.

(2) Let Γ_t be the result of applying $\sigma^-(m_t)$ to Γ_t^*; that is, if we ignore multiplicities,

$$\Gamma_t = \{m_t\} \cup ((\Gamma_t^* \cap [1 \mathinner{.\,.} m_t]) - 1) \cup (\Gamma_t^* \cap [m_t + 1 \mathinner{.\,.} d - 1]).$$

The initial cache contents C_0 do not significantly affect the behavior of the algorithm, since all residual effects of C_0 have disappeared after each d-git has appeared at least once. Thus if f_t and f_t' denote the probability of failure at time t under the assumption of two different initial conditions C_0 and C_0', we have

$$|f_t - f_t'| < q_t,$$

where q_t is the probability that the sequence $(a_1, \dots, a_{t-1})$ does not contain all d of the possible d-gits. From the well-known theory of "coupon collecting" (see, for example, [6, exercise 3.3.2–8]), the generating function for q_t is

$$\sum_{t \geq 1} q_t z^t = \frac{1}{1-z}\left(z - z^{d+1}\left(\frac{d-1}{d-z}\right)\left(\frac{d-2}{d-2z}\right) \cdots \left(\frac{1}{d-(d-1)z}\right)\right).$$

This function is analytic for $|z| < d/(d-1)$, so q_t converges exponentially to zero. We are therefore justified in assuming that C_0 is chosen in any convenient way.

The rules of optimum caching define a Markov process on the set of $\binom{d}{h}$ possible states Γ_t. From each state Γ_{t-1} there are d equally likely transitions to successor states Γ_t according to rules (1) and (2) above, depending on the value of m_t. This Markov process has a steady state in which each set Γ occurs with probability $p(\Gamma)$. Instead of choosing C_0 in any particular way, let us assume that Γ_0 takes on each particular value Γ with probability $p(\Gamma)$; then the steady state is achieved immediately and f_t is independent of t. Indeed, the probability of failure at time t is

$$\sum \{p(\Gamma) \mid 0 \notin \Gamma\}.$$

Let us represent state Γ by the binary string $c_0 c_1 \ldots c_{d-1}$, where $c_x = 1$ if $x \in \Gamma$, otherwise $c_x = 0$. For example, if d is ten and Γ is $\{2, 3, 5, 7\}$ the binary string is 0011010100. In this state, a failure occurs, and $\Gamma^* = 1011010000$ according to rule (1); the ten possible successors corresponding to $m_t \in \{0, 1, \ldots, 9\}$ in rule (2) are

1011010000	0110110000
0111010000	0110101000
0111010000	0110100100
0111010000	0110100010
0110110000	0110100001.

We can find the steady-state probabilities by solving $\binom{d}{h}$ simultaneous equations in $\binom{d}{h}$ unknowns.

If two states Γ have the same value of Γ^*, they are equivalent as far as rule (2) is concerned, so we can combine them. Notice that we can deduce the full set of probabilities $p(\Gamma)$ from the steady states $p^*(\Gamma^*)$, if we want to. This reduces the number of equations and variables to $\binom{d-1}{h-1}$.

For example, let $d = 5$ and $h = 3$. The possible values of Γ^* are 11100, 11010, 11001, 10110, 10101, 10011. We obtain the following equations, by considering the action of rule (2) followed by rule (1):

$$p^*_{11100} = \tfrac{3}{5} p^*_{11100} \qquad\qquad\qquad\qquad + \tfrac{4}{5} p^*_{10110} + \tfrac{2}{5} p^*_{10101}$$
$$p^*_{11010} = \tfrac{1}{5} p^*_{11100} + \tfrac{2}{5} p^*_{11010} \qquad\qquad\qquad + \tfrac{2}{5} p^*_{10101} + \tfrac{1}{5} p^*_{10011}$$
$$p^*_{11001} = \tfrac{1}{5} p^*_{11100} \qquad\quad + \tfrac{2}{5} p^*_{11001}$$
$$p^*_{10110} = \qquad\qquad\quad \tfrac{2}{5} p^*_{11010} \qquad\quad + \tfrac{1}{5} p^*_{10110} \qquad\qquad\quad + \tfrac{3}{5} p^*_{10011}$$
$$p^*_{10101} = \qquad\qquad\quad \tfrac{1}{5} p^*_{11010} + \tfrac{1}{5} p^*_{11001} \qquad\qquad + \tfrac{1}{5} p^*_{10101}$$
$$p^*_{10011} = \qquad\qquad\qquad\qquad\quad \tfrac{2}{5} p^*_{11001} \qquad\qquad\qquad\qquad\quad + \tfrac{1}{5} p^*_{10011}$$

These equations are slightly redundant, since their sum is a trivial identity; but the additional relation $p^*_{11100} + \cdots + p^*_{10011} = 1$ yields the unique steady state solution

$$p^*_{11100} = \frac{120}{317}, \qquad p^*_{11010} = \frac{64}{317}, \qquad p^*_{11001} = \frac{40}{317},$$

$$p^*_{10110} = \frac{47}{317}, \qquad p^*_{10101} = \frac{26}{317}, \qquad p^*_{10011} = \frac{20}{317}.$$

It is not difficult to see that the limiting value of f_t is

$$f(h, d) = \frac{d-1}{d} \sum \{p^*(\Gamma^*) \mid 1 \notin \Gamma^*\},$$

hence $f(3, 5) = \frac{4}{5}(p^*_{10110} + p^*_{10101} + p^*_{10011}) = \frac{372}{1585}$.

3. Special Cases

The formulas in Section 2 can be solved for $h = 2$ and all $d \geq 2$ in the following way. Let $X_k = \{0, k\}$ and $x_k = p^*(X_k)$ for $1 \leq k < d$. Applying rule (2) to $\Gamma^* = X_k$ gives the equiprobable successor states $\{0, k\}, \{1, k\}, \ldots, \{k-1, k\}, \{k-1, k\}, \{k-1, k+1\}, \ldots, \{k-1, d-1\}$; following this by rule (1) gives no change if $k = 1$, otherwise it yields $X_k, X_1, \ldots, X_{k-2}$, and $d - k + 1$ copies of X_{k-1}. Thus we obtain the equations

$$
\begin{aligned}
dx_1 &= 2x_1 + (d-1)x_2 + & x_3 + & x_4 + \cdots + x_{d-1} \\
dx_2 &= x_1 + & x_2 + (d-2)x_3 + & x_4 + \cdots + x_{d-1} \\
dx_3 &= x_1 & + & x_3 + (d-3)x_4 + \cdots + x_{d-1} \\
&\ \ \vdots \\
dx_{d-2} &= x_1 & & + x_{d-2} + 2x_{d-1} \\
dx_{d-1} &= x_1 & & + x_{d-1}
\end{aligned}
$$

and $x_1 + x_2 + \cdots + x_{d-1} = 1$. We have $f(2, d) = (1 - x_1)(d - 1)/d$, so it suffices to compute x_1.

The calculations will be demonstrated for $d = 5$, since the same pattern works for all d. We have

$$
\begin{pmatrix}
-4 & 3 & 1 & 1 \\
0 & -4 & 2 & 1 \\
0 & 0 & -4 & 1 \\
1 & 1 & 1 & 1
\end{pmatrix}
\begin{pmatrix}
x_2 \\
x_3 \\
x_4 \\
x_1
\end{pmatrix}
=
\begin{pmatrix}
0 \\
0 \\
0 \\
1
\end{pmatrix};
$$

these equations can be solved by adding multiples of rows 1, 2, and 3 to row 4. The successive contents of row 4 will be

$$
\begin{array}{cccc}
y_1 & 1 & 1 & 1 \\
0 & y_2 & 1 + y_1/4 & 1 + y_1/4 \\
0 & 0 & y_3 & 1 + y_1/4 + y_2/4 \\
0 & 0 & 0 & y_4
\end{array}
$$

where $y_1 = 1$, $y_2 = 1 + 3y_1/4$, $y_3 = 1 + y_1/4 + 2y_2/4$, and $y_4 = 1 + y_1/4 + y_2/4 + y_3/4$. If we set $y_0 = 0$, we see that

$$
y_2 - y_1 = \frac{3}{4}(y_1 - y_0), \quad y_3 - y_2 = \frac{2}{4}(y_2 - y_1), \quad y_4 - y_3 = \frac{1}{4}(y_3 - y_2);
$$

hence $y_4 x_1 = 1$, where

$$
y_4 = 1 + \frac{3}{4} + \frac{3}{4}\cdot\frac{2}{4} + \frac{3}{4}\cdot\frac{2}{4}\cdot\frac{1}{4} = Q(4).
$$

Here

$$
Q(n) = 1 + \frac{n-1}{n} + \frac{n-1}{n}\frac{n-2}{n} + \cdots
$$

is Ramanujan's function studied in [5, Section 1.2.11.3]. For general d, a similar derivation gives $x_1 = 1/Q(d-1)$, so we have

$$
f(2, d) = \frac{d-1}{d}\left(1 - \frac{1}{Q(d-1)}\right).
$$

This formula is surprising on two counts. In the first place, the probability $1 - f(2, d)$ of nonfailure is

$$
\frac{d-1}{dQ(d-1)} + \frac{1}{d},
$$

which is $\sqrt{2/(\pi d)} + O(1/d)$ by [5, equation 1.2.11.3–(25)]. This is roughly $\sqrt{d}$ times the nonfailure probability obtained without a clairvoyant cache, even though our cache has only two entries, so the small cache is doing unexpectedly well on random data. In the second place, the formula for $f(2, d)$ is rather simple, so it calls for a simpler proof.

A somewhat simpler proof can be contrived by looking more closely at what optimal caching does when $h = 2$. Given $(a_1, a_2, \ldots)$, the cache scores a "lucky hit" at time t whenever $a_t = a_{t-1}$. Let us delete all such a_t from the sequence, since their effect is easily accounted for. We are left with a sequence $(a'_1, a'_2, \dots)$ which is random except for the fact that $a'_t \neq a'_{t-1}$; hence each a'_t now has $d-1$ equally likely possibilities instead of d. In the residual sequence, optimal caching with $h = 2$ scores a "real hit" when the first a'_t occurs that equals a'_k for some $k < t$. The expected value of t can be shown to equal $1 + Q(d-1)$. After this, the algorithm essentially proceeds in the same way on the sequence $(a'_{t-1}, a'_t, \dots)$, so the failure probability on $(a'_1, a'_2, a'_3, \dots)$ turns out to be $1 - 1/Q(d-1)$.

However, neither of these proofs for $h = 2$ seems to generalize to $h = 3$. It appears that there is no simple formula for $f(h, d)$ when $h \geq 3$ and d is arbitrary, although of course the author would like to be proved wrong on this point. Can the value of $f(\lfloor d/2 \rfloor, d)$ be calculated exactly for large values of d, without requiring exponential time and space?

There is at least one more special case that can be solved exactly, namely when $h = d - 1$. In this case failures are quite rare, of course. We may assume that C_0 contains the first $d - 1$ elements that appear in $(a_1, a_2, \dots)$; the first failure is then at time t when the dth distinct element enters the picture. Then the same process continues with respect to $(a_t, a_{t+1}, \dots)$, because the first $d-1$ elements of this residual sequence are now present in the cache when the optimal strategy is being used. Hence the failure rate $f(d-1, d)$ is $1/(E_d - 1)$, where E_d is the expected value of the first failure time t. The value of E_d is well known from the analysis of coupon collecting to be dH_d (see [6, exercise 3.3.2–8]); hence

$$f(d-1, d) = \frac{1}{dH_{d-1}} \sim \frac{1}{d \ln d}.$$

4. A Lower Bound

In this section we shall prove that $f(h, d)$ cannot be lower than $1 - O(\sqrt{h/d})$, because even a clairvoyant caching strategy cannot be more efficient than this when it is faced with a completely random sequence.

The lower bound we shall consider is based on a simple idea: No matter what the contents of the cache are at time t, if the sequence $(a_{t+1}, \dots, a_{t+s})$ has r distinct d-gits, it must cause at least $r - h$ failures. Therefore if E_{rd} is the expected length of time before r distinct d-gits occur in a random d-ary sequence, the value of $f(h, d)$ must be at least $(r - h)/E_{rd}$. (This follows because we will have approximately $n(r - h)$ or more failures at time nE_{rd}, when n is large.)

Once again the theory of coupon collecting comes to our aid; we have

$$E_{rd} = \frac{d}{d} + \frac{d}{d-1} + \dots + \frac{d}{d-r+1} = (H_d - H_{d-r})d,$$

since it takes $d/(d-k)$ steps on the average to obtain a new d-git after k distinct d-gits have already appeared.

We get the best lower bound by choosing r so that $(r-h)/E_{rd}$ is maximized. If we set $(r-h)/E_{rd} \approx (r+1-h)/E_{(r+1)d}$, in an attempt to find the best value of r, we find that

$$\frac{r-h}{d-r} \approx H_d - H_{d-r}.$$

Let $x = r/d$ and $y = h/d$; then we have $(r-h)/(d-r) = (x-y)/(1-x)$, and $H_d - H_{d-r} = \ln(1/(1-x)) + O(x(1-x)^{-1}d^{-1})$. The solution to $(x-y)/(1-x) = \ln(1/(1-x))$ is $x = \sqrt{2y} + O(y)$ as $y \to 0$; therefore when $h \ll d$ the best choice of r is approximately equal to $\sqrt{2hd}$.

Suppose $h \leq \frac{1}{8}d$, and set $r = \lceil \sqrt{2hd} \rceil$, so that $r \leq \frac{1}{2}d$. We have

$$E_{rd} = (H_d - H_{d-r})d = d \cdot \ln\left(\frac{d}{d-r}\right) + O\left(\frac{r}{(d-r)d}\right)$$

$$= r + \frac{r^2}{2d} + O\left(\frac{r^3}{d^2}\right),$$

since H_n lies between $\ln n + \gamma$ and $\ln n + \gamma + 1/(12n)$. Therefore

$$1 - f(h,d) \leq \frac{E_{rd}-r+h}{E_{rd}} \leq \frac{E_{rd}-r+h}{r}$$

$$= \frac{2h + O(r^3/d^2) + O(r/d)}{r} = \sqrt{\frac{2h}{d}} + O\left(\frac{h}{d}\right).$$

Furthermore when $h \geq \frac{1}{8}d$ we obviously have $1 - f(h,d) \leq 1 \leq \sqrt{2h/d} + 4h/d$, so the asymptotic relation

$$1 - f(h,d) \leq \sqrt{\frac{2h}{d}} + O\left(\frac{h}{d}\right)$$

holds uniformly for $1 \leq h \leq d$.

5. An Upper Bound

Since the optimum caching strategy is optimum, we can obtain an upper bound on $f(h,d)$ by analyzing any particular caching strategy. The trick is to find a near-optimum strategy that has a reasonably simple analysis.

We shall study the following scheme: "Look ahead in the sequence until finding the first time t that the sequence $(a_1, a_2, \ldots, a_t)$ contains exactly $t - h + 1$ distinct d-gits, that is, $h - 1$ duplicates. This sequence can obviously be allocated to a cache of size h in such a way that only $t - h + 1$ failures occur, using up to $h - 1$ cache positions for repeated elements and using the other cache position for all the others. Then repeat the same process on $(a_{t+1}, a_{t+2}, \ldots)$." If T_{hd} is the expected value of t, we will have $t - n(h - 1)$ failures when t is approximately nT_{hd}, hence we obtain the upper bound

$$f(h, d) \leq 1 - \frac{h - 1}{T_{hd}}.$$

In order to analyze this strategy, we need to count the number of sequences $(a_1, a_2, \ldots, a_t)$ having the necessary property. Such sequences are characterized by two conditions: (i) exactly $t - h + 1$ distinct d-gits appear, and (ii) the final d-git a_t appears at least twice. The number of ways to partition a set of size t into $t - h + 1$ parts is $\left\{{t \atop t-h+1}\right\}$, from which we subtract the $\left\{{t-1 \atop t-h}\right\}$ partitions in which the final element is a singleton. (Here $\left\{{n \atop k}\right\}$ denotes a signless Stirling number of the second kind; see, for example, exercise 1.2.6–64 of [5].) Multiplying by $d(d - 1) \ldots (d - t + h)$, to convert partitions into sequences, we obtain the desired number of $(a_1, a_2, \ldots, a_t)$, namely

$$\frac{d!}{(d - t + h - 1)!} \left(\left\{{t \atop t - h + 1}\right\} - \left\{{t - 1 \atop t - h}\right\} \right).$$

Dividing by d^t gives the probability that a particular value of t occurs. Using the identity

$$\left\{{n \atop m}\right\} = m \left\{{n - 1 \atop m}\right\} + \left\{{n - 1 \atop m - 1}\right\},$$

we can put the formulas into slightly simpler form. Let $p_{hd}(k)$ be the probability that $t = h - 1 + k$. Then

$$p_{hd}(k) = \frac{k}{d^{h-k+1}} \frac{d!}{(d - k)!} \left\{{h + k - 2 \atop k}\right\},$$

$$T_{hd} = h - 1 + \sum_{k=1}^{d} k p_{hd}(k).$$

6. Q-Algebra

One way to estimate the value of T_{hd}, and thereby to complete the analysis in Section 5, is to develop a theory about sums of the form

$$Q(a_1, a_2, a_3, \dots) = a_1 + a_2 \frac{n-1}{n} + a_3 \frac{n-1}{n} \frac{n-2}{n} + \cdots$$

$$= \sum_{k \geq 1} a_k \frac{n!}{n^k (n-k)!}.$$

Here n is an understood parameter, so that $Q(a_1, a_2, a_3, \dots)$ is actually a function of n; but the coefficients a_k are independent of n. Such sums have arisen in connection with quite a variety of algorithms, for example, in the study of random mappings [6, exercises 3.1–12 and 3.1–14], hashing [7, exercise 6.4–50], interleaved memory [8], and sorting in place [14]. Therefore it seems useful to study their properties more closely.

When all the a_i equal 1, we have the function $Q(1, 1, 1, \dots) = Q(n)$ for which Ramanujan [11] derived the asymptotic series

$$Q(n) = \frac{n! \, e^n}{2 n^n} - \frac{1}{3} - \frac{4}{135 n} + \frac{8}{2835 n^2} + \frac{16}{8505 n^3} + O(n^{-4})$$

$$= \sqrt{\frac{\pi n}{2}} - \frac{1}{3} + \frac{1}{12} \sqrt{\frac{\pi}{2n}} - \frac{4}{135 n} + \frac{1}{288} \sqrt{\frac{\pi}{2 n^3}} + O(n^{-2}).$$

This function $Q(n)$ shows up in unexpected places; for example, Cauchy [2] proved that

$$\frac{1}{n^n} \sum_k \binom{n}{k} k^k (n-k)^{n-k} = 1 + Q(n).$$

Most of the properties of Q-functions can be derived from two identities that are not difficult to establish:

$$r Q(a_1, a_2, \dots) + s Q(b_1, b_2, \dots) = Q(r a_1 + s b_1, r a_2 + s b_2, \dots);$$

$$Q(a_1, 2a_2, 3a_3, \dots) = n Q(a_1, a_2 - a_1, a_3 - a_2, \dots).$$

We can use these basic identities to deduce, for example, that

$$Q(1, 2, 3, \dots) = n Q(1, 0, 0, \dots) = n;$$

$$Q(1^2, 2^2, 3^2, \dots) = n Q(1, 1, 1, \dots) = n Q(n);$$

$$Q(1^3, 2^3, 3^3, \dots) = n Q(1, 3, 5, \dots) = n \big(2 Q(1, 2, 3, \dots) - Q(1, 1, 1, \dots) \big)$$

$$= 2 n^2 - n Q(n).$$

In general, there exist coefficients q_{mk} such that

$$Q(1^m, 2^m, 3^m, \ldots) = q_{m0}Q^{(m)} - q_{m1}Q^{(m-1)} + q_{m2}Q^{(m-2)} - \cdots,$$

where $Q^{(m)}$ is a "semi-polynomial" in n:

$$Q^{(m)} = \begin{cases} n^{(m+1)/2} & \text{if } m \text{ is odd}; \\ n^{m/2}Q(n) & \text{if } m \text{ is even}. \end{cases}$$

The coefficients q_{mk} are integers satisfying the recurrence

$$q_{mk} = \binom{m-1}{1}q_{m-2,k} + \binom{m-1}{2}q_{m-3,k-1} + \binom{m-1}{3}q_{m-4,k-2} + \cdots$$

for $m \geq 2$, and $q_{1k} = q_{0k} = \delta_{k0}$. Thus we have the following triangle of coefficients:

$m = 2$	1							
$m = 3$	2	1						
$m = 4$	3	3	1					
$m = 5$	8	10	4	1				
$m = 6$	15	35	25	5	1			
$m = 7$	48	105	109	56	6	1		
$m = 8$	105	413	490	294	119	7	1	
$m = 9$	384	1260	2300	1918	734	246	8	1
$m = 10$	945	5445	9450	10518	6825	1749	501	9	1

Notice that the value of q_{m0} is the product $(m-1)(m-3)\ldots(2 \text{ or } 1)$, which is sometimes denoted by double factorial notation '$(m-1)!!$'.

Conversely, there is an inverse triangle that specifies polynomials P_m such that

$$Q(P_m(1), P_m(2), P_m(3), \ldots) = Q^{(m)}.$$

Our derivation in Section 5 actually tells us what the inverse coefficients $P_m(k)$ are, in the case that $m = 2r - 1$ is odd, since the probabilities $P_{hd}(k)$ defined in that section must sum to 1. We obtain the identity

$$Q\left(\left\{{r \atop 1}\right\}, 2\left\{{r+1 \atop 2}\right\}, 3\left\{{r+2 \atop 3}\right\}, \ldots\right) = n^r$$

by setting $n = d$ and $r = h - 1$. This identity can also be verified directly by using the recurrences for the Stirling numbers and for $Q(a_1, a_2, \ldots)$.

Digression: It is natural to seek similar coefficients for the even values of m; let us regard these as Stirling numbers with half-integer entries, and define them by the formula

$$Q\left(\left\{{r+\frac{1}{2} \atop 1}\right\}, 2\left\{{r+\frac{3}{2} \atop 2}\right\}, 3\left\{{r+\frac{5}{2} \atop 3}\right\}, \ldots\right) = n^r Q(n).$$

We have $\left\{{r+1/2 \atop r}\right\} = r$ and $\left\{{r+1/2 \atop 1}\right\} = 1$ for all positive integers r, and the other values come from the Stirling recurrence

$$\left\{{r + \tfrac{1}{2} \atop k}\right\} = k\left\{{r - \tfrac{1}{2} \atop k}\right\} + \left\{{r - \tfrac{1}{2} \atop k - 1}\right\}.$$

Here is a table of such half-integer Stirling numbers $\left\{{r+1/2 \atop k}\right\}$:

	$k = 1$	$k = 2$	$k = 3$	$k = 4$	$k = 5$	$k = 6$	$k = 7$	$k = 8$
$r = 1$	1							
$r = 2$	1	2						
$r = 3$	1	5	3					
$r = 4$	1	11	14	4				
$r = 5$	1	23	53	30	5			
$r = 6$	1	47	182	173	55	6		
$r = 7$	1	95	593	874	448	91	7	
$r = 8$	1	191	1874	4089	3114	994	140	8

They have the generating function

$$\sum_{k \geq n} \left\{{k + \tfrac{1}{2} \atop n}\right\} z^{k-n} = \frac{1}{1 - nz} + \frac{1}{(1 - nz)(1 - (n - 1)z)}$$

$$+ \cdots + \frac{1}{(1 - nz)(1 - (n - 1)z)\ldots(1 - z)}.$$

When r is near k, special formulas exist for $\left\{{r \atop k}\right\}$. We have

$$\left\{{k \atop k}\right\} = 1,$$

$$\left\{{k + \tfrac{1}{2} \atop k}\right\} = k,$$

$$\left\{{k + 1 \atop k}\right\} = \binom{k + 1}{2},$$

$$\left\{{k + \tfrac{3}{2} \atop k}\right\} = \binom{k + 2}{3} + \binom{k + 1}{3},$$

$$\left\{{k + 2 \atop k}\right\} = \binom{k + 3}{4} + 2\binom{k + 2}{4},$$

$$\left\{{k + \tfrac{5}{2} \atop k}\right\} = \binom{k + 4}{5} + 5\binom{k + 3}{5} + 2\binom{k + 2}{5},$$

and in general $\left\{{k+m/2 \atop k}\right\}$ is a polynomial in k of the form $k^m/m!! + O(k^{m-1})$; this polynomial is zero when k is an integer in the range $-m/2 \le k \le 0$, except when $m = 0$. Such formulas can be derived by using the fact that

$$\left\{{r+k \atop k}\right\} = k\left\{{r-1+k \atop k}\right\} + (k-1)\left\{{r-1+k-1 \atop k-1}\right\}$$
$$+ (k-2)\left\{{r-1+k-2 \atop k-2}\right\} + \cdots .$$

The coefficients of this expansion have been given an interesting combinatorial interpretation by Gessel and Stanley [4], in the case that $m = 2l$ is even: The multiset $\{1, 1, 2, 2, \dots, l, l\}$ has $(m-1)!!$ permutations $a_1 \dots a_m$ such that if $u < v < w$ and $a_u = a_w$ then $a_v > a_w$; and the coefficient of $\binom{k+m-1-j}{m}$ in the expansion of $\left\{{k+m/2 \atop k}\right\}$ is the number of such permutations for which the inequality $a_i > a_{i+1}$ occurs exactly j times. Stanley has observed [15] that the same property holds when $m = 2l - 1$ is odd, if half-integer Stirling numbers are defined as above; in this case the relevant multiset is $\{1, 2, 2, \dots, l, l\}$. For example, when $m = 5$, the eight permutations

$$12233, \quad 12332, \quad 13322, \quad 33122, \quad 22133, \quad 22331, \quad 23321, \quad 33221$$

have respectively 0, 1, 1, 1, 1, 1, 2, 2 occurrences of $a_i > a_{i+1}$; hence the coefficients of the expansion of $\left\{{k+5/2 \atop k}\right\}$ are 1, 5, 2.

7. An Upper Bound (continued)

Returning to the analysis in Section 5, we want to compute the expected value $\sum_{k \ge 0} k p_{hd}(k)$, which can be expressed as

$$n^{-r} Q\left(1^2 \left\{{r \atop 1}\right\}, 2^2 \left\{{r+1 \atop 2}\right\}, 3^2 \left\{{r+2 \atop 3}\right\}, \dots\right)$$

if we let $r = h - 1$ and $n = d$. It appears difficult to evaluate this sum in closed form, but we can deduce the asymptotic behavior for fixed r by noting that it has the form

$$n^{-r} Q(P(1), P(2), P(3), \dots),$$

where $P(k) = k^2 \left\{{r-1+k \atop k}\right\} = k^{2r}/(2r-2)!! + O(k^{2r-1})$ is a polynomial. Thus

$$Q(P(1), P(2), P(3), \dots) = q_{(2r)0} \frac{Q^{(2r)}}{(2r-2)!!} + O(Q^{(2r-1)})$$

$$= \frac{(2r-1)!!}{(2r-2)!!} n^r Q(n) + O(n^r).$$

The coefficient $(2r-1)!!/(2r-2)!! = (r-\frac{1}{2})(r-\frac{3}{2})\ldots\frac{3}{2}/(r-1)! = \Gamma(r+\frac{1}{2})/(\Gamma(r)\Gamma(\frac{3}{2}))$ is asymptotic to $2\sqrt{r/\pi} + O(r^{-1/2})$; let us denote it by $2\sqrt{h/\pi}\alpha_h^{-1}$, so that $\alpha_h = 1 + O(1/h)$. In this notation, we have proved that

$$T_{hd} = h - 1 + \sum_{k \geq 0} kp_{hd}(k) = \frac{2}{\alpha_h}\sqrt{h/\pi}\,Q(d) + O(1),$$

where the constant implied by the O depends on h but not on d. Our upper bound $f(h,d) \leq 1 - (h-1)/T_{hd}$ now translates into

$$1 - f(h,d) \geq \alpha_h\sqrt{h/2d} + O(h/d)$$

for fixed h as $d \to \infty$. Since $\alpha_h \to 1$, the right-hand side is about half of the uniform bound

$$1 - f(h,d) \leq \sqrt{2h/d} + O(h/d)$$

that we derived in Section 4. It can be shown that α_h decreases when h increases.

Andrei Broder has discovered that the quantity T_{hd} arises also in another context. Let f be a random mapping from $\{0,\ldots,d-1\}$ to $\{0,\ldots,d-1\}$, and let $(a_1, a_2, \ldots, a_s)$ be a random s-tuple of d-gits. Then the average number of elements reachable from the a_j under f, namely the average cardinality of the set

$$\{f^k(a_j) \mid k \geq 0, 1 \leq j \leq s\},$$

is precisely $T_{s+1,d} - s$. Here is a sketch of Broder's elegant (unpublished) proof: Each of the d^{d+s} equally likely choices of f and $(a_1, \ldots, a_s)$ can be encoded as the sequence of $(d+s)$ d-gits

$$(f^0(a_1), f^1(a_1), \ldots, f^{k_1}(a_1), f^0(a_2), \ldots, f^{k_2}(a_2), \ldots,$$
$$f^0(a_s), \ldots, f^{k_s}(a_s), f(b_1), \ldots, f(b_q)),$$

where k_j is the smallest iterate of f such that $f^{k_j}(a_j)$ is equal to a previous element of the sequence, and where $b_1 < \cdots < b_q$ are the elements that do not occur in $\{f^k(a_j)\}$ for any j and k. For example, if $d = 10$ and $s = 3$, the mapping and sequence defined by

$$(f(0), \ldots, f(9)) = (3,1,4,1,5,9,2,6,5,3), \qquad (a_1, a_2, a_3) = (2,7,1)$$

would be encoded as

$$(2, 4, 5, 9, 3, 1, 1, 7, 6, 2, 1, 3, 5);$$

it is clearly possible to invert this code, reconstructing the mapping and the sequence. If the cardinality of $\{f^k(a_j)\}$ is m, the number t of d-gits in the encoded sequence before s duplicates have occurred is $m + s$. Hence Broder's problem is equivalent to the problem we have been discussing.

Our estimate of T_{hd} has been proved above only for fixed h as $d \to \infty$, but a similar result can be shown to hold when h and d both approach infinity simultaneously. Boris Pittel [10] has proved that a set of m distinct elements almost always leads to approximately $\pi(m, d)$ elements after iteration of a random mapping, where

$$\left(1 - \frac{\pi(m, d)}{d}\right) e^{\pi(m,d)/d} = 1 - \frac{m}{d}.$$

It can be shown that $\pi(m, d)/d = U\left(\sqrt{2m/d}\right)$, where

$$U(z) = z - \frac{1}{3}z^2 + \frac{11}{72}z^3 - \frac{43}{540}z^4 + \frac{769}{17280}z^5 - \frac{221}{8505}z^6 + \cdots$$

satisfies the relation

$$(1 - U(z))e^{U(z)} = 1 - \tfrac{1}{2}z^2.$$

This power series converges for $-\sqrt{2} < z \le \sqrt{2}$; hence we have

$$\pi(m, d) = \sqrt{2md} + O(m)$$

uniformly for $m \le (1 - \epsilon)d$, where the constant in the O depends on ϵ. Now the average number of distinct elements in a random sequence $(a_1, \ldots, a_s)$ is $d - d(1 - 1/d)^s = d(1 - e^{-s/d}) + O(1)$, and the variance is of order d; see, for example [7, exercise 5.2.5–5 (or exercise 5.2.5–6 in the second edition)]. With high probability, the relevant values of m in the calculation of T_{nd} by Broder's method will be $(1 - e^{-h/d})d + O(1)$, and we obtain the estimate

$$T_{hd} = \sqrt{2hd} + O(h)$$

when $d \ge h \to \infty$.

8. A Nonuniform Model

Instead of considering completely random sequences $(a_1, a_2, \ldots)$, let us assume that a probability distribution $(p_1, p_2, \ldots, p_d)$ has been given such that, at each time t, the element a_t has probability p_k of being the "kth least recently used" element. In other words, p_1 is the probability that $a_t = a_{t-1}$; p_2 is the probability that a_t is the most recent element different from a_{t-1} (thus $a_t = a_s \neq a_{s+1} = \cdots = a_{t-1}$); and so on. This definition does not work when t is so small that the d-gits have not all appeared as yet; to resolve this ambiguity, we assume that a random permutation of $\{0, 1, \ldots, d-1\}$ has been prefixed to the sequence at time 0. The effect of changing this initial permutation is simply to permute all of the entries $(a_1, a_2, \ldots)$; thus if π is any permutation of $\{0, 1, \ldots, d-1\}$, the sequences $(a_1, a_2, \ldots)$ and $(\pi(a_1), \pi(a_2), \ldots)$ are equally likely.

We can generate such sequences in the following way: Start with a random permutation $(\rho_1(0), \rho_1(1), \ldots, \rho_1(d-1))$. At time t, set $a_t \leftarrow \rho_t(m_t)$, where m_t is selected at random with probability p_k that $m_t = k - 1$. Then set

$$(\rho_{t+1}(0), \rho_{t+1}(1), \ldots, \rho_{t+1}(d-1))$$
$$= (\rho_t(m_t), \rho_t(0), \ldots, \rho_t(m_t - 1), \rho_t(m_t + 1), \ldots, \rho_t(d-1)),$$

and do the same thing at time $t+1$. Note that $\rho_t(k-1)$ is the kth least recently used element preceding time t.

This construction, which generates a_t based on past history, is similar to the construction of Section 2, which generates a_t based on the future. Yet the two methods are quite different (unless $m_t = 0$ or 1), since we have $\rho_{t+1} = \sigma^-(m_t)\rho_t$ now while we had $\rho_{t+1} = \sigma(m_t)\rho_t$ in Section 2. Both random processes have $d!$ states, represented by the permutation $\sigma^-(m_t)\rho_t$ at time t, but there is no way to map the states of one process into the states of the other.

Let us therefore consider also a nonuniform model like that of Section 2, where m_t receives the value $k - 1$ with probability p_k. This is a futuristic model in which a_t has probability p_k of being the "kth most remotely used" element.

It turns out that both of these models are identical, even though they treat time in completely opposite ways. In order to see why this is true, we shall show that each subsequence $(a_1, a_2, \ldots, a_t)$ is equally likely in both models. The proof is easiest to understand by considering an example: Suppose $d = 10$, and let $(a_1, a_2, \ldots, a_t)$ be the sequence

$$(3, 1, 4, 1, 5, 9, 2, 6, 5, 3, 5, 8, 9, 7, 9, 3).$$

The probability of obtaining this sequence in the least-recently-used model is

$$q_1\, q_2\, q_3\, p_2\, q_4\, q_5\, q_6\, q_7\, p_4\, p_7\, p_2\, q_8\, p_6\, q_9\, p_2\, p_5\,,$$

where q_k denotes the probability that a particular element is making its first appearance, after $k-1$ elements are present; we have $q_k = (p_k + \cdots + p_n)/(n-k+1)$. The probability of obtaining this sequence in the most-remotely-used model is

$$p_7\, p_2\, q_9\, q_8\, p_4\, p_6\, q_7\, q_6\, p_2\, p_5\, q_5\, q_4\, p_2\, q_3\, q_2\, q_1\,,$$

where q_k is used here for the probability that the kth last element has a particular value; again $q_k = (p_k + \cdots + p_n)/(n-k+1)$. Both of these products of probabilities have the same value. The reason is that if we look at any particular d-git, say 9, we can count how many distinct d-gits occur between its consecutive appearances; in this case the counts for 9 are 5 and 1, since $\{2, 6, 5, 3, 5, 8\}$ has five distinct elements and $\{7\}$ has 1. The contribution of the 9's to the product in the LRU model is therefore $q_x p_6 p_2$, and in the MRU model the contribution is $p_6 p_2 q_y$, for some x and y. Thus the two products have the same p's, in permuted order; and they also clearly have the same q's, so the probabilities are identical.

Historians tell us that the future is like the past, and the mathematical proof in the preceding paragraph might be what they have in mind. At any rate, the fact that both models agree is good grounds to believe that this nonuniform model is of potential interest in studies of algorithms that deal with sequences. Furthermore, the identity of the two models makes it feasible to study the optimum caching strategy, which looks into the future, when it is applied to LRU data, which is based on the past.

For example, let us consider the case $h = 2$ in the nonuniform model. The methods of Section 3 apply without change; we simply generalize the formulas in the obvious way. The matrix

$$\begin{pmatrix} -4 & 3 & 1 & 1 \\ 0 & -4 & 2 & 1 \\ 0 & 0 & -4 & 1 \\ 1 & 1 & 1 & 1 \end{pmatrix} \quad \text{becomes} \quad \begin{pmatrix} -q_2 & q_3 & p_3 & p_3 \\ 0 & -q_2 & q_4 & p_4 \\ 0 & 0 & -q_2 & q_5 \\ 1 & 1 & 1 & 1 \end{pmatrix},$$

where we define

$$q_k = p_k + p_{k+1} + \cdots + p_d.$$

Triangularizing the matrix as before now yields

$$y_2 - y_1 = \frac{q_3}{q_2}(y_1 - y_0), \qquad y_3 - y_2 = \frac{q_4}{q_2}(y_2 - y_0), \qquad y_4 - y_3 = \frac{q_5}{q_2}(y_3 - y_4),$$

and we obtain the general formula

$$f(2, d) = q_2 \left(1 - \frac{1}{1 + r_3 + r_3 r_4 + \cdots + r_3 r_4 \ldots r_d} \right), \qquad r_k = q_k/q_2,$$

for the failure rate of optimum caching in the nonuniform model. The steady state probabilities $x_k = p^*(\Gamma^*)$ for $\Gamma^* = \{0, k\}$ are given by the general formulas

$$x_k = (z_k - z_{k+1})x_1, \qquad z_k = r_{k+1} + r_{k+1}r_{k+2} + r_{k+1}r_{k+2}r_{k+3} + \cdots.$$

Of course, the fact that "the future is like the past" does not mean that a caching-strategy based on replacing the least-recently-used item will be optimum with respect to lookahead. The failure rate in our nonuniform model will be simply $q_{h+1} = p_{h+1} + \cdots + p_d$ if the least-recently-used strategy is employed, since this strategy keeps the h most recently used elements in the cache.

The nonuniform model considered here has been the subject of an extensive literature, beginning with [12]; it is generally called the *LRU stack model*. See [13] for a survey of other results about this model, including a derivation of the expected "working set" size.

9. Open Problems

Many interesting questions about optimum caching are still waiting to be answered. For example, the lower bounds derived here do not quite match the upper bounds.

The behavior of $f(h, d)$ when $h \geq 3$ in the nonuniform model should also prove to be interesting, in connection with various probability distributions. For theoretical purposes it makes sense to drop the parameter d and to work with a possibly infinite probability distribution $(p_1, p_2, \ldots)$. If $p_d \neq 0$ and $p_k = 0$ for all $k > d$, we obtain the nonuniform model for finite d as a special case of this infinite model. Furthermore the formulas for the infinite model will be reasonable approximations to the finite models.

For example, it makes sense to study a geometric probability distribution $(p, qp, q^2p, \ldots)$ in this way. The failure probability when $h = 2$, according to the formula in Section 8, involves an elliptic function when this distribution is assumed; the value turns out to be

$$q(1 - 1/(1 + q + q^3 + q^6 + q^{10} + \cdots)).$$

This research was supported in part by the National Science Foundation and the Office of Naval Research.

References

[1] L. A. Belady, "A study of replacement algorithms for a virtual-storage computer," *IBM Systems Journal* **5** (1966), 78–101.

[2] A. Cauchy, "Application du calcul des résidus à la sommation de plusieurs suites," *Exercices de Mathématiques* (Paris: 1826), 62–73. Reprinted in *Œuvres Complètes d'Augustin Cauchy* (2) **6** (Paris: Gauthier–Villars, 1887), 62–73.

[3] David R. Fuchs and Donald E. Knuth, "Optimal font caching," *ACM Transactions on Programming Languages and Systems* **7** (1985), 62–79.

[4] Ira Gessel and Richard P. Stanley, "Stirling polynomials," *Journal of Combinatorial Theory* (A) **24** (1978), 24–33.

[5] Donald E. Knuth, *Fundamental Algorithms*, Volume 1 of *The Art of Computer Programming* (Reading, Massachusetts: Addison–Wesley, 1968).

[6] Donald E. Knuth, *Seminumerical Algorithms*, Volume 2 of *The Art of Computer Programming* (Reading, Massachusetts: Addison–Wesley, 1969).

[7] Donald E. Knuth, *Sorting and Searching*, Volume 3 of *The Art of Computer Programming* (Reading, Massachusetts: Addison–Wesley, 1973).

[8] Donald E. Knuth and Gururaj S. Rao, "Activity in an interleaved memory," *IEEE Transactions on Computers* **C-24** (1975), 943–944. [Reprinted as Chapter 8 of the present volume.]

[9] R. L. Mattson, J. Gecsei, D. R. Slutz, and I. L. Traiger, "Evaluation techniques for storage hierarchies," *IBM Systems Journal* **9** (1970), 78–117.

[10] Boris Pittel, "On distributions related to transitive closures of random finite mappings," *Annals of Probability* **11** (1983), 428–441.

[11] S. Ramanujan, "Questions for solution, number 294," *Journal of Indian Mathematical Society* **3** (1911), 128; **4** (1912), 151–152. Reprinted in *Collected Papers of Srinivasa Ramanujan* (Cambridge: 1927), 323–324.

[12] J. E. Shemer and G. A. Shippey, "Statistical analysis of paged and segmented computer systems," *IEEE Transactions on Electronic Computers* **EC-15** (1966), 855–863.

[13] Jeffrey R. Spirn, *Program Behavior: Models and Measurements* (New York: Elsevier, 1977).

[14] Stanford Computer Science Department, Qualifying examination in the analysis of algorithms (April 1981).

[15] Richard P. Stanley, personal communication (July 1981).

Addendum

When I wrote this paper in 1985, I had high hopes that the half-integer Stirling numbers $\left\{r+1/2 \atop k\right\}$ introduced in Section 6 would turn out to agree with the "true" values of $\left\{r+1/2 \atop k\right\}$ as soon as a definitive way to extend Stirling numbers to noninteger arguments was discovered, except perhaps for a constant factor like $\sqrt{\pi}$. But alas, mathematics does not appear to be unreasonably effective in this instance: Philippe Flajolet and Helmut Prodinger have found an excellent (and probably optimum) way to extend the classical definition of Stirling numbers ["On Stirling numbers for complex arguments and Hankel contours," *SIAM Journal on Discrete Mathematics* **12** (1999), 155–159], but their definition gives

$$\left\{k+\tfrac{1}{2} \atop k\right\} = \frac{1}{k!}\left(k^{k+\frac{1}{2}} - \binom{k}{1}(k-1)^{k+\frac{1}{2}} + \cdots + (-1)^k\binom{k}{k}1^{k+\frac{1}{2}}\right),$$

not k.

Chapter 18

A Trivial Algorithm Whose Analysis Isn't

[Written with Arne T. Jonassen. Originally published in Journal of Computer and System Sciences **16** *(1978), 301–322.]*

Very few theoretical results have been obtained to date about the behavior of information retrieval algorithms under random deletions, as well as random insertions. The present paper offers a possible explanation for this dearth of results, by showing that one of the simplest such algorithms already requires a surprisingly intricate analysis. Even when the data structure never contains more than three items at a time, the expected performance of the standard tree search/insertion/deletion algorithm involves Bessel functions and the solution of bivariate integral equations. A step-by-step expository analysis of this problem is given, and it is shown how the difficulties arise and can be surmounted.

1. Introduction

An algorithm known as "tree search and insertion" has become one of the most commonly used methods for maintaining a dynamically growing dictionary or symbol table (see [3]). This algorithm was discovered independently by several people during the 1950s, and in 1962 Thomas N. Hibbard [1] showed that entries could also be deleted dynamically without difficulty. At that time Hibbard proved one of the first results that might be called a theorem of "pure computer science," because it was one of the first results ever to be proved about data structure manipulations: He showed that a random deletion from a random tree, using his deletion algorithm, leaves a random tree. Although the statement may seem self-evident when stated in this way, it was in fact a surprising result, because the deletion algorithm was necessarily asymmetric while random trees are symmetric. Hibbard's theorem can be stated more precisely as follows: "If $n + 1$ items are inserted into an initially

257

empty binary tree, in random order, and if one of those items (selected at random) is deleted, the probability that the resulting binary tree has a given shape is the same as the probability that this tree shape would be obtained by inserting n items into an initially empty tree, in random order." It took great foresight even to conjecture such a result in 1962; people rarely *proved* things about computer programs in those days, unless perhaps numerical analysis was involved, and binary trees were not well understood. Furthermore, the proof was not simple.

Ten years later, Gary D. Knott proved a much deeper result [2]: "If n items are inserted into an initially empty binary tree, in random order, and if the first k items inserted are subsequently deleted by Hibbard's algorithm, in the same order as they were inserted, the resulting binary tree is random." (In other words, the probability that the resulting tree has a given shape is the same as the probability that this shape would be obtained if $n - k$ items had been inserted into an initially empty tree in random order.) The theorems of Hibbard and Knott seemed to settle the question of deletions, since they proved stability of the tree distribution under a wide variety of deletion disciplines.

However, Knott also discovered a surprising paradox: Although Hibbard's theorem establishes that $n + 1$ random insertions followed by a random deletion produces a tree whose shape has the distribution of n random insertions, we cannot conclude that a subsequent random insertion yields a tree whose shape has the distribution of $n + 1$ random insertions! For ten years it had been believed that Hibbard's theorem proved the stability of the algorithms under repeated insertions and deletions (see [1, page 5] and [3, first printing, pages 429–432]); the discovery of a subtle fallacy in this reasoning therefore came as a shock.

In order to understand the paradox, we need to know only what Hibbard's algorithm does to binary search trees with one, two, or three elements. The five binary search trees on three elements $x < y < z$ are

$$A(x,y,z) \qquad B(x,y,z) \qquad C(x,y,z) \qquad D(x,y,z) \qquad E(x,y,z)$$

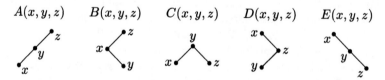

and the two possibilities on two elements $x < y$ are

$$F(x,y) \qquad\qquad\qquad G(x,y)$$

The standard insertion algorithm produces the following binary search tree when inserting element z into a tree containing x and y, with $x < y$:

Initial tree	Result if $z < x$	Result if $x < z < y$	Result if $y < z$
$F(x,y)$	$A(z,x,y)$	$B(x,z,y)$	$C(x,y,z)$
$G(x,y)$	$C(z,x,y)$	$D(x,z,y)$	$E(x,y,z)$

In other words, z is simply attached "at the bottom" where it fits. Hibbard's deletion algorithm operates as follows on a 3-element tree:

Initial tree	Delete x	Delete y	Delete z
$A(x,y,z)$	$F(y,z)$	$F(x,z)$	$F(x,y)$
$B(x,y,z)$	$F(y,z)$	$F(x,z)$	$G(x,y)$
$C(x,y,z)$	$G(y,z)$	$F(x,z)$	$F(x,y)$
$D(x,y,z)$	$G(y,z)$	$G(x,z)$	$G(x,y)$
$E(x,y,z)$	$G(y,z)$	$G(x,z)$	$G(x,y)$

If we insert three elements $x < y < z$ in random order, we get a tree of shape A, B, C, D, E with the respective probabilities $1/6$, $1/6$, $2/6$, $1/6$, $1/6$; then a random deletion leaves us with the following six possibilities and probabilities:

$F(x,y)$	$F(x,z)$	$F(y,z)$	$G(x,y)$	$G(x,z)$	$G(y,z)$
$3/18$	$4/18$	$2/18$	$3/18$	$2/18$	$4/18$

The probability of shape F at this point is $9/18 = 1/2$, in accord with Hibbard's theorem.

But now comes another random insertion, say w. The probability is $1/4$ that w is the smallest of $\{w,x,y,z\}$; and the other three cases $x < w < y < z$, $x < y < w < z$, $x < y < z < w$ also occur with probability $1/4$. Thus the tree $F(x,y)$ becomes $A(w,x,y)$, $B(x,w,y)$, or $C(x,y,w)$ with respective probabilities $1/4$, $1/4$, $1/2$; and the other cases $F(x,z)$, $\ldots$, $G(y,z)$ can be worked out similarly. We find that the insertion of w produces a tree of shape A, B, C, D, E with the respective probabilities

$$\frac{3+4+4}{72}, \quad \frac{3+8+2}{72}, \quad \frac{6+4+2+3+2+8}{72}, \quad \frac{3+4+4}{72}, \quad \frac{6+2+4}{72},$$

namely

$$11/72, \quad 13/72, \quad 25/72, \quad 11/72, \quad 12/72. \tag{1.1}$$

A random deletion now produces a tree of shape F with probability

$$\frac{11}{72} + \frac{2}{3} \cdot \frac{13}{72} + \frac{2}{3} \cdot \frac{25}{72} = \frac{109}{216} > \frac{1}{2}.$$

A study of this example shows where the fallacy occurred: The "random" tree shape after a deletion is not independent of the "random" values remaining. For example, when x is deleted (relatively large values remaining), the tree tends to be of shape G, but when z is deleted (relatively small values remaining) the tree shape is not biased towards F or G.

Fortunately the deviation from randomness occurs in the right direction here: The trees actually tend to get *better*, in the sense that the balanced shape C (which requires less search time) becomes more probable. Extensive empirical studies by Knott [2] give overwhelming support to the conjecture that random deletions do not degrade the average search time; but no proof has yet been found.

More precisely, Knott's conjecture is this: Consider a pattern of $n + k$ insertions and n deletions, in some order, where the number of deletions never exceeds the number of insertions. For example, one of the patterns with $n = 4$ and $k = 4$ is $IIIDIIDIIIDD$.

To do each insertion, put a new random element into the tree, say a uniform random number between 0 and 1; to do each deletion, choose a random element uniformly from among those present. All of these random choices are to be independent. Then for each fixed pattern of I's and D's, the average path length of the resulting tree is conjectured to be at most equal to the average path length of the pattern consisting solely of k I's.

In attempting to explore this conjecture, it is natural to investigate the simple case of patterns

$$III, \quad IIIDI, \quad IIIDIDI, \quad \ldots, \quad III(DI)^n, \quad \ldots$$

for $k = 3$. Such patterns never require us to deal with more than three elements in the tree at any time; so all we must do is study the following trivial procedure.

T1. [Insert two.] Let x and y be independent uniform random numbers. Insert x into an empty tree, then insert y. (If $x < y$, we get the tree $G(x, y)$, otherwise we get $F(y, x)$.)

T2. [Insert one.] Insert a new independent uniform random number into the tree.

T3. [Delete one.] Choose one of the three elements in the tree at random, each with probability 1/3, and delete it using Hibbard's method.

T4. [Repeat.] Return to step T2.   □

At the beginning of the $(n + 1)$st occurrence of step T3, we have a tree of shape A, B, C, D, or E, with certain probabilities a_n, b_n, c_n, d_n, e_n; we want to show that these probabilities approach a "steady state." According to the conjecture, c_n should be $> 1/3$, because only shape C has a path length smaller than the other shapes. The first two times we get to step T3, we have seen that $(a_n, b_n, c_n, d_n, e_n)$ are respectively

$$\left(\frac{1}{6}, \frac{1}{6}, \frac{2}{6}, \frac{1}{6}, \frac{1}{6}\right) \qquad \text{and} \qquad \left(\frac{11}{72}, \frac{13}{72}, \frac{25}{72}, \frac{11}{72}, \frac{12}{72}\right).$$

What do these probabilities look like after n deletions have been made, for large n? This is the problem we shall investigate in the following pages.

It turns out that this problem is not as simple as it might appear at first, in spite of the triviality of the algorithm; in fact, the analysis ranks among the more difficult of the exact analyses of all algorithms that have been carried out to date, although it is "elementary" in the sense that no deep theorems of analysis are required. From the form of the answers we shall derive, it will be clear that the problem itself is *intrinsically difficult* — no really simple derivation would be able to produce such a complicated answer, and the answer is correct! Since the difficulties we will encounter are interesting and instructive, the solution will be presented here in a motivated way, explaining how it was found.

One might ask why the exact analysis of this process should be carried out at all, given that the answer is hard to determine; in other words, what is the point of this work? The authors first began to study the problem simply because the mathematics was challenging — surprisingly intricate yet not quite impossible — and because the problem continued to lead to interesting subproblems. The form of the final solution demonstrates that nontrivial mathematics is sometimes necessary to understand programs that are very simple; and the solution procedure shows how to develop the techniques of algorithmic analysis in the new direction that was needed.

Indeed, when the problem was finally solved, the result proved to be even more interesting than expected, since the simplicity of the program combined with the difficulty of the analysis made it necessary to investigate the fundamentals of algorithmic analysis more carefully than before. The simplifications that apply in other successful analyses are missing here, so a new basic approach to studying the average behavior of algorithms using multidimensional integrals became necessary. Further work is now in progress to develop this integral-oriented approach, since it has the potential of leading to automated analysis of algorithms, extending the present techniques of automated proofs of algorithms.

2. The Recurrences to be Solved

The behavior of the trivial algorithm depends only on the relative order of the elements inserted, and on the particular choice made at each deletion step. Therefore one way to analyze the situation after the pattern $III(DI)^n$ is to consider $(n + 3)! \, 3^n$ configurations to be equally likely, reflecting the relative order of the $n + 3$ elements inserted together with the n three-way choices of which element to delete. For example, when $n = 1$ there are 72 equally likely possibilities, and our analysis of this case in (1.1) essentially considered them all.

However, such a discrete approach leads to great complications. The following continuous approach, which follows the algorithm more closely, turns out to be much simpler. Let $f_n(x, y) \, dx \, dy$ be the differential probability that the tree is $F(X, Y)$ at the beginning of step T2, after n elements have been deleted, where

$$x \leq X < x + dx \qquad \text{and} \qquad y \leq Y < y + dy;$$

and let $g_n(x, y) \, dx \, dy$ be the corresponding probability that it is $G(X, Y)$. Let

$$a_n(x, y, z) \, dx \, dy \, dz, \quad \ldots, \quad e_n(x, y, z) \, dx \, dy \, dz$$

be the respective probabilities that the tree is $A(X, Y, Z), \ldots, E(X, Y, Z)$ at the beginning of step T3, for some $x \leq X < x + dx$, $y \leq Y < y + dy$, and $z \leq Z < z + dz$. Then we can write down recurrence relations for these differential probabilities by translating the algorithm directly into mathematical formalism. First we have

$$
\begin{aligned}
a_n(x, y, z) &= f_n(y, z), \\
b_n(x, y, z) &= f_n(x, z), \\
c_n(x, y, z) &= f_n(x, y) + g_n(y, z), \\
d_n(x, y, z) &= g_n(x, z), \\
e_n(x, y, z) &= g_n(x, y),
\end{aligned}
\qquad (2.1)
$$

for $0 \leq x < y < z \leq 1$, by considering the six possible actions of step T2. (These probabilities are, of course, zero when $x < 0$, $x > y$, $y > z$, or $z > 1$; at the boundaries where $x = 0$, $x = y$, $y = z$, or $z = 1$ there may be discontinuities, and we can define the functions there in any way we like.) Secondly we have

$$
\begin{aligned}
f_{n+1}(x, y) = \frac{1}{3} &\int_0^x \big(a_n(t, x, y) + b_n(t, x, y)\big)\, dt \\
+ \frac{1}{3} &\int_x^y \big(a_n(x, t, y) + b_n(x, t, y) + c_n(x, t, y)\big)\, dt \\
+ \frac{1}{3} &\int_y^1 \big(a_n(x, y, t) + c_n(x, y, t)\big)\, dt,
\end{aligned}
$$

$$
\begin{aligned}
g_{n+1}(x, y) = \frac{1}{3} &\int_0^x \big(c_n(t, x, y) + d_n(t, x, y) + e_n(t, x, y)\big)\, dt \\
+ \frac{1}{3} &\int_x^y \big(d_n(x, t, y) + e_n(x, t, y)\big)\, dt \\
+ \frac{1}{3} &\int_y^1 \big(b_n(x, y, t) + d_n(x, y, t) + e_n(x, y, t)\big)\, dt,
\end{aligned}
\tag{2.2}
$$

for $0 \le x < y \le 1$, by considering the possible actions of step T3. Inserting (2.1) into (2.2) and applying obvious simplifications yields the fundamental recurrences

$$
\begin{aligned}
f_{n+1}(x, y) = \frac{1}{3}\bigg(&f_n(x, y) + \int_0^y f_n(t, y)\, dt + \int_x^y f_n(x, t)\, dt \\
&+ \int_x^y g_n(t, y)\, dt + \int_y^1 f_n(y, t)\, dt + \int_y^1 g_n(y, t)\, dt \bigg),
\end{aligned}
$$

$$
\begin{aligned}
g_{n+1}(x, y) = \frac{1}{3}\bigg(&g_n(x, y) + \int_0^x f_n(t, x)\, dt + \int_0^x g_n(t, y)\, dt \\
&+ \int_0^x g_n(t, x)\, dt + \int_x^1 g_n(x, t)\, dt + \int_y^1 f_n(x, t)\, dt \bigg);
\end{aligned}
\tag{2.3}
$$

consideration of step T1 also leads to the obvious initial conditions

$$
f_0(x, y) = g_0(x, y) = 1. \tag{2.4}
$$

Both (2.3) and (2.4) hold for $0 \le x < y \le 1$.

We have now transformed the algorithm mechanically into a set of equations that describe the distribution of its behavior quite precisely. The quantities of interest to us are

$$a_n = \int_0^1 \int_0^z \int_0^y a_n(x, y, z) \, dx \, dy \, dz, \quad \ldots,$$

$$e_n = \int_0^1 \int_0^z \int_0^y e_n(x, y, z) \, dx \, dy \, dz, \qquad (2.5)$$

namely the respective probabilities that a tree of shape $A, \ldots, E$ occurs after the insertion/deletion pattern $III(DI)^n$. We can also compute

$$f_n = \int_0^1 \int_0^y f_n(x, y) \, dx \, dy \quad \text{and} \quad g_n = \int_0^1 \int_0^y g_n(x, y) \, dx \, dy, \quad (2.6)$$

the probabilities that the tree shape is F or G after the pattern $II(ID)^n$. Hibbard's theorem for trees of size 2 states that $f_1 = f_0$ and $g_1 = g_0$.

3. Simplification of the Recurrences

What can we do with such formidable recurrences (2.3)–(2.4)? In the first place we can look for invariant relations that might be used to simplify them.

When the algorithm reaches step T2, it is clear that the two numbers X and Y in its tree are random, except for the condition that $X < Y$. Thus we must have

$$f_n(x, y) + g_n(x, y) = 2, \qquad \text{for } 0 \le x < y \le 1 \text{ and } n \ge 0. \qquad (3.1)$$

(The sum is 2, not 1, since the probability that $x \le X < x + dx$ and $y \le Y < y + dy$ given that $X < Y$ is $2 \, dx \, dy$.) This formula could also be proved directly from (2.3) and (2.4), by induction on n.

Relation (3.1) means that we really have only one function to worry about, namely $f_n(x, y)$. Let us rewrite (2.3) and (2.4) to take account of this fact:

$$f_0(x, y) = 1;$$

$$f_{n+1}(x, y) = \frac{1}{3} \left(2 - 2x + f_n(x, y) + \int_0^x f_n(t, y) \, dt + \int_x^y f_n(x, t) \, dt \right), \quad (3.2)$$

for $n \ge 0$. Henceforth we shall avoid mentioning the side condition $0 \le x < y \le 1$, for if we use (3.2) to define $f_n(x, y)$ for *all* real numbers x and y it will agree with the true $f_n(x, y)$ when $0 \le x < y \le 1$.

We have obtained a much simpler recurrence than (2.3)–(2.4), but relation (3.2) still has some undesirable features. Before proceeding any further, we can at least use (3.2) to check what we have done so far, by computing the first few cases of f_n:

$$f_1(x,y) = 1 - \frac{2}{3}x + \frac{1}{3}y, \qquad\qquad f_1 = \frac{1}{2};$$

$$f_2(x,y) = 1 - \frac{8}{9}x + \frac{4}{9}y + \frac{1}{18}(x-y)^2, \qquad f_2 = \frac{109}{216}.$$

Good.

We are hoping that the process converges for large n, and in this case the limiting distribution $f(x,y) = f_\infty(x,y)$ will have to satisfy the integral equation

$$f(x,y) = \frac{1}{3}\left(2 - 2x + f(x,y) + \int_0^x f(t,y)\,dt + \int_x^y f(x,t)\,dt\right). \quad (3.3)$$

Before going on to find a solution to this equation, let us verify that $f_n(x,y)$ will indeed converge to $f(x,y)$ if $f(x,y)$ exists: Subtracting (3.3) from (3.2) yields

$$r_{n+1}(x,y) = \frac{1}{3}\left(r_n(x,y) + \int_0^x r_n(t,y)\,dt + \int_x^y r_n(x,t)\,dt\right),$$

where $r_n(x,y) = f_n(x,y) - f(x,y)$. Now if $|r_n(x,y)| \le \alpha$ for $0 \le x < y \le 1$, we will have

$$|r_{n+1}(x,y)| \le \frac{1}{3}\left(\alpha + \int_0^x \alpha\,dt + \int_x^y \alpha\,dt\right) = \frac{1+y}{3}\alpha \le \frac{2}{3}\alpha.$$

Therefore if $f(x,y)$ exists, so that $r_0(x,y)$ is bounded, the remainder $r_n(x,y) = O\big((2/3)^n\big)$ converges rapidly to zero, regardless of the initial distribution $f_0(x,y)$.

It remains to determine $f(x,y)$, whose defining equation (3.3) can be rewritten

$$f(x,y) = 1 - x + \frac{1}{2}\left(\int_0^x f(t,y)\,dt + \int_x^y f(x,t)\,dt\right). \quad (3.4)$$

The coefficient $1/2$ can be removed from this relation by letting

$$q(x,y) = f(2x, 2y),$$

so that

$$q(x,y) = 1 - 2x + \int_0^x q(t,y)\,dt + \int_x^y q(x,t)\,dt. \quad (3.5)$$

What is this function $q(x,y)$? (It is suggested that the reader might enjoy trying to find it before reading on.)

4. Solving the Integral Equation

When attempting to solve (3.5), perhaps the first thing we might try is differentiation. Let $q'(x, y) = \partial q(x, y)/\partial x$, and $q_{\prime}(x, y) = \partial q(x, y)/\partial y$; then

$$q'(x, y) = -2 + q(x, y) + \int_x^y q'(x, t)\, dt - q(x, x), \qquad (4.1)$$

$$q_{\prime}(x, y) = \int_0^x q_{\prime}(t, y)\, dt + q(x, y), \qquad (4.2)$$

$$q_{\prime}'(x, y) = q_{\prime}(x, y) + q'(x, y). \qquad (4.3)$$

If we postulate that q has a power series expansion

$$q(x, y) = \sum_{m,n \geq 0} q_{m,n} \frac{x^m}{m!} \frac{y^n}{n!} \qquad (4.4)$$

we find

$$q'(x, y) = \sum_{m,n \geq 0} q_{m+1,n} \frac{x^m}{m!} \frac{y^n}{n!},$$

$$q_{\prime}(x, y) = \sum_{m,n \geq 0} q_{m,n+1} \frac{x^m}{m!} \frac{y^n}{n!},$$

$$q_{\prime}'(x, y) = \sum_{m,n \geq 0} q_{m+1,n+1} \frac{x^m}{m!} \frac{y^n}{n!}. \qquad (4.5)$$

Therefore (4.3) yields the simple relation

$$q_{m+1,n+1} = q_{m,n+1} + q_{m+1,n}, \qquad \text{for } m, n \geq 0, \qquad (4.6)$$

from which it is possible to determine all the $q_{m,n}$ in terms of the boundary values $q_{0,n}$ and $q_{m,0}$.

Setting $x = 0$ in (3.5) yields

$$q(0, y) = 1 + \int_0^y q(0, t)\, dt; \qquad (4.7)$$

hence $q(0, y) = e^y$ and

$$q_{0,n} = 1, \qquad \text{for } n \geq 0. \qquad (4.8)$$

Now comes a tricky manipulation, which was found while playing around trying to determine $q(x, 0)$. If we apply (4.1) with x and y interchanged, and add the two results, we get

$$q'(x, y) + q'(y, x) = -4 + q(x, y) + q(y, x) - q(x, x) - q(y, y)$$

$$+ \int_x^y (q'(x, t) - q'(y, t))\, dt$$

$$= -4 + \int_x^y (q'(t, x) - q'(t, y))\, dt$$

$$+ \int_x^y (q'(x, t) - q'(y, t))\, dt.$$

Let $s(x, y)$ be the symmetric function $q'(x, y) + q'(y, x)$; we have just proved that

$$s(x, y) = -4 + \int_x^y \big(s(x, t) - s(y, t)\big)\, dt. \tag{4.9}$$

But this equation implies that $s(x, y) = -4$, identically! Let

$$s(x, y) = \sum_{m,n \geq 0} s_{m,n} \frac{x^m\, y^n}{m!\, n!}, \qquad s_{m,n} = q_{m+1,n} + q_{n+1,m}. \tag{4.10}$$

The coefficients $s_{m,n}$ for $m + n = k > 0$ on the left-hand side of (4.9) all arise as homogeneous linear combinations of the coefficients $s_{m,n}$ for $m + n = k - 1$, since

$$\int_x^y (x^m t^n - y^m t^n)\, dt = \frac{x^m y^{n+1} + x^{n+1} y^m - x^{m+n+1} y^0 - x^0 y^{m+n+1}}{n + 1};$$

hence we can prove by induction on k that $s_{m,n} = 0$ whenever $m + n = k > 0$. It follows that

$$q_{m+1,n} = -q_{n+1,m}, \qquad \text{for } m, n \geq 0 \text{ and } m + n > 0. \tag{4.11}$$

When $m = n = 0$ we have $-4 = s_{0,0} = q_{1,0} + q_{1,0}$, hence $q_{1,0} = -2$; relations (4.6) and (4.8) imply that $q_{1,n} = n - 2$ for all $n \geq 0$, and (4.11) with $n = 0$ yields

$$q_{m,0} = -q_{1,m-1} = 3 - m \qquad \text{for } m \geq 2. \tag{4.12}$$

We have found the desired boundary conditions, and it remains to deduce the general formula using (4.6). The binomial coefficient

$$\binom{m + n + a}{m + b}$$

satisfies (4.6) for all integers a and b, so it suffices to find a linear combination of these binomial coefficients, subject to the condition that the known values of $q_{m,n}$ are obtained whenever $m = 0$ or $n = 0$. The solution in this form is not unique, because of identities between binomial coefficients; probably the most elegant way to express it is

$$q_{m,n} = \binom{m+n-3}{m} - \binom{m+n-3}{m-4}. \tag{4.13}$$

Our derivation has proved that $q_{m,n}$ must have this value if the power series $q(x,y)$ postulated in (4.4) satisfies (3.5). Conversely, it is clear that a power series solution to (3.5) exists, since the set of values $q_{m,n}$ with $m + n = k$ defines the set of values with $m + n = k + 1$ after integration. Therefore the function

$$q(x,y) = \sum_{m,n \geq 0} \left(\binom{m+n-3}{m} - \binom{m+n-3}{m-4} \right) \frac{x^m \, y^n}{m! \, n!} \tag{4.14}$$

solves (3.5). Note that $|q_{m,n}| \leq 2^{m+n}$, hence the power series is absolutely convergent for all x and y; (4.14) is the only power series solution.

Finally let us try to express $q(x,y)$ in terms of simpler functions, possibly even "known" ones. The following somewhat surprising identity is especially useful for functions of this type:

$$e^{-x-y} \sum_{m,n \geq 0} \binom{m+n+a}{m+b} \frac{x^m \, y^n}{m! \, n!}$$

$$= \sum_{j,k,m,n \geq 0} (-1)^{j+k} \binom{m+n+a}{m+b} \frac{x^{j+m} \, y^{k+n}}{j! \, m! \, k! \, n!}$$

$$= \sum_{M,N \geq 0} \frac{x^M \, y^N}{M! \, N!} \sum_{j,k \geq 0} (-1)^{j+k} \binom{M}{j}\binom{N}{k}\binom{M+N-j-k+a}{M-j+b}$$

$$= \sum_{M,N \geq 0} \frac{x^M \, y^N}{M! \, N!} \sum_{j,k \geq 0} (-1)^{M+b+k} \binom{M}{j}\binom{N}{k}\binom{-N+k-a+b-1}{M-j+b}$$

$$= \sum_{M,N \geq 0} \frac{x^M \, y^N}{M! \, N!} \sum_{k \geq 0} (-1)^{M+b+k} \binom{N}{k}\binom{M-N+k-a+b-1}{M+b}$$

$$= \sum_{M,N \geq 0} \frac{x^M \, y^N}{M! \, N!} (-1)^{M+N+b} \binom{M-N-a+b-1}{M-N+b}$$

$$= \sum_{M,N \geq 0} \frac{x^M \, y^N}{M! \, N!} \binom{a}{M-N+b}. \tag{4.15}$$

When $M - N$ has a fixed value, the terms of this sum are readily expressed in terms of modified Bessel functions of the first kind, defined as usual by the formula

$$I_r(2z) = \sum_{k \geq \max(0,-r)} \frac{z^{2k+r}}{k!\,(k+r)!}. \qquad (4.16)$$

For example, if $a \geq 0$ all terms vanish except those for $0 \leq M - N + b \leq a$, hence (4.15) reduces to a finite sum

$$\sum_r \binom{a}{r} \sum_{\substack{M,N \geq 0 \\ M+b=N+r}} \frac{x^M\,y^N}{M!\,N!} = \sum_r \binom{a}{r} \left(\left(\frac{x}{y}\right)^{1/2} \right)^{r-b} I_{r-b}(2(xy)^{1/2}).$$

On the other hand, if $a < 0$ (as it unfortunately is in our case), another function is apparently required.

Let $h(x,y)$ be the double power series

$$\sum_{m \geq n \geq 0} \frac{x^m\,y^n}{m!\,n!}, \qquad (4.17)$$

which converges absolutely for all x and y. We have

$$h(x,y) = \sum_{m,n \geq 0} \frac{x^{m+n}}{(m+n)!} \frac{y^n}{n!} = \sum_{m \geq 0} \left(\frac{x}{y}\right)^{m/2} I_m(2(xy)^{1/2}). \qquad (4.18)$$

Furthermore

$$h(x,y) = e^y \sum_{m \geq 0} \frac{x^m}{m!} \left(1 - \frac{1}{m!} \int_0^y e^{-t} t^m \, dt \right)$$

$$= e^{x+y} - e^y \int_0^y e^{-t} \left(\sum_{m \geq 0} \frac{t^m x^m}{m!^2} \right) dt$$

$$= e^{x+y} - e^y \int_0^y e^{-t} I_0 (2(tx)^{1/2}) \, dt; \qquad (4.19)$$

so $h(x,y)$ can be expressed in at least two ways in terms of Bessel functions. But it does not seem to have any simpler expressions in "closed form." The definition of $h(x,y)$ is already sufficiently simple that we can consider it a known function; we will express $q(x,y)$ in terms of $h(x,y)$ and Bessel functions.

By (4.14) and (4.15),

$$e^{-x-y}q(x,y) = \sum_{m,n\geq0} \frac{x^m\,y^n}{m!\,n!}(-1)^{m+n}\left(\binom{m-n+2}{m-n} - \binom{m-n-2}{m-n-4}\right)$$

$$= \sum_{m\geq n\geq0} \frac{x^m\,y^n}{m!\,n!}(-1)^{m+n}(4m-4n-2+3\delta_{mn}+\delta_{m(n+1)})$$

$$= 4xy i_1(xy) - 4xh(-x,-y) + 4yh(-x,-y) - 4y i_0(xy)$$
$$- 2h(-x,-y) + 3i_0(xy) - x i_1(xy)$$

where $i_r(z) = \sum_{k\geq0} z^k/(k!\,(k+r)!)$. This formula yields the steady-state density function $f(x,y) = f_\infty(x,y)$ of the trivial algorithm, if we replace x and y by $x/2$ and $y/2$:

$$f(x,y) = e^{(x+y)/2}\left((2y-2x-2)h\left(-\frac{x}{2},-\frac{y}{2}\right) + (3-2y)I_0\left((xy)^{1/2}\right)\right.$$
$$\left. + \frac{(2y-1)x}{(xy)^{1/2}}I_1\left((xy)^{1/2}\right)\right), \tag{4.20}$$

for $0 \leq x < y \leq 1$.

5. An Explicit Formula

Now that the limiting behavior has been found, we can look back at the original recurrence (3.2) and see that it does not appear so formidable any more. Let us define a sequence of polynomials as follows:

$$p_0(x,y) = 1, \tag{5.1}$$
$$p_1(x,y) = y - 2x, \tag{5.2}$$
$$p_{k+1}(x,y) = \int_0^x p_k(t,y)\,dt + \int_x^y p_k(x,t)\,dt, \quad \text{for } k \geq 1. \tag{5.3}$$

Thus $p_2(x,y) = (x-y)^2/2$, $p_3(x,y) = y^3/6$, etc.; it is easy to see that each term of $p_k(x,y)$ has total degree k.

These polynomials handle the complicated parts of recurrence (3.2). If we assume that $f_n(x,y)$ is a linear combination of the p's, say

$$f_n(x,y) = \sum_{k\geq0} \varphi_{n,k}\,p_k(x,y) \tag{5.4}$$

with $\varphi_{n,0} = 1$, relations (3.2) and (5.3) imply that $f_{n+1}(x, y)$ also has such a representation, namely

$$f_{n+1}(x,y) = \frac{1}{3}\left(2 - 2x + f_n(x, y) + y + \sum_{k \geq 1} \varphi_{n,k}p_{k+1}(x, y)\right)$$

$$= 1 + \frac{1}{3}\left(\sum_{k \geq 1} \varphi_{n,k}p_k(x, y) + \sum_{k \geq 0} \varphi_{n,k}p_{k+1}(x, y)\right).$$

Hence (5.4) holds for all n if the coefficients $\varphi_{n,k}$ satisfy

$$\varphi_{n+1,0} = 1,$$
$$\varphi_{n+1,k+1} = (\varphi_{n,k+1} + \varphi_{n,k})/3, \quad \text{for } n \geq 0 \text{ and } k \geq 0. \quad (5.5)$$

Since $\varphi_{0,k} = 0$ for all $k \geq 1$, this recurrence is easy to solve, and we have

$$\varphi_{n,k} = \sum_{j=1}^{n} \binom{j-1}{k-1} 3^{-j}, \quad \text{for } n \geq 0 \text{ and } k \geq 1. \quad (5.6)$$

Equation (5.4) would now be a fairly explicit formula for $f_n(x, y)$, if we only knew $p_k(x, y)$.

Let $n \to \infty$; then

$$\varphi_{\infty,k} = \sum_{j=1}^{\infty} \binom{j-1}{k-1} 3^{-j} = 2^{-k}, \quad \text{for } k \geq 1. \quad (5.7)$$

Since $f(2x, 2y) = q(x, y)$, and since all the terms of $p_k(x, y)$ have total degree k, we must have

$$q(x, y) = \sum_{k \geq 0} p_k(x, y). \quad (5.8)$$

Therefore we can find $p_k(x, y)$ by selecting the terms of total degree k in (4.14), namely

$$p_k(x, y) = \frac{1}{k!}\sum_{j}\binom{k}{j}\left(\binom{k-3}{j} - \binom{k-3}{j-4}\right)x^j y^{k-j}. \quad (5.9)$$

We may also express $p_k(x, y)$ in "closed form," in terms of the Jacobi polynomials defined by

$$(x - y)^n P_n^{(\alpha,\beta)}\left(\frac{x+y}{x-y}\right) = \sum_{j}\binom{n+\alpha}{j}\binom{n+\beta}{n-j}x^j y^{n-j}; \quad (5.10)$$

the result is

$$p_k(x, y) = \frac{1}{k!}\left((x-y)^k P_k^{(-3,0)}\left(\frac{x+y}{x-y}\right) - x^4(x-y)^{k-4}P_{k-4}^{(1,4)}\left(\frac{x+y}{x-y}\right)\right).$$
$$(5.11)$$

6. Approach to the Answers

We have shown that the trivial algorithm leads to a (nontrivial) limiting distribution. What we really want to know is the limiting probabilities of the various tree shapes that arise, namely the quantities a_n, b_n, c_n, d_n, e_n, f_n, and g_n defined by the integrals in (2.5) and (2.6), as $n \to \infty$.

We clearly have

$$a_n + b_n + c_n + d_n + e_n = 1, \tag{6.1}$$

$$f_n + g_n = 1. \tag{6.2}$$

Furthermore since $b_n(x, y, z) + d_n(x, y, z) = 2$ by (2.1) and (3.1), we have

$$b_n + d_n = 1/3. \tag{6.3}$$

Another relation, slightly more subtle, also holds. We have

$$a_n = \iiint\limits_{0 \le x \le y \le z \le 1} f_n(y, z)\,dx\,dy\,dz = \iint\limits_{0 \le x \le y \le 1} x f_n(x, y)\,dx\,dy;$$

$$b_n = \iiint\limits_{0 \le x \le y \le z \le 1} f_n(x, z)\,dx\,dy\,dz = \iint\limits_{0 \le x \le y \le 1} (y - x) f_n(x, y)\,dx\,dy;$$

$$\frac{1}{3} - e_n = \iiint\limits_{0 \le x \le y \le z \le 1} f_n(x, y)\,dx\,dy\,dz = \iint\limits_{0 \le x \le y \le 1} (1 - y) f_n(x, y)\,dx\,dy.$$

Therefore

$$a_n + b_n + 1/3 - e_n = f_n. \tag{6.4}$$

And still another relation, even more subtle, can be obtained by looking more closely. If we integrate both sides of (3.2) over $0 \le x \le y \le 1$ we find

$$3f_{n+1} = \frac{2}{3} + f_n + \iint\limits_{0 \le x \le y \le 1} \int_0^x f_n(t, y)\,dt + \iint\limits_{0 \le x \le y \le 1} \int_x^y f_n(x, t)\,dt$$

$$= \frac{2}{3} + f_n + b_n + \frac{1}{3} - e_n.$$

Combining this with (6.4) yields the somewhat surprising formula

$$a_n + 3f_{n+1} = 2/3 + 2f_n. \tag{6.5}$$

For example, we know that $a_1 = 11/72$, $f_1 = 1/2$, and $f_2 = 109/216$; everything checks out beautifully.

From relations (6.1)–(6.5) we can determine all of a_n, b_n, c_n, d_n, e_n, f_n, and g_n knowing only the values of b_n and f_n for all n. Let us first look at f_n, and especially at the component involving $p_k(x, y)$:

$$
\iint\limits_{0 \le x \le y \le 1} p_k(x, y)\, dx\, dy = \frac{1}{k!} \sum_j \binom{k}{j} \left(\binom{k-3}{j} - \binom{k-3}{j-4} \right) \frac{1}{j+1} \frac{1}{k+2}
$$

$$
= \frac{1}{(k+2)!} \sum_j \binom{k+1}{j+1} \left(\binom{k-3}{j} - \binom{k-3}{j-4} \right)
$$

$$
= \frac{1}{(k+2)!} \left(\binom{2k-2}{k} - \binom{2k-2}{k-4} \right). \qquad (6.6)
$$

Similarly we have

$$
\iint\limits_{0 \le x \le y \le 1} (y - x) p_k(x, y)\, dx\, dy
$$

$$
= \frac{1}{k!} \sum_j \binom{k}{j} \left(\binom{k-3}{j} - \binom{k-3}{j-4} \right) \frac{1}{j+1} \frac{1}{j+2} \frac{1}{k+3}
$$

$$
= \frac{1}{(k+3)!} \sum_j \binom{k+2}{j+2} \left(\binom{k-3}{j} - \binom{k-3}{j-4} \right)
$$

$$
= \frac{1}{(k+3)!} \left(\binom{2k-1}{k} - \binom{2k-1}{k-4} \right). \qquad (6.7)
$$

These quantities are nonnegative for all $k \ge 0$, and since the coefficients $\varphi_{n,k}$ in (5.4) and (5.6) are monotone nondecreasing with n, it follows that

$$
f_{n+1} \ge f_n \qquad \text{and} \qquad b_{n+1} \ge b_n \qquad \text{for } n \ge 0. \qquad (6.8)
$$

(A similar argument shows that $e_{n+1} \ge e_n$ for all n.)

Let us now look at the limiting behavior. We have

$$
f_\infty(x, y) = f(x, y) = \sum_{k \ge 0} \frac{1}{2^k} p_k(x, y)
$$

by (5.7); hence by (6.6) and (6.7) the probabilities f_n and b_n increase to the limits

$$
f_\infty = \sum_{k \ge 0} \frac{1}{2^k (k+2)!} \left(\binom{2k-2}{k} - \binom{2k-2}{k-4} \right),
$$

$$
b_\infty = \sum_{k \ge 0} \frac{1}{2^k (k+3)!} \left(\binom{2k-1}{k} - \binom{2k-1}{k-4} \right). \qquad (6.9)
$$

7. Evaluation of the Final Sums

The formulas in (6.9) converge rapidly, so we could compute them and be done; but of course we would like to express the results in terms of "known" mathematical quantities, for if there is a simple answer we want to know about it. In order to get a cleaner sum to work with, let us consider the similar series

$$s_r(x) = \sum_{k \geq 0} \frac{(x/2)^k}{(k+r)!} \binom{2k}{k},\tag{7.1}$$

which converges absolutely for all x. Differentiation yields

$$\begin{aligned}
s'_r(x) &= \sum_{k \geq 1} \frac{(x/2)^{k-1}}{(k+r)!}(2k-1)\binom{2k-2}{k-1}\\
&= \sum_{k \geq 0} \frac{(x/2)^k}{(k+r+1)!}(2k+1)\binom{2k}{k}\\
&= \sum_{k \geq 0} \frac{(x/2)^k}{(k+r+1)!}\bigl(2(k+r+1)-(2r+1)\bigr)\binom{2k}{k}\\
&= 2s_r(x) - (2r+1)s_{r+1}(x).\tag{7.2}
\end{aligned}$$

Thus if we define

$$t_r(x) = e^{-2x}s_r(x),\tag{7.3}$$

we have

$$t'_r(x) = -(2r+1)t_{r+1}(x).\tag{7.4}$$

According to this relation, we obtain all $t_r(x)$ by starting with $t_0(x)$ and differentiating.

A curious thing happens when we look at $t_0(x)$: We have

$$\begin{aligned}
e^{-2x}s_0(x) &= \sum_{k \geq 0} \frac{(x/2)^k}{k!}\binom{2k}{k}\sum_{j \geq 0}\frac{(-2x)^j}{j!}\\
&= \sum_{m \geq 0} \frac{(-2x)^m}{m!}\sum_k \binom{m}{k}\frac{(-1)^k}{4^k}\binom{2k}{k}\\
&= \sum_{m \geq 0} \frac{(-2x)^m}{m!}\sum_k \binom{m}{m-k}\binom{-1/2}{k}\\
&= \sum_{m \geq 0} \frac{(-2x)^m}{m!}\binom{m-1/2}{m}\\
&= \sum_{m \geq 0} \frac{(-x/2)^m}{m!}\binom{2m}{m} = s_0(-x),
\end{aligned}$$

using the familiar identities

$$(-1)^m \binom{-1/2}{m} = \binom{m-1/2}{m} = 4^{-m} \binom{2m}{m}. \tag{7.5}$$

In other words, $t_0(x) = s_0(-x)$, and $e^{-x} s_0(x) = e^x s_0(-x)$ is an *even* function! This coincidence deserves looking into; let us write

$$e^{-x} s_0(x) = \sum_{k \geq 0} \frac{(x/2)^k}{k!} \binom{2k}{k} \sum_{j \geq 0} \frac{(-x)^j}{j!} = \sum_{m \geq 0} \frac{(-x)^m}{m!} u_m$$

where

$$u_m = \sum_k \binom{m}{k} \frac{(-1)^k}{2^k} \binom{2k}{k}. \tag{7.6}$$

After a few moments of playing with this sum, an experienced binomial-coefficientologist might come up with the following elementary approach:

$$\begin{aligned}
u_m &= u_{m-1} + \sum_k \binom{m-1}{k-1} \frac{(-1)^k}{2^k} \binom{2k}{k} \\
&= u_{m-1} - \sum_k \binom{m-1}{k} \frac{(-1)^k}{2^{k+1}} \binom{2k+2}{k+1} \\
&= u_{m-1} - \sum_k \binom{m}{k+1} \frac{(-1)^k}{2^k} \binom{2k}{k} \frac{2k+1}{m} \\
&= u_{m-1} - \sum_k \binom{m}{k+1} \frac{(-1)^k}{2^k} \binom{2k}{k} \frac{2k+2}{m} \\
&\quad + \sum_k \binom{m}{k+1} \frac{(-1)^k}{2^k} \binom{2k}{k} \frac{1}{m} \\
&= u_{m-1} - 2u_{m-1} + \frac{1}{m} \sum_k \binom{m}{k+1} \frac{(-1)^k}{2^k} \binom{2k}{k};
\end{aligned}$$

hence

$$m(u_m + u_{m-1}) = \sum_k \binom{m}{k+1} \frac{(-1)^k}{2^k} \binom{2k}{k},$$

$$\begin{aligned}
(m-1)(u_{m-1} + u_{m-2}) &= \sum_k \binom{m-1}{k+1} \frac{(-1)^k}{2^k} \binom{2k}{k} \\
&= \sum_k \binom{m}{k+1} \frac{(-1)^k}{2^k} \binom{2k}{k} - u_{m-1}.
\end{aligned}$$

Subtracting these equations yields

$$mu_m = (m-1)u_{m-2}.$$

Now $u_0 = 1$ and $u_1 = 0$, hence $u_{2m+1} = 0$, as we knew; and

$$u_{2m} = \left(\frac{2m-1}{2m}\right)\left(\frac{2m-3}{2m-2}\right)\cdots\left(\frac{1}{2}\right) = \binom{m-1/2}{m} = \frac{1}{4^m}\binom{2m}{m}. \quad (7.7)$$

(Is there a simpler elementary proof of this formula?) We have shown that

$$e^{-x}s_0(x) = \sum_{m\geq 0}\frac{(-x)^{2m}}{(2m)!}u_{2m} = \sum_{m\geq 0}\frac{(x/2)^{2m}}{m!\,m!} = I_0(x); \quad (7.8)$$

so our friend the modified Bessel function has appeared again. The formulas above now yield the identities

$$s_r(x) = e^{2x}t_r(x) = e^{2x}\frac{(-1)^r}{1\cdot 3\cdot\,\ldots\,\cdot(2r-1)}\frac{d^r}{dx^r}(e^{-x}I_0(x)),$$

from which we have

$$s_0(x) = e^x I_0(x),$$
$$s_1(x) = e^x(I_0(x) - I_0'(x)),$$
$$s_2(x) = \tfrac{1}{3}e^x(I_0(x) - 2I_0'(x) + I_0''(x)), \qquad (7.9)$$
$$s_3(x) = \tfrac{1}{15}e^x(I_0(x) - 3I_0'(x) + 3I_0''(x) - I_0'''(x)),$$

and so on. It is easy to see from definition (4.16) that

$$I_0'(x) = I_1(x), \qquad I_1'(x) = I_0(x) - x^{-1}I_1(x); \quad (7.10)$$

hence we can express each $s_r(x)$ in terms of $I_0(x)$ and $I_1(x)$.

Finally to get f_∞ and b_∞ we need to express the sums of (6.9) in terms of $s_r(x)$ for various r. The problem boils down to expressing the binomial coefficient $\binom{2n+m}{n}$ as a linear combination of binomial coefficients that have the form $\binom{2n+2k}{n+k}$. For $m = 0$ this is no problem, and for $m = 1$ we have

$$\binom{2n+1}{n} = \frac{1}{2}\binom{2n+2}{n+1} \qquad \text{if } n \geq 0.$$

For $m \geq 2$ we can reduce the problem to the cases $m - 1$ and $m - 2$, since

$$\binom{2n+m}{n} = \binom{2n+2+(m-1)}{n+1} - \binom{2n+2+(m-2)}{n+1}.$$

Iterating this idea leads us to the desired identity,

$$\binom{2n+m}{n} = \frac{1}{2}\sum_{k=1}^{m}(-1)^{m-k}\binom{2n+2k}{n+k}\binom{k}{m-k}\frac{m}{k}, \qquad (7.11)$$

valid for $m \geq 1$ and $n \geq -m/2$. In particular we find

$$\binom{2n-2}{n} = \binom{2n-2}{n-2} + \delta_{n0} = \frac{1}{2}\binom{2n}{n} - \binom{2n-2}{n-1} + \frac{1}{2}\delta_{n0},$$

$$\binom{2n-2}{n-4} = \frac{1}{2}\binom{2n+4}{n+2} - 3\binom{2n+2}{n+1} + \frac{9}{2}\binom{2n}{n} - \binom{2n-2}{n-1} - \frac{3}{2}\delta_{n0},$$

$$\binom{2n-1}{n} = \frac{1}{2}\binom{2n}{n} + \frac{1}{2}\delta_{n0},$$

$$\binom{2n-1}{n-4} = \frac{1}{2}\binom{2n+6}{n+3} - \frac{7}{2}\binom{2n+4}{n+2} + 7\binom{2n+2}{n+1} - \frac{7}{2}\binom{2n}{n} + \frac{1}{2}\delta_{n0},$$

for all $n \geq 0$.

Letting s_r stand for $s_r(1)$, we can now rewrite (6.9) as

$$f_\infty = \frac{1}{2}s_2 - \frac{1}{2}s_3 + \frac{1}{4} - \frac{4}{2}\left(s_0 - 1 - \frac{2}{2}\right) + 3 \cdot 2(s_1 - 1) - \frac{9}{2}s_2 + \frac{1}{2}s_3 + \frac{3}{4}$$

$$= -1 - 2s_0 + 6s_1 - 4s_2$$

$$= \frac{4}{3}eI_0(1) - 2eI_1(1) - 1; \qquad (7.12)$$

$$b_\infty = \frac{1}{2}s_3 + \frac{1}{12} - \frac{8}{2}\left(s_0 - 1 - \frac{2}{2} - \frac{6}{8}\right) + \frac{7 \cdot 4}{2}\left(s_1 - 1 - \frac{1}{2}\right)$$

$$\qquad - 7 \cdot 2\left(s_2 - \frac{1}{2}\right) + \frac{7}{2}s_3 - \frac{1}{12}$$

$$= -3 - 4s_0 + 14s - 14s_2 + 4s_3$$

$$= 2eI_0(1) - \frac{12}{5}eI_1(1) - 3. \qquad (7.13)$$

The Bessel function values we need are readily computed to be

$$I_0(1) = 1.26606\,58777\,52008\,33559\,82446\,25214\,71753\,76077-, \quad (7.14)$$
$$I_1(1) = 0.56515\,91039\,92485\,02720\,76960\,27609\,86330\,73289-. \quad (7.15)$$

Finally therefore we have the answers:

$$a_\infty = 2/3 - f_\infty \quad \approx 0.15049\,16196\,41488\,77320, \quad (7.16)$$
$$b_\infty \quad \approx 0.19601\,96040\,80347\,57536, \quad (7.17)$$
$$c_\infty = f_\infty - e_\infty \quad \approx 0.35250\,55369\,95186\,10505, \quad (7.18)$$
$$d_\infty = 1/3 - b_\infty \quad \approx 0.13731\,37292\,52985\,75797, \quad (7.19)$$
$$e_\infty = 1 + b_\infty - 2f_\infty \approx 0.16366\,95100\,29991\,78842, \quad (7.20)$$
$$f_\infty \quad \approx 0.51617\,50470\,25177\,89347, \quad (7.21)$$
$$g_\infty = 1 - f_\infty \quad \approx 0.48382\,49529\,74822\,10653. \quad (7.22)$$

The average internal path length of the tree just before the $(n+1)$st deletion is $3a_n + 3b_n + 2c_n + 3d_n + 3e_n = 3 - c_n$. We have proved that c_n converges to c_∞, which is greater than $c_0 = 1/3$; this is consistent with the conjecture that deletions do not make the path length larger than pure insertions do. However, it is interesting to note that the convergence of c_n to c_∞ is *not* monotonic:

$$c_0 = \frac{1}{3} \qquad \approx 0.33333$$

$$c_1 = \frac{25}{72} \qquad \approx 0.34722$$

$$c_2 = \frac{19}{54} \qquad \approx 0.35185$$

$$c_3 = \frac{143}{405} \qquad \approx 0.35309$$

$$c_4 = \frac{3004}{8505} \qquad \approx 0.35320$$

$$c_5 = \frac{1152983}{3265920} \qquad \approx 0.35303$$

$$c_6 = \frac{4667107}{13226976} \qquad \approx 0.35285$$

$$c_7 = \frac{699791131}{1984046400} \qquad \approx 0.35271$$

Therefore random deletions do not always enhance the average path length; the pattern $IIIDIDIDIDI$ leads to a better average search time than does the same pattern followed by DI, and an argument that does not rely on such monotonicity will be necessary to prove Knott's conjecture.

8. Modified Deletions

To complete our study of this process we should also look at what happens if we use the "improved" deletion algorithm discussed in [3, shortly before 6.2.2–(11)]. Here a new "step D1$\frac{1}{2}$" is introduced, to simplify the deletion of nodes having an empty left subtree.

The modified algorithm changes only one thing with respect to trees with three or fewer nodes: The deletion of x from $D(x, y, z)$ now produces $F(y, z)$ instead of $G(y, z)$. The net effect is that the integral

$$\int_0^x g_n(t, y)\, dt$$

moves from the sum for $g_{n+1}(x, y)$ to the sum for $f_{n+1}(x, y)$ in (2.3).

Fortunately this change makes the analog of (3.2) much simpler than before; we now have

$$f_0(x, y) = 1,$$
$$f_{n+1}(x, y) = \frac{1}{3}\left(2 + f_n(x, y) + \int_x^y f_n(x, t)\, dt\right), \quad \text{for } n \geq 0, \quad (8.1)$$

since (3.1) remains valid. The relation corresponding to (3.3) reduces to

$$f(x, y) = 1 + \frac{1}{2}\int_x^y f(x, t)\, dt \qquad (8.2)$$

and by arguing as before (but with considerably fewer complications) we can deduce the solution

$$f_\infty(x, y) = e^{(y-x)/2}. \qquad (8.3)$$

In fact, it is not difficult to establish the general formula

$$f_n(x, y) = \sum_{k=0}^n \frac{(y-x)^k}{k!} \sum_{t=k}^n \left(\frac{1}{3}\right)^t \binom{t-1}{t-k} \qquad \text{for } n \geq 0. \qquad (8.4)$$

Since $f(x, y)$ now has such a simple form, we can easily determine the limiting integrals corresponding to (2.5) and (2.6):

$$a_\infty = 8e^{1/2} - 13 \quad \approx 0.18977, \tag{8.5}$$

$$b_\infty = 20 - 12e^{1/2} \approx 0.21534, \tag{8.6}$$

$$c_\infty = 1/3 \quad\quad\quad \approx 0.33333, \tag{8.7}$$

$$d_\infty = 1/3 - b_\infty \quad \approx 0.11799, \tag{8.8}$$

$$e_\infty = 1/3 - a_\infty \quad \approx 0.14356, \tag{8.9}$$

$$f_\infty = 4e^{1/2} - 6 \quad \approx 0.59489, \tag{8.10}$$

$$g_\infty = 7 - 4e^{1/2} \quad \approx 0.40511. \tag{8.11}$$

As expected, there is now a stronger bias towards the F tree. The unexpected result is that c_∞ has such a simple form compared to the others; in fact it turns out that

$$c_n = 1/3 \quad \text{for all } n \geq 0, \tag{8.12}$$

so the average internal path length is the same as that of a random tree built up from three insertions! Equation (8.12) follows easily from (8.4) and the fact that

$$\iiint\limits_{0 \leq x \leq y \leq z \leq 1} \left((y - x)^k - (z - y)^k\right) dx\, dy\, dz = 0 \quad \text{for } k \geq 0.$$

Since the values of c_n in the unmodified algorithm are *greater* than $1/3$, for $n \geq 1$, the average internal path length actually turns out to be worse when we use the "improved" algorithm. On the other hand, Knott's empirical data in [2] indicate that the modified algorithm does indeed lead to an improvement when the trees are larger.

The preparation of this paper was supported in part by the Norwegian Research Council for Science and the Humanities, by the United States National Science Foundation, and by the United States Office of Naval Research. Some of the calculations were performed using MACSYMA, supported by the Defense Advanced Research Projects Agency.

References

[1] Thomas N. Hibbard, "Some combinatorial properties of certain trees with applications to searching and sorting," *Journal of the Association for Computing Machinery* **9** (1962), 13–28.

[2] Gary Don Knott, *Deletion in Binary Storage Trees*, Computer Science Technical Report STAN-CS-75-491 (Ph.D. thesis, Stanford University, 1975), 93 pages.

[3] Donald E. Knuth, *Sorting and Searching*, Volume 3 of *The Art of Computer Programming* (Reading, Massachusetts: Addison-Wesley, 1973).

[4] Donald E. Knuth, "Deletions that preserve randomness," *IEEE Transactions on Software Engineering* **SE-3** (1977), 351–359. [Reprinted as Chapter 19 of the present volume.]

Addendum

There are indeed simpler ways to deduce (7.7) from (7.6): See Helmut Prodinger, "Knuth's old sum — a survey," *Bulletin of the European Association for Theoretical Computer Science (EATCS)* **54** (October 1994), 232–245.

See also Ricardo A. Baeza-Yates, "A trivial algorithm whose analysis is not: A Continuation," *BIT* **29** (1989), 378–394, for further development of the topics above, including the case of four elements.

Knott's conjecture turns out to be false — indeed, astonishingly false — when larger search trees are considered. Jeffrey L. Eppinger ["An empirical study of insertion and deletion in binary search trees," *Communications of the ACM* **26** (1983), 663–669; corrigendum, **27** (1984), 235] made empirical studies of random trees formed by the insertion/deletion sequence $I^N(DI)^n$, for fixed N and for $n = 1, 2, 3,$ .... He found that the path length initially decreased, as predicted by the conjecture, but then it started to increase again until reaching a steady state when n was approximately N^2; this steady state was actually *worse* than the initial path length for $n = 0$ when N was larger than about 128. In fact, Joseph Culberson and J. Ian Munro have given good grounds to believe that the expected steady state path length is asymptotic to $N\sqrt{2N/9\pi}$, while a random insertion-only tree has an average path length of only $2N \ln N + O(N)$ [see "Explaining the behaviour of binary search trees under prolonged updates: A model and simulations," *The Computer Journal* **32** (1989), 68–75; "Analysis of the standard deletion algorithms in exact fit domain binary search trees," *Algorithmica* **5** (1990), 295–311]. On the other hand, Eppinger found that a symmetrical strategy, in which Hibbard's deletion algorithm alternates with its left-right dual, does apparently lead to a steady state better than trees formed by insertions only. His empirical approach still awaits theoretical confirmation.

The Ph.D. thesis of Lyle Ramshaw [*Formalizing the Analysis of Algorithms*, Computer Science Technical Report STAN-CS-79-741 (Stanford University, 1979), 115 pages] explains how to transform programs mechanically into recurrence relations and integrals that describe their quantitative behavior.

Chapter 19

Deletions That Preserve Randomness

[Originally published in IEEE Transactions on Software Engineering **SE-3** *(1977), 351–359.]*

This paper discusses dynamic properties of data structures under insertions and deletions. It is shown that, in certain circumstances, the result of n random insertions and m random deletions will be equivalent to n − m random insertions, under various interpretations of the word "random" and under various constraints on the order of insertions and deletions.

1. Introduction

When we try to analyze the average behavior of algorithms that operate on dynamically varying data structures, we typically find it much easier to deal with structures that merely grow in size than to deal with structures that can both grow and shrink. In other words, the study of insertions into data structures has proved to be much simpler than the study of insertions mixed with deletions. One instance of this phenomenon is described in [5], where what looks like an especially simple problem turns out to require manipulations with Bessel functions, although the data structure being considered never contains more than three elements at a time.

Occasionally an analysis of mixed insertions and deletions turns out to be workable because we can prove some sort of invariance property; if we can show that deletions preserve "randomness" of the structure, in some sense, the analysis reduces to a study of structures built by random insertions. The purpose of this note is to investigate some simple properties that imply various kinds of insensitivity to deletions.

Let us say that a *data organization* is a class of data structures together with associated algorithms for operating on those structures;

for example, we might have binary search trees together with algorithms for searching them, inserting into them, and deleting from them. We shall restrict attention to data organizations that depend only on the relative order of the keys of items being inserted and deleted. In other words, if we consider the two data structures formed by the sequence of operations

$$A_1(x_1), \; A_2(x_2), \; \ldots, \; A_n(x_n)$$
$$A_1(y_1), \; A_2(y_2), \; \ldots, \; A_n(y_n)$$

where each $A_k(x)$ means either "insert an element with key x" or "delete an element with key x," the two sequences should produce isomorphic data structures if $x_i < x_j$ holds whenever $y_i < y_j$, for all i and j. Such data organization schemes are quite common: Binary search trees with or without height balancing or weight balancing [7], 2-3 trees [1], leftist trees [7], and binomial queues [8] all have this property because they operate entirely by making comparisons on keys.

2. Preliminary Definitions

Let $I(x)$ denote the operation "insert an element with key x" and let $D(x)$ mean "delete an element with key x." We shall be dealing with sequences of operations

$$A_1(x_1), \; A_2(x_2), \; \ldots, \; A_n(x_n)$$

where each A_i is I or D, and where each insertion $I(x_j)$ introduces an element x_j that is distinct from $x_1, \ldots, x_{j-1}$ with probability 1. Furthermore $D(x_j)$ will make sense only if x_j has previously been inserted and not yet deleted; in particular, the number of D's must never exceed the number of I's, counting from left to right.

Since we are assuming that the relative order of keys is all that matters, not their precise value, it suffices to restrict attention to keys $\{1, 2, \ldots, n\}$ when there have been n insertions. If $y_1, y_2, \ldots, y_n$ is any sequence of n distinct keys, let

$$\rho(y_1 y_2 \ldots y_n)$$

be the canonically reordered permutation of $\{1, 2, \ldots, n\}$ obtained by mapping the jth smallest key into the number j. For example,

$$\rho(8 \; \pi \; e \; \sqrt{29}) = 4\,2\,1\,3.$$

If $x_1 x_2 \ldots x_n$ is a permutation of $\{1, 2, \ldots, n\}$, we write

$$S(x_1 x_2 \ldots x_n)$$

for the data structure obtained after the sequence of insertion operations

$$I(x_1)\, I(x_2)\, \ldots\, I(x_n).$$

Finally we write

$$R(x_1 x_2 \ldots x_n \backslash j) = y_1 \ldots y_{n-1}$$

if the operation of deleting j from $S(x_1 x_2 \ldots x_n)$ and renumbering yields the structure $S(y_1 \ldots y_{n-1})$, where $x_1 x_2 \ldots x_n$ is a permutation of $\{1, 2, \ldots, n\}$, $y_1 \ldots y_{n-1}$ is a permutation of $\{1, \ldots, n-1\}$, and $1 \le j \le n$.

It is possible for several input permutations to yield the same structure; in other words we might have $S(x_1 x_2 \ldots x_n) = S(x_1' x_2' \ldots x_n')$ although $x_1 x_2 \ldots x_n \ne x_1' x_2' \ldots x_n'$. In this case the R notation is not uniquely defined, since any permutation $y_1 \ldots y_{n-1}$ yielding $S(y_1 \ldots y_{n-1})$ could be used as the value of $R(x_1 x_2 \ldots x_n \backslash j)$. However, we will assume that a particular $y_1 \ldots y_{n-1}$ has been selected in each case. Thus, if $S(x_1 x_2 \ldots x_n) = S(x_1' x_2' \ldots x_n')$ we might wish to define $R(x_1 x_2 \ldots x_n \backslash j) \ne R(x_1' x_2' \ldots x_n' \backslash j)$ even though it will be true that $S(R(x_1 x_2 \ldots x_n \backslash j)) = S(R(x_1' x_2' \ldots x_n' \backslash j))$. Some of these definitions of R will be better than others; a typical theorem to be proved below states that deletions will preserve a certain kind of randomness if it is possible to define an R function with certain properties.

The R function can be used to define a deletion operation on permutations of arbitrary keys in the following way. Let π be any permutation of n distinct elements (not necessarily integers), and let u be the jth smallest element of π. Then we define $\pi \backslash u$ (with respect to a given R function) to be the unique permutation of the elements of π other than u such that

$$\rho(\pi \backslash u) = R(\rho(\pi) \backslash j).$$

For example, let $\pi = 8\,3\,2\,5$ and $R(4\,2\,1\,3 \backslash 2) = 1\,3\,2$; then $\pi \backslash 3 = 2\,8\,5$.

3. Examples

Perhaps the simplest kind of data structure is an unordered linear list, where an insertion is done by simply appending the new element at the right of the list and a deletion is done by deleting the element and closing up the space it occupied. Then $S(x_1x_2\ldots x_n)$ is the linear list $\langle x_1, x_2, \ldots, x_n\rangle$, and $R(x_1x_2\ldots x_n\backslash j) = \rho(x_1\ldots x_{k-1}x_{k+1}\ldots x_n)$ where $x_k = j$. In this system the representation preserves all information about the order of insertion.

At the other extreme we might consider a sorted linear list, in which $S(x_1x_2\ldots x_n) = \langle 1, 2, \ldots, n\rangle$ for all permutations $x_1x_2\ldots x_n$ of $\{1, 2, \ldots, n\}$. In such a system $R(x_1x_2\ldots x_n\backslash j)$ can be defined to be any permutation of $\{1, \ldots, n-1\}$ that we wish, as a function of $x_1x_2\ldots x_n$ and j.

In between these extremes lie many other regimens, and binary search trees provide a simple but interesting example. This system defines $S(x_1x_2\ldots x_n)$ as the empty binary tree if $n = 0$, otherwise $S(x_1x_2\ldots x_n)$ consists of a root and two subtrees; the left subtree is $S(\rho(y_1\ldots y_m))$ and the right subtree is $S(\rho(y_1'\ldots y_{n-1+m}'))$, where $(y_1\ldots y_m)$ and $(y_1'\ldots y_{n-1-m}')$ are respectively obtained from $x_1\ldots x_n$ by striking out all elements $\geq x_1$ and $\leq x_1$. Furthermore $R(x_1x_2\ldots x_n\backslash j) = \rho(x_1\ldots x_{k-1}x_{k+1}\ldots x_n)$ or $\rho(x_1\ldots x_{l-1}x_{l+1}\ldots x_n)$, where $x_k = j$ and $x_l = j+1$ if $j < n$; here x_k is deleted if $j = n$ or $l < k$, otherwise x_l is deleted. For example,

$$S(1\,2\,3) = \diagdown \,, \qquad S(1\,3\,2) = \diagup\!\!\!\!\diagdown \,,$$
$$S(2\,1\,3) = S(2\,3\,1) = \diagup\!\!\!\!\diagdown \,,$$
$$S(3\,1\,2) = \diagdown\!\!\!\!\diagup \,, \qquad S(3\,2\,1) = \diagup \,;$$

and deletion is defined as follows when $n = 3$:

$$R(1\,2\,3\backslash 1) = 1\,2, \quad R(1\,2\,3\backslash 2) = 1\,2, \quad R(1\,2\,3\backslash 3) = 1\,2;$$
$$R(1\,3\,2\backslash 1) = 1\,2, \quad R(1\,3\,2\backslash 2) = 1\,2, \quad R(1\,3\,2\backslash 3) = 1\,2;$$
$$R(2\,1\,3\backslash 1) = 1\,2, \quad R(2\,1\,3\backslash 2) = 2\,1, \quad R(2\,1\,3\backslash 3) = 2\,1;$$
$$R(2\,3\,1\backslash 1) = 1\,2, \quad R(2\,3\,1\backslash 2) = 2\,1, \quad R(2\,3\,1\backslash 3) = 2\,1;$$
$$R(3\,1\,2\backslash 1) = 2\,1, \quad R(3\,1\,2\backslash 2) = 2\,1, \quad R(3\,1\,2\backslash 3) = 1\,2;$$
$$R(3\,2\,1\backslash 1) = 2\,1, \quad R(3\,2\,1\backslash 2) = 2\,1, \quad R(3\,2\,1\backslash 3) = 2\,1.$$

This particular rule for deletion corresponds to that of Hibbard [3]; a more elaborate method is given in [7].

4. Deletion Sensitivity and Insensitivity

From an intuitive standpoint, we wish to show that certain data organizations satisfy theorems of the following general character: "The result of n random insertion operations combined in some order with m random deletion operations is a random data structure on $n - m$ elements; that is, the result has the same probability distribution as we would have obtained by doing $n - m$ random insertions."

The first such theorem was proved by T. N. Hibbard [3], who showed that binary search trees have the following property: Suppose we create a binary tree by inserting n distinct elements in random order, then we delete one of the elements chosen at random (each being equally likely). The resulting tree shapes will have the same probability distribution as we would have generated by inserting $n - 1$ distinct elements in random order. We shall call this *one-step deletion insensitivity*, abbreviated I^*D_r. (The motivation for this abbreviation will come later; it essentially means "any number of random insertions followed by one random deletion.")

Our definitions have the following immediate consequence.

Lemma 0. *A data organization has the I^*D_r property if and only if its R function can be defined in such a way that, for each n, the $n \cdot n!$ values of $R(x_1 x_2 \ldots x_n \backslash j)$ comprise each of the $(n - 1)!$ permutations $y_1 \ldots y_{n-1}$ exactly n^2 times.*

For example, the tableau above for binary search trees with $n = 3$ shows '1 2' and '2 1' each occurring nine times.

Proof. The "if" part is obvious. Conversely, consider a data structure σ that is equal to $S(y_1 \ldots y_{n-1})$ for exactly s different permutations $y_1 \ldots y_{n-1}$ of $\{1, \ldots, n - 1\}$. The I^*D_r property states that n random insertions followed by one random deletion should produce this data structure with relative frequency s; in other words, the $n \cdot n!$ values of $S(R(x_1 x_2 \ldots x_n \backslash j))$ as $x_1 x_2 \ldots x_n$ ranges over the $n!$ essentially different insertions and the n essentially different deletions should include the given structure σ exactly $n^2 s$ times. By redefining $R(x_1 x_2 \ldots x_n \backslash j)$ if necessary when the I^*D_r property holds, we can ensure that each of the s permutations $y_1 \ldots y_{n-1}$ occurs exactly n^2 times. $\square$

The I^*D_r property might seem to be all that one needs to guarantee insensitivity to any number of deletions, when they are intermixed with insertions in any order. At least, many people (including the present author when writing the first edition of [7]) believed this, and the subtle fallacy in such reasoning was apparently first pointed out by G. D. Knott in his thesis [6]. Before we proceed to study stronger forms of deletion insensitivity, it is important to understand why the problem is not entirely trivial, so we should look at binary trees more closely.

Consider the following process.

Step 1: Create a binary search tree by starting with the empty tree and inserting three independent random real numbers, uniformly distributed between 0 and 1.

Step 2: Delete one of these three numbers, selected at random. (In other words, each is selected with probability $\frac{1}{3}$.)

Step 3: Insert a fourth independent random real number uniformly distributed between 0 and 1.

Since the binary search tree organization has the I^*D_r property, we know that the tree remaining after Step 2 will be like a random tree after two insertions; that is, ⟋ and ⟍ will be equally likely. Furthermore it is easy to verify that the element x inserted in Step 3 is equally likely to be smaller than, between, or larger than the two elements remaining after Step 2. For example, the probability that x will be the smallest remaining element is $\frac{1}{3}$. Therefore the insertion in Step 3 would seem to behave as the random insertion of a third element into a random two-element tree.

Yet when we analyze carefully what happens after Steps 1, 2, and 3 have been performed, we find that the tree ⟋⟍ is obtained with probability $\frac{25}{72}$, *not* $\frac{1}{3}$. (See [5] for a detailed study of this process.)

The fallacy comes from the fact that the probabilities for the result of Step 2 and the relative position of x in Step 3 are not independent. If we are *given* the fact that the result of Step 2 was ⟍, the conditional probability for element x to be smaller than the two remaining elements turns out to be $\frac{13}{36}$, not $\frac{1}{3}$, since this arises when x is the smallest of all four elements (probability $\frac{1}{4}$) and when x was second smallest but the smallest was deleted (probability $\frac{1}{4}$ times $\frac{4}{9}$, since exactly four of the nine cases with $R(x_1x_2x_3\backslash j) = 1\,2$ have $j = 1$). Therefore, inserting a random element of the interval $[0\mathbin{..}1]$ is not equivalent to inserting a number with probability $\frac{1}{3}$ of being smaller than the two remaining, even though a random element in $[0\mathbin{..}1]$ does have (unconditional) probability $\frac{1}{3}$ of being smaller than the two remaining.

5. Further Definitions

The example just given shows that deletion insensitivity is not as simple as it may seem at first, so we need to be somewhat careful in our treatment. In this section we shall define several types of insertions and deletions that lead to various types of insensitivity that seem to be of importance. The following shorthand notations will prove to be convenient.

I_r Insertion of a random real number from some continuous distribution; for example, the distribution might be uniform on the interval $[0 \mathinner{\ldotp\ldotp} 1]$. Each random number inserted is assumed to have the same distribution, and it is to be independent of all previously inserted numbers. Thus, if we look at n such random numbers $(x_1, x_2, \ldots x_n)$, the $n!$ possible orderings $\rho(x_1 x_2 \ldots x_n)$ are equally likely, and the particular distribution involved has no effect on the behavior of the data organization.

I_o Insertion of a random number by order, in the sense that the new number is equally likely to fall into any of the $d+1$ intervals defined by the d numbers still present as keys after previous insertions and deletions; this is to be independent of the history by which those d numbers were actually obtained. The example in the previous section shows that I_o is a different concept from I_r. It is a somewhat artificial kind of random insertion, but it may be a sufficiently good approximation to reality in some applications, and it agrees with I_r before any deletions have taken place.

I_b "Biased" insertion of a random real number obtained as follows: Generate an independent random number X with the exponential distribution, so that $1 - e^{-x}$ is the probability that $X \le x$; then insert the number $X + t$, where t denotes the key most recently deleted (or 0 if there have been no prior deletions). Such insertions arise naturally in priority queue disciplines, where the element with smallest remaining key is always chosen for deletion. The keys can be thought of as specific moments of time when events take place; in this interpretation the exponential deviate X represents a random "waiting time," so that $X + t$ is the time when a newly inserted event will be deleted if the most recent deletion occurred at time t. (Another way to produce biased insertions is to generate a uniform real number X in $[0 \mathinner{\ldotp\ldotp} 1]$ and to *multiply* it by the most recently deleted key, or by 1 if there were no prior deletions. This corresponds to the stated distribution if the *largest* key is always deleted, since it is essentially isomorphic under the mapping $f(x) = -\log x$.)

D_r Random deletion, in the sense that if d keys are present each is chosen for deletion with probability $1/d$.

D_o Deletion by relative order or rank, in the sense that if d keys are present and if some number j between 1 and d is specified, the jth smallest element is deleted. Such a j is specified in advance for each deletion.

D_q "Priority queue" deletion, the special case of D_o in which j is always equal to 1.

D_a Deletion by relative age, in the sense that if d keys are present and if some number k between 1 and d is specified, the kth oldest element (the one that has been present kth longest) is deleted. Such a k is specified in advance for each deletion.

D_f "FIFO" deletion, the special case of D_a in which k is always equal to 1.

D_l "LIFO" deletion, the special case of D_a in which k is always equal to the current value of d.

Using these abbreviations we shall talk about four different kinds of deletion insensitivity:

I^*D Any number of insertions followed by one deletion.

I^*D^* Any number of insertions followed by any number of deletions.

I^*DI^* Any number of insertions, followed by one deletion, followed by any number of insertions.

$(I, D)^*$ Any number of insertions and deletions, arbitrarily intermixed.

(Of course we also require that deletions never outnumber insertions.) The I's and D's will have subscripts to identify their type; for example, $(I_r, D_f)^*$ stands for any number of insertions of random uniform numbers intermixed with FIFO deletions. In the first two cases I^*D and I^*D^*, however, no subscript will be given to the I's, since I_r, I_o, and I_b are obviously equivalent until the first deletion has occurred.

We would like to say that a data organization has the $(I_r, D_f)^*$ *property* if operations $(I_r, D_f)^*$ always produce an essentially random data structure; a data organization might similarly have the I^*D_r property, and so on. These intuitive notions can be formalized as follows, in terms of the R function for that data organization: Consider a sequence of operations

$$A_1(u_1), A_2(u_2), \ldots, A_{m+n}(u_{m+n})$$

that includes n insertions and m deletions; each $A_i(u_i)$ is an insertion or deletion of a given type (for example, an I_r or a D_f). We define a permutation π_i of the u's remaining after i steps as follows:

π_0 is the null permutation;

if $A_i(u_i)$ is an insertion, π_i is π_{i-1} followed by u_i;

if $A_i(u_i)$ is a deletion, π_i is the permutation $\pi_{i-1} \backslash u_i$ defined in Section 2.

In other words the R function gives us a way to convert deletions on the given data structures to deletions on permutations of the keys. Each permutation π_i has the property that the data structure obtained after i steps is exactly the same as the structure that would be created by inserting the elements of π_i in order from left to right (without deletions).

For example, consider the operation sequence

$$I(0.5), \ I(0.2), \ I(0.6), \ D(0.5), \ I(0.4)$$

on binary search trees; then we have

$$\pi_3 \ = \ 0.5 \ 0.2 \ 0.6, \qquad \pi_4 \ = \ 0.6 \ 0.2, \qquad \pi_5 = 0.6 \ 0.2 \ 0.4,$$

since $\rho(\pi_4) = R(2\,1\,3\backslash 2) = 2\,1$.

After n insertions and m deletions we will obtain some permutation π_{m+n} of the remaining $n - m$ elements. An R function will be called *insensitive* to deletions if the elements of π_{m+n} are in random order after such a sequence of random insertions and deletions, that is, if the resulting permutations $\rho(\pi_{m+n})$ of $\{1, \ldots, n - m\}$ are uniformly distributed.

According to this formal definition, it should be clear for example that a data organization has the I^*D_r property if and only if it has an R function that is I^*D_r deletion insensitive. On the other hand our definition uses only the R function, not the S function, so we are actually distinguishing between different permutations that might yield the same data structure after insertion; we are therefore talking about rather strong forms of deletion insensitivity. This aspect of our model is discussed further in Section 10.

6. Reducing the Number of Cases

With three types of insertion, six types of deletion, and four ways to combine them, we have defined $6+6+18+18 = 48$ types of deletion insensitivity, namely I^*D_r, I^*D_o, $\ldots$; $I^*D_r^*$, $I^*D_o^*$, $\ldots$; $I_r^*D_rI_r^*$, $\ldots$, $I_b^*D_lI_b^*$; $(I_r, D_r)^*$, $(I_r, D_o)^*$, $\ldots$, $(I_b, D_l)^*$. But many of these are uninteresting, since (for example) biased insertions I_b are probably meaningful only in connection with priority queue deletions, type D_q.

It is well known that the exponential distribution is "memoryless," in the sense that if X is an exponential deviate and if we are told that $X \geq x_0$, the conditional distribution of $X - x_0$ given this knowledge is again exponential. This suggests that $(I_b, D_q)^*$ is actually equivalent to $(I_o, D_q)^*$, a fact first proved rigorously by Jonassen and Dahl in their study of priority queue algorithms (see [4]). Therefore we need not consider I_b any further; we can replace it by I_o.

A sequence of random operations with insertions of real numbers can be converted to a discrete probability space in a simple way, because our data organization is assumed to depend only on comparisons between distinct keys. If there are n insertion operations of type I_r, we can assume without loss of generality that the numbers inserted are the integers $\{1, 2, \ldots, n\}$ in some order, and that each of the $n!$ permutations is equally likely. On the other hand, suppose that the insertions are of type I_o, where the structure contains respectively $d_1, d_2, \ldots, d_n$ elements just before each insertion; then the number of equiprobable cases to consider is $(d_1 + 1)(d_2 + 1) \ldots (d_n + 1)$. Furthermore, if we are doing m random deletions of type D_r, with respectively $d'_1, \ldots, d'_m$ elements present before the deletions, we should multiply the number of equally probable types of insertions by $d'_1 \ldots d'_m$, the number of different ways to specify the deleted keys.

For example, consider again the sequence of operations $I_r I_r I_r D_r I_r$ discussed in Section 3. We have $n = 4$, $m = 1$, and $d'_1 = 3$, so the number of equally probable ways the algorithm might behave is $n! \times d'_1 \ldots d'_m = 24 \times 3 = 72$. In 25 of these ways the resulting data structure is ⌃, agreeing with our claim that the probability of this tree is $\frac{25}{72}$. Furthermore, it turns out that the final permutation $\rho(\pi_5)$ will be $2\,3\,1$ in 13 cases; this confirms that the probability of obtaining ⌃, given that the tree after the deletion was ⌐ (that is, given the 36 cases with $\rho(\pi_4) = 1\,2$) is $\frac{13}{36}$. On the other hand if the operations had been $I_o I_o I_o D_r I_o$, we would have had $n = 4$, $d_1 d_2 d_3 d_4 = 0\,1\,2\,2$, $m = 1$, and $d'_1 = 3$, so the number of equally probable ways the algorithm might behave would have been $1 \cdot 2 \cdot 3 \cdot 3 \times d'_1 \ldots d'_m = 54$. Under the latter model (which corresponds to the fallacy discussed in Section 3), the tree ⌃ occurs with probability $\frac{1}{3}$; in fact, it is not difficult to prove that the R function given for binary search trees is $(I_o, D_r)^*$ deletion insensitive, by writing down the reasoning that might have led us to believe (fallaciously) that it was $(I_r, D_r)^*$ deletion insensitive.

An R function cannot be $I_r^* D_q I_r^*$ deletion insensitive. In fact, this is obvious, for the operations $I_r I_r D_q I_r$ lead to six equiprobable values of π_4 (namely $2\,3$, $3\,2$, $2\,3$, $3\,1$, $3\,2$, and $3\,1$), hence $\rho(\pi_4) = 1\,2$ with probability $\frac{1}{3}$ and $\rho(\pi_4) = 2\,1$ with probability $\frac{2}{3}$. This holds for all R functions, since $R(x_1 x_2 \backslash j)$ is forced to equal 1. Since D_q is a special case of D_o, no R function can be $I_r^* D_o I_r^*$ deletion insensitive either, much less $(I_r, D_o)^*$. Fortunately such types of insensitivity do not seem to be very important in applications.

The fact that I^*D specifies a smaller class of operations than I^*D^* or I^*DI^*, and that these in turn are smaller than $(I, D)^*$, means for example that

$$(I_r, D_r)^* \implies I^*D_r^* \implies I^*D_r;$$

any R function that is $(I_r, D_r)^*$ insensitive is also $I^*D_r^*$, etc. Similarly, the fact that D_q is a special case of D_o means that insensitivity under D_o implies insensitivity under D_q; and insensitivity under D_a implies insensitivity under both D_f and D_l. Furthermore, insensitivity under either D_o or D_a implies insensitivity under D_r, since D_r corresponds to a sum of disjoint cases with the j_i's or k_i's varying in all d_i' possible ways.

Thus there are many obvious implications between the various types of deletion insensitivity that remain to be investigated; and we will find that many of these are actually equivalent to each other.

The first equivalence result is, in fact, obvious:

Lemma 1. Let D be D_r, D_o, or D_q. Then

$$(I_o, D)^* \iff I_o^*DI_o^* \iff I^*D^* \iff I^*D.$$

Proof. Since $(I_o, D)^* \implies I^*D^* \implies I^*D$, and $(I_o, D)^* \implies I^*DI_o^* \implies I^*D$, it remains to show that $I_o^*D \implies (I_o, D)^*$; that is, we need only prove that one-step deletion insensitivity implies full $(I_o, D)^*$ insensitivity. But this is obvious since we can prove that $\rho(\pi_i)$ is uniformly distributed after an I_o insertion if $\rho(\pi_{i-1})$ was, and one-step insensitivity implies that $\rho(\pi_i)$ is uniformly distributed after deletion if $\rho(\pi_{i-1})$ was. Thus $\rho(\pi_i)$ is uniformly distributed for all i. $\square$

Similarly, when D is D_a, D_f, or D_l we have $I^*D \iff I_o^*DI_o^*$. But I^*D^* need not be equivalent to these, since the first deletion might "confuse" the ages of the remaining elements. For example, the reader should have little difficulty constructing R functions that are I^*D_l insensitive but not $I^*D_l^*$ insensitive.

7. Necessary and Sufficient Conditions

We can make further progress in understanding deletion insensitivity if we convert the definitions into properties of the R function. Let P_n be the set of all permutations of $\{1, 2, \ldots, n\}$; and if x is such a permutation, let x_k be its kth element, from left to right, for $1 \le k \le n$. If $x \in P_n$ and $y \in P_{n-1}$, we write

$$[x \backslash j = y]$$

for the function of x, j, and y that is 1 if $R(x \backslash j) = y$, otherwise 0. In terms of this notation, the following lemma is an immediate consequence of the definitions:

Lemma 2. *An R function is*

a) *I^*D_r insensitive if and only if $\sum_{j=1}^{n}\sum_{x\in P_n}[x\backslash j=y]=n^2$, for all $y\in P_{n-1}$ and $n\geq 1$;*

b) *I^*D_o insensitive if and only if $\sum_{x\in P_n}[x\backslash j=y]=n$, for all $y\in P_{n-1}$ and $n\geq j\geq 1$;*

c) *I^*D_q insensitive if and only if $\sum_{x\in P_n}[x\backslash 1=y]=n$, for all $y\in P_{n-1}$ and $n\geq 1$;*

d) *I^*D_a insensitive if and only if $\sum_{x\in P_n}[x\backslash x_k=y]=n$, for all $y\in P_{n-1}$ and $n\geq k\geq 1$;*

e) *I^*D_f insensitive if and only if $\sum_{x\in P_n}[x\backslash x_1=y]=n$, for all $y\in P_{n-1}$ and $n\geq 1$;*

f) *I^*D_l insensitive if and only if $\sum_{x\in P_n}[x\backslash x_n=y]=n$, for all $y\in P_{n-1}$ and $n\geq 1$.*　□

Clearly (b) $\Longrightarrow$ (c), (d) $\Longrightarrow$ (e) and (f), and (b) or (d) $\Longrightarrow$ (a), as we already knew. Furthermore, it is easy to see that these are the *only* implications between the six types; we might have (e) and (f) and (c) but not (a), etc.

The next result is less obvious, possibly even surprising, since it states that a comparatively weak form of deletion insensitivity is equivalent to a comparatively strong property.

Theorem 1. $I^*D_o \iff I_r^*D_rI_r^* \iff (I_r, D_r)^*$.

Proof. Since $(I_r, D_r)^* \Longrightarrow I_r^*D_rI_r^*$, we must only show that $I_r^*D_rI_r^* \Longrightarrow I^*D_o$ and $I^*D_o \Longrightarrow (I_r, D_r)^*$.

Assume first that a given R function is $I_r^*D_rI_r^*$ deletion insensitive, and consider the sequence of operations $I_r^n D_r I_r$ for some fixed n. Any of the $n \cdot (n+1)!$ equally probable realizations of such operations defines a sequence of permutations $\pi_1, \ldots, \pi_{n+2}$ such that $\rho(\pi_{n+2})$ is a uniformly distributed permutation of $\{1, 2, \ldots, n\}$; hence every possible permutation $\rho(\pi_{n+2})$ occurs $n(n+1)$ times. Let $\rho(\pi_{n+2}) = y_1 \ldots y_{n-1}y_n$ and $\pi_{n+2} = y_1' \ldots y_{n-1}'y_n'$, where $y_n = j$, and suppose that t is the element missing from $y_1' \ldots y_n'$, where $1 \leq t \leq n+1$; then $y_i = y_i'$ or $y_i' - 1$ according as $y_i' < t$ or $y_i' > t$. The number of ways to obtain $\rho(\pi_{n+2}) = y_1 \ldots y_{n-1}y_n$ is

$$\sum_{x\in P_n}\left(\sum_{t=1}^{j}[x\backslash t=\rho(y_1\ldots y_{n-1})] + \sum_{t=j+1}^{n+1}[x\backslash(t-1)=\rho(y_1\ldots y_{n-1})]\right)$$

$$= \sum_{x\in P_n}\sum_{t=1}^{n}[x\backslash t=\rho(y_1\ldots y_{n-1})] + \sum_{x\in P_n}[x\backslash j=\rho(y_1\ldots y_{n-1})].$$

This is

$$n^2 + \sum_{x \in P_n} [x \backslash j = \rho(y_1 \ldots y_{n-1})]$$

by Lemma 2(a), since R is $I^* D_r$ deletion insensitive; and it equals $n(n+1)$ by assumption. Therefore R is $I^* D_o$ deletion insensitive by Lemma 2(b).

Now assume that a given R function is $I^* D_o$ deletion insensitive, and consider any given sequence of operations $A_1(u_1), \ldots, A_{m+n}(u_{m+n})$ corresponding to n I_r's and m D_r's, where there are respectively $d_1', \ldots, d_m'$ elements present before the deletions. Any of the $n! \, d_1' \ldots d_m'$ equally probable realizations of such operations defines a sequence of permutations $\pi_1, \ldots, \pi_{m+n}$, where the keys inserted are $\{1, 2, \ldots, n\}$ in some order, and we wish to prove that each of the $(n-m)!$ possible values of $\rho(\pi_{m+n})$ occurs $n! \, d_1' \ldots d_m'/(n-m)!$ times. Let $z_1, \ldots, z_m$ be the elements deleted, so that $\pi_{m+n} z_1 \ldots z_m$ is a permutation of the n elements inserted. We will prove that each of these $n!$ permutations occurs exactly $d_1' \ldots d_m'$ times.

In order to avoid cumbersome notations, a single example should suffice to explain the basic idea. Suppose the sequence is

$$I_r I_r I_r I_r I_r D_r I_r D_r D_r I_r I_r$$

so that $n = 8$, $m = 3$, and $d_1' d_2' d_3' = 5\,5\,4$; and suppose we want to count how many realizations will yield $\pi_{11} = 5\,1\,6\,3\,7$ and $z_1 z_2 z_3 = 8\,2\,4$. Working backwards, we must have $\pi_9 = 5\,1\,6$, $\pi_8 = $ a permutation of $\{1, 4, 5, 6\}$ such that $\pi_8 \backslash 4 = \pi_9$, $\pi_7 = $ a permutation $x_1 x_2 x_3 x_4 x_5$ of $\{1, 2, 4, 5, 6\}$ such that $\pi_7 \backslash 2 = \pi_8$, and $\pi_5 = $ a permutation of $\{x_1, x_2, x_3, x_4, 8\}$ such that $\pi_5 \backslash 8 = x_1 x_2 x_3 x_4$. By Lemma 2(b) the number of choices for π_8 is 4, and for each π_8 there are 5 suitable π_7's, and for each π_7 there are 5 suitable π_5's; hence there are $d_1' d_2' d_3'$ solutions. It should be clear that this method of proof is completely general. □

Theorem 1 completes a characterization of deletion insensitivity involving D_r, D_o, and D_q: We have three classes

$$\text{A. } (I_o, D_r)^* \iff I_o^* D_r I_o^* \iff I^* D_r^* \iff I^* D_r$$

$$\text{B. } (I_o, D_o)^* \iff I_o^* D_o I_o^* \iff I^* D_o^* \iff I^* D_o$$

$$\iff I_r^* D_r I_r^* \iff (I_r, D_r)^*$$

$$\text{C. } (I_o, D_q)^* \iff I_o^* D_q I_o^* \iff I^* D_q^* \iff I^* D_q$$

where B $\Longrightarrow$ A and B $\Longrightarrow$ C, and it is impossible for any R function to be insensitive with respect to $(I_r, D_o)^*$, $(I_r, D_q)^*$, $I_r^* D_o I_r^*$, or $I_r^* D_q I_r^*$.

8. Age-Sensitive Deletions

Let us now consider D_a more closely.

Theorem 2. *An R function is $I_r^* D_a I_r^*$ deletion insensitive if and only if, for $1 \leq j, k \leq n$ and all $y \in P_{n-1}$, there exists a unique $x \in P_n$ such that $x_k = j$ and $R(x \backslash j) = y$.*

Proof. Assume first that a given R function is $I_r^* D_a I_r^*$ deletion insensitive, and consider the sequence of operations $I_r^n D_a I_r$ for some fixed n, where the deletion operation removes the kth element inserted. Any of the $(n + 1)!$ equally probable realizations of such operations defines a sequence of permutations $\pi_1, \ldots, \pi_{n+2}$ such that $\rho(\pi_{n+2})$ is a uniformly distributed permutation of $\{1, 2, \ldots, n\}$; hence every possible permutation $\rho(\pi_{n+2})$ occurs $n + 1$ times. Now argue as in Theorem 1 with the extra restriction that $x \in P_n$ is such that x_k is the element being deleted. Using Lemma 2(d) we find that the number of ways to obtain $\rho(\pi_{n+2}) = y_1 \ldots y_{n-1} y_n$ is

$$n + \sum_{\substack{x \in P_n \\ x_k = j}} [x \backslash j = \rho(y_1 \ldots y_{n-1})]$$

when $y_n = j$; hence the condition in Theorem 2 is necessary.

Conversely, assume that the stated condition holds, and consider a given sequence of operations $I_r^p D_a I_r^{n-p}$ where D_a deletes the kth element inserted. For example, the sequence might be $I_r I_r I_r I_r I_r D_a I_r I_r$ with $n = 7$, $p = 5$, and $k = 4$. The number of realizations that yield $\pi_8 = 3\,1\,4\,5\,7\,2$ is the number of permutations x of $\{1, 3, 4, 5, 6\}$ such that $x_4 = 6$ and $x \backslash 6 = 3\,1\,4\,5$; and by hypothesis there is just one such x. There are seven choices of π_8 with $\rho(\pi_8) = 3\,1\,4\,5\,6\,2$, and every such choice occurs once. This argument clearly generalizes to prove that R is $I_r^* D_a I_r^*$ deletion insensitive. □

Corollary. $I_r^* D_a I_r^* \Longrightarrow (I_r, D_r)^*$.

Proof. The condition of Theorem 2 is much stronger than the condition for $I^* D_o$ in Lemma 2(b), since the latter requires only that the equation $R(x \backslash j) = y$ have exactly n solutions when j and y are given. Now apply Theorem 1. □

The condition of Theorem 2 is not strong enough to prove $(I_r, D_a)^*$ insensitivity, which seems to be very strong property indeed. The author has been unable to construct any R functions that are $(I_r, D_a)^*$ insensitive except those that satisfy the following strong requirement.

Condition Q: For each $1 \leq k \leq n$ there exists a permutation $q_1 \ldots q_{n-1}$ of $\{1, \ldots, k-1, k+1, \ldots, n\}$ such that $R(x_1 x_2 \ldots x_n \backslash x_k) = \rho(x_{q_1} \ldots x_{q_{n-1}})$. In other words, deletion of the kth element inserted will permute the other elements in a way depending only on k, not on their values.

This condition may not be necessary, but it is at least sufficient to prove what we want.

Theorem 3. *An R function that satisfies Condition Q is $(I_r, D_a)^*$ deletion insensitive.*

Proof. Consider the operation sequence

$$I_r I_r I_r I_r I_r D_a I_r D_a D_a I_r I_r$$

where the three D_a's respectively have $k = 2$, 3, 4, and let us count how many realizations will yield $\pi_{11} = 5\,1\,6\,3\,7$ after deleting the elements $8\,2\,4$ in this order. Suppose the eight insertions are $z_1 z_2 z_3 z_4 z_5 z_6 z_7 z_8$ respectively, a permutation of $\{1, 2, \ldots, 8\}$; we will show that the z's are uniquely determined by these assumptions. For concreteness, let us suppose that some of the permutations implied by Condition Q are $x_1 x_2 x_3 x_4 x_5 \backslash x_2 = x_3 x_1 x_5 x_4$, $x_1 x_2 x_3 x_4 x_5 \backslash x_4 = x_2 x_5 x_3 x_1$, and $x_1 x_2 x_3 x_4 \backslash x_2 = x_3 x_1 x_4$. Then we know that $\pi_5 = z_1 z_2 z_3 z_4 z_5$, $z_2 = 8$, $\pi_6 = z_3 z_1 z_5 z_4$, $\pi_7 = z_3 z_1 z_5 z_4 z_6$, $z_4 = 2$, $\pi_8 = z_1 z_6 z_5 z_3$, $z_6 = 4$, $\pi_9 = z_5 z_1 z_3$, $\pi_{11} = z_5 z_1 z_3 z_7 z_8 = 5\,1\,6\,3\,7$; hence $z_1 \ldots z_8 = 1\,8\,6\,2\,5\,4\,3\,7$. This argument clearly generalizes to prove the theorem, since there is always a unique realization for each choice of π_{m+n} and the sequence of elements deleted, for each choice of k's in the D_a operations.   □

There is an interesting way to weaken Condition Q to obtain a somewhat weaker kind of deletion insensitivity, yet one that is stronger than the condition of Lemma 2(d):

Condition Q_o: For each $1 \leq k \leq n$ there exists a sequence of n permutations $(q_{1,1} \ldots q_{1,n-1}), \ldots, (q_{n,1} \ldots q_{n,n-1})$ of $\{1, \ldots, k-1, k+1, \ldots, n\}$ with the following property: For all $y \in P_{n-1}$ there exists a permutation $p_1 \ldots p_n$ of $\{1, \ldots, n\}$, possibly depending on y, such that

$$\rho(x_1 \ldots x_{k-1} x_{k+1} \ldots x_n) = y \quad \text{and} \quad x_k = j \quad \text{implies}$$
$$R(x_1 \ldots x_n \backslash x_k) = \rho(x_{q_{p_j,1}} \ldots x_{q_{p_j,n-1}}).$$

In other words, when we delete the kth element inserted the result is one of n specified permutations of the remaining elements; and if the remaining elements are held fixed, while x_k runs through all n possible values relative to them, the results run through these n specified permutations in some order. Condition Q implies Condition Q_o, since the n specified permutations might be identical.

This rather peculiar condition seems to be just what is needed to prove the following slightly weakened form of Theorem 3.

Theorem 4. *An R function that satisfies Condition Q_o is $(I_o, D_a)^*$ deletion insensitive.*

Proof. As in the previous proofs, it is most convenient to consider a more-or-less random example that is sufficiently general to be convincing without the introduction of elaborate notation. Consider the operation sequence

$$I_o I_o I_o I_o I_o D_a I_o D_a D_a I_o I_o$$

where the three D_a's have $k = 2, 4, 4$, respectively. There are $1 \cdot 2 \cdot 3 \cdot 4 \cdot 5 \cdot 5 \cdot 4 \cdot 5$ realizations of this sequence; we will show that $5 \cdot 5 \cdot 4$ of them will yield any given value of $\rho(\pi_{11})$. For example, suppose $\rho(\pi_{11}) = 3\,1\,4\,2\,5$. There are five choices for the q permutation in the first deletion; let us choose one of these, and assume for example that the deletion takes $\pi_5 = z_1 z_2 z_3 z_4 z_5$ into $\pi_6 = z_1' z_2' z_3' z_4' = z_3 z_1 z_5 z_4$. In other words, one of the q permutations for $n = 5$ and $k = 2$ is assumed to be $3\,1\,5\,4$. (If $3\,1\,5\,4$ occurs as two or more of the q permutations we also choose the subscript j such that $3\,1\,5\,4 = q_{j,1} q_{j,2} q_{j,3} q_{j,4}$; thus, five distinct choices are possible even when the q permutations are not distinct.) Then if $\pi_7 = z_1' z_2' z_3' z_4' z_5'$ we must delete the fourth oldest element, which is z_3' (since it equals z_5); again we have five q permutations to choose from, and let us suppose that the q permutation for the second deletion yields $\pi_8 = z_1'' z_2'' z_3'' z_4'' = z_4' z_1' z_5' z_2'$; we similarly shall choose one of the four q permutations now available for the last deletion and suppose that it yields $\pi_9 = z_1''' z_2''' z_3''' = z_2'' z_4'' z_1''$.

To make $\rho(\pi_{11}) = 3\,1\,4\,2\,5$ we now can work backwards and identify the relative sizes of various elements: Since $\rho(\pi_9) = 2\,1\,3$, we know that $\rho(z_1'' z_2'' z_4'') = 3\,2\,1$. This value of y together with Condition Q_o allows us to determine $\rho(\pi_8)$, since each possible value of z_3' relative to z_1'', z_2'', and z_4'' corresponds to one of the predetermined choices of q permutation once $\rho(z_1'' z_2'' z_4'')$ is known. In our case $\rho(\pi_8)$ must be $4\,3\,1\,2$, $4\,3\,2\,1$, $4\,2\,3\,1$, or $3\,2\,4\,1$, and our choice of q-permutation subscript tells us which of these occurs, say $4\,2\,3\,1$. Then $\rho(z_1' z_2' z_4' z_5') = 2\,1\,4\,3$ and we can similarly reconstruct $\rho(\pi_7)$, which might be $2\,1\,3\,5\,4$. In the same way $\rho(\pi_6) = 2\,1\,3\,4$ implies that $\rho(z_1 z_3 z_4 z_5) = 1\,2\,4\,3$; and we can use this knowledge to find $\rho(\pi_5)$, say $2\,1\,3\,5\,4$. Each I_o insertion has now been characterized. Thus each of our $5 \cdot 5 \cdot 4$ choices has led to a unique realization such that $\rho(\pi_{11}) = 3\,1\,4\,2\,5$. $\square$

Although I_o is a somewhat artificial type of random insertion, Theorem 4 is interesting because $(I_o, D_a)^*$ insensitivity implies $I^* D_a^*$ insensitivity, and this special case is not artificial.

Let us conclude our theoretical investigations by considering briefly the FIFO and LIFO deletion types, D_f and D_l. If the R function satisfies

$$R(x_1 x_2 \ldots x_n \backslash x_1) = \rho(x_2 \ldots x_n)$$

it is obviously $(I_r, D_f)^*$ insensitive. (Notice that this condition might hold even though neither Condition Q nor Q_o is satisfied; in fact the weak condition of Lemma 2(a) might not even hold.)   On the other hand when the R function does not satisfy the stated formula, there do not appear to be any interesting conditions that guarantee $I^* D_f^*$ insensitivity, other than the condition Q_o we have already discussed. (We might have, say, $R(x_1 x_2 \ldots x_n \backslash x_1) = \rho(x_3 x_2 x_4 \ldots x_n)$ and $R(x_1 x_2 \ldots x_n \backslash x_2) = \rho(x_1 x_3 \ldots x_n)$; these conditions lead to $(I_r, D_f)^*$ insensitivity without the full generality of Condition Q but they do not seem to be very interesting.) Essentially the same remarks hold also for LIFO deletions, if R does or does not satisfy

$$R(x_1 \ldots x_{n-1} x_n \backslash x_n) = \rho(x_1 \ldots x_{n-1}).$$

9. Applications

Let us finally apply these theorems to some important data organizations. Sorted and unsorted linear lists have every possible type of insensitivity to deletions, but this is obvious without a fancy theory.

Binary search trees provide what is perhaps the most interesting application. We have already mentioned that Hibbard [3] originated this theory by essentially proving that the R function defined in Section 2 is $I^* D_r$ insensitive. Knuth [7, answer to exercise 6.2.2–13] observed that it is in fact $I^* D_a$ insensitive; then Knott [6] went much further, proving that Hibbard's R function is $(I_o, D_a)^*$ insensitive. In particular, if we do n random insertions, followed by $m < n$ FIFO deletions, the resulting tree has the shape distribution of a binary tree after $n - m$ random insertions. This is a difficult theorem to prove, perhaps the "deepest" result about a data structure that had been obtained by anyone before 1975.

It is possible to establish Knott's theorem using the theory above; in fact, much of that theory was motivated by what he did. We want to show that the binary search tree organization satisfies Condition Q_o. Let $k \leq n$ be given, and for $1 \leq l \leq n$ let

$$q_{l,1} \ldots q_{l,n-1} = \begin{cases} 1 \ldots (k-1)(k+1) \ldots n, & \text{if } l \leq k; \\ 1 \ldots (k-1)\, l\, (k+1) \ldots (l-1)(l+1) \ldots n, & \text{if } l > k. \end{cases}$$

Let $y = y_1 \ldots y_{n-1} \in P_{n-1}$ be given, and let $z_1 \ldots z_{n-1}$ be the inverse permutation, so that $y_{z_j} = j$. It is not difficult to verify that Condition Q_o holds with the permutation defined by

$$P_j = \begin{cases} z_j, & \text{if } z_j < k; \\ z_j + 1, & \text{if } z_j \geq k; \\ k, & \text{if } j = n. \end{cases}$$

Thus binary search trees are $(I_o, D_a)^*$ insensitive to deletions using Hibbard's method. On the other hand we have seen that they are not $(I_r, D_r)^*$ insensitive, so by Theorem 1 they are not even $I^* D_o$ insensitive.

Suppose we define deletion in a different way, essentially by interchanging left and right in Hibbard's method: Let $R(x_1 x_2 \ldots x_n \backslash j) = \rho(x_1 \ldots x_{k-1} x_{k+1} \ldots x_n)$ or $\rho(x_1 \ldots x_{l-1} x_{l+1} \ldots x_n)$ where $x_k = j$ and $x_l = j - 1$ if $j > 1$, and where x_k is deleted if $j = 1$ or $l < k$, otherwise x_l is deleted. (For example, this changes $R(1\,3\,2 \backslash 1)$ and $R(3\,1\,2 \backslash 3)$ to $2\,1$ in the table of Section 3; it also changes $R(2\,1\,3 \backslash 2)$ and $R(2\,3\,1 \backslash 2)$ to $1\,2$.) Like Hibbard's function, this one is $(I_o, D_a)^*$ insensitive to deletions; and it also satisfies Lemma 2(c), so it is $(I_b, D_q)^*$ insensitive as well. Furthermore, like Hibbard's function it possesses $(I_r, D_l)^*$ insensitivity. We can also verify (I_b, D_q, D_l) insensitivity, if the I_b insertions are biased by the most recent D_q (not D_l) deletion. (Is it $(I_b, D_q, D_a)^*$ insensitive in this sense?)

J. Vuillemin [8] has recently defined a useful type of data organization that he calls binomial queues, and M. R. Brown [2] has shown that they are highly insensitive to deletions. In fact, Brown proved that the corresponding R function satisfies Condition Q, hence binomial queues are $(I_r, D_a)^*$ and $(I_r, D_r)^*$ insensitive.

The leftist tree structures developed in 1971 by C. Crane (see [7, Section 5.2.3]) unfortunately do not share such nice properties. In fact, the corresponding function $R(x_1 x_2 x_3 x_4 \backslash j)$ has a pronounced bias towards $3\,2\,1$ and $2\,3\,1$ except when $j = 1$, and the function $R(x_1 x_2 x_3 x_4 x_5 \backslash 1)$ is extremely biased. Therefore leftist trees are quite sensitive to deletions, and it will probably be very difficult to analyze them. In fact, the analysis for pure insertions is already very formidable. Similar remarks apply to balanced trees.

10. Degeneracy

We have defined deletion insensitivity only in terms of the R function. But when many different permutations lead to the same data structure (that is, if they yield the same S value) it might be possible to have deletion insensitivity that cannot be "lifted" back to any R function for the organization. For example, when the data structure consists of a sorted linear list, the S function is essentially constant, so we trivially have $(I_r, D_o)^*$ insensitivity; but we have observed that no R function can have this property.

In other words, the conditions we have derived in Theorems 1 and 2 are sufficient but not necessarily necessary for insensitivity. An example can be given of a data organization that is $I_r^* D_r I_r^*$ insensitive when the S equivalences are considered, yet it is not $I^* D_o$ insensitive: Let $R(x_1 \ldots x_n \backslash x_k) = \rho(x_1 \ldots x_{k-1} x_{k+1} \ldots x_n)$ for $n \neq 3$, $R(x_1 x_2 x_3 \backslash 1) = 1\,2$, $R(x_1 x_2 x_3 \backslash 2) = 2\,1$, $R(1\,2\,3 \backslash 3) = R(1\,3\,2 \backslash 3) = R(2\,3\,1 \backslash 3) = 1\,2$, $R(2\,1\,3 \backslash 3) = R(3\,1\,2 \backslash 3) = R(3\,2\,1 \backslash 3) = 2\,1$; and let $S(x_1 \ldots x_n) = S(y_1 \ldots y_n)$ if and only if $x_1 \ldots x_n = y_1 \ldots y_n$ or $n \geq 3$ and $x_4 \ldots x_n = y_4 \ldots y_n$ and $S(\rho(x_1 x_2 x_3)) = S(\rho(y_1 y_2 y_3))$, where $S(1\,3\,2) = S(2\,3\,1)$ and $S(3\,1\,2) = S(3\,2\,1)$. The operations $III D_q$ leave a nonrandom result; but $I_r^n D_r I_r^m$ clearly produces a random structure when $n \neq 3$, and this can be verified also for $n = 3$. Thus Theorem 1 is not true when we take the S equivalences into account.

It appears unlikely that any conditions weaker than those discussed in the lemmas and theorems above will be useful for proving deletion insensitivity in practice. Furthermore, the existence of an R function satisfying the six respective conditions in Lemma 2 is, in fact, easily seen to be both necessary and sufficient for the six corresponding kinds of $I^* D$ insensitivity. (We proved this for $I^* D_r$ in Section 4.)

By generalizing the methods of this paper to n-tuples of numbers from $\{1, 2, \ldots, m\}$ instead of permutations, it would be possible to study whether or not various hash table algorithms are sensitive to deletions.

Acknowledgments

I wish to thank Mark Brown and Gary Knott for their comments on the first draft of this paper.

References

[1] A. V. Aho, J. Hopcroft, and J. D. Ullman, The Design and Analysis of Computer Algorithms (Reading, Massachusetts: Addison–Wesley, 1974).

[2] Mark R. Brown, "Implementation and analysis of binomial queue algorithms," *SIAM Journal on Computing* **7** (1978), 298–319.

[3] Thomas N. Hibbard, "Some combinatorial properties of certain trees with applications to searching and sorting," *Journal of the Association for Computing Machinery* **9** (1962), 13–28.

[4] A. Jonassen, "The stationary p-tree forest," Computer Science Technical Report STAN-CS-76-573 (Stanford University, 1976), 88 pages.

[5] Arne T. Jonassen and Donald E. Knuth, "A trivial algorithm whose analysis isn't," *Journal of Computer and System Sciences* **16** (1978), 301–322. [Reprinted as Chapter 18 of the present volume.]

[6] Gary Don Knott, "Deletion in binary storage trees," Computer Science Technical Report STAN-CS-75-491 (Ph.D. thesis, Stanford University, 1975), 93 pages.

[7] Donald E. Knuth, *Sorting and Searching*, Volume 3 of *The Art of Computer Programming* (Reading, Massachusetts: Addison–Wesley, 1973).

[8] Jean Vuillemin, "A data structure for manipulating priority queues," *Communications of the ACM* **21** (1978), 309–315.

This research was supported in part by the National Science Foundation, the Office of Naval Research, and IBM Corporation.

Addendum

Some of the interesting sequels to this paper known to the author are:

[9] Jeffrey Scott Vitter, "Deletion algorithms for hashing that preserve randomness," *Journal of Algorithms* **3** (1982), 261–275.

[10] W. C. Chen and J. S. Vitter, "Deletion algorithms for coalesced hashing," *The Computer Journal* **29** (1986), 436–450.

[11] J. Françon, B. Randrianarimanana, and R. Schott, "Analysis of dynamic algorithms in Knuth's model," *Theoretical Computer Science* **72** (1990), 147–167.

[12] G. Louchard, B. Randrianarimanana, and R. Schott, "Dynamic algorithms in D. E. Knuth's model: a probabilistic analysis," *Theoretical Computer Science* **93** (1992), 201–225.

[13] G. Louchard, Claire Kenyon, and R. Schott, "Data structures' maxima," *SIAM Journal on Computing* **26** (1997), 1006–1042.

Chapter 20

Analysis of a Simple Factorization Algorithm

*[Written with Luis Trabb Pardo. Originally published in Theoretical Computer Science **3** (1976), 321–348.]*

The probability that the kth largest prime factor of a number n is at most n^x is shown to approach a limit $F_k(x)$ as $n \to \infty$. Several interesting properties of $F_k(x)$ are explored, and numerical tables are given. These results are applied to the analysis of an algorithm commonly used to find all prime factors of a given number. The average number of digits in the kth largest prime factor of a random m-digit number is shown to be asymptotically equivalent to the average length of the kth longest cycle in a random permutation of m objects.

0. Introduction

Perhaps the simplest way to discover the prime factorization of an integer n is to try dividing it by 2, 3, 4, 5, ... and to "cast out" each factor that is discovered; we stop when the trial divisor exceeds the square root of the remaining unfactored part.

The speed of this method obviously depends on the size of the prime factors of n. For example, if n is prime, the number of trial divisions is approximately $n^{1/2}$; but if n is a power of 2, the number of divisions is only about $\log n$. In this paper we shall analyze the algorithm when n is a "random" integer, determining the approximate probability that the number of trial divisions is $\leq n^x$ when x is a given number between 0 and 1/2. One of the results we shall prove is that the number of trial divisions will be at most $n^{0.35}$, about half of the time.

In order to carry out the analysis, we shall study the distribution of the kth largest prime factor of a random integer. This problem is of independent interest in number theory, and for $k > 1$ it does not appear to have been studied before. (Wunderlich and Selfridge [17] gave a heuristic argument that the second-largest prime factor will tend to be roughly $(n^{1-0.61})^{0.61} \approx n^{0.24}$ because the median value of the largest prime factor is $\approx n^{0.61}$; besides their remark, which stimulated the present investigation, the authors are not aware of any published study of the second-largest prime factor. John M. Pollard [private communication] has independently investigated the distribution of second-largest prime factors, and his computed values agree with those presented below.)

Section 1 of this paper presents the factorization algorithm in detail and proves its correctness. Quantitative analysis begins in Section 2, where the two frequency counts involved in the running time are interpreted in terms of the size of the largest two prime factors.

The distribution of kth largest prime factors is investigated heuristically in Section 3, somewhat as a physicist might do the analysis. A rigorous derivation of this distribution, somewhat as a mathematician might do the analysis, is presented in Section 4. Sections 5 and 6 continue the mathematical play by deriving interesting identities and asymptotic formulas satisfied by these distributions. Section 7 comes back to the factorization procedure and applies the ideas to the results of Sections 1 and 2, somewhat as a computer scientist might do the analysis.

Section 8 discusses the particular theoretical model used in these analyses, and explains why the traditional "mean and variance" approach is inappropriate for algorithms such as this. Numerical tables and empirical confirmation of the theory appear in Section 9. Finally, Section 10 discusses a rather surprising connection between prime factors of random m-digit integers and the cycle lengths of random permutations of m objects.

Although we shall deal with a very simple approach to factoring, the results and methods of this paper apply to many other algorithms as well. The paper is self-contained, and includes several examples suitable for classroom exposition of asymptotic methods.

1. The Algorithm

Here is the standard "divide and factor" algorithm that we shall analyze in detail. A proof of its validity follows immediately from the following invariant assertions governing the variables used:

$$n \geq 2; \tag{1.1}$$

$$n = p_1 \ldots p_t m; \tag{1.2}$$

$$p_1, \ldots, p_t \text{ are prime numbers}; \tag{1.3}$$

$$m \geq d; \tag{1.4}$$

all prime factors of m are $\geq d.$ (1.5)

Since our goal is to analyze a simple algorithm rather than to present it in optimized form ready for extensive use, we shall simply consider the following informal ALGOL-like description:

```
t := 0;  m := n;  d := 2;                          1
while d² ≤ m do                                  D + 1
begin Increase d or decrease m:
    if d divides m then                            D
       begin
          t := t + 1;  p_t := d;  m := m/d        T − 1
       end
    else d := d + 1                             D − T + 1
end;
t := t + 1;  p_t := m;  m := 1;  d := 1;           1
```

The invariant assertions hold after each line of this program. The expressions in the right-hand column specify the number of times the operations in a particular line will be performed, where

D is the number of trial divisions performed; (1.6)

T is the number of prime factors of n (counting multiplicity). (1.7)

The usual refinements of this algorithm, which avoid a lot of nonprime trial divisors by making d run through only values of the form $6k \pm 1$ when $d > 3$, have the effect of dividing D by a constant. Therefore our analysis of this simple case will apply also with minor variations to the more complicated cases.

2. Preliminary Analysis

Let n_k be the kth largest prime factor of n; thus $n_k = p_{T+1-k}$ after the algorithm terminates, for $1 \leq k \leq T$. If n has fewer than k prime factors (counting multiplicities), let $n_k = 1$. We also let $n_0 = \infty$ for convenience in what follows.

The **while** loop in the algorithm can terminate in three different ways, depending on how we last encounter it:

Case 1. $n < 4$. Then $D = 0$.

Case 2. $n \geq 4$ and the Dth trial division succeeds. Then the final trial division was by $d = n_2$, where $d^2 > n_1$. Since d is initially 2 and the statement $d := d + 1$ is performed $D - T + 1$ times, we have

$$D = n_2 + T - 3, \qquad n_2^2 > n_1. \tag{2.1}$$

Case 3. $n \geq 4$ and the Dth trial division fails. Then the final trial division was by d, where $n_2 \leq d$ and $d^2 < n_1$ and $(d+1)^2 > n_1$. (Note that if we set $p_0 := 1$ we have $d \geq p_{t-1}$ throughout the **while** loop.) Thus we have

$$D = \lceil \sqrt{n_1} \rceil + T - 3, \qquad n_2^2 < n_1. \tag{2.2}$$

In all three cases we have the formula

$$D = \max(n_2, \lceil \sqrt{n_1} \rceil) + T - 3. \tag{2.3}$$

Clearly D is the dominant factor in the running time, so most of our analysis will be devoted to it. However, it turns out that the analysis of T is also very interesting; for large random n, the number T of prime factors can be regarded as a normally-distributed random variable with mean $\ln \ln n + 1.03$ and standard deviation $\sqrt{\ln \ln n}$ (see Appendix A).

3. The kth Largest Prime Factor

In order to analyze D, we shall first analyze the distributions of n_1 and n_2 (and n_k in general). This analysis will be of interest in itself, since one of the common improvements to the simple algorithm in Section 1 is to test m for primality (by another method) whenever a new factor has been cast out; then the running time for factorization is essentially governed by n_2 alone, rather than by $\max(n_2, \sqrt{n_1})$.

Let $P_k(x, N)$ be the number of integers n in the range $1 \leq n \leq N$ such that

$$n_k \leq N^x, \tag{3.1}$$

where x is any number ≥ 0. Thus $P_k(x, N)/N$ is the probability that a random integer between 1 and N will have its kth largest prime factor $\leq N^x$. We will prove that this probability tends to a limiting distribution

$$\lim_{N \to \infty} \frac{P_k(x, N)}{N} = F_k(x), \tag{3.2}$$

where $F_k(x)$ has interesting properties discussed below.

Before we establish (3.2) rigorously, it will be helpful to give a heuristic derivation analogous to that given by Dickman [4], who was the first to study this question in the case $k = 1$. Let us consider $P_k(t + dt, N) - P_k(t, N)$, the number of $n \leq N$ such that n_k lies between N^t and N^{t+dt}, when dt is very small. To count the number of such n, we take all primes p lying between N^t and N^{t+dt}, and multiply by all numbers $m \leq N^{1-t}$ such that $m_k \leq p$ and $m_{k-1} \geq p$. Now if $n = mp$ we have $n \leq N$ and $n_k = p$; conversely every $n \leq N$ with n_k between N^t and N^{t+dt} will have the form $n = mp$ where p and m have the stated form. Note that the number of $m \leq N^{1-t}$ such that $m_k \leq p$ is approximately $P_k(t/(1-t), N^{1-t})$, and the unwanted subset consisting of those m with $m_{k-1} < p$ has approximately $P_{k-1}(t/(1-t), N^{1-t})$ members. Hence the number of m with $mp \leq N$ and $m_k \leq p$ and $m_{k-1} \geq p$ is $P_k(t/(1-t), N^{1-t}) - P_{k-1}(t/(1-t), N^{1-t})$, ignoring second-order terms, and we have

$$P_k(t + dt, N) - P_k(t, N)$$
$$\approx \left(\pi(N^{t+dt}) - \pi(N^t)\right)\left(P_k\left(\frac{t}{1-t}, N^{1-t}\right) - P_{k-1}\left(\frac{t}{1-t}, N^{1-t}\right)\right). \quad (3.3)$$

The π function in this formula denotes, as usual, the quantity

$$\pi(x) = \text{the number of primes not exceeding } x. \quad (3.4)$$

According to the prime number theorem we have $\pi(x) \approx x/\ln x$, hence

$$\pi(N^{t+dt}) - \pi(N^t) \approx N^t \, dt/t. \quad (3.5)$$

Plugging this into (3.3) and dividing by N yields

$$\frac{P_k(t + dt, N) - P_k(t, N)}{N}$$
$$\approx \left(\frac{P_k(t/(1-t), N^{1-t})}{N^{1-t}} - \frac{P_{k-1}(t/(1-t), N^{1-t})}{N^{1-t}}\right)\frac{dt}{t}; \quad (3.6)$$

when $N \to \infty$ we have the differential equation

$$F_k'(t) \, dt = \left(F_k\left(\frac{t}{1-t}\right) - F_{k-1}\left(\frac{t}{1-t}\right)\right)\frac{dt}{t}. \quad (3.7)$$

Since $F_k(0) = 0$, we may integrate (3.7) to deduce the formula

$$F_k(x) = \int_0^x \left(F_k\left(\frac{t}{1-t}\right) - F_{k-1}\left(\frac{t}{1-t}\right)\right)\frac{dt}{t}. \quad (3.8)$$

According to our convention $n_0 = \infty$, we define

$$F_0(x) = 0 \qquad \text{for all } x. \quad (3.9)$$

We also must have

$$F_k(x) = 1 \qquad \text{if } x \geq 1 \text{ and } k \geq 1. \quad (3.10)$$

Now it is easy to see that (3.8), (3.9), and (3.10) define $F_k(x)$ uniquely for $0 \leq x \leq 1$, since we have

$$F_k(x) = 1 - \int_x^1 \left(F_k\left(\frac{t}{1-t}\right) - F_{k-1}\left(\frac{t}{1-t}\right)\right)\frac{dt}{t}, \quad (3.11)$$

and this relation defines $F_k(x)$ in terms of its values at points $> x$.

4. Proof Without Handwaving

Our discussion in the previous section was only quasi-rigorous, but it showed that *if* the limiting relationship (3.2) holds then $F_k(x)$ had better be the function defined by (3.8), (3.9), and (3.10). Now that we have a formula for F_k, let us try to prove the limiting formula (3.2).

It is more convenient to work with the functions ρ_k defined by

$$\rho_k(\alpha) = F_k(1/\alpha); \qquad (4.1)$$

the equations of Section 3 transform into the somewhat simpler recurrence formulas

$$\rho_k(\alpha) = 1 - \int_1^\alpha \big(\rho_k(t-1) - \rho_{k-1}(t-1)\big)\,\frac{dt}{t}, \quad \text{for } \alpha > 1,\ k \geq 1; \quad (4.2)$$

$$\rho_k(\alpha) = 1 \qquad \text{for } 0 < \alpha \leq 1 \text{ and } k \geq 1; \qquad (4.3)$$

$$\rho_k(\alpha) = 0 \qquad \text{for } \alpha \leq 0 \text{ or } k = 0. \qquad (4.4)$$

Furthermore we let $S_k(x, y)$ be the set of positive integers $n \leq x$ such that $n_k \leq y$, and we let $\Psi_k(x, y) = \|S_k(x, y)\|$ be its cardinality, so that

$$P_k(x, N) = \Psi_k(N, N^x). \qquad (4.5)$$

We will show that

$$\Psi_k(N^\alpha, N) = \rho_k(\alpha)N^\alpha + O(N^\alpha/\log N^\alpha), \qquad (4.6)$$

and it follows that a stronger form of (3.2) is true:

$$\frac{P_k(x, N)}{N} = F_k(x) + O\left(\frac{1}{\log N}\right). \qquad (4.7)$$

Indeed, we will prove a result even stronger than (4.6), namely

$$\Psi_k(x^\alpha, x) = \rho_k(\alpha)x^\alpha + \sigma_k(\alpha)x^\alpha/\ln x^\alpha + O(x^\alpha/(\log x)^2) \qquad (4.8)$$

as $x \to \infty$ for all fixed $\alpha > 1$, where $\sigma_k(\alpha)$ will be defined appropriately below. In principle, the approach we shall use could be extended to obtain an asymptotic formula for $\Psi_k(x^\alpha, x)$ that is good to $O(x^\alpha/(\log x)^r)$ for any fixed r; the method is based on ideas of de Bruijn [1], who went on to find extremely precise asymptotic expansions of $\Psi_1(N^\alpha, N)$ in an elegant way using Stieltjes integration by parts. (*Note:* When $k = 1$, the limiting formula (3.2) was first established by Ramaswami [13]; Norton [11, pages 9–27] has given a comprehensive survey of the literature relating to this important special case.)

We shall use a strong form of the prime number theorem due to de La Vallée Poussin [3]:

$$\pi(x) = L(x) + O(xe^{-C\sqrt{\log x}}), \tag{4.9}$$

where C is a positive constant and

$$L(x) = \int_2^x \frac{dt}{\ln t}. \tag{4.10}$$

Now to the proof, which will be "elementary" except for our use of (4.9). Letting p range over primes and n over positive integers, we have

$$\lfloor x^\alpha \rfloor - \Psi_k(x^\alpha, x) = \sum_{x < p \leq x^\alpha} \|\{n \leq x^\alpha \mid n_k = p\}\|$$

$$= \sum_{x < p \leq x^\alpha} \|\{m \leq x^\alpha/p \mid m_k \leq p \text{ and } m_{k-1} \geq p\}\|$$

$$= \sum_{x < p \leq x^\alpha} \left(\Psi_k(x^\alpha/p, p) - \Psi_{k-1}(x^\alpha/p, p - \epsilon)\right)$$

where ϵ is a small positive number and $\Psi_0(x, y) = 0$. The key idea in our derivation will be to replace the sum $\sum_{x < p \leq x^\alpha} \Psi_k(x^\alpha/p, p)$ by the integral $\int_x^{x^\alpha} \Psi_k(x^\alpha/y, y)\, dy/\ln y$, when $\alpha > 1$, using the "density" function for primes suggested by (4.10). To justify this, we have

$$\left(\sum_{x < p \leq x^\alpha} \Psi_k\left(\frac{x^\alpha}{p}, p\right)\right) - \int_x^{x^\alpha} \Psi_k\left(\frac{x^\alpha}{y}, y\right) \frac{dy}{\ln y}$$

$$= \left(\sum_{x < p \leq x^\alpha} \sum_{n \in S_k(x^\alpha/p, p)} 1\right) - \int_x^{x^\alpha} \left(\sum_{n \in S_k(x^\alpha/y, y)} 1\right) \frac{dy}{\ln y}$$

$$= \sum_{\substack{1 \leq n \leq x^{\alpha-1} \\ n_k \leq x^\alpha/n}} \left(\left(\sum_{\substack{n_k \leq p \leq x^\alpha/n \\ x < p}} 1\right) - \int_{\max(n_k, x)}^{x^\alpha/n} \frac{dy}{\ln y}\right)$$

$$= \sum_{\substack{1 \leq n \leq x^{\alpha-1} \\ n_k \leq x^\alpha/n}} \left(\pi(x^\alpha/n) - \pi(\max(n_k, x))\right)$$

$$\qquad + O(1) - L(x^\alpha/n) + L(\max(n_k, x))\Big)$$

$$= \sum_{\substack{1 \leq n \leq x^{\alpha-1} \\ n_k \leq x^\alpha/n}} O\left(\frac{x^\alpha}{n} e^{-C\sqrt{\log x}}\right) = O(x^\alpha(\log x^\alpha)e^{-C\sqrt{\log x}}). \tag{4.11}$$

A similar estimate applies to $\sum_{x < p \le x^\alpha} \Psi_{k-1}(x^\alpha/p, p - \epsilon)$, so we have

$$\Psi_k(x^\alpha, x) = x^\alpha - \int_x^{x^\alpha} \left(\Psi_k \left(\frac{x^\alpha}{y}, y \right) - \Psi_{k-1} \left(\frac{x^\alpha}{y}, y \right) \right) \frac{dy}{\ln y}$$

$$+ O \left(\frac{\alpha x^\alpha}{(\log x)^r} \right) \qquad (4.12)$$

as $x \to \infty$, for all fixed $r \ge 0$. This is the formula we shall use for $\alpha > 1$; when $0 \le \alpha \le 1$ we have $\Psi_k(x^\alpha, x) = \lfloor x^\alpha \rfloor$. The brackets $\lfloor \; \rfloor$ in the latter formula turn out to be important, since the integral (4.12) is sensitive to $O(1)$ terms in the vicinity of $y = x^\alpha$.

Our proof of (4.8) will be by induction on k, and for fixed k by induction on $\lceil \alpha \rceil$. Actually the first case $(k = 1, \lceil \alpha \rceil = 2)$ is the most delicate; when $1 < \alpha \le 2$ we have

$$\int_x^{x^\alpha} \Psi_1 \left(\frac{x^\alpha}{y}, y \right) \frac{dy}{\ln y} = \int_x^{x^\alpha} \left(\frac{x^\alpha}{y} - \left\{ \frac{x^\alpha}{y} \right\} \right) \frac{dy}{\ln y}$$

$$= x^\alpha \int_x^{x^\alpha} d \ln \ln y - \int_1^{x^{\alpha-1}} \frac{\{u\} \, du}{u^2 \ln(x^\alpha/u)}$$

$$= x^\alpha \ln \alpha - \frac{x^\alpha}{\ln x^\alpha} \int_1^{x^{\alpha-1}} \frac{\{u\} \, du}{u^2}$$

$$- \frac{x^\alpha}{\ln x^\alpha} \int_1^{x^{\alpha-1}} \frac{\{u\} \ln u \, du}{u^2 \ln(x^\alpha/u)},$$

where $\{x\}$ denotes $x - \lfloor x \rfloor$. Now

$$\int_1^{x^{\alpha-1}} \frac{\{u\} \, du}{u^2} = \sum_{1 \le n < \lfloor x^{\alpha-1} \rfloor} \int_n^{n+1} \frac{(u - n) \, du}{u^2} + \int_{\lfloor x^{\alpha-1} \rfloor}^{x^{\alpha-1}} \frac{\{u\} \, du}{u^2}$$

$$= \sum_{1 \le n < \lfloor x^{\alpha-1} \rfloor} \left(\left(\ln \frac{n+1}{n} \right) - \frac{1}{n-1} \right) + O(x^{1-\alpha})^2$$

$$= \left(\ln \lfloor x^{\alpha-1} \rfloor \right) - \left(H_{\lfloor x^{\alpha-1} \rfloor} - 1 \right) + O(x^{1-\alpha})^2$$

$$= 1 - \gamma + O(x^{1-\alpha}),$$

where γ is Euler's constant. Also

$$\int_1^{x^{\alpha-1}} \frac{\{u\} \ln u \, du}{u^2 \ln(x^\alpha/u)} \le \int_1^{x^{\alpha-1}} \frac{\{u\} \ln u \, du}{u^2 \ln x}$$

$$\le \int_1^\infty \frac{\{u\} \ln u \, du}{u^2 \ln x} \le \int_1^\infty \frac{\ln u \, du}{u^2 \ln x} = \frac{1}{\ln x}.$$

Therefore by (4.12) we have

$$\Psi_1(x^\alpha, x) = x^\alpha - \int_x^{x^\alpha} \Psi_1\left(\frac{x^\alpha}{y}, y\right) \frac{dy}{\ln y} + O\left(\frac{\alpha x^\alpha}{(\log x)^3}\right)$$

$$= x^\alpha(1 - \ln \alpha) + \frac{x^\alpha}{\ln x^\alpha}(1 - \gamma)$$

$$+ O\left(\frac{x}{\log x}\right) + O\left(\frac{x^\alpha}{(\log x)^2}\right) \qquad (4.13)$$

for $1 < \alpha \le 2$. For any fixed value of $\alpha > 1$ we could absorb the error estimate $O(x/\log x)$ in the other term $O(x^\alpha/(\log x)^2)$; however, the derivation below needs uniform bounds in which the constants implied by O notation do not depend on x or α.

We will establish (4.8) by proving the formula

$$\Psi_k(x^\alpha, x) = x^\alpha \rho_k(\alpha) + \frac{x^\alpha}{\ln x^\alpha} \sigma_k(\alpha) + O\left(\frac{x}{\log x}\right) + O\left(\frac{x^\alpha}{(\log x)^2}\right) \qquad (4.14)$$

for $1 < \alpha \le m$, where the bounding constants implied by the O's depend only on k and m. Equation (4.13) says that (4.14) holds for $k = 1$ and $m = 2$ if we set $\sigma_1(\alpha) = 1 - \gamma$ for $1 < \alpha \le 2$, because $\rho_1(\alpha)$ is equal to $1 - \ln \alpha$ in this range by (4.2), (4.3), and (4.4). If (4.14) holds for $k = 1$ and $1 < \alpha \le m$, we can increase m by considering the range $m < \alpha \le m + 1$, when we have

$$\int_x^{x^\alpha} \Psi_1\left(\frac{x^\alpha}{y}, y\right) \frac{dy}{\ln y} = \int_1^\alpha \Psi_1(x^{\alpha(t-1)/t}, x^{\alpha/t}) x^{\alpha/t} \frac{dt}{t}$$

$$= \int_1^2 \lfloor x^{\alpha(t-1)/t} \rfloor x^{\alpha/t} \frac{dt}{t}$$

$$+ x^\alpha \int_2^\alpha \left(\rho_1(t-1) + \frac{\sigma_1(t-1)}{\ln x^{\alpha(t-1)/t}}\right) \frac{dt}{t}$$

$$+ \int_2^\alpha O\left(\frac{x^{2\alpha/t}}{\log x^{\alpha/t}}\right) \frac{dt}{t}$$

$$+ \int_2^\alpha O\left(\frac{x^\alpha}{(\log x^{\alpha/t})^2}\right) \frac{dt}{t}$$

by substituting $x^{\alpha/t}$ for y. We can deal with all four integrals as follows. First,

$$\int_1^2 \lfloor x^{\alpha(t-1)/t} \rfloor x^{\alpha/t} \frac{dt}{t} = \int_1^2 x^\alpha \frac{dt}{t} - x^\alpha \int_1^2 \{x^{\alpha(t-1)/t}\} x^{\alpha/t} \frac{dt}{t}$$

$$= x^\alpha \int_1^2 \rho_1(t-1) \frac{dt}{t} - x^\alpha \int_1^{x^{\alpha/2}} \frac{\{u\} \, du}{u^2 \ln(x^\alpha/u)},$$

and we also have

$$\int_1^{x^{\alpha/2}} \frac{\{u\}\, du}{u^2 \ln(x^\alpha/u)} = \frac{1}{\ln x^\alpha}\left(1 - \gamma + O\left(\frac{1}{\log x}\right)\right) \tag{4.15}$$

for $\alpha > 2$ by arguing as we did earlier. Next,

$$\int_2^\alpha \frac{\sigma_1(t-1)}{\ln x^{\alpha(t-1)/t}} \frac{dt}{t} = \frac{1}{\ln x^\alpha}\int_1^{\alpha-1} \frac{\sigma_1(t)\, dt}{t}\,;$$

$$\int_2^\alpha \frac{1}{(\log x^{\alpha/t})^2} \frac{dt}{t} = O\left(\frac{1}{(\log x)^2}\right).$$

And finally,

$$\int_2^\alpha \left(\frac{x^{2\alpha/t}\, dt}{t \log x^{\alpha/t}}\right) = \frac{1}{\log x}\int_2^\alpha x^{2/\alpha}\, dt$$

$$= \frac{1}{\log x}\int_{2/\alpha}^1 \frac{x^{\alpha u}\, du}{u^2}$$

$$= \frac{1}{\log x}\int_{2/\alpha}^1 O(x^{\alpha u})\, du = O\left(\frac{1}{(\log x)^2}\right).$$

This establishes (4.14) for $m < \alpha \le m+1$, by (4.12), if we define

$$\sigma_1(\alpha) = 1 - \gamma - \int_1^{\alpha-1} \sigma_1(t) \frac{dt}{t} \tag{4.16}$$

for $\alpha > 2$.

A similar but simpler derivation applies when $k \ge 2$. Assuming that (4.14) holds for $1 < \alpha \le m$, we extend this to $m < \alpha \le m+1$ by noting that

$$\int_x^{x^\alpha} \left(\Psi_k\left(\frac{x^\alpha}{y}, y\right) - \Psi_{k-1}\left(\frac{x^\alpha}{y}, y\right)\right) \frac{dy}{\ln y}$$

$$= \int_1^\alpha \left(\Psi_k(x^{\alpha(t-1)/t}, x^{\alpha/t}) - \Psi_{k-1}(x^{\alpha(t-1)/t}, x^{\alpha/t})\right) x^{\alpha/t} \frac{dt}{t}$$

$$= x^\alpha \int_2^\alpha \left(\rho_k(t-1) - \rho_{k-1}(t-1)\right) \frac{dt}{t}$$

$$\quad + \frac{x^\alpha}{\ln x^\alpha}\int_2^\alpha \left(\sigma_k(t-1) - \sigma_{k-1}(t-1)\right) \frac{dt}{t-1}$$

$$\quad + O\left(\frac{x^\alpha}{(\log x)^2}\right)$$

when $\alpha > 2$, and it is zero when $\alpha \leq 2$. Thus the desired relation follows for $k \geq 2$ provided that we define

$$
\sigma_k(\alpha) = \begin{cases} 0, & \text{if } \alpha \leq 2; \\ -\int_2^\alpha \big(\sigma_k(t-1) - \sigma_{k-1}(t-1)\big)\dfrac{dt}{t-1}, & \text{if } \alpha > 2. \end{cases} \tag{4.17}
$$

It follows that

$$
\sigma_k(\alpha) = (1 - \gamma)\big(\rho_k(\alpha - 1) - \rho_{k-1}(\alpha - 1)\big) \tag{4.18}
$$

for all $k \geq 1$.

5. Identities Satisfied by ρ_k

The functions $\rho_k(a)$ defined by (4.2), (4.3), and (4.4) possess many surprising properties, and we shall examine some of them in this section.

Our first goal is to express the ρ_k in terms of some special polylogarithm functions L_k, defined by

$$
L_0(\alpha) = 0 \quad \text{for } \alpha \leq 0, \qquad L_0(\alpha) = 1 \quad \text{for } \alpha > 0; \tag{5.1}
$$

$$
L_k(\alpha) = \int_1^\alpha L_{k-1}(t - 1)\frac{dt}{t}. \tag{5.2}
$$

Thus $L_1(\alpha) = \ln \alpha$ for $\alpha \geq 1$, $L_2(\alpha) = \int_2^\alpha \ln(t - 1)\, dt/t$ for $\alpha \geq 2$, and $L_k(\alpha) = 0$ for $\alpha \leq k$. In general, $L_k(\alpha)$ can be expressed as $1/k!$ times the integral of $(dx_1 \ldots dx_k)/(x_1 \ldots x_k)$ over all points $(x_1, \ldots, x_k)$ in the simplex defined by $x_1, \ldots, x_k \geq 1$ and $x_1 + \cdots + x_k \leq \alpha$. For example, $L_3(\alpha)$ can be expressed as

$$
\int_1^{\alpha/3} \frac{dx}{x} \int_x^{(\alpha-x)/2} \frac{dy}{y} \int_y^{(\alpha-x-y)/1} \frac{dz}{z} = \int_3^\alpha \frac{dt}{t} \int_2^{t-1} \frac{du}{u} \int_1^{u-1} \frac{dv}{v}
$$

if we let $t = \alpha/x$, $u = (\alpha - x)/y$, and $v = (\alpha - x - y)/z$.

By iterating the recurrence for ρ_k we find

$$
1 - \rho_1(\alpha) = L_1(\alpha) - L_2(\alpha) + L_3(\alpha) - L_4(\alpha) + L_5(\alpha) - \cdots, \tag{5.3}
$$

$$
1 - \rho_2(\alpha) = \qquad L_2(\alpha) - 2L_3(\alpha) + 3L_4(\alpha) - 4L_5(\alpha) + \cdots, \tag{5.4}
$$

for $\alpha > 0$, and in general

$$
1 - \rho_k(\alpha) = \sum_n \binom{-k}{n} L_{n+k}(\alpha). \tag{5.5}
$$

These infinite sums are actually finite for any particular value of α.

Now let us examine several auxiliary functions:

$$S_k(\alpha, \beta) = \int_0^\alpha \frac{\rho_k(t-1)\, dt}{\beta - t} \qquad \text{for } \beta > \alpha \text{ or } \beta < 0; \tag{5.6}$$

$$S_k(\alpha) = S_k(\alpha, \alpha + 1); \tag{5.7}$$

$$I_k(\alpha) = \int_0^\alpha \frac{\rho_k(t-1)}{t} \ln(t+1)\, dt; \tag{5.8}$$

$$\sigma_k(\alpha) = \int_0^\alpha \frac{\rho_k(t-1)}{t}\, dt; \tag{5.9}$$

$$e_k(x) = \int_0^\infty \rho_k(t)e^{-tx}\, dt, \qquad x > 0. \tag{5.10}$$

(Equation (5.9) defines a different function $\sigma_k(\alpha)$ from the one in Section 4.) It follows immediately from the definition $\rho_k(\alpha) = 1 - \sigma_k(\alpha) + \sigma_{k-1}(\alpha)$ that

$$\sigma_k(\alpha) = k - \rho_1(\alpha) - \cdots - \rho_k(\alpha). \tag{5.11}$$

Integration by parts enables us to evaluate $I_k(\alpha)$ as follows:

$$I_k(\alpha) - I_{k-1}(\alpha) = -\rho_k(t)\ln(t+1)\Big|_0^\alpha + \int_0^\alpha \frac{\rho_k(t)\, dt}{t+1}$$

$$= -\rho_k(\alpha)\ln(\alpha+1) + \sigma_k(\alpha+1). \tag{5.12}$$

Thus in particular we have

$$I_1(\alpha) = -\rho_1(\alpha)\ln(\alpha+1) + 1 - \rho_1(\alpha+1), \tag{5.13}$$

$$I_2(\alpha) = -\rho_1(\alpha)\ln(\alpha+1) - \rho_2(\alpha)\ln(\alpha+1)$$
$$+ 3 - 2\rho_1(\alpha+1) - \rho_2(\alpha+1), \tag{5.14}$$

etc. A somewhat surprising consequence of this relation is that $I_k(\infty) = k(k+1)/2$, while $\sigma_k(\infty) = k$; in particular, $I_1(\infty) = \sigma_1(\infty)$.

Integration by parts applied to $S_k(\alpha, \beta)$ yields

$$S_k(\alpha, \beta) - S_{k-1}(\alpha, \beta) = -\frac{t\rho_k(t)}{\beta - t}\Big|_0^\alpha + \beta \int_0^\alpha \frac{\rho_k(t)\, dt}{(\beta - t)^2}$$

$$= -\frac{\alpha\rho_k(\alpha)}{\beta - \alpha} + \beta \int_1^{\alpha+1} \frac{\rho_k(t-1)\, dt}{(\beta + 1 - t)^2}. \tag{5.15}$$

Also, differentiating the integral that defines $S_k(\alpha) = S_k(\alpha, \alpha + 1)$ with respect to α leads to a formula that can be combined with this one:

$$S_k'(\alpha) = \rho_k(\alpha - 1) - \int_1^\alpha \frac{\rho_k(t-1)\,dt}{(\alpha + 1 - t)^2}$$

$$= \rho_k(\alpha - 1) - \frac{1}{\alpha}\big((\alpha - 1)\rho_k(\alpha - 1) + S_k(\alpha - 1) - S_{k-1}(\alpha - 1)\big)$$

$$= \frac{1}{\alpha}\big(\rho_k(\alpha - 1) + S_{k-1}(\alpha - 1) - S_k(\alpha - 1)\big). \tag{5.16}$$

Now we are ready to prove an important relation that expresses ρ_{k+1} in terms of ρ_k and ρ_{k-1}:

Lemma 5.1. *For all $k \geq 1$ and all $\alpha > 0$ we have*

$$\rho_{k+1}(\alpha) = \rho_k(\alpha) + \frac{1}{k}\big(S_k(\alpha) - S_{k-1}(\alpha)\big). \tag{5.17}$$

Proof. Since $\rho_{k+1}(\alpha) = \rho_k(\alpha) = 1$ and $S_k(\alpha) = S_{k-1}(\alpha) = 0$ for $0 < \alpha \leq 1$, the result holds for $\lceil \alpha \rceil = 1$; we will show that the derivatives agree, by induction on $\lceil \alpha \rceil$. Since

$$(\alpha + 1)\rho_{k+1}'(\alpha + 1) = \rho_k(\alpha) - \rho_{k+1}(\alpha) = \big(S_{k-1}(\alpha) - S_k(\alpha)\big)/k,$$

$$(\alpha + 1)\rho_k'(\alpha + 1) = \rho_{k-1}(\alpha) - \rho_k(\alpha),$$

$$(\alpha + 1)S_k'(\alpha + 1) = \rho_k(\alpha) + S_{k-1}(\alpha) - S_k(\alpha),$$

$$(\alpha + 1)S_{k-1}'(\alpha + 1) = \rho_{k-1}(\alpha) + S_{k-2}(\alpha) - S_{k-1}(\alpha),$$

the desired result is equivalent to

$$\frac{k-1}{k}\rho_k(\alpha) = \frac{k-1}{k}\rho_{k-1}(\alpha) + \frac{1}{k}\big(S_{k-1}(\alpha) - S_{k-2}(\alpha)\big).$$

For $k = 1$ this is obvious, otherwise it holds by induction.   □

By iterating the recurrence in the lemma, it follows that

$$\rho_{k+1}(\alpha) = \rho_1(\alpha) + \frac{1}{2 \cdot 1}S_1(\alpha) + \cdots + \frac{1}{k(k-1)}S_{k-1}(\alpha) + \frac{1}{k}S_k(\alpha). \tag{5.18}$$

Finally let us consider the functions $e_k(x)$ defined in (5.10). Somewhat surprisingly, these can actually be expressed in closed form:

Theorem 5.2. Let $E(x) = E_1(x)$ be the exponential integral function

$$E(x) = \int_x^\infty e^{-t}\frac{dt}{t} = \int_1^\infty e^{-xt}\frac{dt}{t}. \tag{5.19}$$

Then

$$e_k(x) = \frac{1}{xe^{E(x)}}\left(1 + \frac{E(x)}{1!} + \cdots + \frac{E(x)^{k-1}}{(k-1)!}\right). \tag{5.20}$$

Proof. Once again we integrate by parts:

$$e_k(x) - e_{k-1}(x) = \int_1^\infty \frac{\rho_k(t-1) - \rho_{k-1}(t-1)}{t} te^{-(t-1)x}\,dt$$

$$= -e^x \int_0^\infty te^{-tx}\,d\rho_k(t)$$

$$= e^x \int_0^\infty \rho_k(t)(e^{-tx} - txe^{-tx})\,dt$$

$$= e^x\bigl(e_k(x) + xe_k'(x)\bigr).$$

If we let $f_k(x) = xe^{E(x)}e_k(x)$, we have therefore

$$f_k'(x) = e^{E(x)}\bigl(e_k(x) + xe_k'(x) - e^{-x}e_k(x)\bigr)$$

$$= -\frac{e^{-x}}{x}f_{k-1}(x) = E'(x)f_{k-1}(x)$$

and it follows by induction on k that

$$f_k(x) = C + \frac{E(x)}{1!} + \cdots + \frac{E(x)^{k-1}}{(k-1)!}.$$

In order to evaluate C, we integrate by parts in the opposite direction:

$$xe_k(x) = -\int_0^\infty \rho_k(t)\,d(e^{-tx})$$

$$= -\rho(t)e^{-tx}\Big|_0^\infty + \int_0^\infty e^{-tx}\,d\rho_k(t)$$

$$= 1 - \int_1^\infty e^{-tx}\bigl(\rho_k(t-1) - \rho_{k-1}(t-1)\bigr)\frac{dt}{t}$$

$$= 1 - \int_x^\infty e^{-u}\left(\rho_k\Bigl(\frac{u}{x} - 1\Bigr) - \rho_{k-1}\Bigl(\frac{u}{x} - 1\Bigr)\right)\frac{du}{u}.$$

Hence $C = \lim_{x\to\infty} xe_k(x) = \lim_{x\to\infty} f_k(x) = 1$. $\square$

Theorem 5.2 now allows us to write down an "explicit" equation for $\rho_k(x)$, instead of a recurrence relation, namely

$$\rho_k(x) = \frac{1}{2\pi} \int_{-\infty}^{\infty} e^{ixt} e_k(it)\, dt, \qquad \text{for } x > 0. \tag{5.21}$$

This follows by Fourier inversion, since equation (5.20) can be extended to all complex x not on the negative real axis, by analytic continuation. (Note that $E(x) = \ln 1/x + O(1)$ as $x \to 0$, hence $e_k(x) = O(\ln(1/x))^{k-1}$ and the integral is convergent at $t = 0$.) The case of $k = 1$ of (5.21) was obtained by de Bruijn in [2].

6. Asymptotic Formulas

In this section we shall study the asymptotic behavior of $\rho_k(\alpha)$ for large α. Our starting point is a simple proof that $\rho_1(\alpha)$ is exponentially small: Let us write $\rho(\alpha)$ for $\rho_1(\alpha)$. Then since

$$1 + \int_2^\alpha \rho(t-1)\, dt = \int_1^\alpha \rho(t-1)\, dt$$

$$= -t\rho(t)\Big|_1^\alpha + \int_1^\alpha \rho(t)\, dt$$

$$= 1 - \alpha\rho(\alpha) + \int_2^{\alpha+1} \rho(t-1)\, dt \tag{6.1}$$

we have

$$\int_\alpha^{\alpha+1} \rho(t-1)\, dt = \alpha\rho(\alpha). \tag{6.2}$$

It follows immediately that $\alpha\rho(\alpha) < \rho(\alpha - 1)$ for all $\alpha > 1$, hence by induction

$$\rho(n) \le 1/n! \tag{6.3}$$

for all integers $n \ge 1$. Considerably more precise formulas have been obtained by de Bruijn [1] and others, and numerical results have been tabulated by Mitchell [10] and by van de Lune and Wattel [15]; but (6.3) suffices for our purposes in this section.

The rapid decrease of $\rho_1(\alpha)$ simplifies the numerical evaluation of integrals and it also leads to a simple treatment of the asymptotic behavior of $\rho_2(\alpha)$:

Theorem 6.1. *For all fixed $r \geq 1$ we have*

$$\rho_2(\alpha) = e^\gamma \left(\frac{c_0}{\alpha} + \frac{c_1}{\alpha^2} + \cdots + \frac{c_{r-1}}{\alpha^r} \right) + O(\alpha^{-r-1}) \qquad (6.4)$$

as $\alpha \to \infty$, where the coefficients c_k are defined by

$$\sum_{k \geq 0} c_k \frac{z^k}{k!} = \exp\left(\int_0^z (e^t - 1) \frac{dt}{t} \right) = \exp\left(\sum_{k \geq 1} \frac{1}{k} \frac{z^k}{k!} \right). \qquad (6.5)$$

Thus

$$\langle c_0, c_1, c_2, \ldots \rangle = \left\langle 1, 1, \frac{3}{2}, \frac{17}{6}, \frac{19}{3}, \frac{81}{5}, \frac{8351}{180}, \frac{184553}{1260}, \frac{52907}{105}, \ldots \right\rangle.$$

Before proving the theorem, we note that (6.5) implies the recurrence formula

$$c_n = \frac{1}{n} \sum_{k=1}^n \binom{n}{k} c_{n-k}, \qquad n \geq 1. \qquad (6.6)$$

Therefore $c_n > ((n-1)/2)c_{n-2}$ for $n \geq 2$, and $c_{2n+1} > n!$; the infinite series $\sum c_k / \alpha^k$ diverges for all α. In other words, (6.4) is strictly an asymptotic formula.

Proof. From Lemma 5.1 and equation (6.3) we have

$$\rho_2(\alpha) = \rho_1(\alpha) + S_1(\alpha)$$

$$= \rho(\alpha) + \int_0^{\alpha-1} \frac{\rho(t)\, dt}{\alpha - t}$$

$$= \sum_{k=0}^r \frac{1}{\alpha^{k+1}} \int_0^{\alpha-1} \rho(t) t^k \, dt + O(\alpha^{-r-1}) \qquad (6.7)$$

since $\int_0^{\alpha-1} \rho(t) t^{r+1}\, dt / (\alpha - t) < \int_0^{\alpha-1} \rho(t) t^{r+1}\, dt < \infty$. Furthermore we have

$$\int_{\alpha-1}^\infty \rho(t) t^k \, dt = O\left(\int_{\alpha-1}^\infty e^{-t} t^k dt \right) = O(e^{-\alpha} \alpha^k) = O(e^{-\alpha/2}) \qquad (6.8)$$

as $\alpha \to \infty$, by making very crude estimates not even as powerful as (6.3); so we can integrate to ∞ in (6.7):

$$\rho_2(\alpha) = \frac{a_0}{\alpha} + \frac{a_1}{\alpha^2} + \cdots + \frac{a_{r-1}}{\alpha^r} + O(\alpha^{-r-1}), \qquad (6.9)$$

where

$$a_k = \int_0^\infty \rho(t) t^k \, dt. \qquad (6.10)$$

It remains to evaluate the coefficients a_k. We have

$$\sum_{k \geq 0} a_k \frac{(-x)^k}{k!} = \int_0^\infty \rho(t) e^{-xt}\, dt = e_1(x) = e^{-E(x) - \ln x} \qquad (6.11)$$

by Theorem 5.2; and it is well known that

$$-E(x) - \ln x = \gamma + \sum_{k \geq 1} \frac{(-x)^k}{k \cdot k!}. \qquad (6.12)$$

(See, for example, [8, exercise 5.2.2–43].) This combines with (6.11) and (6.5) to prove that $a_k = e^\gamma c_k$. □

Incidentally, a similar method can be used to prove the identity

$$\int_1^\infty \left(\rho_2(t) - e^\gamma / t \right) dt = e^\gamma - 1. \qquad (6.13)$$

The coefficients c_k have the curious property that

$$\rho_2(\alpha) = e^\gamma \left(\frac{c_0}{\alpha + 1} + \frac{2c_1}{(\alpha + 1)^2} + \cdots + \frac{r c_{r-1}}{(\alpha + 1)^r} \right) + O(\alpha^{-r-1}) \quad (6.14)$$

is also an asymptotic expansion of ρ_2, but not as accurate when truncated. Another series,

$$\rho_2(\alpha) = e^\gamma \left(\frac{c_0}{\alpha - 1} + \frac{c_1 - c_0}{2(\alpha - 1)^2} + \frac{c_2 - c_1 + c_0}{3(\alpha - 1)^3} + \cdots \right) + O(\alpha^{-r-1})$$

is, in turn, more accurate than (6.4). These series are obtainable from one another using the relation $\rho_2(\alpha) = -(\alpha + 1)\rho_2'(\alpha + 1) + \rho_1(\alpha)$.

For larger values of k we shall content ourselves with establishing the leading term in the asymptotic expansion of ρ_k, namely

$$\rho_k(\alpha) = \frac{e^\gamma (\ln \alpha)^{k-2}}{(k-2)! \, \alpha} + O\left(\frac{(\ln \alpha)^{k-3}}{\alpha} \right), \qquad \text{for } k \geq 3. \qquad (6.15)$$

[Appendix B contains an asymptotic expansion of ρ_3.] Consider first

$$S_2(\alpha) = \int_1^\alpha \left(\frac{e^\gamma}{t} + O\left(\frac{1}{t^2} \right) \right) \frac{dt}{\alpha + 1 - t} \qquad (6.16)$$

and note that

$$\int_1^\alpha \frac{dt}{t(\alpha+1-t)} = \frac{1}{\alpha+1}\left(\int_1^\alpha \frac{dt}{t} + \int_1^\alpha \frac{dt}{\alpha+1-t}\right) = \frac{2\ln\alpha}{\alpha+1},$$

$$\int_1^\alpha \frac{dt}{t^2(\alpha+1-t)} = \frac{1}{\alpha+1}\int_1^\alpha \frac{dt}{t^2} + \frac{1}{\alpha+1}\int_1^\alpha \frac{dt}{t(\alpha+1-t)}$$

$$= \frac{1}{\alpha+1}\left(1 - \frac{1}{\alpha}\right) + \frac{2\ln\alpha}{(\alpha+1)^2} = O(\alpha^{-1}). \quad (6.17)$$

Hence $S_2(\alpha) = 2e^\gamma \alpha^{-1}\ln\alpha + O(\alpha^{-1})$, and $\rho_3(\alpha) = e^\gamma \alpha^{-1}\ln\alpha + O(\alpha^{-1})$ by (5.18). In order to use this approach for larger k, we note that

$$\int_1^\alpha \frac{(\ln t)^k\, dt}{t(\alpha+1-t)} = \frac{1}{\alpha+1}\int_1^\alpha \frac{(\ln t)^k\, dt}{t} + \frac{1}{\alpha+1}\int_1^\alpha \frac{(\ln t)^k\, dt}{\alpha+1-t}$$

$$= \frac{1}{(\alpha+1)}\frac{(\ln\alpha)^{k+1}}{(k+1)} + \frac{k}{\alpha+1}\int_1^\alpha \frac{(\ln t)^{k-1}\ln(\alpha+1-t)\, dt}{t}$$

$$= \frac{1}{(\alpha+1)}\frac{(\ln\alpha)^{k+1}}{(k+1)} + \frac{\ln(\alpha+1)}{\alpha+1}(\ln\alpha)^k$$

$$+ \frac{k}{\alpha+1}\int_1^\alpha (\ln t)^{k-1}\ln\left(1 - \frac{t}{\alpha+1}\right)\frac{dt}{t}.$$

Now $\ln(1-x) = -xf(x)$, where f is a function satisfying

$$1 < f\left(\frac{t}{\alpha+1}\right) \le f\left(\frac{\alpha}{\alpha+1}\right) = \frac{\alpha+1}{\alpha}\ln(\alpha+1) \qquad (6.18)$$

when $1 \le t \le \alpha$; hence

$$\int_1^\alpha \frac{(\ln t)^{k-1}}{t}\ln\left(1 - \frac{t}{\alpha+1}\right)dt = \frac{1}{\alpha+1}\int_1^\alpha (\ln t)^{k-1}O(\log\alpha)\, dt$$

$$= O(\log\alpha)^k. \qquad (6.19)$$

We have now proved the estimate

$$\int_1^\alpha \frac{(\ln t)^k dt}{t(\alpha+1-t)} = \frac{k+2}{k+1}\frac{(\ln\alpha)^{k+1}}{\alpha} + O\left(\frac{(\ln\alpha)^k}{\alpha}\right), \qquad (6.20)$$

for all $k \ge 0$. Formula (6.15) follows by induction, using (5.18) together with

$$S_k(\alpha) = \frac{e^\gamma k(\ln\alpha)^{k-1}}{(k-1)!\,\alpha} + O\left(\frac{(\ln\alpha)^{k-2}}{\alpha}\right). \qquad (6.21)$$

7. Application to Factoring

The distributions $F_k(x) = \rho_k(1/x)$ can be used to estimate the running time of various algorithms for factorization. For example, Pollard's important new Monte Carlo method [12] takes about $\sqrt{n_2}$ steps, where n_2 is the second-largest prime factor of n, so we can use a table of F_2 to state that Pollard's method will complete the factorization in $O(n^{0.106})$ steps at most, about half of the time.

For the simple algorithm of Section 1, we need to analyze the distribution of $\max(n_2, \sqrt{n_1})$, and this quantity does not appear to be expressible directly as an algebraic function of the F_k. However, we can readily carry out the analysis by using the techniques above. Let $G(x)$ be the limiting probability that $\max(n_2, \sqrt{n_1}) \leq N^x$, when n is a random integer between 1 and N. Then $G(x) = F_1(x) + G_1(x) = F_2(x) - G_2(x)$, where $G_1(x)$ is the probability that $N^x \leq n_1 \leq N^{2x}$ and $n_2 \leq N^x$, and $G_2(x)$ is the probability that $n_1 > N^{2x}$ and $n_2 \leq N^x$. Arguing as above, we find

$$G_1(x) = \int_x^{2x} \frac{dt}{t} F_1\left(\frac{x}{1-t}\right) = \int_x^{2x} \frac{dt}{t} \rho\left(\frac{1-t}{x}\right); \qquad (7.1)$$

$$G_1\left(\frac{1}{\alpha}\right) = \int_{1/\alpha}^{2/\alpha} \rho((1-t)\alpha) \frac{dt}{t} = \int_{\alpha-1}^{\alpha} \frac{\rho(u-1)\,du}{\alpha+1-u}; \qquad (7.2)$$

$$G_2(x) = \int_{2x}^1 \frac{dt}{t} F_1\left(\frac{x}{1-t}\right) = \int_{2x}^1 \frac{dt}{t} \rho\left(\frac{1-t}{x}\right); \qquad (7.3)$$

$$G_2\left(\frac{1}{\alpha}\right) = \int_{2/\alpha}^1 \rho((1-t)\alpha) \frac{dt}{t} = \int_1^{\alpha-1} \frac{\rho(u-1)\,du}{\alpha+1-u}. \qquad (7.4)$$

(Notice that $G_1(1/\alpha) + G_2(1/\alpha) = S_1(\alpha) = F_2(1/\alpha) - F_1(1/\alpha)$, in agreement with Lemma 5.1.) It is clear from our asymptotic results that $G_1(1/\alpha)$ decreases exponentially for large α, hence it is numerically better to use the formula $G(x) = F_1(x) + G_1(x)$ than to use $F_2(x) - G_2(x)$; furthermore the integration is over a limited range. On the other hand for $2 \leq \alpha \leq 3$ it is most convenient to use G_2, since $G_2(1/\alpha) = \ln(\alpha/2)$ in this range.

8. Remarks About the Model

The probability considerations above are for random n between 1 and N, and for relations such as $n_k \leq N^x$; but from an intuitive standpoint we might rather ask for the probability of a relation such as $n_k \leq n^x$, without considering N. Actually it is easy to convert from one model to the other, since most numbers between 1 and N are large.

More precisely, consider how many numbers n between $\frac{1}{2}N$ and N have $n_k \leq N^x$; this is $P_k(x, N) - P_k(x, \frac{1}{2}N) = \frac{1}{2}NF_k(x) + O(N/\log N)$, since $P_k(x, N) = N \cdot F_k(x) + O(N/\log N)$. Furthermore, consider how many of these n have $n^x < n_k \leq N^x$: The latter relation implies $N^x \geq n_k > (\frac{1}{2}N)^x = N^{x - \log 2/\log N}$, and $F_k(x - \log 2/\log N) = F_k(x) + O(1/\log N)$, since F_k is differentiable; so the number of such n is at most $P_k(x, N) - P_k(x - \log 2/\log N, N) = O(N/\log N)$. (The constant implied by the O in (4.7) will be independent of x in a bounded region about x.)

We have shown that $F_k(x) + O(1/\log N)$ of all n between $\frac{1}{2}N$ and N satisfy $n_k \leq n^x$. Therefore if $Q_k(x, N)$ denotes the total number of $n \leq N$ such that $n_k \leq n^x$, we have

$$Q_k(x, N) = \sum_{j=1}^{\lg \log N} \left(F_k(x) + O\left(\frac{1}{\log(N/2^j)}\right) \right) \frac{N}{2^j} + O\left(\frac{N}{\log N}\right)$$

$$= NF_k(x) + O\left(\frac{N}{\log N}\right), \tag{8.1}$$

by dividing the range $N/\log N \leq n \leq N$ into $\lg \log N$ parts.

It is customary to define the "probability" of a statement $S(n)$ about the positive integer n by the formula

$$\Pr(S(n)) = \lim_{N \to \infty} \frac{1}{N}\left(\text{number of } n \leq N \text{ such that } S(n) \text{ is true}\right), \tag{8.2}$$

when this limit exists. Thus, we can state well-known facts such as the following: $\Pr(n \text{ is odd}) = 1/2$; $\Pr(n \text{ is prime}) = 0$; $\Pr(n \text{ is squarefree}) = 6/\pi^2$. Equation (8.1) now yields another result of this type:

$$\Pr(n_k \leq n^x) = F_k(x), \tag{8.3}$$

for all fixed x.

Another important observation should also be made about the theoretical model we have used to study the factorization algorithm in this paper. We have stated our results in terms of the probability that the running time is $\leq N^x$ (or, if we prefer, $\leq n^x$); this contrasts with the customary approach to the study of average running time, which derives mean values and the standard deviation. The reason for abandoning the traditional approach is that the mean and standard deviation are particularly uninformative for this algorithm. This phenomenon is apparent when we consider that the mean running time over all $n \leq N$ will be relatively near the worst case $n^{0.5}$, but in more than 70 percent of all cases the actual running time will be less than $n^{0.4}$.

In order to understand this rather anomalous situation more fully, let us calculate the asymptotic mean and standard deviation of the largest prime factor n_1, when all integers $1 \leq n \leq N$ are considered equally likely. Let $\Phi(t)$ be the probability that $n_1 \leq t$, when n is in this range. Then the analysis of $\Psi_1(t)$ in Section 4 allows us to conclude that

$$\Phi(t) = 1 + \ln \ln t - \ln \ln N + \frac{1}{\ln N} \int_1^{N/t} \frac{\{u\} \, du}{u^2} + O\left(\frac{1}{\log N}\right)^2, \quad (8.4)$$

for $\sqrt{N} \leq t \leq N$.

We shall now calculate the asymptotic behavior of the kth moment of this distribution, namely the asymptotic expected value of n_1^k. [Incidentally, our derivation will provide a good example of the use of Stieltjes integration.] The kth moment is

$$\mathrm{E}(n_1^k) = \int_1^N t^k \, d\Phi(t), \quad (8.5)$$

and since the integral from 1 to $\sqrt{N}$ is $O\left(N^{k/2} \int_1^{\sqrt{N}} d\Phi(t)\right) = O(N^{k/2})$ it can safely be ignored. We are left with

$$\int_{\sqrt{N}}^N t^k d\left(1 + \ln \ln t - \ln \ln N + \frac{1}{\ln N} \int_1^{N/t} \frac{\{u\} \, du}{u^2} + O\left(\frac{1}{\log N}\right)^2\right)$$

$$= \int_{\sqrt{N}}^N t^k d \ln \ln t - \frac{1}{\ln N} \int_1^{\sqrt{N}} \left(\frac{N}{v}\right)^k d \int_1^v \frac{\{u\} \, du}{u^2} + O\left(\frac{N^k}{(\log N)^2}\right), \quad (8.6)$$

by replacing t by N/v in the second integral. [The O estimate here is justified by the following general lemma: Let $\int_a^b f(t) \, dg(t)$ and $\int_a^b f(t) \, dh(t)$ exist, where $h(t) = O(g(t))$, and where both f and g are positive monotone functions on $[a \mathinner{.\,.} b]$. Then it is easy to see that

$$\int_a^b f(t) \, dh(t) = O(f(a)g(a)) + O(f(b)g(b)) + O\left(\int_a^b f(t) \, dg(t)\right),$$

if we integrate by parts twice.] The first integral in (8.6) is

$$\int_{\sqrt{N}}^N \frac{t^{k-1} dt}{\ln t} = N^k \int_1^{\sqrt{N}} \frac{dv}{v^{k+1}(\ln N - \ln v)}$$

$$= \frac{N^k}{\ln N} \left(\int_1^{\sqrt{N}} \frac{dv}{v^{k+1}} + \int_1^{\sqrt{N}} \frac{\ln v \, dv}{v^{k+1}(\ln N - \ln v)}\right)$$

$$= \frac{N^k}{k \ln N} + O\left(\frac{N^k}{(\log N)^2}\right).$$

The second integral is $-N^k/\ln N$ times the integral $\int_1^{\sqrt{N}}\{v\}\,dv/v^{k+2}$, which is within $O(N^{-(k+1)/2})$ of

$$\int_1^\infty \frac{\{v\}\,dv}{v^{k+2}} = \sum_{j\geq 1}\int_j^{j+1}\frac{(v-j)\,dv}{v^{k+2}}$$

$$= \sum_{j\geq 1}\left(\frac{1}{k}\left(\frac{1}{j^k}-\frac{1}{(j+1)^k}\right)-\frac{j}{k+1}\left(\frac{1}{j^{k+1}}-\frac{1}{(j+1)^{k+1}}\right)\right)$$

$$= \sum_{j\geq 1}\left(\frac{1}{k(k+1)}\left(\frac{1}{j^k}-\frac{1}{(j+1)^k}\right)-\frac{1}{k+1}\frac{1}{(j+1)^{k+1}}\right)$$

$$= \frac{1}{k(k+1)}-\frac{1}{k+1}(\zeta(k+1)-1)=\frac{1}{k}-\frac{\zeta(k+1)}{k+1}.$$

Thus we have shown that

$$\mathrm{E}(n_1^k)=\frac{\zeta(k+1)}{k+1}\frac{N^k}{\ln N}+O\left(\frac{N^k}{(\log N)^2}\right). \tag{8.7}$$

It follows that the mean value of n_1 is asymptotically $(\pi^2/12)N/\ln N$, and the standard deviation is $(\zeta(3)/3)^{1/2}N/\sqrt{\ln N}$, to within a factor of $1+O(1/\log N)$. In particular, the ratio

$$\frac{\text{standard deviation}}{\text{mean}}\to\infty \tag{8.8}$$

as $N\to\infty$; this fact demonstrates the unsuitability of a traditional "mean and variance" approach to the analysis of such algorithms.

9. Numerical Results

The differential-difference equations for ρ_k are conveniently suited to numerical integration. For example, given internal arrays containing $\rho_1(m+k/n)$, $\rho_2(m+k/n)$, and $\rho_3(m+k/n)$ for $0\leq k\leq n+t$, where m is some fixed integer and $\delta=1/n$ is the step size and t depends on the method of integration, one pass over these arrays serves to increase m by 1. When m reaches a suitably large value, the asymptotic formulas derived above provide an excellent check on the accuracy of the calculations. Another excellent check comes from the formula

$$e^\gamma=\int_0^\infty \rho(t)\,dt=\rho(1)+2\rho(2)+3\rho(3)+\cdots, \tag{9.1}$$

α	$\rho_1(\alpha)$	$\rho_2(\alpha)$	$\rho_3(\alpha)$	$G(1/\alpha)$
1.0	1.000000 000000	1.000000 000000	1.000000 000000	1.000000 000000
1.5	0.594534 891892	1.000000 000000	1.000000 000000	1.000000 000000
2.0	0.306852 819440	1.000000 000000	1.000000 000000	1.000000 000000
2.5	0.130319 561832	0.953389 706294	1.000000 000000	0.730246 154979
3.0	0.048608 388291	0.852779 323041	1.000000 000000	0.447314 214932
3.5	0.016229 593243	0.733481 165219	0.997526 273042	0.223819 493955
4.0	0.004910 925648	0.623681 059959	0.985113 653272	0.096399 005935
4.5	0.001370 117741	0.533652 572034	0.960975 011157	0.036573 065077
5.0	0.000354 724700	0.463222 186987	0.927859 653628	0.012413 482748
6.0	0.000019 649696	0.365217 751694	0.851107 195638	0.001092 266742
7.0	0.000000 874567	0.301786 010308	0.777229 329492	0.000071 391673
8.0	0.000000 032321	0.257435 710831	0.712844 794121	0.000003 662651
9.0	0.000000 001016	0.224592 162720	0.657959 581954	0.000000 153284
10.0	0.000000 000028	0.199248 208994	0.611115 997540	0.000000 005383
12.0	0.000000 000000	0.162638 856635	0.535865 613616	0.000000 000004
14.0	0.000000 000000	0.137437 368144	0.478221 749442	0.000000 000000
16.0	0.000000 000000	0.119016 453035	0.432642 865532	0.000000 000000
18.0	0.000000 000000	0.104958 753569	0.395653 753569	0.000000 000000
20.0	0.000000 000000	0.093875 845625	0.364991 546696	0.000000 000000
25.0	0.000000 000000	0.074277 803044	0.307069 057805	0.000000 000000
30.0	0.000000 000000	0.061453 736517	0.266170 912880	0.000000 000000
40.0	0.000000 000000	0.045683 813582	0.211838 770538	0.000000 000000
50.0	0.000000 000000	0.036356 095670	0.177085 969207	0.000000 000000
60.0	0.000000 000000	0.030192 055732	0.152778 425203	0.000000 000000

TABLE 1. Values computed by numerical integration.

which follows from (6.2), (6.4), and (6.10). (Incidentally, identity (9.1) appears to be new, although an equivalent result was recently found independently by van Rongen [16]. It was discovered empirically, after noticing that the results of numerical integration seemed to resemble a "familiar" constant. This particular constant came as a surprise, since e^γ usually occurs only in connection with infinite products, while (9.1) is an infinite *sum*. After the proof of (9.1) was found, Theorem 5.2 followed rather quickly. Thus, numerical results indeed suggest theorems.)

Table 1 gives representative values of ρ_1, ρ_2, ρ_3, and G to 12 decimal places, and Table 2 shows percentage points of the distributions F_1, F_2, F_3. For example, the probability is only 10 percent that $n_3 > n^{0.18616}$. (Karl Dickman published 8-digit values of $\rho_1(\alpha)$ for integer $\alpha \leq 8$ in 1930 [4]; his figures were correct except that $\rho_1(7)$ was said to be 0.0000 0088.)

p	$F_1^{-1}(p)$	$F_2^{-1}(p)$	$F_3^{-1}(p)$
0.01	0.26974	0.00558	0.00068
0.02	0.29341	0.01110	0.00149
0.03	0.31004	0.01656	0.00239
0.04	0.32341	0.02196	0.00334
0.05	0.33483	0.02730	0.00435
0.10	0.37851	0.05308	0.00995
0.15	0.41288	0.07741	0.01629
0.20	0.44304	0.10033	0.02327
0.25	0.47068	0.12191	0.03079
0.30	0.49656	0.14216	0.03882
0.40	0.54881	0.17892	0.05636
0.50	0.60653	0.21172	0.07584
0.60	0.67032	0.24267	0.09745
0.70	0.74082	0.27437	0.12165
0.75	0.77880	0.29153	0.13506
0.80	0.81873	0.31035	0.14972
0.85	0.86071	0.33201	0.16627
0.90	0.90484	0.35899	0.18616
0.95	0.95123	0.39672	0.21377
0.96	0.96079	0.40681	0.22141
0.97	0.97045	0.41850	0.23054
0.98	0.98020	0.43268	0.24224
0.99	0.99005	0.45169	0.25954
1.00	1.00000	0.50000	0.33333

TABLE 2. Percentiles for the largest three prime factors.

Figure 1 shows these distributions graphically, and illustrates the derivative values $F_1'(0) = G'(0) = F_2'(\frac{1}{2}) = F_3'(\frac{1}{3}) = 0$, $F_2'(0) = e^\gamma$, $G'(\frac{1}{2}) = 2$, $F_1'(1) = 1$, $F_3'(0) = \infty$. Although the graphs of F_1, F_2, and F_3 are qualitatively different, the graphs of F_k for $k \geq 4$ resemble that of F_3 (but they rise ever more steeply).

Empirical confirmation of the theory is illustrated in Figure 2, which shows exact empirical distribution functions corresponding to Figure 1 for the 100 numbers $n = 10^{10} - m$, $1 \leq m \leq 100$. As expected, the deviation from $F_k(x)$ is most pronounced for $k = 1$ and $x > \frac{1}{2}$, but the deviations are not severe. This set of numbers contains three primes $(10^{10} - 33, 10^{10} - 57, 10^{10} - 71)$, and ten products of two primes. The smallest values of n_1 occurred for $10^{10} - 100 = 137 \cdot 101 \cdot 73 \cdot 11 \cdot 5^2 \cdot 3^2 \cdot 2^2$, $10^{10} - 64 = 463 \cdot 431 \cdot 29 \cdot 3^3 \cdot 2^6$; the largest values of n_2 occurred for $10^{10} - 69 = 456767 \cdot 21893$, $10^{10} - 22 = 85021 \cdot 19603 \cdot 3 \cdot 2$; the largest

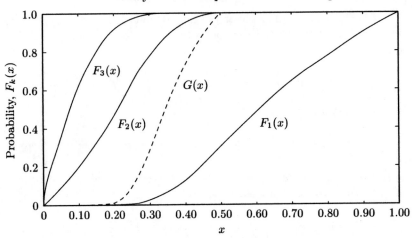

FIGURE 1. Distributions of the three largest prime factors of a random integer and the distribution of the simple factorization time.

values of n_3 occurred for $10^{10} - 51 = 88301 \cdot 421 \cdot 269$, $10^{10} - 73 = 13879 \cdot 359 \cdot 223 \cdot 3^2$. The smallest values of $\max(\sqrt{n_1}, n_2)$ occurred for $10^{10} - 100 = 137 \cdot 101 \cdot 73 \cdot 11 \cdot 5^2 \cdot 3^2 \cdot 2^2$, $10^{10} - 25 = 2857 \cdot 113 \cdot 59 \cdot 7 \cdot 5^2 \cdot 3$ (so these would be the easiest numbers in the given range to factor by the simple algorithm); the smallest values of n_1 for which $\sqrt{n_1} > n_2$ occurred for $10^{10} - 66 = 59417 \cdot 103 \cdot 43 \cdot 19 \cdot 2$, $10^{10} - 68 = 77201 \cdot 53 \cdot 47 \cdot 13 \cdot 2^2$.

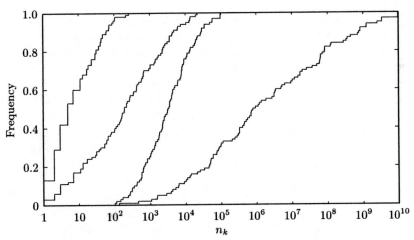

FIGURE 2. Empirical distribution functions corresponding to Figure 1, based on the factors of the largest 100 10-digit numbers.

In Dickman's original paper [4], he calculated the "average" value of x such that $n_1 = n^x$, namely the expected value of $\log n_1 / \log n$. This equals

$$D_1 = \int_0^1 x \, dF_1(x) = -\int_1^\infty \rho'(t) \frac{dt}{t} = \int_1^\infty \rho(t-1) \frac{dt}{t^2} \qquad (9.2)$$

and by (5.14) we also have

$$\int_1^\infty \rho(t-1) \frac{dt}{t^2} = -S_1(\infty, -1) = \int_1^\infty \rho(t-1) \frac{dt}{t+1}. \qquad (9.3)$$

In a similar way we can determine the expected value of $\log n_k / \log n$, a number that can be expressed in several ways, namely

$$D_k = \int_0^1 x \, dF_k(x) = \int_1^\infty \left(\rho_k(t-1) - \rho_{k-1}(t-1) \right) \frac{dt}{t^2}$$

$$= \int_1^\infty \left(\rho_k(t-1) - 2\rho_{k-1}(t-1) + \rho_{k-2}(t-1) \right) \frac{dt}{t+1}$$

$$= 1 - \int_1^\infty \rho_k(t) \frac{dt}{t^2}. \qquad (9.4)$$

Numerical evaluation (using the asymptotic formulas for ρ_2 and ρ_3) gives

$$D_1 \approx 0.62432\,99885; \qquad (9.5)$$

$$D_2 \approx 0.20958\,08743; \qquad (9.6)$$

$$D_3 \approx 0.08831\,60989. \qquad (9.7)$$

(Dickman's value for D_1 was 0.624329998. Note that D_2 is not equal to $D_1(1 - D_1)$, although n_2 is the largest prime factor of n/n_1.)

The average value of a logarithm may seem at first to be of limited practical interest, by comparison with the median and other percentiles; however, we can interpret it meaningfully by saying that $D_k m$ is the *asymptotic average number of digits* in the kth largest prime factor of an m-digit number. Dickman's constant D_1 arises also in an unexpected way in connection with our simple factoring algorithm: The probability that $n_2 < \sqrt{n_1}$, namely the probability that the algorithm needs to divide by all numbers up to $\sqrt{n_1}$, is

$$\int_0^1 \frac{dt}{t} F_1 \left(\frac{t}{2(1-t)} \right) = \int_0^1 \frac{dt}{t} \rho \left(\frac{2(1-t)}{t} \right) = \int_1^\infty \rho(u-1) \frac{du}{u+1} \qquad (9.8)$$

by substituting $u = 2/t - 1$. So this probability equals D_1! In the empirical tests that led to Figure 2, exactly 61 of the 100 numbers had $n_2 < \sqrt{n_1}$.

10. Relation to Permutations

The numerical value of D_1 in (9.5) leads again to a feeling of *déjà vu*; and sure enough, Dickman's constant turns out to be the same as "Golomb's constant," which has been evaluated to 53 places in [10]. Golomb's constant λ is defined to be $\lim_{n\to\infty} l_n/n$, where l_n is the average length of the longest cycle in a random n-permutation. In Golomb's original analysis [6] of this combinatorial problem — which is not obviously related to prime factors at all! — he independently defined a function essentially identical to $\rho(\alpha)$, and he computed $\lambda = \int_1^\infty \rho(t-1)\,dt/t^2$ numerically. Another expression $\lambda = \int_1^\infty \exp(-x - E(x))\,dx$ was found later by Shepp and Lloyd [14].

In Table 1 of their paper, Shepp and Lloyd also list the limiting values $l^{(k)}/n \to \int_0^\infty E(t)^{k-1}\exp(-t-E(t))\,dt/(k-1)!$ for the average length of the kth longest cycle; and their values agree numerically with D_k for $1 \le k \le 3$. In fact, the Shepp–Lloyd formula yields D_k for all k, since (5.20) implies that

$$
\int_0^\infty \frac{E(t)^{k-1}}{(k-1)!} \frac{dt}{e^{t+E(t)}} = \int_0^\infty te^{-t}\big(e_k(t) - e_{k-1}(t)\big)\,dt
$$

$$
= \int_0^\infty te^{-t} \int_0^\infty \big(\rho_k(u) - \rho_{k-1}(u)\big)e^{-tu}\,du\,dt
$$

$$
= \int_1^\infty \big(\rho_k(u-1) - \rho_{k-1}(u-1)\big) \int_0^\infty te^{-tu}\,dt\,du
$$

$$
= \int_1^\infty \big(\rho_k(u-1) - \rho_{k-1}(u-1)\big)\frac{du}{u^2}. \tag{10.1}
$$

Therefore *the distribution of the number of digits in the prime factors of a random m-digit number is approximately the same as the distribution of the cycle lengths in a random permutation of m elements.* (Notice that there are approximately $\ln m$ factors, and approximately $\ln m$ cycles.)

There is a fairly simple explanation for the fact that $\rho_k(\alpha)$ turns up in the study of cycles in permutations. Let $Q_k(n,r)$ be the number of permutations of n objects having fewer than k cycles of length exceeding r. Then, by considering the permutations of $n+1$ elements $\{0, 1, \dots, n\}$ and considering the $n!/(n-m)!$ possible cycles in which 0 appears with m different elements, we have

$$
Q_k(n+1,r) = \sum_{m=0}^{r-1} \frac{n!}{(n-m)!}Q_k(n-m,r) + \sum_{m=r}^{n} \frac{n!}{(n-m)!}Q_{k-1}(n-m,r).
$$

Therefore if $q_k(n, r) = Q_k(n, r)/n!$ is the probability that the kth largest cycle has length $\leq r$, we have

$$(n + 1)q_k(n + 1, r) = \sum_{m=0}^{r-1} q_k(n - m, r) + \sum_{m=r}^{n} q_{k-1}(n - m, r); \quad (10.2)$$

replacing n by $n - 1$ yields

$$nq_k(n, r) = \sum_{m=0}^{r-1} q_k(n - 1 - m, r) + \sum_{m=r}^{n-1} q_{k-1}(n - 1 - m, r). \quad (10.3)$$

Subtracting these two equations, we have

$$(n+1)\big(q_k(n+1, r) - q_k(n, r)\big) = q_{k-1}(n-r, r) - q_k(n-r, r), \quad (10.4)$$

and this is analogous to the differential equation

$$\alpha\rho_k'(\alpha) = \rho_{k-1}(\alpha - 1) - \rho_k(\alpha - 1). \quad (10.5)$$

The connection between the two problems is completed by showing that $q_k(n, r) = \rho_k(n/r) + O(1/r)$.

A similar distribution is obtained for the degrees of the factors of a random polynomial of degree n, over a finite field: The average degree of the kth "largest" irreducible factor will tend to be approximately $D_k n$.

Let us close by stating an open problem: Are the functions ρ_k algebraically independent? They are linearly independent, because of (5.5).

Acknowledgments

We wish to thank N. G. de Bruijn, Roger Eggleton, Karl K. Norton, John Pollard, and Marvin Wunderlich for correspondence relating to early drafts of this paper. A letter received from Nathan J. Fine in June 1965 regarding Golomb's problem was also very helpful for this research.

Appendix A. The Number of Prime Factors

Following the notation of Hardy and Wright [7], let $\omega(n)$ be the number of distinct prime factors of n, and let $\Omega(n)$ be the total number of prime factors including multiplicity. Thus, $\Omega(n)$ is the quantity T in the analysis of the algorithm above. Clearly $1 \leq \Omega(n) \leq \lg n$, and both of these limits are obtained for infinitely many n; similarly $\omega(n)$ can get as large as $\ln n / \ln \ln n$. On the other hand these extreme values are relatively rare, and the number of factors is usually near $\ln \ln n$.

Erdős and Kac [5] proved that the number of n in the range $1 \leq n \leq N$ such that $\omega(n) < \ln \ln N + c\sqrt{\ln \ln N}$ is

$$\left(\frac{1}{\sqrt{2\pi}} \int_{-\infty}^{c} e^{-t^2/2} dt \right) N + o(N); \qquad (A.1)$$

hence, for example, the probability that $|\omega(n) - \ln \ln N| < c\sqrt{\ln \ln N}$ for fixed $c > 0$ approaches the limiting value

$$\frac{1}{\sqrt{2\pi}} \int_{-c}^{c} e^{-t^2/2} dt. \qquad (A.2)$$

We might say that $\omega(n)$ behaves essentially like a normally distributed random variable with mean and variance $\ln \ln n$, when n is large.

Erdős and Kac remarked that their methods, which were based on the idea that residues modulo distinct primes are independent, could be extended to the case of prime factors with multiplicities included, but they did not state what the resulting theorem would be. Fortunately it is easy to deduce the asymptotic behavior of $\Omega(n)$ from that of $\omega(n)$, using a method like that in [7]. Let $k(N)$ be the number of n in $1 \leq n \leq N$ such that

$$\omega(n) < \ln \ln N + c\sqrt{\ln \ln N} \qquad (A.3)$$

and let $K(N)$ be the number such that

$$\Omega(n) < \ln \ln N + c\sqrt{\ln \ln N} + \ln \ln \ln N. \qquad (A.4)$$

Then $|k(N) - K(N)|$ is at most the number of n that satisfy (A.3) but not (A.4), or (A.4) but not (A.3), and both of these quantities are $o(N)$: If n satisfies (A.3) but not (A.4), we have $\Omega(n) - \omega(n) > \ln \ln \ln N$; and the number of such n is $O(N/\ln \ln \ln N)$, because

$$\sum_{n=1}^{N} (\Omega(n) - \omega(n)) = O(N) \qquad (A.5)$$

by [7, Theorem 430]. If n satisfies (A.4) but not (A.3), then

$$\ln \ln N + c\sqrt{\ln \ln N} \leq \omega(n) < \ln \ln N + \left(c + \frac{\ln \ln \ln N}{\sqrt{\ln \ln N}} \right) \sqrt{\ln \ln N},$$

and this is $o(N)$ by the theorem of Erdős and Kac.

We have proved that the number of n in the range $1 \leq n \leq N$ such that $\Omega(n) < \ln \ln N + c\sqrt{\ln \ln N}$ is asymptotically given by the normal distribution (A.1). But this estimate is insensitive to $O(1)$ terms, so the "average order" [7, Theorem 430] is also relevant:

$$\lim_{N \to \infty} \frac{1}{N} \sum_{n=1}^{N} (\omega(n) - \ln \ln N)$$

$$= \gamma + \sum_{p \text{ prime}} \left(\ln \left(1 - \frac{1}{p} \right) + \frac{1}{p} \right)$$

$$= \gamma + \sum_{n=2}^{\infty} \frac{\ln \zeta(n) \mu(n)}{n}$$

$$\approx 0.26149\,72128\,47642\,78375\,54268\,38608\,69585\,90516- ; \quad \text{(A.6)}$$

$$\lim_{N \to \infty} \frac{1}{N} \sum_{n=1}^{N} (\Omega(n) - \ln \ln N)$$

$$= \gamma + \sum_{p \text{ prime}} \left(\ln \left(1 - \frac{1}{p} \right) + \frac{1}{p-1} \right)$$

$$= \gamma + \sum_{n=2}^{\infty} \frac{\ln \zeta(n) \varphi(n)}{n}$$

$$\approx 1.03465\,38818\,97437\,91161\,97942\,98464\,63825\,46703+ . \quad \text{(A.7)}$$

The number in (A.6) is sometimes called Mertens's constant (see [9, equation (17)]); the slightly larger number in (A.7) is more relevant to our factorization algorithm.

Let $S = \{10^{10} - m \mid 1 \leq m \leq 100\}$ be the numbers used to construct Figure 2 above. For $n \in S$ we have $\ln \ln n \approx 3.1366$, and the following table shows the actual distribution of $\omega(n)$ and $\Omega(n)$.

k	1	2	3	4	5	6	7	8	9	10	11	12
$\|\{n \in S \mid \omega(n) = k\}\|$	3	14	36	29	14	3	1	0	0	0	0	0
$\|\{n \in S \mid \Omega(n) = k\}\|$	3	10	27	23	15	11	5	3	1	1	0	1

The respective mean values are 3.50 and 4.27. The number of squarefree n (those with $\omega(n) = \Omega(n)$) was 61, compared to the expected value $600/\pi^2 = 60.793$.

Appendix B. An Asymptotic Formula for ρ_3

In this appendix we shall sketch the derivation of an asymptotic expression for $\rho_3(\alpha)$ as $\alpha \to \infty$. Our starting point is the formula

$$
S_2(\alpha) = \int_0^{\alpha-1} \frac{\rho_2(t)\,dt}{\alpha - t}
$$

$$
= \sum_{k=0}^{r} \frac{1}{\alpha^{k+1}} \int_0^{\alpha-1} \rho_2(t) t^k \, dt + \frac{1}{\alpha^{r+1}} \int_0^{\alpha-1} \frac{\rho_2(t) t^{r+1} dt}{\alpha - t}; \quad \text{(B.1)}
$$

we replace the final term by its asymptotic value

$$
\frac{e^\gamma}{\alpha^{r+1}} \int_0^{\alpha-1} \frac{(c_0 t^r + \cdots + c_{r-1} t)\,dt}{\alpha - t} + O\left(\frac{1}{\alpha^{r+1}} \int_0^{\alpha-1} \frac{dt}{\alpha - t} \right), \quad \text{(B.2)}
$$

so that the remainder is $O(\alpha^{-r-1} \log \alpha)$. The main integral in (B.2) is a linear combination of integrals having the form

$$
\int_0^{\alpha-1} \frac{t^k dt}{\alpha - t} = \int_1^{\alpha} \frac{(\alpha - t)^k dt}{t}
$$

$$
= \alpha^k (\ln \alpha - H_k) - \sum_{j=1}^{k} \binom{k}{j} (-1)^j \frac{\alpha^{k-j}}{j}, \quad \text{(B.3)}
$$

and it remains to evaluate $\int_0^{\alpha-1} \rho_2(t) t^k \, dt$ to $O(\alpha^{k-r} \log \alpha)$. Since $\rho_2 = S_1 + \rho_1$, we have

$$
\int_0^{\alpha} \rho_2(t) t^k \, dt = \int_0^{\alpha} t^k \, dt \left(\int_1^{t} \frac{\rho(u-1)\,du}{t+1-u} + \rho(t) \right)
$$

$$
= \left(\int_1^{\alpha} \rho(u-1)\,du \int_u^{\alpha} \frac{t^k \, dt}{t+1-u} \right) + a_k + O(\alpha^{-r-1})
$$

$$
= \sum_{j=1}^{k} \binom{k}{j} \frac{1}{j} \int_1^{\infty} \rho(u-1)(u-1)^{k-j} \left((\alpha+1-u)^j - 1 \right) du
$$

$$
+ \int_1^{\alpha} \rho(u-1)(u-1)^k \ln(\alpha+1-u)\, du + a_k + O(\alpha^{-r-1})
$$

$$
= \sum_{j=1}^{k} \left(\alpha^j - \binom{k}{j} \right) \frac{a_{k-j}}{j} + (\ln \alpha - H_k + 1) a_k
$$

$$
- \sum_{j=1}^{r} \alpha^{-j} \frac{a_{k+j}}{j} + O(\alpha^{-r-1}), \quad \text{(B.4)}
$$

where $a_k = \int_0^\infty \rho(t) t^k dt = e^\gamma c_k$. If we sum appropriate multiples of equations (B.3) and (B.4), replacing α by $\alpha - 1$ in the latter, we get

$$S_2(\alpha) = (2\ln\alpha + 1)\rho_2(\alpha) - \frac{2b_0}{\alpha} - \frac{2b_1}{\alpha^2} - \cdots - \frac{2b_{r-1}}{\alpha^r} + O(\alpha^{-r-1}), \quad \text{(B.5)}$$

where

$$b_k = H_k a_k + \sum_{j=1}^{k} \binom{k}{j} \frac{a_{k-j}}{j}. \qquad \text{(B.6)}$$

In particular,

$$\langle b_0, b_1, b_2, \ldots \rangle = e^\gamma \left\langle 0, 2, \frac{19}{4}, \frac{415}{36}, \frac{551}{18}, \frac{13391}{150}, \frac{1023289}{3600}, \ldots \right\rangle.$$

Since $\rho_3 = \frac{1}{2}(\rho_1(\alpha) + \rho_2(\alpha) + S_2(\alpha))$, we have the desired asymptotic series,

$$\rho_3(\alpha) = (\ln\alpha + 1)\rho_2(\alpha) - \frac{b_0}{\alpha} - \cdots - \frac{b_{r-1}}{\alpha^r} + O(\alpha^{-r-1}). \qquad \text{(B.7)}$$

Incidentally, it can be shown as in Section 6 that

$$\int_1^\infty \left(\rho_3(t) - \frac{e^\gamma (1 + \ln t)}{t} \right) dt = e^\gamma \left(1 + \frac{\pi^2}{12} + \frac{3\gamma^2}{2} \right) - 1. \qquad \text{(B.8)}$$

This research was supported in part by the National Science Foundation, the Office of Naval Research, and IBM Corporation. Some of the computations and formula manipulation were done with the MACSYMA system supported by the Advanced Research Projects Agency (ARPA).

References

[1] N. G. de Bruijn, "On the number of positive integers $\leq x$ and free of prime factors $> y$," *Indagationes Mathematicæ* **13** (1951), 50–60.

[2] N. G. de Bruijn, "The asymptotic behaviour of a function occurring in the theory of primes," *Journal of the Indian Mathematical Society* (A) **15** (1951), 25–32.

[3] Charles de La Vallée Poussin, "Sur la fonction $\zeta(s)$ de Riemann et le nombre des nombres premiers inférieurs à une limite donnée," *Mémoires Couronnés et Mémoires des Savants Étrangers Publies par l'Académie royale des Sciences, des Lettres et des Beaux-Arts de Belgique* **59** (1899), 1–74.

[4] Karl Dickman, "On the frequency of numbers containing prime factors of a certain relative magnitude," *Arkiv för Matematik, Astronomi och Fysik* **22A**, 10 (1930), 1–14.

[5] P. Erdös and M. Kac, "The Gaussian law of errors in the theory of additive number theoretic functions," *American Journal of Mathematics* **62** (1940), 738–742.

[6] S. W. Golomb, L. R. Welch, and R. M. Goldstein, "Cycles from nonlinear shift registers," *Progress Report Number 20-389* (Pasadena, California: Jet Propulsion Laboratory, California Institute of Technology, 1959).

[7] G. H. Hardy and E. M. Wright, *An Introduction to the Theory of Numbers*, 4th edition (Oxford: Clarendon Press, 1960).

[8] Donald E. Knuth, *Sorting and Searching*, Volume 3 of *The Art of Computer Programming* (Reading, Massachusetts: Addison–Wesley, 1973).

[9] F. Mertens, "Ein Beitrag zur analytischen Zahlentheorie," *Journal für die reine und angewandte Mathematik* **78** (1874), 46–62.

[10] W. C. Mitchell, "An evaluation of Golomb's constant," *Mathematics of Computation* **22** (1968), 411–415.

[11] Karl K. Norton, "Numbers with small prime factors, and the least kth power non-residue," *Memoirs of the American Mathematical Society* **106** (1971), 1–106.

[12] J. M. Pollard, "A Monte Carlo method for factorization," *BIT* **15** (1975), 331–334.

[13] V. Ramaswami, "The number of positive integers $\leq x$ and free of prime divisors $> x^c$, and a problem of S. S. Pillai," *Duke Mathematical Journal* **16** (1949), 99–109.

[14] L. A. Shepp and S. P. Lloyd, "Ordered cycle lengths in a random permutation," *Transactions of the American Mathematical Society* **121** (1966), 340–357.

[15] J. van de Lune and E. Wattel, "On the numerical solution of a differential-difference equation arising in analytic number theory," *Mathematics of Computation* **23** (1969), 417–421.

[16] J. B. van Rongen, "On the largest prime divisor of an integer," *Indagationes Mathematicæ* **37** (1975), 70–76.

[17] M. C. Wunderlich and J. L. Selfridge, "A design for a number theory package with an optimized trial division routine," *Communications of the ACM* **17** (1974), 272–276.

Addendum

When this paper was written in 1975, the authors were unaware of any prior work on the distribution of kth largest prime factors. But Patrick Billingsley had already derived important results about the *joint distribution* of the k largest prime factors ["On the distribution of large prime divisors," *Periodica Mathematica Hungarica* **2** (1972), 283–289]. Using methods completely different from those of the present paper, Billingsley showed that the probability density function for $n_1 = n^{x_1}$, $n_2 = n^{x_2}$, $\ldots$, $n_k = n^{x_k}$ is

$$\frac{dx_1\, dx_2\, \ldots\, dx_k}{x_1 \ldots x_{k-1}\,(1 - x_1 - \cdots - x_{k-1})}\, f\!\left(\frac{x_k}{1 - x_1 - \cdots - x_{k-1}}\right)$$

when $x_1 \geq x_2 \geq \cdots \geq x_k \geq 0$, where $f(x) = F_1'(x) = \rho(1/x - 1)/x$ is the density function for the case $k = 1$ considered by Dickman. (See Figure 3.) For example, the differential probability that $n_1 = n^x$ and $n_2 = n^y$ is the interesting surface

$$\frac{1}{x(1 - x)}\, f\!\left(\frac{y}{1 - x}\right), \qquad 1 \geq x \geq y \geq 0.$$

Further results about this joint distribution were subsequently obtained by A. M. Vershik ["Асимптотическое распределение разложений натуральных чисел но простые делители," *Doklady Akademii Nauk SSSR* **289** (1986), 269–272; English translation, "The asymptotic distribution of factorizations of natural numbers into prime divisors," *Soviet Mathematics — Doklady* **34** (1987), 57–61], who noted that it occurs not only in connection with factoring and with cycle lengths in permutations, but also in models of biological processes [G. A. Watterson, "The stationary distribution of the infinitely-many neutral alleles diffusion model," *Journal of Applied Probability* **13** (1976), 639–651, 897; J. F. C. Kingman, "The population structure associated with the Ewens sampling formula," *Theoretical Population Biology* **11** (1977), 274–283]. As a result of these other applications it has become known to statisticians as the Poisson–Dirichlet distribution with parameter 1.

An elegant new way to derive the distribution of prime factor lengths, based on listing the factors in *random* order weighted by their logarithms instead of listing them in decreasing order, was discovered by Peter Donnelly and Geoffrey Grimmett ["On the asymptotic distribution of large prime factors," *Journal of the London Mathematical Society* (2)

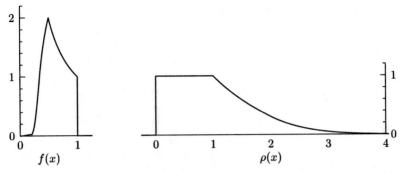

FIGURE 3. The probability density function $f(x) = \rho(1/x - 1)/x$ for the quantity $(\log n_1)/(\log n)$, the number of digits in the largest prime factor of a random integer n.

47 (1993), 395–404]. This order corresponds to listing the cycles of a permutation by first taking the cycle that contains the smallest element, then the cycle that contains the smallest element not in the first cycle, etc., essentially ordering the cycles by their "cycle leaders."

James Lee Hafner and Kevin S. McCurley ["On the distribution of running times of certain integer factoring algorithms," *Journal of Algorithms* **10** (1989), 531–556] proved that

$$\frac{P_2(1/\alpha, N)}{N} = \rho_2(\alpha)\left(1 + O\left(\frac{\alpha}{\lg N}\right)\right),$$

uniformly for $1 \le \alpha \le \lg N$, and used this result to analyze other algorithms for factoring. [See also Carl Pomerance and Jonathan Sorenson, "Counting the integers factorable via cyclotomic methods," *Journal of Algorithms* **19** (1995), 250–265.]

Results of a different nature were found by János Galambos ["The sequences of prime divisors of integers," *Acta Arithmetica* **31** (1976), 213–218] who showed that if k approaches infinity with n but remains $o(\log \log n)$, then $\log n_k / \log n$ almost surely lies between $e^{-(1+\epsilon)k}$ and $e^{-(1-\epsilon)k}$. He also considered the probability that exactly m of the prime factors satisfy $\log n_k / \log n_{k+1} > x \ln \ln n$, given $x > 1$, showing that this probability approaches $x^{-m}e^{-1/x}/m!$ as $n \to \infty$ ["Extensions of some extremal properties of prime divisors to Poisson limit theorems," *Contemporary Mathematics* **143** (1993), 363–369].

Further properties of the remarkable functions $\rho_k(\alpha)$ almost certainly remain to be discovered.

Persi Diaconis [personal communication] has used the methods of Bahman Saffari ["Sur quelques applications de la 'méthode de l'hyperbole' de Dirichlet à la théorie des nombres premiers," *L'Enseignement Mathématique* **14** (1968), 205–224] and Hubert Delange ["Sur des formules de Atle Selberg," *Acta Arithmetica* **19** (1971), 105–146] to derive precise asymptotic formulas for the mean and variance of the quantity $T = \Omega(n)$, the number of prime factors of n (counting multiplicity):

$$\frac{1}{N} \sum_{n=1}^{N} \Omega(n) \sim \ln \ln N + \sum_{k=0}^{\infty} \frac{a_k}{(\ln N)^k};$$

$$\frac{1}{N} \sum_{n=1}^{N} \left(\Omega(n) - \frac{1}{N} \sum_{n=1}^{N} \Omega(n) \right)^2 \sim \ln \ln N + \sum_{k=0}^{\infty} \frac{c_k}{(\ln N)^k}.$$

Here a_0 is the constant in (A.7), and

$$a_k = -\int_1^{\infty} \frac{\{t\}}{t^2} (\ln t)^{k-1} \, dt$$

$$= (k-1)! \left(\frac{\gamma_0}{0!} + \cdots + \frac{\gamma_{k-1}}{(k-1)!} - 1 \right) \qquad \text{for } k \geq 1,$$

where γ_m is the "Stieltjes constant" defined by either of the formulas

$$\gamma_m = \lim_{n \to \infty} \left(\sum_{k=1}^{n} \frac{(\ln k)^m}{k} - \frac{(\ln n)^{m+1}}{m+1} \right);$$

$$\zeta(1-z) + \frac{1}{z} = \sum_{m=0}^{\infty} \gamma_m \frac{z^m}{m!}.$$

Also

$$c_0 = a_0 - \frac{\pi^2}{6} + \sum_{p \text{ prime}} \frac{1}{(p-1)^2};$$

$$c_1 = \gamma - 1 - 2 \sum_{p \text{ prime}} \frac{\ln p}{(p-1)^2};$$

and the expressions for the remaining coefficients c_k are too complicated to reproduce here. The sums appearing in c_0 and c_1 are respectively equal to

$$\sum_{\substack{p \text{ prime}}} \frac{1}{(p-1)^2} = \sum_{n=2}^{\infty} \frac{\varphi_2(n) - \varphi(n)}{n} \ln \zeta(n)$$

$$\approx 1.37506\,49947\,48635\,28791\,72531\,30522\,43969\,91796-,$$

$$\sum_{\substack{p \text{ prime}}} \frac{\ln p}{(p-1)^2} = -\sum_{n=2}^{\infty} \varphi(n) \frac{\zeta'(n)}{\zeta(n)}$$

$$\approx 1.22696\,88056\,53470\,00596\,56625\,68745\,76256\,29883-;$$

the first of these formulas uses the function $\varphi_2(n)$ defined by

$$\frac{\varphi_2(n)}{n^2} = \prod_{\substack{p \backslash n \\ p \text{ prime}}} \left(1 - \frac{1}{p^2}\right), \qquad \frac{\zeta(s-2)}{\zeta(s)} = \sum_{n=1}^{\infty} \frac{\varphi_2(n)}{n^s}.$$

Chapter 21

The Expected Linearity of a Simple Equivalence Algorithm

[Written with Arnold Schönhage. Originally published in Theoretical Computer Science **6** *(1978), 281–315.]*

The average time needed to form unions of disjoint equivalence classes, using an algorithm suggested by Aho, Hopcroft, and Ullman, is shown to be linear in the total number of elements, thereby establishing a conjecture of Yao. The analytic methods used to prove this result are of interest in themselves, as they are based on extensions of Stepanov's approach to the study of random graphs. Several refinements of Yao's analyses of related algorithms are also presented, based on a "repertoire" approach to the solution of recurrence relations.

0. Introduction

The problem of maintaining a representation of equivalence classes or partitions of a set arises in many applications. Aho, Hopcroft, and Ullman [1, Chapter 4] have called this the UNION-FIND problem, and they begin their exposition by introducing the following simple data organization:

Let $R[x]$ be the name of the equivalence class containing element x.

Let $N[s]$ be the number of elements in equivalence class s.

Let $L[s]$ designate a linked list containing the elements of class s.

To merge disjoint equivalence classes s and t, where $N[s] \leq N[t]$, set $R[x] \leftarrow t$ for all x in $L[s]$, append $L[s]$ to $L[t]$, add $N[s]$ to $N[t]$, and call the new equivalence class t.

Initially all classes have size 1, and they are merged into larger and larger classes as the algorithm proceeds.

This strategy allows us to find the equivalence class containing a given element in constant time; and the cost of replacing two classes by their union is essentially proportional to the size of the smaller class, that is, to the number of times $R[x]$ is changed. If there are n elements in all, it is easy to see that $R[x]$ is changed at most $\lg n$ times for each x, since the class containing x must at least double in size whenever $R[x]$ changes. Therefore it will take at most $O(n \log n)$ units of time to do all the union operations.

In this paper we shall prove that the *average* amount of time to do all unions by the stated method is only $O(n)$, thereby establishing a conjecture of Yao [12]. The probability distribution on the set of possible input sequences, under which such "average" behavior occurs, can be defined in several equivalent ways corresponding to the conventional notion of a random graph; in essence, the probability that classes s and t will be merged at any particular step is proportional to $N[s]N[t]$.

Section 1 describes a convenient way to deal with large random graphs, by analogy with the treatment of large systems of particles in statistical mechanics, an approach that was first suggested by Stepanov [10]. Section 2 develops several estimates useful in the study of this probability model, and Section 3 explains how to apply the resulting formulas to the above algorithm. The proof of linearity is completed in Sections 4, 5, and 6.

Following Yao [12], we shall call the stated algorithm QFW, for "quick find weighted"; one can quickly find the equivalence class containing x by simply looking at $R[x]$, and the class sizes or weights $N[s]$ are used to decide how the updating is done. QFW is a refinement of the unweighted algorithm QF, which dispenses with the $N[s]$ table and simply updates one of the two classes selected with equal probability. In Section 7 the QF algorithm is shown to require $\sim n^2/8$ updates on the average. Empirical experiments on QF and QFW, confirming this theory, appear in Section 8.

Section 9 discusses another probability model under which we might wish to study the average behavior of QF and QFW, based on the hypothesis that the actual unions to be performed take place in random order. Recurrence relations that arise in this model are studied in Sections 10, 11, and 12, culminating in detailed exact or asymptotic calculations of the average cost.

Finally, Section 13 discusses the distribution of "union trees" associated with equivalence algorithms, and relates such trees to two other algorithms (QM and QMW) described by Yao, in addition to QF and QFW. Several open problems conclude the paper.

1. Connectivity of Random Graphs

Let us imagine that each of the $(n^2-n)/2$ pairs of distinct elements $\{x, y\}$ has been associated in some manner with $(n^2 - n)/2$ independent equal-sized samples of some radioactive substance like radium, where there is probability e^{-t} that any particular sample of radium has emitted no α particles between time 0 and time t. When the radium associated with $\{x, y\}$ fires off its first particle, we immediately draw a line between x and y; at any time $t > 0$ the lines drawn in this way define an undirected graph on the n given elements.

Let $P_n(t)$ be the probability that the random graph defined in this way is connected at time t; thus $P_n(t)$ is an increasing function that approaches 1 as $t \to \infty$. It is easy to verify, for example, that

$$P_1(t) = 1;$$
$$P_2(t) = 1 - e^{-t};$$
$$P_3(t) = 1 - 3e^{-2t} + 2e^{-3t};$$
$$P_4(t) = 1 - 4e^{-3t} - 3e^{-4t} + 12e^{-5t} - 6e^{-6t}.$$

Another way to define a random graph is to say that each of the $(n^2 - n)/2$ edges is independently present with probability p and absent with probability $q = 1 - p$; then $P_n(t)$ is the probability of connectedness if we set $q = e^{-t}$. This definition was introduced by Gilbert [3], who wrote, for example, '$P_3 = 1 - 3q^2 + 2q^3$'; but we shall see that Stepanov's physical interpretation tends to be more suggestive in developing the theory.

Incidentally, $P_n(t)$ may be regarded as a generating function for two types of discrete quantities associated with random graphs: If $C(n, m)$ denotes the number of connected graphs on n labeled vertices having m edges, we have

$$P_n(t) = \sum_{m \geq 0} C(n, m)(1 - e^{-t})^m\, e^{-t((n^2-n)/2-m)}$$
$$= e^{-(n^2-n)t/2} \sum_{m \geq 0} C(n, m)(e^t - 1)^m; \tag{1.1}$$

and if $A(n, m)$ denotes the number of ordered sequences of edges $\{x_1, y_1\}$, $\{x_2, y_2\}$, $\ldots$, $\{x_m, y_m\}$ defining a connected graph, where $x_i \neq y_i$ but duplicate edges $\{x_i, y_i\} = \{x_j, y_j\}$ are allowed, we have

$$P_n(t) = e^{-(n^2-n)t/2} \sum_{m \geq 0} A(n, m)\, t^m/m!\,, \tag{1.2}$$

since $e^t t^k / k!$ is the probability that a given edge has "fired" exactly k times. The sum in (1.1) can, of course, be restricted to the range $n - 1 \le m \le (n^2 - n)/2$, since $C(n, m) = 0$ when $m < n - 1$; similarly, we can replace "$m \ge 0$" by "$m \ge n - 1$" in (1.2). Equations (1.1) and (1.2) are both equivalent to the formal power series identity

$$\ln \sum_{n=0}^{\infty} e^{n(n-1)t/2} \frac{z^n}{n!} = \sum_{n=0}^{\infty} e^{n(n-1)t/2} P_n(t) \frac{z^n}{n!}, \qquad (1.3)$$

using the well-known generating function for connected graphs [3].

It is easy to compute the functions $P_n(t)$ for $n = 1, 2, \ldots$ by using the recurrence formula

$$\sum_{k \ge 1} \binom{n-1}{k-1} P_k(t) e^{-k(n-k)t} = 1; \qquad (1.4)$$

this formula follows immediately from the fact that the kth term of the sum is the probability that a particular point x is connected to exactly k points (including itself) at time t. Identity (1.4) has a remarkable corollary,

$$\sum_{k \ge 1} \binom{n-1}{k-1} P_k(t) (e^{-kt} + z)^{n-k} = (1 + z)^{n-1}, \qquad (1.5)$$

which holds for all z; the coefficient of z^m on the left-hand side of (1.5) can be shown to equal the coefficient on the right, using (1.4).

Stepanov [9] discovered two nonlinear identities

$$P_n(t) = \sum_{k \ge 1} \binom{n-2}{k-1} P_k(t) P_{n-k}(t) (e^{-k(n-1-k)t} - e^{-k(n-k)t}), \qquad (1.6)$$

$$P_n'(t) = \frac{n(n-1)}{2} \sum_{k \ge 1} \binom{n-2}{k-1} P_k(t) P_{n-k}(t) e^{-k(n-k)t}, \qquad (1.7)$$

for which he gave rather lengthy algebraic and analytic proofs. His first formula can be proved more directly by observing that the kth term in the sum is the probability of a connected graph in which a particular point x would be connected to exactly k points if another particular point y were removed. There are $\binom{n-2}{k-1}$ ways to choose the $k - 1$ other points, and the graph restricted to x and those other points must be connected, as must the graph restricted to the remaining $n - k$ points including y; and there must be at least one edge from the k points to y, but none from the k points to the remaining $n-1-k$. Stepanov's second formula can be proved by noting that $P_n(t)\,dt$ is the probability that the graph becomes connected at time t (that is, between times t and $t+dt$); this is the number of ways to choose an edge $\{x,y\}$, times the number of ways to divide the n points into a set of k elements containing x and a set of $n-k$ elements containing y, times the probability that the k points and the $n-k$ points are already connected, times the probability e^{-t} that the edge $\{x,y\}$ has just "fired," times the probability that the other $k(n-k)-1$ edges between the two sets have not yet fired.

2. Bounds on the Probability of Connectedness

If we set $z = e^{-nt}$ in (1.5), we find

$$P_n(t) = (1 - e^{-nt})^{n-1} - \sum_{k=1}^{n-1} \binom{n-1}{k-1} P_k(t)(e^{-kt} - e^{-nt})^{n-k}, \quad (2.1)$$

hence (see [10])

$$P_n(t) \le (1 - e^{-nt})^{n-1}. \quad (2.2)$$

In fact, a similar argument proves the sharper upper bound

$$P_n(t) \le (1 - e^{-(n-1)t})^{n-1},$$

but we will not need this improvement. When t is large, the bound in (2.2) is very good because the correction terms dropped from (2.1) become exponentially small; but when t is near zero, we can squeeze another factor of n out of the upper bound, since

$$P_n(t) \le n^{n-2}(1 - e^{-t})^{n-1}. \quad (2.3)$$

(See [11, page 228].) This formula follows because a connected graph must contain a spanning tree as a subgraph; there are n^{n-2} spanning trees on n labeled points and $(1 - e^{-t})^{n-1}$ is the probability that any particular spanning tree is present.

A simple lower bound for $P_n(t)$ can be obtained by considering only the term for $m = n - 1$ in (1.1):

$$P_n(t) \ge n^{n-2}(1 - e^{-t})^{n-1}(e^{-(n-2)t/2})^{n-1}. \quad (2.4)$$

Relations (2.3) and (2.4) combine to give the formula

$$P_n(t) = n^{n-2}\,t^{n-1}(1 - O(n^2 t)). \quad (2.5)$$

(Here and in the sequel we shall use O notation to stand for functions bounded by absolute constants, depending only on specified conditions. For example, in (2.5) the $O(n^2 t)$ stands for any function of n and t whose absolute value is at most $Cn^2 t$ for some C, when $n \geq 1$ and $t \geq 0$.)

We shall be especially concerned with values of $P_n(t)$ for $t \ll 1/n$, and the upper bound (2.2) shows that $P_n(t)$ is exponentially small in this range. In order to understand more easily what is going on, let us magnify the values by defining

$$\omega_n(t) = P_n(t)/(1 - e^{-nt})^{n-1}. \tag{2.6}$$

If we apply formula (1.7), together with formula (1.6) both as it stands and with k replaced by $n - k$, we obtain

$$\omega_n'(t) = \left((1 - e^{-nt})P_n'(t) - n(n-1)e^{-nt}P_n(t)\right)/(1 - e^{-nt})^n$$

$$= \frac{n(n-1)}{2} \sum_{k \geq 1} \binom{n-2}{k-1} \frac{P_k(t)P_{n-k}(t)}{(1 - e^{-nt})^n} e^{-k(n-k)t}$$

$$\times \left(1 - e^{-nt} - e^{-nt}(e^{kt} - 1 + e^{(n-k)t} - 1)\right)$$

$$= \frac{n(n-1)}{2} \sum_{k \geq 1} \binom{n-2}{k-1} \omega_k(t)\omega_{n-k}(t)e^{-k(n-k)t}$$

$$\times \left(\frac{1 - e^{-kt}}{1 - e^{-nt}}\right)^k \left(\frac{1 - e^{-(n-k)t}}{1 - e^{-nt}}\right)^{n-k}; \tag{2.7}$$

hence $\omega_n(t)$ satisfies a surprisingly simple differential difference equation

$$\omega_n'(t) = \frac{1}{2} \sum_k \binom{n}{k} \frac{\theta_k(t)\theta_{n-k}(t)}{\sinh(nt/2)^n}, \tag{2.8}$$

where $\theta_n(t) = n\omega_n(t) \sinh(nt/2)^n$ (see [10]). It follows in particular that $\omega_n(t)$ is monotone increasing. Our bounds on $P_n(t)$ imply that

$$\omega_n(t) = \frac{1}{n}(1 + O(n^2 t)) \qquad \text{for } t = O(n^{-2}); \tag{2.9}$$

$$\frac{1}{n} \leq \omega_n(t) \leq 1. \tag{2.10}$$

We can also obtain a recurrence for $\omega_n(t)$ analogous to (1.4) and (2.7), using (1.5) with $z = -e^{-nt}$:

$$\sum_{k \geq 1} \binom{n-1}{k-1} \omega_k(t)e^{-k(n-k)t} \left(\frac{1-e^{-kt}}{1-e^{-nt}}\right)^{k-1} \left(\frac{1-e^{-(n-k)t}}{1-e^{-nt}}\right)^{n-k} = 1. \tag{2.11}$$

We shall make several uses of the following estimate for $\omega_n(t)$, which is of particular interest when $t < n^{-3/2}$:

Lemma 1. $\omega_n(t) \leq (1/n) \exp(cn^{3/2}t)$, where $c = \sqrt{\pi/8} \approx 0.62666$.

Proof. It is easy to verify that $\sinh(at)/\sinh(bt) \leq a/b$ when $0 < a \leq b$ and $t \geq 0$, hence (2.8) implies

$$\omega'_n(t) \leq \frac{1}{2} \sum_k \binom{n}{k} k\omega_k(t)(n-k)\omega_{n-k}(t)\left(\frac{k}{n}\right)^k \left(\frac{n-k}{n}\right)^{n-k}. \quad (2.12)$$

Note that equality holds when $t = 0$. Let us now consider the quantity

$$\phi(n,k) = \binom{n}{k}\left(\frac{k}{n}\right)^k \left(\frac{n-k}{n}\right)^{n-k}$$

which appears in this sum. Euler's summation formula implies that

$$\ln n! = n \ln n - n + \ln\sqrt{2\pi n} + \int_n^\infty t^{-2} h(t)\, dt,$$

where $h(t) = \{t\}\{1 - t\}/2$ and $\{t\}$ denotes $t - \lfloor t \rfloor$, the fractional part of t. Consequently

$$\ln \phi(n,k) = \ln\sqrt{\frac{n}{2\pi k(n-k)}} - \left(\int_k^n + \int_{n-k}^\infty\right) t^{-2} h(t)\, dt,$$

and we obtain the bound

$$\sum_{0 < k < n} \phi(n,k) \leq \sqrt{\frac{n}{2\pi}} \sum_{0 < k < n} \frac{1}{\sqrt{k(n-k)}}$$

$$< \sqrt{\frac{n}{2\pi}} \int_0^1 \frac{dx}{\sqrt{x(1-x)}} = \sqrt{\frac{n}{2\pi}} B\left(\frac{1}{2}, \frac{1}{2}\right) = \sqrt{\frac{\pi n}{2}}.$$

By induction we have

$$k\omega_k(t) \cdot (n-k)\omega_{n-k}(t) \leq \exp(c(k^{3/2} + (n-k)^{3/2})t) \leq \exp(cn^{3/2}t),$$

so (2.12) yields

$$\omega'_n(t) \leq \sqrt{\frac{\pi n}{8}} \exp(cn^{3/2}t),$$

$$\omega_n(t) \leq \frac{1}{n} + c\sqrt{n} \int_0^1 \exp(cn^{3/2}t)\, du = \frac{1}{n} \exp(cn^{3/2}t). \quad \square$$

Incidentally, it can be shown that

$$\omega'_n(0) = \tfrac{1}{2}(Q(n) - 1), \tag{2.13}$$

where

$$Q(n) = 1 + \frac{n-1}{n} + \frac{n-1}{n}\frac{n-2}{n} + \cdots$$
$$= \sqrt{\frac{\pi n}{2}} - \frac{1}{3} + \frac{1}{12}\sqrt{\frac{\pi}{2n}} - \frac{4}{135n} + O(n^{-3/2}), \tag{2.14}$$

by using "Abel identities"; see [8, Section 1.5] and [4, Section 1.2.11.3]. Therefore the constant c in Lemma 2.1 is best possible.

3. Connection to the Equivalence Algorithm

When the radium associated with edge $\{x, y\}$ emits an α-particle, we can imagine invoking the equivalence algorithm at that instant, merging classes $R[x]$ and $R[y]$ if they are distinct. Then the equivalence classes at any time will be the same as the connected components of the random graph. The probability that two edges fire simultaneously is zero; and as $t \to \infty$ the graph becomes connected with probability 1. In effect we are considering a random execution of the equivalence algorithm where the classes to be merged at each stage are selected by choosing uniformly among all pairs (x, y) of elements that are not already equivalent. This seems to be the most natural way to define the average behavior of the process.

When $R[x]$ is a class of size k and $R[y]$ is a class of size m, let us say that the algorithm does a (k, m)-merge; the cost of such a merge is $\min(k, m)$. Therefore the average running time to do $n - 1$ unions that connect the graph is

$$\sum_{k=1}^{n-1}\sum_{m=1}^{n-k} \min(k, m) E_{n,k,m}, \tag{3.1}$$

where $E_{n,k,m}$ is the average number of (k, m)-merges performed. In more intuitive terms, the average number of times the firing of an α-particle causes a component of size k to be joined to a component of size m is $E_{n,k,m} + E_{n,m,k}$, when $k \neq m$.

Given any fixed way to partition the n elements into sets (A, B, C) of respective sizes $(k, m, n-k-m)$, the probability that the random process will at some time do a (k, m)-merge with A and B as the respective classes is

$$\frac{1}{2} \int_0^\infty P_k(t) P_m(t) e^{-(k+m)(n-k-m)t} \, d(1 - e^{-kmt}), \qquad (3.2)$$

since $1 - e^{-kmt}$ is the distribution function for the firing of at least one of the km edges between A and B, while $P_k(t) P_m(t) e^{-(k+m)(n-k-m)t}$ is the probability that A and B are internally connected but not joined to C at time t. (The factor $\frac{1}{2}$ in (3.2) accounts for the probability that x instead of y belongs to class A when the edge $\{x, y\}$ fires, since we may regard (x, y) and (y, x) as equally probable.) By considering all possible choices of A, B, and C, we have

$$E_{n,k,m} = \frac{n!}{2 \cdot k! \, m! \, (n - k - m)!}$$
$$\times \int_0^\infty P_k(t) P_m(t) kme^{-kmt} e^{-(k+m)(n-k-m)t} \, dt. \quad (3.3)$$

For example, consider the simplest case $k = m = 1$: The expected number of times we form a class of size 2 is

$$E_{n,1,1} = \frac{n(n-1)}{2} \int_0^\infty e^{-(2n-3)t} \, dt = \frac{n(n-1)}{4n - 6} \approx n/4. \qquad (3.4)$$

It follows that about $n/2$ singletons are built into pairs, while the other $n/2$ elements begin their interactions by being hooked to larger components.

Similar formulas hold for other small values of k and m. For example, we have

$E_{n,1,2} = n(n-1)[n \neq 2]/(18n - 42);$

$E_{n,1,3} = 3n(n-1)(n-2)(n-3)/((8n-20)(4n-13)(4n-11));$

$E_{n,2,2} = n(n-1)(n-2)[n \neq 3]/((16n-40)(4n-11));$

$E_{n,1,4} = 2(20n-69)n(n-1)(n-2)[n \neq 3](n-4)/(5(5n-16)^3(5n-21));$

$E_{n,2,3} = 3(15n-53)n(n-1)(n-2)[n \neq 3](n-4)/(10(5n-16)^4).$

But no simple pattern is evident. The denominator of $E_{n,k,m}$ always consist of factors that are linear in n, for all fixed k and m, but the numerator of $E_{n,1,5}$ does not resolve into linear factors.

When k and m are fixed, we can deduce the asymptotic behavior of $E_{n,k,m}$ as $n \to \infty$ by using only the comparatively weak estimate (2.5), since the important contribution to the integral occurs when t is very small. Let

$$l = k + m; \qquad (3.5)$$

then

$$E_{n,k,m} = \frac{1}{2} \binom{n}{l} \binom{l}{k} k^{k-1} m^{m-1}$$

$$\times \int_0^\infty t^{l-2} (1 - O(k^2 t))(1 - O(m^2 t)) e^{-(nl - l^2 + km)t} \, dt$$

and the integral is

$$\frac{(l-2)!}{(nl - l^2 + km)^{l-1}} - O(n^{-l}) \qquad \text{as } n \to \infty.$$

It follows that

$$E_{n,k,m} = \binom{k+m-2}{k-1} \frac{k^{k-2} m^{m-2}}{2(k+m)^{k+m-1}} n + O(1) \qquad (3.6)$$

when k and m are fixed.

4. Preparations for the Estimations

Our main goal is to prove that the QFW algorithm has linear expected time, namely that the sum (3.1) is $O(n)$. Since $E_{n,k,m}$ does not seem to have a simple formula we must content ourselves with approximate values.

Stirling's approximation applied to (3.6) indicates that we might expect the estimate

$$E_{n,k,m} = O\left(\frac{n}{k^{3/2} m^{3/2} (k+m)^{1/2}}\right) \qquad (4.1)$$

to be valid. If such a uniform bound could be proved, we would be done, since it implies that

$$\sum_{k=1}^{n-1} \sum_{m=1}^{n-k} \min(k, m) E_{n,k,m} \le \sum_{1 \le k \le m < n} k(E_{n,k,m} + E_{n,m,k})$$

$$= \sum_{1 \le k \le m < n} O\left(\frac{n}{k^{1/2} m^2}\right)$$

$$= \sum_{1 \le m < n} O\left(\frac{n m^{1/2}}{m^2}\right) = O(n). \qquad (4.2)$$

Actually (4.1) is *not* true when $k = 1$ and $m = n-1$, as we shall see later; however, the methods we shall discuss below are strong enough to prove (4.1) in the special cases

$$k, m \leq n^{2/3} \quad \text{or} \quad k, m > n^{2/3}. \tag{4.3}$$

Fortunately this suffices to prove the desired result, since the "uncontrolled" terms have a sum bounded by n: We have

$$\sum_{1 \leq k \leq n^{2/3}} \sum_{n^{2/3} < m < n} k(E_{n,k,m} + E_{n,m,k}) \leq n, \tag{4.4}$$

since the left-hand side is less than the average number of times the QFW algorithm changes $R[x]$ while including x for the first time in a class of size $> n^{2/3}$, and this can happen at most once for any element.

By (3.3), (2.6), and Lemma 1 our mission will be accomplished if we can prove that

$$\frac{n!}{k!\,m!\,(n-k-m)!} \int_0^\infty (1 - e^{-kt})^{k-1}(1 - e^{-mt})^{m-1}$$
$$\times \exp\big(c(k^{3/2}+m^{3/2})t - kmt - (k+m)(n-k-m)t\big)\,dt$$
$$= O\left(\frac{n}{k^{3/2}m^{3/2}(k+m)^{1/2}}\right) \tag{4.5}$$

under condition (4.3). In other words we are interested in integrals of the form

$$I(k, m, w) = \int_0^\infty (1 - e^{-kt})^{k-1}(1 - e^{-mt})^{m-1}e^{-wt}\,dt. \tag{4.6}$$

5. Estimate of the Integral

Using the identity

$$1 - e^{-\alpha t} = \alpha \int_0^1 t e^{-x_1 \alpha t}\,dx_1 \tag{5.1}$$

repeatedly in (4.6), we can express $I(k, m, w)$ in the form

$$k^{k-1}m^{m-1} \int_0^\infty \underbrace{\int_0^1 \cdots \int_0^1}_{k-1+m-1 \text{ times}} \exp\big(-wt - k(x_1 + \cdots + x_{k-1})t$$
$$- m(y_1 + \cdots + y_{m-1})t\big)\,dx\,dy\,dt,$$

where $dx = dx_1 \dots dx_{k-1}$ and $dy = dy_1 \dots dy_{m-1}$. Hence

$$I(k,m,w) = k^{k-1}m^{m-1}(k+m-2)! \int_0^1 \dots \int_0^1 \frac{dx\,dy}{(w+k\xi+m\eta)^{k+m-1}}, \quad (5.2)$$

where $\xi = x_1 + \dots + x_{k-1}$ and $\eta = y_1 + \dots + y_{m-1}$. Let us now translate the domain of integration, writing

$$I(k,m,w) = k^{k-1}m^{m-1}(k+m-2)!\, J\left(k,m,w + \binom{k}{2} + \binom{m}{2}\right), \quad (5.3)$$

$$J(k,m,w) = \int_{-1/2}^{+1/2} \dots \int_{-1/2}^{+1/2} \frac{dx\,dy}{(w+k\xi+m\eta)^{k+m-1}}. \quad (5.4)$$

We wish to estimate $J(k,m,w)$, but first let us try the same kind of operations on a similar but simpler integral:

$$\int_0^\infty (1-e^{-\alpha t})^{k-1} e^{-wt}\, dt$$

$$= \alpha^{k-1}(k-1)! \int_{-1/2}^{+1/2} \dots \int_{-1/2}^{+1/2} \frac{dx}{(w+\alpha(k-1)/2+\alpha\xi)^k}.$$

The integral in this case can be evaluated exactly as a Beta function,

$$\int_0^\infty (1-e^{-\alpha t})^{k-1} e^{-wt}\, dt = \frac{1}{\alpha} \int_0^1 (1-u)^{k-1} u^{w/\alpha-1}\, du = \frac{1}{\alpha} \frac{\Gamma(k)\,\Gamma(w/\alpha)}{\Gamma(k+w/\alpha)};$$

hence we have derived the rather remarkable formula

$$\int_{-1/2}^{+1/2} \dots \int_{-1/2}^{+1/2} \frac{dx}{(w+\alpha\xi)^k} = \frac{1}{\alpha^k} \frac{\Gamma(w/\alpha - (k-1)/2)}{\Gamma(w/\alpha + (k+1)/2)}$$

$$= \frac{1}{\left(w - \alpha\dfrac{k-1}{2}\right)\left(w - \alpha\dfrac{k-3}{2}\right) \dots \left(w + \alpha\dfrac{k-3}{2}\right)\left(w + \alpha\dfrac{k-1}{2}\right)}. \quad (5.5)$$

Incidentally, (5.5) may be regarded as a consequence of the considerably more general identity

$$\Delta^n f(w) = \sum_j \binom{n}{j} (-1)^{n-j} f(w+j)$$

$$= \int_0^1 \dots \int_0^1 f^{(n)}(w + t_1 + \dots + t_n)\, dt_1 \dots dt_n \quad (5.6)$$

used in interpolation theory.

Proof. Let k and m satisfy (4.3) and $k + m \leq n$; we may assume that $k \leq m$. Let

$$w = (k+m)n - (k+m)^2 + km - c(k^{3/2} + m^{3/2}), \tag{6.1}$$

where c is the constant of Lemma 1, so that

$$E_{n,k,m} \leq \frac{n!}{k!\, m!\, (n-k-m)!}\, I(k,m,w). \tag{6.2}$$

We wish to apply Lemma 2 to estimate $I(k,m,w)$; so we must check that $m(k+m) \leq 2w + m(m-1)$, namely that

$$2c(k^{3/2} + m^{3/2}) \leq 2(k+m)(n-k-m) + (k-1)m. \tag{6.3}$$

If $k \leq m \leq n^{2/3}$ this certainly holds for all sufficiently large n; and when $n^{1/2} \ln n \leq k \leq m$ we obtain (6.3) for all large n by the estimates $2c(k^{3/2}+m^{3/2}) \leq 4cm^{3/2} \leq m^{3/2} \ln n - m \leq (n^{1/2} \ln n - 1)m \leq (k-1)m$. (We really only need to consider $k > n^{2/3}$ in this argument, but the more general estimate will be useful in the proof of Theorem 2 below.)

In order to simplify the formulas obtained after applying Lemma 2 in (6.2), we shall write

$$y = n - (k+m-1)/2,$$
$$z = \left(w + \binom{k}{2} + \binom{m}{2}\right) \Big/ (k+m), \tag{6.4}$$

noting that

$$y = z + 1 + c\frac{k^{3/2} + m^{3/2}}{k+m} \leq z + 1 + c\sqrt{m}. \tag{6.5}$$

The factor $n!/(n-k-m)!$ in (6.2) can be rewritten as

$$\left(y - \frac{k+m-1}{2}\right)\left(y - \frac{k+m-3}{2}\right) \cdots \left(y + \frac{k+m-1}{2}\right) = O\!\left(y^{k+m} e^{-f(k+m,y)}\right)$$

by (5.8); hence (6.2) and Lemma 2 imply that

$$E_{n,k,m} = O\!\left(\frac{k^{k-1} m^{m-1}(k+m-2)!\, y^{k+m}}{k!\, m!\, (k+m)^{k+m-1} z^{k+m-1}}\right) e^{Q}$$
$$= O\!\left(\frac{n}{k^{3/2} m^{3/2}(k+m)^{1/2}}\right) e^{R}, \tag{6.6}$$

where

$$Q = f\!\left(m, z - \frac{k(k-1)}{2(k+m)}\right) + f(k,z) - f(k+m,y),$$
$$R = Q + O\!\left(m \log \frac{y}{z}\right). \tag{6.7}$$

The proof of Theorem 1 will be complete if we can show that R is bounded above, since we have already noted that Theorem 1 follows from (4.1) under condition (4.3).

Relations (6.4) and (6.5) make it clear that $z \geq n/3$ for all large n; hence

$$\frac{y}{z} = 1 + O\left(\frac{m^{1/2}}{n}\right). \tag{6.8}$$

Furthermore it is clear from (5.9) that

$$f(m, v + d) = f(m, v) + O(md/v),$$

and that

$$f(k + m, y) - f(k, y) \geq f(k + m, u) - f(k, u) \qquad \text{when } y \leq u.$$

Let us set

$$u = \frac{k + m}{m}\left(y - \frac{k(k - 1)}{2(k + m)}\right). \tag{6.9}$$

Then $y \leq u \leq 2y$, and we can simplify R as follows:

$$R = f\left(m, y - \frac{k(k - 1)}{2(k + m)}\right) + O\left(\frac{m^{3/2}}{y}\right) + f(k, y) + O\left(\frac{km^{1/2}}{y}\right)$$
$$\qquad - f(k + m, y) + O\left(\frac{m^{3/2}}{n}\right)$$
$$= f\left(m, \frac{m}{k + m}u\right) + f(k, y) - f(k + m, y) + O\left(\frac{m^{3/2}}{n}\right)$$
$$\leq f\left(m, \frac{m}{k + m}u\right) + f(k, u) - f(k + m, u) + O\left(\frac{m^{3/2}}{n}\right). \tag{6.10}$$

Since

$$f\left(m, \frac{m}{k + m}u\right) + f(k, u) - f(k + m, u)$$
$$= \sum_{j \geq 1} \frac{1}{2j(2j + 1)(2u)^{2j}}\left(m(k + m)^{2j} + k^{2j+1} - (k + m)^{2j+1}\right)$$
$$= -\sum_{j \geq 1} \frac{k((k + m)^{2j} - k^{2j})}{2j(2j + 1)(2u)^{2j}} < -\frac{km^2}{24u^2} < -\frac{km^2}{96n^2}, \tag{6.11}$$

the remainder R is surely bounded when $k \le m \le n^{2/3}$. On the other hand when $n^{2/3} < k \le m$, let $g(n) = m^{3/2}/n$; then

$$R \le -\frac{km^2}{96n^2} + O\left(\frac{m^{3/2}}{n}\right) \le -\frac{m^2}{96n^{4/3}} + O\left(\frac{m^{3/2}}{n}\right)$$

$$= -\frac{1}{96}g(n)^{4/3} + O(g(n))$$

is less than some absolute constant.   □

This proof of Theorem 1 shows that $E_{n,k,m}$ is extremely small when $m \ge k \ge n^{2/3+\epsilon}$ and also in certain other cases (for example, when $k = n^{1/2+\epsilon}$ and $m = n^{1-\epsilon}$). Thus the algorithm almost never merges two large classes; one way to state this is

Theorem 2. *The probability that the equivalence algorithm merges two classes of sizes k and m, with*

$$\frac{n \ln n}{\sqrt{m}} \le k \le m, \tag{6.12}$$

is superpolynomially small; that is, it is $O(n^{-b})$ for all constants b.

Proof.   The argument used to prove Theorem 1 shows that

$$E_{n,k,m} = O\left(\frac{n}{k^{3/2}m^{3/2}(k+m)^{1/2}}\right)\exp\left(-\frac{km^2}{96n^2} + O\left(\frac{m^{3/2}}{n}\right)\right);$$

this is superpolynomially small since

$$-\frac{km^2}{96n^2} + O\left(\frac{m^{3/2}}{n}\right) \le \frac{m^{3/2}}{n}\left(-\frac{\ln n}{96} + O(1)\right)$$

and $m^{3/2}/n \ge \ln n$. Summing over all k and m leaves a superpolynomially small result.   □

7. The Unweighted Algorithm

If the QFW algorithm had not used the array $N[s]$, so that unions would be done by renaming the elements in the larger class with probability $\frac{1}{2}$, its average running time would be significantly greater. Let $E_{n,k}$ be the average number of equivalence classes of size k formed during a random execution of the algorithm, namely the average number of components of size k that appear, as the edges of the random graph appear in random order. The average running time of the "unweighted" algorithm can be expressed as

$$\frac{1}{2}\sum_{k=1}^{n-1} k\,E_{n,k}\,, \tag{7.1}$$

since the elements of each component of size $< n$ have a 50-50 chance of being renamed.

As in Equation (3.3), we can write down an integral for $E_{n,k}$, this time more easily than before:

$$E_{n,k} = \binom{n}{k}\int_0^\infty P_k(t)\,d(1-e^{-k(n-k)t})$$

$$= \binom{n}{k}k(n-k)\int_0^\infty P_k(t)e^{-k(n-k)t}\,dt, \tag{7.2}$$

for $1 \le k < n$. We can now argue as before to obtain satisfactory estimates of $E_{n,k}$ when $k \le n^{2/3}$ or when k is sufficiently large:

Theorem 3.

a) $\dfrac{n}{k^2} \le E_{n,k} \le \dfrac{n}{k^2}\exp\left(\dfrac{ck^{3/2}}{n-k-c\sqrt{k}}\right),\qquad$ for $n > k + c\sqrt{k}$,

  where c is the constant of Lemma 1;

b) $E_{n,k} = 1 - \dfrac{n-k}{k}(H_n - H_{n-k}) + O\left(\dfrac{\log n}{n}\right),\qquad$ for $\epsilon \le k/n < 1$,

  where the constant implied by the O may depend on ϵ.

Proof. Since $\omega_k(t) \ge 1/k$ we have

$$E_{n,k} \ge \binom{n}{k}(n-k)\int_0^\infty (1-e^{-kt})^{k-1}e^{-k(n-k)t}\,dt$$

$$= \binom{n}{k}\frac{n-k}{k}\int_0^1 (1-x)^{k-1}x^{n-k-1}\,dx = \frac{n}{k^2},$$

on setting $x = e^{-kt}$ and using well known properties of the Beta function. The upper bound follows in a similar manner,

$$E_{n,k} \le \binom{n}{k}(n-k)\int_0^\infty (1-e^{-kt})^{k-1}e^{ck^{3/2}t-k(n-k)t}\,dt$$

$$= \binom{n}{k}\frac{n-k}{k}\int_0^1 (1-x)^{k-1}x^{n-k-c\sqrt{k}-1}\,dx$$

$$= \frac{n}{k^2}\frac{n-1}{(n-c\sqrt{k}-1)}\frac{n-2}{(n-c\sqrt{k}-2)}\cdots\frac{n-k}{(n-c\sqrt{k}-k)}$$

$$\le \frac{n}{k^2}\exp\left(c\sqrt{k}\left(\frac{1}{n-c\sqrt{k}-1}\cdots\frac{1}{n-c\sqrt{k}-k}\right)\right)$$

since $x/(x-y) \leq e^{y/(x-y)}$.

To prove (b) we use Stepanov's theorem [10] that

$$\omega_n(t) = \left(1 - (1+nt)e^{-kt}\right)\left(1 + o(1)\right) \tag{7.3}$$

uniformly for $t \geq y_0/n$; by careful analysis of his proof we can replace the $o(1)$ term by $O(\log n/n)$, where the constant implied by this O depends on y_0. Thus

$$E_{n,k} = \binom{n}{k}k(n-k)\int_0^\infty (1 - (1+kt)e^{-kt})(1 - e^{-kt})^{k-1}e^{-k(n-k)t}\,dt$$

$$\times \left(1 + O\left(\frac{\log n}{\epsilon n}\right)\right)$$

$$+ O\left(\binom{n}{k}k(n-k)\int_0^{y_0/k} (1 - e^{-kt})^{k-1}e^{-k(n-k)t}\,dt\right)$$

$$= \binom{n}{k}(n-k)\int_0^1 (1 - (1 - \ln x)x)(1 - x)^{k-1}x^{n-k-1}\,dx$$

$$\times \left(1 + O\left(\frac{\log n}{\epsilon n}\right)\right)$$

$$+ O\left(\binom{n}{k}(n-k)\int_{1-z_0}^1 (1 - x)^{k-1}x^{n-k-1}\,dx\right)$$

where $1 - z_0 = \exp(-y_0)$. The latter integral is clearly less than z_0^k, and by choosing z_0 sufficiently small as a function of ϵ we can ensure that

$$z_0^k \leq z_0^{\epsilon n} = 3^{-n};$$

this is small enough to wipe out the contribution from $\binom{n}{k}(n-k)$, so the correction term is negligible. The main term is

$$\int_0^1 (1 - x)^k x^{n-k-1}\,dx + \int_0^1 (1 - x)^{k-1}x^{n-k}\ln x\,dx$$

$$= \frac{k!\,(n-k-1)!}{n!} + \frac{d}{dn}\int_0^1 (1 - x)^{k-1}x^{n-k}\,dx$$

$$= \frac{k!\,(n-k-1)!}{n!} - \frac{(k-1)!\,(n-k)!}{n!}(H_n - H_{n-k}). \quad \square$$

Part (a) of this theorem implies that

$$E_{n,k} \sim n^{1-2\alpha} \qquad \text{for } k = n^\alpha, \quad \alpha < \tfrac{2}{3}; \tag{7.4}$$

this is rather striking when $\frac{1}{2} < \alpha < \frac{2}{3}$, since it approaches $n^{-1/3}$. The connected components of a random graph apparently tend to grow quite rapidly once they get to this size range; they must move quickly past such values of k.

The approximation for $E_{n,k}$ in part (b) of the theorem,

$$1 - \frac{n-k}{k}(H_n - H_{n-k}) = 1 + \left(\frac{n}{k} - 1\right)\ln\left(1 - \frac{k}{n}\right) + O\left(\frac{1}{k}\right)$$

$$= \frac{k}{2n} + O\left(\frac{k^2}{n^2} + \frac{1}{k}\right),$$

has the right order of growth when $k = n^{2/3}$, but it has been proved only for $k \geq \epsilon n$. At any rate we can determine the asymptotic value of (7.1) without knowing too much about $E_{n,k}$ in the middle range of k. The sum of $kE_{n,k}$ for $k < \epsilon n$ is at most ϵn^2, since it is obvious that $E_{n,k} \leq \lfloor n/k \rfloor$ for all k. (All components of size k formed during the algorithm are disjoint, so there are never more than $\lfloor n/k \rfloor$ of them.) The sum of $kE_{n,k}$ for $k \geq \epsilon n$ differs from $n^2/4$ by at most $\epsilon n^2 + O(n \log n)$, since

$$\sum_{k=1}^{n-1}\left(k - (n-k)(H_n - H_{n-k})\right) = \frac{1}{2}\binom{n}{2} \tag{7.5}$$

and each term in this sum is less than n. Thus

$$\left(\frac{1}{8} - \delta\right)n^2 \leq \frac{1}{2}\sum_{k=1}^{n-1} kE_{n,k} \leq \left(\frac{1}{8} + \delta\right)n^2 \tag{7.6}$$

for all $\delta > 0$ and all sufficiently large n; the running time is asymptotically $n^2/8$, a factor of order n times what it was in the weighted case. It is tempting to conjecture that a stronger result actually holds, namely

$$\frac{1}{2}\sum_{k=1}^{n-1} kE_{n,k} = \frac{1}{8}n^2 + \frac{1}{3}n \ln n + O(n), \tag{7.7}$$

since $\sum_{1 \leq k < n^{2/3}} kE_{n,k} \sim \frac{2}{3}n \ln n$.

A comparison of formulas (3.3) and (7.2) shows that $E_{n,n-1} = 2E_{n,1,n-1}$; and indeed this relation is obvious by the nature of the equivalence algorithm, since any component of size $n-1$ must be merged with the remaining singleton element. Theorem 3(b) now yields

$$E_{n,1,n-1} = \frac{1}{2} + O\left(\frac{\log n}{n}\right), \tag{7.8}$$

hence (4.1) does not hold in general.

8. Numerical Results

Some Monte Carlo experiments were made to test the theory above; for each value of n, random edges $\{x, y\}$ were generated until the corresponding graph was connected, and this process was repeated ten times. Here are the results (with "$\pm$" indicating one unit of standard deviation):

n	Cost, QFW	Cost, QF	$\frac{1}{8}n^2 + \frac{1}{3}n \ln n$
2	1.0 ± 0.0	1.0 ± 0.0	0.96
4	3.4 ± 0.2	4.3 ± 0.1	3.85
8	8.5 ± 0.2	15.7 ± 0.3	13.55
16	20.2 ± 0.8	50.8 ± 2.4	46.79
32	45.6 ± 0.9	178.4 ± 5.7	164.97
64	99.0 ± 1.9	638 ± 19	600.72
128	212.3 ± 4.4	2375 ± 71	2255.02
256	451.2 ± 7.7	8609 ± 153	8665.19
512	936 ± 13	33938 ± 590	33832.67
1024	1941 ± 15	133012 ± 972	133437.94
2048	3955 ± 39	532637 ± 5969	529493.07
4096	7927 ± 49	2130655 ± 11233	2108508.52

Notice that the values in the weighted case seem to be less than $1.95n$, and the values in the unweighted case conform well to the predicted asymptotic behavior.

We can calculate exact values without great difficulty if n is small. For example, when $n = 4$ we readily find

$$E_{4,1,1} = \frac{6}{5}, \qquad E_{4,1,2} = E_{4,1,3} = \frac{2}{5}, \qquad E_{4,2,2} = \frac{1}{5};$$

hence the true average costs of the weighted and unweighted algorithms are respectively 3.2 and 4.4.

Table 1 shows the exact values of $E_{n,k,m}$ when $n = 8$. The average costs are $12265252/1448655 \approx 8.47$ and $16290696/1062347 \approx 15.3$, respectively.

Table 2 shows $E_{n,k,m}$ and $E_{n,m}$ when $n = 16$ and $k \leq m$. Notice that the values of $E_{n,k,m}$ are not convex in general; for example, $E_{16,2,12} < E_{16,2,13} > E_{16,2,14}$. The true average costs for $n = 16$ are 20.332 and 51.120; thus the Monte Carlo results appear to be valid. Incidentally, all of the denominators in Table 1 are products of prime numbers ≤ 23. The numbers $E_{16,k,m}$ in Table 2 are decimal approximations to rational numbers whose denominators are products of primes ≤ 113.

	$m = 1$	$m = 2$	$m = 3$	$m = 4$	$m = 5$	$m = 6$	$m = 7$
$k = 1$	$\frac{28}{13}$	$\frac{28}{51}$	$\frac{60}{209}$	$\frac{5096}{24035}$	$\frac{3046}{15249}$	$\frac{168}{715}$	$\frac{1929822}{5311735}$
$k = 2$		$\frac{2}{11}$	$\frac{134}{1265}$	$\frac{74}{897}$	$\frac{13054}{167739}$	$\frac{66958}{838695}$	
$k = 3$			$\frac{292}{4485}$	$\frac{9472}{187473}$	$\frac{214482}{5311735}$		
$k = 4$				$\frac{30881}{937365}$			

TABLE 1.   Exact values of $E_{8,k,m}$.

	$k = 1$	$k = 2$	$k = 3$	$k = 4$	$k = 5$	$k = 6$	$k = 7$	$k = 8$	$E_{n,m}$
$m = 1$	4.138								16.000
$m = 2$	0.976	0.294							4.138
$m = 3$	0.449	0.148	0.079						1.951
$m = 4$	0.274	0.095	0.052	0.035					1.191
$m = 5$	0.198	0.071	0.039	0.027	0.020				0.846
$m = 6$	0.160	0.058	0.033	0.022	0.017	0.014			0.665
$m = 7$	0.141	0.052	0.029	0.020	0.014	0.011	0.008		0.565
$m = 8$	0.133	0.049	0.027	0.018	0.013	0.009	0.006	0.002	0.511
$m = 9$	0.133	0.048	0.026	0.017	0.011	0.006	0.003		0.487
$m = 10$	0.140	0.050	0.026	0.015	0.008	0.003			0.486
$m = 11$	0.156	0.053	0.026	0.013	0.004				0.505
$m = 12$	0.182	0.058	0.024	0.008					0.543
$m = 13$	0.224	0.061	0.017						0.604
$m = 14$	0.290	0.056							0.692
$m = 15$	0.407								0.814

TABLE 2. Performance of QFW and QF when $n = 16$.

9. Another Model for Average Cost

We might also wish to study the average behavior of an equivalence algorithm under the assumption that the operations consist of the edges of a *random spanning tree* in random order; thus, we assume that the $n^{n-2}(n-1)!$ possible sequences of union operations of the form

$$\text{merge}\{R[x_1], R[y_1]\}; \ldots; \text{merge}\{R[x_{n-1}], R[y_{n-1}]\}$$

are equally likely.

The difference between this model and the previous one can be seen in the case $n = 4$: There are 12 spanning trees that form a Hamiltonian path (type 1), and 4 that form a "star" (type 2). After creating the first component $\{a, b\}$ of size 2, the new model will create a disjoint second component $\{c, d\}$ with probability $\frac{1}{3}$ if the tree is to be type 1, and never if it is to be type 2, hence the overall probability is $\frac{1}{4}$ that two disjoint components of size 2 are formed. The random process we have studied in Sections 1–8, however, will create $\{c, d\}$ with probability $\frac{1}{5}$, since $\{c, d\}$ is only one of five inequivalent pairs that might happen to fire next. The new model is qualitatively different from the old because it makes the merging of two large components significantly more probable; thus, we would not expect the weighted rule to give such a substantial improvement over the unweighted rule when using this model.

In the next few sections we shall use the symbols $E_{n,k,m}$ and $E_{n,k}$ to represent quantities in the new model analogous to those in the old; in other words, $E_{n,k}$ again denotes the expected number of classes of size k formed during the algorithm, and $E_{n,k,m}$ denotes the expected number of times we merge a class $R[x]$ of size k with a class $R[y]$ of size m. Note that we must have

$$E_{n,l} = \sum_{k=1}^{l-1} E_{n,k,l-k} \qquad \text{for } 1 < l \leq n \qquad (9.1)$$

in both models, since every class of size > 1 is obtained by merging.

In the new model the ratio $E_{n,k,l-k}/E_{n,l}$ is independent of n, since the $l - 1$ unions that form a class of size l do not affect the behavior of other unions. More precisely, consider any subset A of l elements, and any sequence of unions in which A is formed. Then we can replace the $l - 1$ unions forming A by any of the $l^{l-2}(l - 1)!$ such sequences, obtaining in this way all sequences of $n - 1$ union operations in which class A is formed and the $n - l$ other unions are held constant. It follows that

$$E_{n,k,l-k}/E_{n,l} = E_{l,k,l-k} \qquad \text{for all } n \geq l. \qquad (9.2)$$

Thus we must only determine the numbers $E_{n,k}$ and $E_{n,k,n-k}$ in the new model in order to deduce all values of $E_{n,k,m}$.

To determine $E_{n,k,n-k}$, consider how many sequences of unions end by merging $R[x]$ with $R[y]$, where class $R[x]$ is a particular set A of size k. There are $k^{k-2}(k - 1)!$ sequences of unions that construct A, $(n - k)^{n-k-2}(n - k - 1)!$ sequences of unions that connect up the other $n - k$ elements, $\binom{n-2}{k-1}$ ways to intermix these sequences, and $k(n - k)$

unions that could come last, hence

$$E_{n,k,n-k} = \binom{n}{k} \frac{k^{k-2}(k-1)!\,(n-k)^{n-k-2}(n-k-1)!}{n^{n-2}(n-1)!} \binom{n-2}{k-1} \frac{k(n-k)}{2}$$

$$= \frac{1}{2(n-1)} \binom{n}{k} \left(\frac{k}{n}\right)^{k-1} \left(\frac{n-k}{n}\right)^{n-k-1}. \tag{9.3}$$

(As in Equation (3.2) we must include a factor of $\frac{1}{2}$ because of the symmetry between x and y.) Notice that for fixed k and l, the asymptotic ratio of $E_{n,k,l-k}/E_{n,l}$ as $n \to \infty$ in our *former* model approaches $E_{l,k,l-k}$, the exact ratio of $E_{n,k,l-k}/E_{n,l}$ in the present model, by Equation (3.6) and Theorem 3(a). Therefore the new model essentially reflects the "local" behavior of the former model on small components. Alternatively we can regard the spanning tree model as an indication of the "early" behavior of the former model, since

$$E_{l,k,l-k} = \lim_{\epsilon \to 0} \frac{E_{n,k,l-k}(\epsilon)}{E_{n,l}(\epsilon)},$$

where the quantities on the right are obtained by substituting ϵ for ∞ in (3.3) and (7.2).

Let $p_{nk} = E_{n,k,n-k}$ be the probability that the final union is a $(k, n - k)$-merge; also let C_n^{QFW} and C_n^{QF} be the average total cost of unions in the weighted and unweighted equivalence algorithms, respectively. The independence argument by which we established (9.2) shows that

$$C_n^{\mathrm{QFW}} = \sum_{0<k<n} p_{nk}\big(\min(k, n - k) + C_k^{\mathrm{QFW}} + C_{n-k}^{\mathrm{QFW}}\big), \tag{9.4}$$

$$C_n^{\mathrm{QF}} = \sum_{0<k<n} p_{nk}\big(k + C_k^{\mathrm{QF}} + C_{n-k}^{\mathrm{QF}}\big), \tag{9.5}$$

because the behavior of the algorithm within the classes of sizes k and $n - k$ is the same as its behavior on classes of total size k and $n - k$. Yao [12] has proved that $C_n^{\mathrm{QFW}} = \Theta(n \log n)$ and $C_n^{\mathrm{QF}} = \Theta(n^{3/2})$, using a different approach to the analysis; by studying recurrences (9.4) and (9.5), we will be able to obtain more precise results.

10. Solution of Recurrences

According to the equations we have just derived, the average behavior of equivalence algorithms in the spanning tree model can be described by recurrence relations of the general form

$$x_n = c_n + \sum_{0 < k < n} p_{nk}(x_k + x_{n-k}) \tag{10.1}$$

where

$$p_{nk} = \frac{1}{2(n-1)} \binom{n}{k} \left(\frac{k}{n}\right)^{k-1} \left(\frac{n-k}{n}\right)^{n-k-1}. \tag{10.2}$$

Before considering this particular recurrence in detail, it will be interesting to deduce properties implied by (10.1) for *any* choice of the p_{nk} such that $\sum_k p_{nk} = 1$, since such recurrences arise also in the solution of several other algorithms (for example, in studies of quicksort and of digital search trees). If $c_1 = 1$ and $c_n = 0$ for all $n > 1$ it is immediate that $x_n = n$ for all n; similarly if $c_1 = 0$ and $c_n = 1$ for all $n > 1$ we have $x_n = n-1$ for all n. In general x_n is a monotone function of $(c_1, \ldots, c_n)$, hence these particular solutions allow us to conclude that

$$c_n = O(1) \quad \text{implies} \quad x_n = O(n). \tag{10.3}$$

Let us now specialize (10.1) to the case that

$$p_{nk} = r(k)r(n-k)/s(n) \tag{10.4}$$

for some functions r and s, where $r(n) = 0$ for $n \leq 0$ and

$$s(n) = \sum_k r(k)r(n-k). \tag{10.5}$$

Clearly (10.2) has this form, with $r(n) = n^{n-1}/n!$ for $n \geq 1$, and $s(n) = 2(n-1)n^{n-2}/n!$. When $p_{nk} = p_{n,n-k}$ we can replace (10.1) by

$$x_n = c_n + 2 \sum_{0 < k < n} p_{nk} x_k. \tag{10.6}$$

If we can find sequences $\langle x_n \rangle$ such that $\sum_k p_{nk} x_k$ has a simple form, we can insert the corresponding values into (10.6) and obtain a sequence $\langle c_n \rangle$ with a known solution $\langle x_n \rangle$; thus we can build up a repertoire of sequences $\langle c_n \rangle$ whose solutions are known. Linear combinations of sequences $\langle c_n \rangle$ in the repertoire can then be used to obtain many further solutions.

The form of (10.4) suggests that we try $x_n = r(n - m)/r(n)$ for some fixed nonnegative integer m; then we have

$$\sum_k p_{nk} x_k = \frac{s(n - m)}{s(n)},$$

hence $x_n^{(m)} = r(n - m)/r(n)$ is the solution to (10.6) when

$$c_n = c_n^{(m)} = \frac{r(n - m)}{r(n)} - 2\frac{s(n - m)}{s(n)}. \tag{10.7}$$

If $r(n) \neq 0$ for all $n \geq 1$, we can obtain *any* sequence as a (possibly infinite) linear combination of the special sequences $\langle c_n^{(m)} \rangle$, since $c_n^{(m)} = 0$ for $n \leq m$ and $c_{m+1}^{(m)} = r(1)/r(m + 1) \neq 0$; the solution to (10.6) will then be the same linear combination of the sequences $\langle x_n^{(m)} \rangle$.

In our case (10.2), we find for example when $m = 1$ that $x_n = (1 - 1/n)^{n-2}$ solves (10.1) when $c_n = (1 - 1/n)^{n-2}(2/(n - 1)^2 - 1)$ for $n \geq 2$. However, this general approach does not seem to lead to sufficiently simple formulas, so we shall now restrict consideration to the particular case (10.2), when more powerful techniques can be used.

11. Solution of the Spanning Tree Recurrence

Let us assume that $c_1 = 0$, since we have already determined the dependence of x_n on c_1. When p_{nk} is given by (10.2), we can multiply both sides of (10.6) by $(n - 1)n^{n-1}/n!$ obtaining

$$\frac{(n - 1)n^{n-1}x_n}{n!} = d_n + n \sum_{0 < k < n} \frac{k^{k-1}x_k}{k!} \frac{(n - k)^{n-k-1}}{(n - k)!}, \tag{11.1}$$

where

$$d_n = (n - 1)n^{n-1}c_n/n!. \tag{11.2}$$

The form of (11.1) suggests that we introduce the generating functions

$$G(z) = \sum_{n \geq 2} \frac{n^{n-1}x_n}{n!} z^n, \tag{11.3}$$

$$T(z) = \sum_{n \geq 1} \frac{n^{n-1}}{n!} z^n, \tag{11.4}$$

$$D(z) = \sum_{n \geq 2} d_n z^n, \tag{11.5}$$

and we obtain the equivalent relation

$$G'(z) - z^{-1}G(z) = z^{-1}D(z) + \frac{d}{dz}(T(z)G(z))$$
$$= z^{-1}D(z) + T'(z)G(z) + T(z)G'(z). \tag{11.6}$$

It is well known that this particular function $T(z)$ satisfies

$$T(z) = ze^{T(z)}; \tag{11.7}$$

see, for example, [4, Equation 2.3.4.4–20]. Hence $T'(z) = T(z)/z + T(z)T'(z)$, and we have

$$T'(z) = \frac{T(z)}{z(1 - T(z))}. \tag{11.8}$$

We can now multiply (11.6) by $1/T(z)$ and rewrite it as

$$\frac{d}{dz}\left(\frac{1 - T(z)}{T(z)}G(z)\right) = \frac{D(z)}{zT(z)}; \tag{11.9}$$

the solution with $c_1 = 0$ is

$$G(z) = \frac{T(z)}{1 - T(z)} \int_0^z \frac{D(w)\,dw}{wT(w)}. \tag{11.10}$$

Let us now imitate the repertoire method of the previous section, finding a set of functions $D_m(w)$ such that the integral in (11.10) has a simple form and then expressing the general case as a linear combination of these special ones. It is natural to set

$$D_m(z) = zT(z)^m T'(z) = T(z)^{m+1}/(1 - T(z)); \tag{11.11}$$

then the corresponding generating function is

$$G_m(z) = \frac{T(z)}{1 - T(z)} \int_0^z T(w)^{m-1}\,dT(w)$$

$$= \frac{T(z)}{1 - T(z)} \cdot \frac{T(z)^m}{m} = \frac{1}{m}D_m(z), \qquad \text{for } m > 0.$$

(In other words, $D_m(z)$ is an eigenfunction of the linear mapping $D \mapsto G$ defined by (11.10), with eigenvalue $1/m$.) To find the power series expansion of $D_m(z)$, we may use Lagrange's general inversion formula, according to which the relations $z = tf(t) = t + f_1t^2 + f_2t^3 + \cdots$ and $1 + w_1z + w_2z^2 + \cdots = g(t) = 1 + g_1t + g_2t^2 + \cdots$ imply that nw_n is the coefficient of t^{n-1} in $g'(t)f(t)^{-n}$. Letting $t = T(z)$, $f(t) = e^{-t}$, and $g(t) = t^{m+1}/(1 - t)$, we obtain $nw_n = \sum_{k=0}^{n-m-1} n^k(n - k)/k! = n^{n-m}/(n - m - 1)!$; hence

$$D_m(z) = \sum_{n>m} \frac{n^{n-m-1}}{(n - m - 1)!}z^n. \tag{11.12}$$

The corresponding c's, according to (11.2), are given by

$$c_n = c_n^{(m)} = \frac{(n - 2)!}{n^{m-1}(n - m - 1)!} = \frac{n - 2}{n} \cdots \frac{n - m}{n}, \tag{11.13}$$

for $n \geq 2$. We have proved the following result:

Lemma 3. *Let m be a positive integer. The solution to the recurrence (10.1) and (10.2) is*

$$x_n = x_n^{(m)} = \frac{n-1}{m} c_n^{(m)}, \qquad (11.14)$$

when $c_n = c_n^{(m)}$ is the sequence defined in (11.13).   □

In order to translate Lemma 3 into a more useful form, let us write

$$Q\langle a_0, a_1, a_2, \dots \rangle(n) = a_0 + a_1 \frac{n-1}{n} + a_2 \frac{n-1}{n} \frac{n-2}{n} + \cdots . \qquad (11.15)$$

(See [6].)   By successively setting $n = 1, 2, 3, \dots$ in this formula we see that *any* function of the positive integer n can be written as $Q\langle a_0, a_1, a_2, \dots \rangle(n)$ for some sequence $\langle a_0, a_1, a_2, \dots \rangle$, and if we are lucky the a's will form a nice pattern.

Suppose $c_n = Q\langle a_0, a_1, a_2, \dots \rangle(n)$ where $a_m = 1$ and all the other a_k are zero. We have

$$\frac{n-1}{n} \frac{n-2}{n} \dots \frac{n-m}{n} = \frac{m}{m+1} c_n^{(m)} + \frac{1}{m+1} c_n^{(m+1)}, \qquad (11.16)$$

so the solution x_n must be

$$\frac{n-1}{m+1} c_n^{(m)} + \frac{n-1}{(m+1)^2} c_n^{(m+1)}$$
$$= \left(\frac{n-1}{n+1} + \frac{n}{(m+1)^2} \right) \frac{n-1}{n} \frac{n-2}{n} \dots \frac{n-m}{n}; \qquad (11.17)$$

note that this works also when $m = 0$. Therefore Lemma 3 can be rephrased as follows:

Corollary. *The solution to the recurrence (10.1) and (10.2) when $c_n = Q\langle a_0, a_1, a_2, \dots \rangle(n)$ is*

$$x_n = (n-1) Q\left\langle \frac{a_0}{1}, \frac{a_1}{2}, \frac{a_2}{3}, \dots \right\rangle(n)$$
$$+ n Q\left\langle \frac{a_0}{1^2}, \frac{a_1}{2^2}, \frac{a_2}{3^2}, \dots \right\rangle(n). \quad □ \qquad (11.18)$$

12. Application to the Spanning Tree Model

Let us now use the results of the previous section to determine the average behavior of the spanning tree model. First we shall study some special cases of the general Q function defined in (11.15). It is not difficult to verify that

$$Q\langle 1, 2, 3, \ldots \rangle(n) = n; \qquad (12.1)$$

furthermore

$$Q\langle 1, 1, 1, \ldots \rangle(n) = Q(n) = \sqrt{\frac{\pi n}{2}} - \frac{1}{3} + O(n^{-1/2}) \qquad (12.2)$$

is the function discussed in (2.14). It is convenient to write $Q_0(n) = n$, $Q_1(n) = Q(n)$, and

$$Q_2(n) = Q\left\langle 1, \frac{1}{2}, \frac{1}{3}, \ldots \right\rangle(n); \qquad (12.3)$$

$$Q_3(n) = Q\left\langle 1, \frac{1}{2^2}, \frac{1}{3^2}, \ldots \right\rangle(n). \qquad (12.4)$$

Kruskal [7] has proved that

$$Q_2(n) = \tfrac{1}{2} \ln n + \tfrac{1}{2}(\gamma + \ln 2) + o(1), \qquad (12.5)$$

and it is obvious that

$$Q_3(n) < 1 + \frac{1}{2^2} + \frac{1}{3^2} + \cdots = O(1).$$

According to Equation (11.18),

$$c_n = Q_j(n) \quad \text{implies} \quad x_n = (n-1)Q_{j+1}(n) + nQ_{j+2}(n). \qquad (12.6)$$

Combining this with (10.3) and the estimates above, we see that

$$c_n = a\sqrt{n} + O(1) \quad \text{implies} \quad x_n = \frac{a}{\sqrt{2\pi}} n \ln n + O(n), \qquad (12.7)$$

for any constant a, since $c_n = (2a/\sqrt{2\pi})Q_1(n) + O(1)$. Similarly we can improve (10.3) to

$$c_n = O(\log n) \quad \text{implies} \quad x_n = O(n). \qquad (12.8)$$

In the unweighted algorithm, we have $c_n = n/2$ for all $n \geq 2$ (see (9.5)), hence the average cost of unweighted unions can be expressed in "closed form" as

$$C_n^{\text{QF}} = \frac{n-1}{2} Q(n) + \frac{n}{2} Q_2(n) - \frac{n}{2}$$

$$= \sqrt{\frac{\pi}{8}} n^{3/2} + \frac{1}{4} n \ln n + O(n). \qquad (12.9)$$

For the weighted algorithm, we must sum

$$c_n = \sum_{0 < k < n} p_{nk} \min(k, n-k), \qquad (12.10)$$

but this does not appear to have a simple closed form. By arguing as in Lemma 1, we have

$$p_{nk} = \frac{1}{2(n-1)} \frac{n}{k} \frac{n}{(n-k)} \phi(n,k)$$

$$= \frac{1}{\sqrt{8\pi}} \frac{n^{3/2}}{k^{3/2}(n-k)^{3/2}} \left(1 + O\left(\frac{1}{k} + \frac{1}{n-k}\right)\right);$$

hence

$$c_n = 2 \sum_{0 < k < n/2} \frac{1}{\sqrt{8\pi}} \frac{n^{3/2}}{k^{1/2}(n-k)^{3/2}} + O(1).$$

Euler's summation formula implies that

$$\sum_{k=1}^{\lfloor n/2 \rfloor} \frac{1}{k^{1/2}(n-k)^{3/2}} = \int_1^{n/2} \frac{dx}{x^{1/2}(n-x)^{3/2}} + O(n^{-3/2})$$

$$+ \frac{1}{2} \int_1^{n/2} \left(\{x\} - \frac{1}{2}\right) \left(\frac{3}{n-x} - \frac{1}{x}\right) \frac{dx}{x^{1/2}(n-x)^{3/2}}$$

$$= \frac{2}{n} \int_1^{n/2} d\left(\frac{x}{n-x}\right)^{1/2} + O(n^{-3/2})$$

$$= \frac{2}{n} + O(n^{-3/2});$$

hence $c_n = \sqrt{2n/\pi} + O(1)$. Relation (12.7) now yields the asymptotic behavior of the algorithm in the weighted case,

$$C_n^{\text{QFW}} = \frac{1}{\pi} n \ln n + O(n). \qquad (12.11)$$

We have proved

Theorem 4. *The average number of times the QFW algorithm changes entries in its R table while doing $n - 1$ set unions, under the spanning tree model, is $\pi^{-1} n \ln n + O(n)$; the (unweighted) QF algorithm makes $(\pi/8)^{1/2} n^{3/2} + \frac{1}{4} n \ln n + O(n)$ such changes, on the average.* □

Here are the results of empirical tests analogous to those in Section 8, using the spanning tree model:

n	Cost, QFW	$\frac{1}{\pi} n \ln n$	Cost, QF	$\sqrt{\pi/8} n^{\frac{3}{2}} + \frac{1}{4} n \ln n$
2	1.0 ± 0	0.4	1.0 ± 0	2.1
4	3.4 ± 0.2	1.8	4.3 ± 0.1	6.4
8	9.0 ± 0.2	5.3	14.3 ± 0.3	18.3
16	22.6 ± 0.6	14.1	44.2 ± 1.9	51.2
32	52.1 ± 2.2	35.3	135 ± 9	141.2
64	121.2 ± 2.7	84.7	343 ± 13	387.4
128	274.6 ± 5.9	197.7	992 ± 47	1062.8
256	580 ± 9	451.9	2980 ± 210	2921.7
512	1350 ± 21	1016.7	7490 ± 520	8058.5
1024	2837 ± 56	2259.3	22450 ± 1765	22308.8
2048	6175 ± 80	4970.5	56637 ± 3980	61983.6
4096	13496 ± 266	10844.7	169628 ± 12930	172791.8

The true values of $(C_n^{\text{QFW}}, C_n^{\text{QF}})$ for $n = 2, 4, 8$, and 16 are respectively $(1, 1)$, $(3.25, 4.375)$, $(8.85, 14.62)$, $(22.09, 44.26)$.

If we set $c_n = \delta_{nk}$ in recurrence (10.1), the resulting value of x_n will be $E_{n,k}$, the average number of classes of size k. Hence the *general* solution to (10.1) and (10.2) can be written

$$x_n = \sum_k c_k E_{n,k}. \tag{12.12}$$

We shall complete our study of the recurrence and the spanning tree model by determining $E_{n,m}$, for fixed $m \geq 2$, using the methods of Section 11.

According to (11.5) and (11.10) we have

$$G(z) = \frac{T(z)}{1 - T(z)} \int_0^z \frac{m^{m-2}}{(m-2)!} \frac{w^{m-1}}{T(w)} \, dw. \tag{12.13}$$

This integral can be evaluated by using the known formula

$$T(z)^r = r \sum_{n \geq r} \frac{n^{n-1-r}}{(n-r)!} z^n, \qquad \text{for } r \neq 0; \tag{12.14}$$

see [4, exercise 2.3.4.4–29]. The integral becomes

$$
-\frac{m^{m-2}}{(m-2)!}\sum_{n\geq-1}\frac{n^n}{(n+1)!}\frac{z^{n+m}}{n+m}
$$

$$
=\frac{1}{m^2}-\frac{m^{m-2}}{(m-2)!}\sum_{n\geq-m}\frac{n^n(n+2)(n+3)\ldots(n+m-1)}{(n+m)!}z^{n+m}. \qquad (12.15)
$$

We wish to write the latter term as a linear combination of the functions $z^m T(z)^{-k}$, for $1\leq k\leq m$; thus, we set

$$
\frac{m^{m-2}}{(m-2)!}\sum_{n\geq-m}\frac{n^n}{(n+m)!}(n+2)\ldots(n+m-1)z^{n+m}
$$

$$
=\sum_{k=1}^{m}b_k z^m T(z)^{-k}
$$

$$
=-\sum_{n\geq-m}\frac{n^n}{(n+m)!}\left(\sum_{k=1}^{m}k b_k n^{k-1}(n+k+1)\ldots(n+m)\right)z^{n+m},
$$

and the b's must satisfy

$$
b_1(n+2)\ldots(n+m)+2b_2 n(n+3)\ldots(n+m)+\cdots
$$
$$
+(m-1)b_{m-1}n^{m-2}(n+m)+mb_m n^{m-1}
$$
$$
=-\frac{m^{m-2}}{(m-2)!}(n+2)(n+3)\ldots(n+m-1)
$$

for all n. Since both sides of this equation are polynomials in n of degree $m-1$, the b's can be determined by successively inserting the values $n=-m,\ldots,n=-1$, and we find without difficulty that

$$
b_{m-j}=m^{j-2}/j!, \qquad \text{for } 0\leq j\leq m-2;
$$
$$
b_1=m^{m-3}/(m-1)!-m^{m-1}/m!. \qquad (12.16)
$$

Now (12.13), (12.14), (12.15), and (11.8) yield

$$
G(z)=\frac{1}{m^2}\frac{T(z)}{1-T(z)}-\sum_{k=1}^{m}b_k z^m T(z)^{-k}z T'(z)
$$

$$
=\sum_{n\geq m}z^n\left(\frac{1}{m^2}\frac{n^n}{n!}+\frac{m^{m-1}}{m!}\frac{(n-m)^{n-m}}{(n-m)!}\right.
$$

$$
\left.-\sum_{j=0}^{m-1}\frac{m^{j-2}(n-m)^{n-j-1}}{j!\,(n-j-1)!}\right).
$$

Hence

$$E_{n,m} = n\left(\frac{1}{m^2} + \frac{m^{m-1}}{m!}\left(1-\frac{m}{n}\right)^{n-1}\frac{(n-1)!}{(n-m)^{m-1}(n-m)!}\right.$$
$$\left. - \sum_{j=0}^{m-1}\frac{m^{j-2}}{j!}\left(1-\frac{m}{n}\right)^{n-1}\frac{(n-1)!}{(n-m)^j(n-j-1)!}\right). \qquad (12.17)$$

In particular,

$$E_{n,2} = \frac{n}{4}\left(1 + \left(1 - \frac{2}{n}\right)^{n-2}\right). \qquad (12.18)$$

For fixed m as $n \to \infty$ we have

$$E_{n,m} \sim \frac{n}{m^2}\left(1 + e^{-m}\left(\frac{m^{m+1}}{m!} - \sum_{j=0}^{m-1}\frac{m^j}{j!}\right)\right)$$
$$= \frac{n}{m^2}\left(1 + \frac{m^m e^{-m}}{m!}(m - Q(m))\right). \qquad (12.19)$$

This coefficient, of order $m^{-3/2}$, is significantly different from our result $E_{n,k} \sim n/k^2$ in the random graph model.

13. Union Trees

In order to analyze a variety of equivalence class algorithms in a variety of models, we can construct an extended binary tree that retains essentially all of the necessary information about the set union operations that caused classes to merge. Given a sequence of ordered pairs (x_1, y_1), ..., (x_{n-1}, y_{n-1}) such that the unordered pairs $\{x_1, y_1\}$, ..., $\{x_{n-1}, y_{n-1}\}$ form a spanning tree on the vertices $\{1, 2, \ldots, n\}$, let the associated *union tree* be defined as follows: For $1 \le j < n$, construct a new node whose left subtree is the union tree for the current component of x_j and whose right subtree is the union tree for the current component of y_j. (By "current component" we mean the connected component defined by the previous edges $\{x_1, y_1\}$, ..., $\{x_{j-1}, y_{j-1}\}$.) The union tree for a component of size 1 is a single terminal node.

Thus, for example, the union tree associated with the sequence $(3, 1)$, $(4, 1)$, $(5, 9)$, $(2, 6)$, $(5, 3)$, $(5, 8)$, $(9, 7)$, $(2, 3)$ is shown in Figure 1. (The labels shown on terminal nodes are not officially part of the tree; they merely help to indicate the manner of construction.) Note that the union tree has been defined for *ordered* pairs (x_j, y_j); if the last pair of the example were $(3, 2)$ instead of $(2, 3)$ the tree would be different.

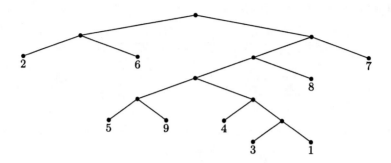

FIGURE 1. A typical union tree.

This convention about ordered pairs avoids complications that would otherwise arise when counting binary trees whose left and right subtrees are isomorphic.

We can extend the models of random behavior used above to obtain definitions of random union trees by assuming that each edge $\{x, y\}$ occurring in the random graph or random spanning tree is equally likely to appear as (x, y) or as (y, x) when the corresponding union tree is being built up. Then each of the $(2n-2)!/n!\,(n-1)!$ possible binary trees with n terminal nodes will occur with a certain probability. For example, when $n = 4$ the five possible union trees (see Figure 2) each occur with probability $1/5$ in the random graph model, while the respective probabilities are $(\frac{3}{16}, \frac{3}{16}, \frac{1}{4}, \frac{3}{16}, \frac{3}{16})$ in the spanning tree model.

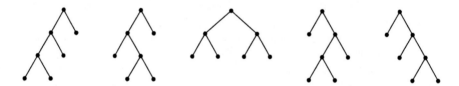

FIGURE 2. The union trees with four terminal nodes.

The probability of a particular tree T can be calculated in the random graph model by considering the probability $P(T, t)$ that T has been formed at time t. Let $|T|$ be the number of terminal nodes of T; and if $|T| > 1$ let T_l and T_r be the respective left and right subtrees of the root, so that $|T_l| + |T_r| = |T|$. When $|T| = 1$ we define $P(T, t) = 1$, otherwise we let

$$P(T,t) = \frac{|T|!}{2(|T_l|-1)!\,(|T_r|-1)!} \int_0^t e^{-|T_l||T_r|u} P(T_l,u) P(T_r,u)\, du. \quad (13.1)$$

Then $P(T,\infty)$ is the probability that T is formed by the algorithm.

For example, when T is the middle tree of Figure 2 we have

$$P(T,t) = \tfrac{1}{5} - 3e^{-4t} + \tfrac{24}{5}e^{-5t} - 2e^{-6t},$$

but for the other four trees we have

$$P(T,t) = \tfrac{1}{5} - e^{-3t} + \tfrac{9}{5}e^{-5t} - e^{-6t}.$$

The sum of $P(T,t)$ over all five trees T is, of course, $P_4(t)$. Although all five trees will occur with probability $\tfrac{1}{5}$, the middle tree tends to occur "faster" when it does occur, since the middle function is $(e^{-t} - e^{-2t})^3$ larger than the others.

Let T_1 be the tree with $|T_1| = 1$, and let T_n be the tree with $|T_n| = n$ whose right subtree is T_{n-1}; thus T_n is a "degenerate" tree, having the longest path length over all trees with n terminal nodes. For these special trees an inductive argument can be used to express the P function as a fairly simple sum,

$$P(T_n,t) = \sum_{k=0}^{n-1} (-1)^k \frac{n!\,(n-1)!\,(2n-1-2k)}{k!\,(2n-1-k)!} e^{-k(2n-1-k)t/2}. \quad (13.2)$$

Curiously we have

$$P(T_n,\infty) = n!\,(n-1)!/(2n-2)!, \quad (13.3)$$

which is the exact reciprocal of the total number of binary trees; in other words, the degenerate tree occurs just as often as it would in a uniform distribution over trees.

Unfortunately the probabilities $P(T,\infty)$ for other trees do not have such simple properties, and for $n > 4$ the distribution becomes far from uniform. Computer calculations for $n = 10$ show that the tree in Figure 3 has maximum probability over all $18!/10!\,9! = 4862$ binary trees with 10 terminal nodes; its probability is $74615232/35942281$ times $1/4862$. The least probable trees are obtained by joining two degenerate T_5's; their probability is only $8515903/27199564$ times $1/4862$. According to

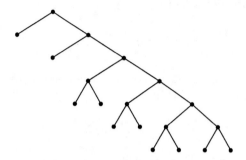

FIGURE 3. The most common union tree with ten terminal nodes.

results we have already derived, a tree whose subtrees both have nearly $n/2$ terminal nodes will almost never occur for large n.

The tree probabilities in the spanning tree model are much simpler. Let $S(T)$ be the set of all $n-1$ nonterminal subtrees of T, when $|T| = n$; then it is not difficult to prove that T occurs in the spanning tree model with probability

$$P(T) = \frac{n!}{(2n)^{n-1}} \prod_{\tau \in S(T)} \frac{|\tau|}{|\tau| - 1}. \tag{13.4}$$

For the probability is clearly

$$\prod_{\tau \in S(T)} p_{|\tau_l||\tau_r|} = \prod_{\tau \in S(T)} \frac{r(|\tau_l|)r(|\tau_r|)}{s(|\tau|)} = \frac{1}{r(n)} \prod_{\tau \in S(T)} \frac{r(|\tau|)}{s(|\tau|)},$$

using the notation of (10.4); and $r(n)/s(n) = n/(2(n - 1))$.

Incidentally, whenever the probability distribution for trees has the "separable" form

$$P(T) = f(|T|) \prod_{\tau \in S(T)} g(|\tau|) \tag{13.5}$$

for some functions f and g, we can use recurrences like (10.1) satisfying property (10.4) to analyze cost functions on the trees. Three examples of such probability distributions appear in [5, exercise 6.3–36].

Once we know the tree probabilities, we can analyze several equivalence algorithms. The cost of tree T in the QFW algorithm is

$$C^{\mathrm{QFW}}(T) = \sum_{\tau \in S(T)} \min(|\tau_l|, |\tau_r|), \tag{13.6}$$

and in the unweighted algorithm it is

$$C^{\mathrm{QF}}(T) = \sum_{\tau \in S(T)} |\tau_l|. \tag{13.7}$$

When the probability model assigns equal probabilities to (x, y) and (y, x), so that all trees obtainable from a given tree by interchanging left and right subtrees are equiprobable, (13.7) can be replaced by one-half the external path length of T_1, i.e.,

$$C^{\mathrm{QF}}(T) = \tfrac{1}{2} \sum_{\tau \in S(T)} |\tau|, \tag{13.8}$$

because $|\tau_l|$ will be $\frac{1}{2}(|\tau_l| + |\tau_r|) = \frac{1}{2}|\tau|$ on the average. The quantity (13.8) will have the same mean as (13.7), but not the same variance.

Yao [12] has analyzed two other algorithms that he calls "quick merge" and "quick merge weighted." It is not difficult to see that we can study the length of "find" operations on the merge steps of these algorithms by considering union trees, using the respective costs

$$C^{\mathrm{QM}}(T) = \sum_{\tau \in S(T)} C^{\mathrm{QF}}(\tau)/|\tau|, \tag{13.9}$$

$$C^{\mathrm{QMW}}(T) = \sum_{\tau \in S(T)} C^{\mathrm{QFW}}(\tau)/|\tau|, \tag{13.10}$$

provided that the probability model we are using assigns equal probability to all sequences $\langle x_1, y_1 \rangle, \ldots, \langle x_{n-1}, y_{n-1} \rangle$ in which $\langle x_j, y_j \rangle$ is replaced by $\langle x'_j, y'_j \rangle$ where x'_j and y'_j are in the same current components as x_j and y_j. Both of the models we are considering have this property; in the random graph model these formulas do not account for "find" operations when a redundant edge is encountered. In the spanning tree model we can obtain the average behavior of these two algorithms by solving the recurrences

$$C_n^{\mathrm{QM}}(T) = \frac{C_n^{\mathrm{QF}}}{n} + 2 \sum_{0 < k < n} p_{nk} C_k^{\mathrm{QM}}, \tag{13.11}$$

$$C_n^{\mathrm{QMW}}(T) = \frac{C_n^{\mathrm{QFW}}}{n} + 2 \sum_{0 < k < n} p_{nk} C_k^{\mathrm{QMW}}, \tag{13.12}$$

as in Section 12 above. From (12.7), (12.8), and Theorem 4 we may conclude that $C_n^{\mathrm{QM}} = \frac{1}{4} n \ln n + O(n)$ and $C_n^{\mathrm{QMW}} = O(n)$, thereby confirming and slightly sharpening Yao's results.

Doyle and Rivest [2] have studied equivalence algorithms under a third probability model, assuming that each union takes place between a random pair of equivalence classes present at the time, regardless of the sizes of these classes. Their model is almost certainly unrealistic, but it does have the curious property that it leads to union trees with the same probability distribution as that of binary search trees (see [5, Section 6.2.2]). For example, the five union trees in Figure 2 have the expected probabilities $(\frac{1}{6}, \frac{1}{6}, \frac{1}{3}, \frac{1}{6}, \frac{1}{6})$ in this model. Since the first union leaves one class of size 2 and $n-2$ classes of size 1, and since the subsequent behavior of the algorithm is to construct a random union tree from these $n-1$ classes, it is clear that random union trees with n terminal nodes are obtained from those with $n-1$ terminals by replacing a random terminal node by a branch node, and this is essentially the same process that produces random binary search trees. We can analyze the four union algorithms in this model by using Equations (9.4), (9.5), (13.11), and (13.12) with the separable probability distribution $p_{nk} = 1/(n-1)$. The resulting solutions are

$$
\begin{aligned}
C_n^{\mathrm{QF}} &= n(H_n - 1) & &= n \ln n + O(n); \\
C_n^{\mathrm{QFW}} &= nH_n - \tfrac{1}{2}nH_{\lfloor n/2 \rfloor} - \lceil n/2 \rceil = \tfrac{1}{2}n \ln n + O(n); \\
C_n^{\mathrm{QM}} &= 2nH_n^{(2)} - 2n - H_n + 1 & &= (\tfrac{1}{3}\pi^2 - 2)n + O(\log n); \\
C_n^{\mathrm{QMW}} &= O(n) & &= O(n).
\end{aligned}
\tag{13.13}
$$

Notice that in this model the union tree tends to be reasonably well-balanced, so the weighted algorithm saves only a factor of 2.

14. Open Problems

We have proved that the QFW algorithm has linear expected running time in the random graph model, and we have analyzed four distinct algorithms in the other models, but several related questions are still waiting to be resolved.

Perhaps the most important problem remaining is to determine the asymptotic behavior of $P_n(t)$ when $n^{-3/2} \leq t \leq n^{-1}$, since our estimates are unsatisfactory in this interval. Such an improvement should help in the analysis of many other algorithms, because the function $P_n(t)$ describes the behavior of random graphs. A detailed knowledge of $P_n(t)$ would probably establish the conjecture (7.7), and perhaps it would also lead to an analytic determination of the constant $\limsup_{n\to\infty}(C_n^{\mathrm{QFW}}/n)$.

Given random input sequences of length l in the random graph model, is it true that the expected running time of algorithm QFW is $O(l)$? Our proof gives $O(l + n)$, which is satisfactory if l is order n at least; and for very small l the individual components almost always have bounded size. But for $l = \Theta(n/\log n)$, say, we do not know how to answer this question.

Another natural problem the authors have not been able to resolve is the estimation of $P(T, \infty)$ for given trees T. This ought to shed further light on equivalence algorithms and the connectivity of random graphs.

This research was supported in part by the National Science Foundation, by the Office of Naval Research, and by IBM Corporation. Computer time was supported by the MACSYMA project of the Defense Advanced Research Projects Agency and by the SUMEX project of the National Institutes of Health.

References

[1] A. V. Aho, J. E. Hopcroft, and J. D. Ullman, *The Design and Analysis of Computer Algorithms* (Reading, Massachusetts: Addison–Wesley, 1974).

[2] Jon Doyle and Ronald L. Rivest, "Linear expected time of a simple Union-Find algorithm," *Information Processing Letters* **5** (1976), 146–148.

[3] E. N. Gilbert, "Random graphs," *Annals of Mathematical Statistics* **30** (1959), 1141–1144.

[4] Donald E. Knuth, *Fundamental Algorithms*, Volume 1 of *The Art of Computer Programming* (Reading, Massachusetts: Addison–Wesley, 1968).

[5] Donald E. Knuth, *Sorting and Searching*, Volume 3 of *The Art of Computer Programming* (Reading, Massachusetts: Addison–Wesley, 1973).

[6] Donald E. Knuth and Gururaj S. Rao, "Activity in an interleaved memory," *IEEE Transactions on Computers* **C-24** (1975), 943–944. [Reprinted as Chapter 8 of the present volume.]

[7] Martin D. Kruskal, "The expected number of components under a random mapping function," *American Mathematical Monthly* **61** (1954), 392–397.

[8] John Riordan, *Combinatorial Identities* (New York: Wiley, 1968).

[9] V. E. Stepanov, "Комбинаторная алгебра и случайные графы," *Teoriiã Veroiãtnosteĭ i ee Primeneniiã* **14** (1969), 393–420. English translation, "Combinatorial algebra and random graphs," *Theory of Probability and Its Applications* **14** (1969), 373–399.

[10] V. E. Stepanov, "О вероятности связности случайного графа $\mathcal{G}_m(t)$," *Teoriíã Veroíãtnosteĭ i ee Primeneniíã* **15** (1970), 56–68. English translation, "On the probability of connectedness of a random graph $\mathcal{G}_m(t)$," *Theory of Probability and Its Applications* **15** (1970), 55–67.

[11] V. E. Stepanov, "Строение случайных графов $\mathcal{G}_m(x|h)$," *Teoriíã Veroíãtnosteĭ i ee Primeneniíã* **17** (1972), 238–252. English translation, "Structure of the random graphs $\mathcal{G}_m(x|h)$," *Theory of Probability and its Applications* **17** (1972), 227–242.

[12] Andrew Chi-chih Yao, "On the average behavior of set merging algorithms (Extended abstract)," *Conference Record of the Eighth Annual ACM Symposium on Theory of Computing* (1976), 192–195.

Addendum

Substantial further progress has been made by Béla Bollobás and Istvan Simon ["Probabilistic analysis of disjoint set union algorithms," *SIAM Journal on Computing* **22** (1993), 1053–1074], who proved that the average running time for QFW under the random graph model studied in Sections 1–6 above is $Cn + o(n/\log n)$, where

$$C = \sum_{m=1}^{\infty} t_m, \qquad t_m = \frac{1}{m} - \frac{m^m}{m!} \sum_{k=1}^{m} \frac{k^{k-1}}{k!} \frac{(k+m-2)!}{(k+m)^{k+m-1}} \frac{1}{1+\delta_{km}}.$$

Here $t_m n$ is the contribution to the running time that corresponds to merging a component of size m with a component of size $\geq m$. More precisely, Bollobás and Simon proved that

$$m\left(E_{n,m,m} + \sum_{k=m+1}^{n-m} (E_{n,m,k} + E_{n,k,m}) \right) = t_m n + o(n^{1/2}),$$

when $m \leq 2(\ln n)^{13}$. (Compare with (3.6).)

It is interesting and instructive to evaluate the Bollobás–Simon constant C numerically. The main task, if we omit the term for $k = m$ in the definition of t_m, is to study the asymptotic behavior of the sum

$$s_m = \sum_{k=1}^{m-1} \frac{k^{k-1}}{k!} \frac{(k+m-2)!}{(k+m)^{k+m-1}}.$$

It is natural to simplify at least one of the factorials by using Stirling's approximation

$$n! \sim \frac{n^n}{e^n}\sqrt{2\pi n}\sum_{j=0}^{\infty}\frac{\sigma_j}{n^j} = \frac{n^n}{e^n}\sqrt{2\pi n}\Big(1+\frac{1}{12n}+\frac{1}{288n^2}-\frac{139}{51840n^3}+\cdots\Big);$$

here the coefficients σ_j are defined by the formal power series

$$\sum_{j=0}^{\infty}\sigma_j z^j = \exp\Big(\sum_{k=1}^{\infty}\frac{B_{2k}z^{2k-1}}{2k(2k-1)}\Big) = \exp\Big(\frac{z}{12}-\frac{z^3}{360}+\frac{z^5}{1260}-\cdots\Big).$$

It follows that

$$s_m = \sum_{k=1}^{m-1}\frac{k^{k-1}}{k!}\frac{(k+m)!}{(k+m)^{k+m}}\frac{1}{(k+m-1)}$$

$$\sim \frac{\sqrt{2\pi}}{e^m}\sum_{k=1}^{m-1}\frac{k^{k-1}e^{-k}}{k!}\frac{\sqrt{k+m}}{k+m-1}\sum_{j=0}^{\infty}\frac{\sigma_j}{(k+m)^j}$$

$$\sim \frac{\sqrt{2\pi m}}{e^m}\sum_{j=1}^{\infty}\frac{\tau_j}{m^j}\sum_{k=1}^{m-1}\frac{k^{k-1}e^{-k}}{k!}\Big(1+\frac{k}{m}\Big)^{\frac{1}{2}-j},$$

where $\tau_j = \sigma_0+\sigma_1+\cdots+\sigma_{j-1}$. Thus we will have an asymptotic series for s_m if we can find an asymptotic series for the simpler sums

$$s_m(\beta) = \sum_{k=1}^{m-1}\frac{k^{k-1}e^{-k}}{k!}\Big(1+\frac{k}{m}\Big)^{-\beta},$$

when $\beta = \frac{1}{2}, \frac{3}{2}, \frac{5}{2}, \ldots$.

The following analysis of $s_m(\beta)$ may not be the simplest possible, but it derives auxiliary information of independent interest. We will find the asymptotic behavior of $s_m(\beta)$ by using the approximation $s_m(\beta) \approx p_m(\beta) + q_m(\beta) - r_m(\beta)$ and finding the behavior of $p_m(\beta)$, $q_m(\beta)$, and $r_m(\beta)$, where

$$p_m(\beta) = \sum_{k=1}^{\infty}\Big(\frac{k^{k-1}e^{-k}}{k!}-\frac{k^{-3/2}}{\sqrt{2\pi}}\sum_{j=0}^{l}(-1)^j\frac{\sigma_j}{k^j}\Big)\Big(1+\frac{k}{m}\Big)^{-\beta};$$

$$q_m(\beta) = \sum_{k=1}^{\infty}\frac{k^{-3/2}}{\sqrt{2\pi}}\sum_{j=0}^{l}(-1)^j\frac{\sigma_j}{k^j}\Big(1+\frac{k}{m}\Big)^{-\beta};$$

$$r_m(\beta) = \sum_{k=m}^{\infty}\frac{k^{-3/2}}{\sqrt{2\pi}}\sum_{j=0}^{l}(-1)^j\frac{\sigma_j}{k^j}\Big(1+\frac{k}{m}\Big)^{-\beta}.$$

Here l is an arbitrary positive integer. This will solve the problem, because we have $\left(1 + \frac{k}{m}\right)^{-\beta} < 1$ and

$$\frac{k^{k-1}e^{-k}}{k!} = \frac{k^{-3/2}}{\sqrt{2\pi}} \sum_{j=0}^{l} (-1)^j \frac{\sigma_j}{k^j} + O(k^{-l-5/2}),$$

hence

$$s_m(\beta) - p_m(\beta) - q_m(\beta) + r_m(\beta) = \sum_{k=m}^{\infty} O(k^{-l-5/2}) = O(m^{-l-3/2}).$$

Let's consider $r_m(\beta)$ first; it is well suited to Euler's summation formula. The general method we will use is typified by a sum such as

$$\sum_{k=m}^{\infty} f\left(\frac{k}{m}\right), \qquad f(x) = x^{-5/2}(1+x)^{-3/2},$$

although in general the exponents $-5/2$ and $-3/2$ will be $-\alpha$ and $-\beta$ where $\alpha - \frac{1}{2}$ and $\beta + \frac{1}{2}$ are positive integers. In the next several formulas, we let $f^{(n)}(x)$ denote the nth derivative of $f(x)$ for all $n \geq 0$, and we also let $f^{(-1)}(x)$ stand for the integral of $f(x)$ with constant chosen so that $f^{(-1)}(\infty) = 0$. In this particular case we have

$$f^{(-1)}(x) = \int_{\infty}^{x} \frac{dx}{x^{5/2}(1+x)^{3/2}}$$

$$= \frac{2x^{1/2}}{(1+x)^{1/2}} + \frac{10}{3} \frac{(1+x)^{1/2}}{x^{1/2}} - \frac{2}{3} \frac{(1+x)^{1/2}}{x^{3/2}} - \frac{16}{3}.$$

Euler's formula yields

$$\sum_{k=m}^{\infty} f\left(\frac{k}{m}\right) = -\sum_{n=0}^{l} \frac{B_n}{n!} \frac{f^{(n-1)}(1)}{m^{n-1}} + O(m^{-l}),$$

because the relation $\alpha + \beta \geq 2$ implies that $f^{(n)}(\infty) = 0$ for all n. The integral can be found in general by starting with the formula

$$\int_{\infty}^{x} \frac{dx}{x^{k+3/2}(1+x)^{1/2}}$$

$$= \sum_{j=0}^{k} (-1)^{j+1} \frac{k^{\underline{j}}}{(k+1/2)^{\underline{j+1}}} \frac{(1+x)^{1/2}}{x^{k-j+1/2}} + (-1)^k \frac{k!}{(k+1/2)^{\underline{k+1}}}$$

and then using integration by parts,

$$\alpha \int_\infty^x \frac{dx}{x^{\alpha+1}(1+x)^\beta} + \beta \int_\infty^x \frac{dx}{x^\alpha(1+x)^{\beta+1}} = \frac{-1}{x^\alpha(1+x)^\beta}$$

to increase β while holding $\alpha + \beta$ constant. We obtain $r_m(\beta)$ by adding together appropriate multiples of $m^{-\alpha} \sum_{k=m}^\infty f(k/m)$ for $f(x) = x^{-\alpha}(1+x)^{-\beta}$ and $\alpha = \frac{3}{2}, \frac{5}{2}, \ldots$.

The sum $q_m(\beta)$ is well suited to Mellin transformation. [See Philippe Flajolet, Xavier Gourdon, and Philippe Dumas, "Mellin transforms and asymptotics: Harmonic sums," *Theoretical Computer Science* **144** (1995), 3–58, Example 13.] Consider, for example, the case

$$\sum_{k=1}^\infty f\left(\frac{k}{m}\right), \qquad f(x) = x^{-5/2}(1+x)^{-3/2}.$$

The Mellin transform is

$$f^*(s) = \int_0^\infty f(x)x^{s-1}\,dx = \int_0^\infty x^{s-7/2}(1+x)^{-3/2}\,dx$$

$$= \int_0^\infty \left(\frac{x}{1+x}\right)^{s-7/2}\left(\frac{1}{1+x}\right)^{3-s}\frac{dx}{(1+x)^2}$$

$$= \int_0^1 y^{s-7/2}(1-y)^{3-s}\,dy = \frac{\Gamma(s-5/2)\Gamma(4-s)}{\Gamma(3/2)}$$

when the real part of s lies between $5/2$ and 4, and analytic continuation extends this to all complex s. Thus

$$\sum_{k=1}^\infty f\left(\frac{k}{m}\right) = \sum_{k=1}^\infty \frac{1}{2\pi i}\int_{c-i\infty}^{c+i\infty} f^*(s)\left(\frac{k}{m}\right)^{-s}\,ds$$

$$= \sum_{k=1}^\infty \frac{1}{2\pi i}\int_{c-i\infty}^{c+i\infty} \frac{\Gamma(s-5/2)\Gamma(4-s)}{\Gamma(3/2)}\frac{m^s}{k^s}\,ds$$

$$= \frac{1}{2\pi i}\int_{c-i\infty}^{c+i\infty} \frac{\Gamma(s-5/2)\Gamma(4-s)m^s\zeta(s)}{\Gamma(3/2)}\,ds$$

if $\frac{5}{2} < c < 4$. We obtain an asymptotic series by decreasing c as far as we like and adding up the residues of poles of the integrand:

$$\sum_{k=1}^\infty f\left(\frac{k}{m}\right) \sim \frac{\Gamma(-3/2)\Gamma(3)}{\Gamma(3/2)}m + \sum_{n=0}^\infty \frac{(-1)^n}{n!}\frac{\Gamma(3/2+n)}{\Gamma(3/2)}m^{5/2-n}\zeta(5/2-n)$$

$$\sim \frac{16}{3}m + \sum_{n=0}^\infty \binom{-3/2}{n}m^{5/2-n}\zeta(5/2-n).$$

In general the critical strip will be $\alpha < c < \alpha + \beta$ and the result will be asymptotically

$$\frac{\Gamma(1-\alpha)\Gamma(\alpha+\beta-1)}{\Gamma(\beta)} m + \sum_{n=0}^{\infty} \binom{-\beta}{n} m^{\alpha-n}\zeta(\alpha-n).$$

The leading term here cancels with part of the term for $n = 0$ in $r_m(\beta)$, namely the constant of integration that makes $f^{(-1)}(\infty) = 0$. Therefore we can ignore both of them when we compute $q_m(\beta) - r_m(\beta)$.

The asymptotics of $p_m(\beta)$ are the most interesting, because they involve additional properties of the tree function $T(z)$ that was considered in Section 11. To deal with $p_m(\beta)$ we will expand the binomial

$$\left(1 + \frac{k}{m}\right)^{-\beta} \sim \sum_{n=0}^{\infty} \binom{-\beta}{n}\left(\frac{k}{m}\right)^n$$

and study the contribution of the terms for $n = 0, 1, \ldots$. The case $n = 0$ is simplest, so we can get oriented by looking at it first: Clearly

$$\sum_{k=1}^{\infty} \left(\frac{k^{k-1}e^{-k}}{k!} - \frac{k^{-3/2}}{\sqrt{2\pi}}\sum_{j=0}^{l}(-1)^j\frac{\sigma_j}{k^j}\right)$$

$$= T\!\left(\frac{1}{e}\right) - \frac{1}{\sqrt{2\pi}}\sum_{j=0}^{l}(-1)^j\sigma_j\zeta(3/2+j)$$

by (11.4). And (11.7) implies that $T(xe^{-x})e^{-T(xe^{-x})} = xe^{-x}$; hence $T(xe^{-x}) = x$ for $0 \le x \le 1$, and we have $T(1/e) = 1$.

Now let's look at the case $n = 3$. We will need to know the value of $\binom{-\beta}{3}m^{-3}$ times the sum

$$\sum_{k=1}^{\infty} \left(\frac{k^{k+2}e^{-k}}{k!} - \frac{1}{\sqrt{2\pi}}\left(\sigma_0 k^{3/2} - \sigma_1 k^{1/2} + \sigma_2 k^{-1/2}\right)\right)$$

$$- \frac{1}{\sqrt{2\pi}}\sum_{j=3}^{l}(-1)^j\sigma_j\zeta(3/2+j-3).$$

By Abel's limit theorem, the sum on k will be

$$\lim_{\epsilon \to 0+} \left(\sum_{k=1}^{\infty} \frac{k^{k+2}e^{-(\epsilon+1)k}}{k!} - \frac{1}{\sqrt{2\pi}}\sum_{k=1}^{\infty} e^{-\epsilon k}\left(\sigma_0 k^{3/2} - \sigma_1 k^{1/2} + \sigma_2 k^{-1/2}\right)\right).$$

A Mellinesque argument allows us to deduce the asymptotic behavior of a polylogarithm function like $\text{Li}_{(-3/2)}(e^{-\epsilon}) = \sum_{k=1}^{\infty} e^{-\epsilon k}/k^{-3/2}$ quite easily: The transform of $f(x) = e^{-\epsilon x}$ is

$$f^*(x) = \int_0^{\infty} e^{-\epsilon x} x^{s-1}\, dx = \Gamma(s)/\epsilon^s$$

when the real part of s is positive; hence

$$\sum_{k=1}^{\infty} e^{-\epsilon k} k^{3/2} = \sum_{k=1}^{\infty} \frac{1}{2\pi i} \int_{c-i\infty}^{c+i\infty} \Gamma(s) \epsilon^{-s} k^{3/2-s}\, ds$$

$$= \frac{1}{2\pi i} \int_{c-i\infty}^{c+i\infty} \Gamma(s) \epsilon^{-s} \zeta(s - 3/2)\, ds$$

if $\Re(s) > \frac{5}{2}$. The asymptotic value is therefore a sum of residues as before:

$$\text{Li}_{(-3/2)}(e^{-\epsilon}) \sim \frac{\Gamma(5/2)}{\epsilon^{5/2}} + \sum_{j=0}^{\infty} \frac{(-1)^j}{j!} \epsilon^j \zeta(-j - 3/2).$$

But what about $\sum_{k=1}^{\infty} k^{k+2} e^{-(\epsilon+1)k}/k!$? We can express this in terms of the tree function, using well-known properties of that function. [See Svante Janson, Donald E. Knuth, Tomasz Luczak, and Boris Pittel, "The birth of the giant component," *Random Structures & Algorithms* 4 (1993), 233–358, Section 4.] The operator

$$\vartheta = z \frac{d}{dz}$$

multiplies the coefficient of z^k in a power series by k; therefore

$$\vartheta^3 T(z) = \sum_{k=1}^{\infty} \frac{k^{k+2} z^k}{k!}.$$

We also have

$$\vartheta T(z) = \frac{T(z)}{1 - T(z)} = \frac{1}{1 - T(z)} - 1,$$

by (11.8). Consequently

$$\vartheta \frac{1}{(1 - T(z))^a} = \frac{a}{(1 - T(z))^{a+2}} - \frac{a}{(1 - T(z))^{a+1}},$$

and we can compute

$$\vartheta^2 T(z) = \frac{1}{(1-T(z))^3} - \frac{1}{(1-T(z))^2};$$

$$\vartheta^3 T(z) = \frac{3}{(1-T(z))^5} - \frac{5}{(1-T(z))^4} + \frac{2}{(1-T(z))^3}.$$

The behavior of $\vartheta^3 T(e^{-\epsilon-1})$ is therefore known if we can deduce the manner in which $T(e^{-\epsilon-1})$ approaches 1 as ϵ decreases to 0.

Suppose variables v and w are related by the law

$$T\left(e^{-w^2/2-1}\right) = 1 - v.$$

Then $1 - v = e^{-w^2/2-1}e^{1-v}$, so we have

$$\frac{w^2}{2} = -v + \ln\frac{1}{1-v} = \frac{v^2}{2} + \frac{v^3}{3} + \frac{v^4}{4} + \cdots;$$

hence

$$w = \left(v^2 + \frac{2}{3}v^3 + \frac{2}{4}v^4 + \cdots\right)^{1/2}.$$

Reverting this series gives v in terms of w, namely

$$v = w - \frac{w^2}{3} + \frac{w^3}{36} + \frac{w^4}{270} + \frac{w^5}{4320} - \frac{w^6}{17010} - \frac{139w^7}{5443200} + \cdots.$$

The desired result now follows if we set $w = \sqrt{2\epsilon}$:

$$T(e^{-\epsilon-1}) = 1-v \qquad = 1 - \sqrt{2\epsilon} + \frac{2\epsilon}{3} - \frac{(2\epsilon)^{3/2}}{36} - \frac{4\epsilon^2}{270} + \cdots,$$

$$\vartheta^3 T(e^{-\epsilon-1}) = \frac{3}{v^5} - \frac{5}{v^4} + \frac{2}{v^3} = \frac{3\epsilon^{-5/2}}{4\sqrt{2}} - \frac{\epsilon^{-3/2}}{24\sqrt{2}} + \frac{\epsilon^{-1/2}}{288\sqrt{2}} - \frac{8}{2835} + O(\epsilon).$$

The terms with negative powers of ϵ cancel with the similar terms from the Mellin analysis:

$$\frac{1}{\sqrt{2\pi}}\left(\sigma_0\frac{\Gamma(5/2)}{\epsilon^{5/2}} - \sigma_1\frac{\Gamma(3/2)}{\epsilon^{3/2}} + \sigma_2\frac{\Gamma(1/2)}{\epsilon^{1/2}}\right) = \frac{3\epsilon^{-5/2}}{4\sqrt{2}} - \frac{\epsilon^{-3/2}}{24\sqrt{2}} + \frac{\epsilon^{-1/2}}{288\sqrt{2}}.$$

(Of course we knew that they would, but this provides a useful check on the computations.) We conclude, by Abel's limit theorem, that the stated sum for $n = 3$ is equal to

$$-\frac{8}{2835} - \frac{1}{\sqrt{2\pi}}\sum_{j=0}^{l}(-1)^j\sigma_j\zeta(3/2 + j - 3).$$

The computations for general n are similar, but tedious if we must apply ϑ repeatedly. Fortunately a beautiful simplification is available:

Lemma. *Let c_n be $(-1)^n n!$ times the coefficient of t^n in $T(e^{-t-1}) = 1 - \sqrt{2t} + \frac{2}{3}t - t^{3/2}/(9\sqrt{2}) + \cdots$. Then*

$$\sum_{k=1}^{\infty} \left(\frac{k^{k+n-1}e^{-k}}{k!} - \frac{k^{n-3/2}}{\sqrt{2\pi}} \sum_{j=0}^{n-1}(-1)^j \frac{\sigma_j}{k^j} \right)$$

$$= c_n - \frac{1}{\sqrt{2\pi}} \sum_{j=0}^{n-1}(-1)^j \sigma_j \zeta(3/2 + j - n).$$

Proof. We use the analog of Taylor's theorem for ϑ in place of $\frac{d}{dz}$:

$$f(se^t) = \sum_{n=0}^{l} \frac{t^n}{n!}\vartheta^n f(s) + \int_0^t \frac{x^l}{l!}\vartheta^{l+1}f(se^{t-x})\,dx;$$

this formula is easily proved by induction. Replacing t by $-t$ and s by $e^{-\epsilon-1}$ tells us that

$$T(e^{-\epsilon-t-1}) \sim \sum_{n=0}^{\infty} \frac{(-t)^n}{n!}\vartheta^n T(e^{-\epsilon-1}),$$

and we can determine the coefficients by setting $w = \sqrt{2(\epsilon + t)}$ in the formula for $1 - v$ above. For example, the term $-w^4/270$ contributes $-4(\epsilon + t)^2/270 = -2\epsilon^2/135 - 4\epsilon t/135 - 2t^2/135$ to the formal power series expansion of $T(e^{-\epsilon-t-1})$, and the term $-w^3/36$ contributes

$$-\frac{\sqrt{2}}{18}\left(\epsilon^{3/2} + \binom{3/2}{1}\epsilon^{1/2}t + \binom{3/2}{2}\epsilon^{-1/2}t^2 + \cdots \right).$$

Negative powers of ϵ occur only when the exponent is a fraction, and those terms cancel out when we apply Abel's limit theorem as we did in the case $n = 3$. Removing those terms and setting $\epsilon = 0$ gives $\sum_{n\geq0}(-t)^n c_n/n!$. □

The first few values are

$$c_0 = 1, \quad c_1 = -\frac{2}{3}, \quad c_2 = -\frac{4}{135}, \quad c_3 = -\frac{8}{2835}, \quad c_4 = \frac{16}{8505}.$$

If these numbers seem familiar it is because they appeared in one of Ramanujan's first publications, except with different signs. Indeed, the asymptotic expansion of Ramanujan's function $Q(N)+1+N$ is obtained from $T(e^{-t-1})$ if each power $t^{k/2}$ is replaced by $(-1)^k\left(\frac{k}{2}\right)!\,N^{1-k/2}$. [See (2.14) and the note by C. C. Rousseau, "A simply obtained asymptotic expansion for the probability that a random mapping is connected," *Applied Mathematics Letters* **2** (1989), 159–161.] Therefore the coefficient of $t^{k/2}$ in $T(e^{-t-1})$ when k is odd must be equal to $-\sqrt{\pi/2}\,\sigma_{(k-1)/2}/(k/2)!$. For example, $1/(9\sqrt{2}) = \sqrt{\pi/2}\cdot\frac{1}{12}\cdot\frac{2}{3}\cdot\frac{2}{1}/\sqrt{\pi}$. The appearance of the prime number 139 in both σ_3 and the coefficient of $t^{7/2}$ is not a coincidence.

Now that we have deduced the asymptotic series for $p_m(\beta)$, $q_m(\beta)$, and $r_m(\beta)$, we are ready to compute the desired series for $s_m(\beta) \sim p_m(\beta) + q_m(\beta) - r_m(\beta)$. Massive cancellation occurs — in fact, all the zeta function constants drop out — and we are left with the following:

$$s_m(\beta) \sim \sum_{n=0}^{\infty} \binom{-\beta}{n}\frac{c_n}{m^n}$$

$$+ \frac{1}{\sqrt{2\pi m}}\sum_{n=0}^{\infty}\frac{1}{m^n}\sum_{j=0}^{n}(-1)^j\sigma_j\frac{B_{n-j}}{(n-j)!}f_{(3/2+j)\beta}^{(n-j-1)}(1).$$

Here $f_{\alpha\beta}(x) = x^{-\alpha}(1+x)^{-\beta}$, and the constant term should be left out of the integral when we compute $f_{\alpha\beta}^{(-1)}(1)$. It is easy to verify that the coefficient of m^{-n} in this expansion is rational, while the coefficient of $m^{-n-1/2}$ is a rational multiple of $\pi^{-1/2}$.

Putting it all together, we have

$$s_m \sim \frac{\sqrt{2\pi m}}{e^m}\sum_{j=1}^{\infty}\frac{\tau_j}{m^j}s_m(j-1/2)$$

$$\sim \frac{\sqrt{2\pi m}}{e^m}\sum_{n=0}^{\infty}\frac{1}{m^{n+1}}\sum_{j=0}^{n}\binom{-1/2-j}{n-j}\tau_{j+1}c_{n-j}$$

$$+ \frac{1}{e^m}\sum_{n=0}^{\infty}\frac{1}{m^{n+1}}\sum_{j=0}^{n}\sum_{k=0}^{n-j}(-1)^j\sigma_j\tau_{k+1}\frac{B_{n-j-k}}{(n-j-k)!}f_{(3/2+j)(1/2+k)}^{(n-j-k-1)}(1)$$

$$\sim \frac{\sqrt{2\pi m}}{e^m}\left(\frac{1}{m} + \frac{17}{12m^2} + \frac{3109}{1440m^3} + \cdots\right)$$

$$- \frac{\sqrt{2}}{e^m}\left(\frac{2}{m} + \frac{32}{9m^2} + \frac{13501}{2880m^3} + \cdots\right).$$

To get t_m, we multiply by $m^m/m!$, subtract the result from $1/m$, and subtract the term for $k = m$ in the definition of t_m. But instead of explicitly subtracting the term for $k = m$, we can save work if we simply modify the formula for s_m, replacing the Bernoulli number B_1 by 0. This yields

$$t_m \sim \frac{1}{\sqrt{\pi m}}\left(\frac{2}{m}+\frac{113}{36m^2}+\frac{37193}{8640m^3}+\cdots\right)-\left(\frac{4}{3m^2}+\frac{92}{45m^3}+\frac{7552}{2835m^3}+\cdots\right).$$

Let a_j denote the coefficient of $m^{-j/2}$ in this expansion. These coefficients initially alternate in sign and have magnitude less than 20 when $j < 40$, but they become somewhat more erratic for larger values of j because Bernoulli numbers begin small but eventually increase superexponentially. For example, $a_3 \approx 1.13$, $a_4 \approx -1.33$, $a_5 \approx 1.77$, $a_6 \approx -2.04$, ..., $a_{40} \approx -11.54$, $a_{41} \approx 4.65$, $a_{42} \approx 2.90$, $a_{43} \approx -58.81$, $a_{44} \approx -11.92$, ..., $a_{55} \approx 168298$, $a_{56} \approx 6606$, $a_{57} \approx -295801$.

Finally, we can evaluate the Bollobás–Simon constant C to high precision by summing the exact values of t_m for $m < 128$, say; then we can use the asymptotic formula up to $O(m^{-57/2})$ for $m \geq 128$, together with the fact that

$$\sum_{k=m}^{\infty}\frac{1}{k^a} = \frac{1}{a-1}\sum_{j=0}^{l}\binom{1-a}{j}\frac{B_j}{m^{a+j-1}}+O(m^{-a-l})$$

when $a > 1$. The result is

$$C = 2.08477\,69048\,47362\,89161\,38698\,79753\,49228\,21989-.$$

Bollobás and Simon also proved that the expected total cost of the first $l = o(n)$ applications of QFW is only $l + o(l)$. Moreover, the expected cost of the first $n/2 - n^{2/3}(\ln n)^{2/3}$ applications of the unweighted algorithm QF is $\frac{1}{3}n\ln n + O(n\log\log n)$, while the expected running time needed to fully connect a graph is $\frac{1}{8}n^2 + O(n(\log n)^2)$. The more precise formula (7.7) remains a conjecture.

Chapter 22

Textbook Examples of Recursion

[Originally published in Artificial Intelligence and Mathematical Theory of Computation: Papers in honor of John McCarthy, edited by Vladimir Lifschitz (New York: Academic Press, 1991), 207–229.]

We discuss properties of recursive schemas related to McCarthy's "91 function" and to Takeuchi's triple recursion. Several theorems are proposed as interesting candidates for machine verification, and some intriguing open questions are raised.

John McCarthy and Ikuo Takeuchi introduced interesting recurrence equations as they were exploring the properties of recursive programs. McCarthy's function [7],

$$f(x) = \text{ if } x > 100 \text{ then } x - 10 \text{ else } f\big(f(x+11)\big),$$

has become known as the "91 function," since it turns out that $f(x) = 91$ for all $x \leq 101$. Takeuchi's "tarai function" [13][14] is a triple recursion,

$$t(x, y, z) = \text{if } x \leq y \text{ then } y$$
$$\text{else } t\big(t(x-1, y, z), \ t(y-1, z, x), \ t(z-1, x, y)\big),$$

which has proved useful for benchmark testing of LISP systems because the recursion terminates only after the definition has been expanded a large number of times (assuming that previously computed values are not remembered). Neither of these functions is of practical importance, because no reasonable programmer would ever want to carry out such recursive computations on a realistic problem. Yet both functions are quite instructive because they illustrate important problems and techniques that arise when we consider the task of verifying computer programs formally. Therefore they make excellent examples for textbooks that discuss recursion.

The purpose of this paper is to obtain new information about $f(x)$ and $t(x, y, z)$ and about some closely related functions. Several of the theorems proved below should provide good test material for automated verification systems. A few open problems are stated, illustrating the fact that extremely simple recursions can lead to quite difficult questions.

1. The 91 Function

It is appropriate to begin by studying the 91 function, because 1991 is the year of John McCarthy's 64th birthday (and because a computer scientist's most significant birthday is the 64th). McCarthy originally wrote down the definition of $f(x)$, as shown above, because he wanted to study a simple recursion whose properties could not be deduced by ordinary mathematical induction. After studying the definition, he was pleasantly surprised to discover that it had the totally unexpected "91 property."

The 91 function certainly belongs to the set of significant textbook examples, because it is mentioned on at least 14 pages of Zohar Manna's well known text, *Mathematical Theory of Computation* [6]. The first published discussions of the function appeared in 1970 [7][9], after it had been investigated extensively at Stanford's Artificial Intelligence Laboratory during 1968 [8].

Instead of using McCarthy's original definition, let's change the specifications a bit and consider the following function (see [6, Problem 5–8]):

$$f(x) = \textbf{if } x > 100 \textbf{ then } x - 10 \textbf{ else } f^{91}(x + 901)$$

where $f^{91}(y)$ stands for $f\big(f\big(\cdots \big(f(y)\big) \cdots\big)\big)$, the 91-times-repeated application of f. According to this new definition, we have

$$f(91) = f^{91}(992) = f^{90}(982) = \cdots = f^2(102) = f(92).$$

And a similar derivation shows that if $90 \le x \le 100$ we have

$$f(x) = f^{91}(x + 901) = \cdots = f^2(x + 11) = f(x + 1);$$

hence

$$f(90) = f(91) = \cdots = f(100) = f(101).$$

And $f(101) = 91$, so we have proved in particular that

$$f(91) = 91.$$

Now let's evaluate $f(x)$ when x is extremely small, say $x = -10^6$. We have

$$f(-1000000) = f^{91}(-999099) = f^{181}(-998198) = \cdots = f^{99811}(-791)$$
$$= f^{99901}(110)$$
$$= f^{99900}(100)$$

and we know that $f(100) = 91$; hence

$$f^{99900}(100) = f^{99899}(91) = f^{99898}(91) = \cdots = f(91) = 91 \,.$$

In general, if x is any integer ≤ 100, let m be the smallest integer such that $x + 901m > 100$, and let n be the smallest integer such that $x + 901m - 10n \leq 100$. Then $m \geq 1$, $n \leq 91$, and

$$f(x) = f^{1+90m}(x+901m) = f^{1+90m-n}(x+901m-10n) = f^{90m-n}(91) \,,$$

where the last step follows since $91 \leq x+901m-10n \leq 100$. We conclude that $f(x) = 91$. (The final step is omitted if $m = 1$ and $n = 91$; that case occurs if and only if $x = 100$.)

How many iterations are needed to compute $f(x)$ by this definition, if we continue to apply the recurrence even when evaluating $f(x)$ for values of x that have already been considered? Let $F(x)$ count the number of times that the test 'if $x > 100$' is performed; then we have

$$F(x) = \textbf{if } x > 100 \textbf{ then } 1$$
$$\textbf{else } 1 + F(x + 901) + F\big(f(x + 901)\big)$$
$$+ F\big(f^2(x + 901)\big) + \cdots + F\big(f^{90}(x + 901)\big) \,.$$

(This is a special case of the general notion of a derived function, which is always jointly recursive with the function from which it has been derived; see McCarthy and Talcott [11] for a general discussion, and see Wegbreit [18] for an early application of the idea to the analysis of running times.) A bit of experimentation reveals that $F(x)$ also reduces to a simple function:

Lemma 1. $F(x) = \textbf{if } x > 100 \textbf{ then } 1 \textbf{ else } 9192 - 91x$.

Proof. If $x < 100$ we have

$$F(x) - F(x + 1) = \sum_{k=0}^{90} \big(F\big(f^k(x + 901)\big) - F\big(f^k(x + 902)\big)\big) \,.$$

Now if $x + 901 \leq 100$, the sum reduces to $F(x + 901) - F(x + 902)$, because the terms for $k > 0$ are $F\big(f^k(x + 901)\big) - F\big(f^k(x + 902)\big) = F(91) - F(91) = 0$. In this case we let $x' = x + 901$. On the other hand if $x + 901 > 100$, let n be minimal such that $x + 901 - 10n \leq 100$. Then $1 \leq n \leq 90$, and $F\big(f^k(x + 901)\big) - F\big(f^k(x + 902)\big) = F(91) - F(91) = 0$ for all $k > n$. We also have $F\big(f^n(x + 901)\big) - F\big(f^n(x + 902)\big) = F(x + 901 - 10n) - F(x + 902 - 10n)$; furthermore $F\big(f^k(x + 902)\big) - F\big(f^k(x + 901)\big) = 1 - 1 = 0$ for all $k < n$. In this case we let $x' = x + 901 - 10n$. In both cases we have found an x' such that

$$F(x + 1) - F(x) = F(x' + 1) - F(x'), \qquad x < x' \leq 100.$$

The proof is therefore complete by induction on $101 - x$ if we simply verify that $F(100) - F(101) = 91$. □

The 91 function suggests that we consider the more general recursive scheme

$$f(x) = \textbf{if } x > a \textbf{ then } x - b \textbf{ else } f^c(x + d),$$

where a is an arbitrary real number, b and d are positive reals, and c is a positive integer.

Theorem 1. *The generalized 91 recursion with parameters (a, b, c, d) defines a total function on the integers if and only if $(c - 1)b < d$. In such a case the values of $f(x)$ also obey the much simpler recurrence*

$$f(x) = \textbf{if } x > a \textbf{ then } x - b \textbf{ else } f\big(x + d - (c - 1)b\big).$$

Proof. It is not difficult to show that any function satisfying the generalized 91 recursion for $c > 1$ must also satisfy

$$f(x) = \textbf{if } x > a \textbf{ then } x - b \textbf{ else } f^{c-1}(x + d - b).$$

For if $x \leq a$, let n be minimal such that $x + nd > a$. Then

$$f^c(x + d) = f^{c+(n-1)(c-1)}(x + nd) = f^{n(c-1)}(x + nd - b);$$
$$f^{c-1}(x + d - b) = f^{c-1+(n-1)(c-1)}\big(x + d - b + (n - 1)d\big);$$

hence $f^c(x + d) = f^{c-1}(x + d - b)$, as desired.

To complete the proof, we use induction on c; and we also need to characterize the parameter settings that cause the given recursive definition to terminate for all x.

If $(c-1)b \geq d$, the expansion of $f(x)$ will not terminate when $a - b < x \leq a$. For if n is minimum such that $x + d - nb \leq a$, we have $n \leq c - 1$, and

$$f(x) = f^c(x+d) = \cdots = f^{c-n}(x + d - nb).$$

Now $c - n > 0$, and $a - b < x + d - nb \leq a$, so this will go on and on.

On the other hand, we can show that no looping will occur if $(c-1)b < d$. Suppose first that $x > a - b$. If $x > a$, obviously $f(x) = x - b$. Otherwise we have $x + d > x + (c-1)b > a + (c-2)b$, hence

$$f(x) = f^c(x+d) = \cdots = f^2\big(x + d - (c-2)b\big) = f\big(x + d - (c-1)b\big).$$

Let $\Delta = d - (c-1)b$, and let m be minimum such that $x + m\,\Delta > a$; then
$$f(x) = f(x + \Delta) = \cdots = f(x + m\,\Delta) = x + m\,\Delta - b.$$

Thus, the expansion of $f(x)$ terminates with a value $> a - b$ whenever $x > a - b$.

Finally, if $x \leq a - b$ and if m is minimal such that $x + md > a - b$, the expansion of
$$f(x) = f^{1+m(c-1)}(x + md)$$

terminates, because we can peel off the f's one by one.   ◻

When the generalized 91 function is total, we can express it in "closed form" as

$$\begin{aligned} f(x) = &\ \textbf{if } x > a \textbf{ then } x - b \\ &\ \textbf{else } a + d - cb - \big((a - x) \bmod (d - (c-1)b)\big). \end{aligned}$$

The special case $c = 2$ of Theorem 1 was first proved by Manna and Pnueli [8].

Open Problem 1. Prove Lemma 1 and Theorem 1 by computer.   ◻

2. The Takeuchi Function

Now we turn to the more complex recurrence

$$\begin{aligned} t(x, y, z) = &\ \textbf{if } x \leq y \textbf{ then } y \\ &\ \textbf{else } t\big(t(x-1, y, z),\ t(y-1, z, x),\ t(z-1, x, y)\big). \end{aligned}$$

John McCarthy observed in unpublished notes [10] that this function can be described more simply as

$$t(x, y, z) = \text{if } x \le y \text{ then } y \text{ else if } y \le z \text{ then } z \text{ else } x\,.$$

If we assume termination, the latter function satisfies the stated recurrence, so it must be identical with the former function.

John had just returned from a conference in Kyoto, and his notes [10] began with a brief comment about the history of this function and its motivation:*

> Ikuo Takeuchi (1978) of the Electrical Communication Laboratory of Nippon Telephone and Telegraph Co. (Japan's Bell Labs) devised a recursive function program for comparing the speeds of LISP systems. It can be made to run a long time without generating large numbers or using much stack.

Takeuchi called his function *tarai*, from the word "taraimawashi," which connotes passing an unpleasant object from one person to another.

At about the same time, John coerced the FOL proof-checking system to construct a 50-step proof that $t(x, y, z)$ has the simple form stated above [10]. This experiment suggested several improvements to FOL.

If we fully expand the definition of $t(x, y, z)$ whenever $x > y$, the proof of termination seems to be nontrivial, because there is no obvious way to impose an order on the set of all arguments (x, y, z) in such a way that no infinitely long dependency chains exist. We shall prove termination as a byproduct of a more general investigation of the total running time needed to evaluate $t(x, y, z)$ by repeated application of the definition.

Let $T(x, y, z)$ be the number of times the **else** clause is invoked when $t(x, y, z)$ is evaluated by ordinary LISP recursion. Then

$$
\begin{aligned}
T(x, y, z) = \ &\text{if } x \le y \text{ then } 0 \\
&\text{else } 1 + T(x - 1, y, z) + T(y - 1, z, x) + T(z - 1, x, y) \\
&\quad + T\big(t(x - 1, y, z),\, t(y - 1, z, x),\, t(z - 1, x, y)\big)\,.
\end{aligned}
$$

---

*Incidentally, [10] was John's first experiment with the use of TEX, a computer typesetting system that the author was developing while sitting in the office next to his. Without his generous provision of computing and printing facilities, TEX would never have existed.

The total number of expansions of the definition will then be $1 + 4T(x, y, z)$, because the latter function $U(x, y, z)$ satisfies the recurrence

$$U(x, y, z) = \textbf{if } x \le y \textbf{ then } 1$$
$$\textbf{else } 1 + U(x - 1, y, z) + U(y - 1, z, x) + U(z - 1, x, y)$$
$$+ U\big(t(x - 1, y, z),\, t(y - 1, z, x),\, t(z - 1, x, y)\big).$$

Before we analyze $T(x, y, z)$, it will be helpful to consider a similar but simpler function,

$$V(x, y, z) = \textbf{if } x \le y \textbf{ then } 0$$
$$\textbf{else } 1 + V(x - 1, y, z) + V(y - 1, z, x) + V(z - 1, x, y).$$

The function $V(x, y, z)$ can be understood as follows. Construct a ternary tree by starting with a simple leaf containing the triple $[x, y, z]$ and then by applying the following operation repeatedly: If any leaf $[x, y, z]$ of the tree-so-far has $x > y$, attach the nodes

$$[x - 1, y, z], \quad [y - 1, z, x], \quad [z - 1, x, y]$$

immediately below it. Then $V(x, y, z)$ will be the number of non-leaf nodes in the final tree. (This function $V(x, y, z)$ has been studied by Ilan Vardi [15]; some of his analysis is reproduced here.)

For example, the tree rooted at $[4, 2, 0]$ is

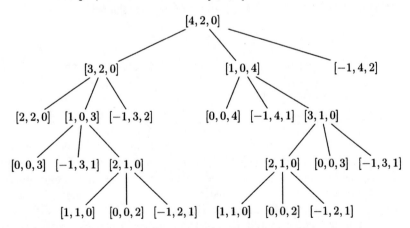

The evaluation of $V(x, y, z)$ is trivial when $x \le y$, and it's also fairly simple when $x > y$ and $x \ge z \ge y$: In that case we have

$$V(x, y, z) = 1 + V(x - 1, y, z) = 1 + x - z + V(z - 1, y, z).$$

A further simplification arises when we realize that the values of $V(x, y, z)$ are invariant if we translate all the parameters by any integer amount:

$$V(x + 1, y + 1, z + 1) = V(x, y, z).$$

Therefore we can shorten our notation and our discussion by assuming that $\min(x, y, z) = 0$.

Suppose the ternary tree has $[x, y, z]$ at the root, where we have either $x > y > z = 0$ or $z > x > y = 0$. Then all of its non-leaf nodes are of two kinds,

$$\begin{aligned} A(a, b) &= [a, b, 0] \\ B(a, b) &= [b, 0, a] \end{aligned} \qquad \text{where } a > b > 0.$$

Below $A(a, b)$ are the three nodes

$$[a - 1, b, 0], \quad [b - 1, 0, a], \quad [-1, a, b]$$

where $[a - 1, b, 0]$ is a leaf if $a = b + 1$, otherwise it is $A(a - 1, b)$; similarly $[b - 1, 0, a]$ is a leaf if $b = 1$, otherwise it is $B(a, b - 1)$; and $[-1, a, b]$ is always a leaf. Below $B(a, b)$ are the same three nodes; they appear in a different order, but that does not matter.

It follows that $V(x, y, 0) = V(y, 0, x)$, for all $x > y > 0$, and that $V(x, y, 0)$ has a simple combinatorial interpretation: It is the number of lattice paths that start at (x, y) and stay within the set

$$\{ (a, b) \mid a > b > 0 \}.$$

(A lattice path is a path in which each step decreases exactly one of the coordinates by unity.) We will say that such a lattice path is *confined*.

Confined lattice paths can be enumerated by using André's well-known reflection principle. (See, for example, [4, exercise 2.2.1–4].) Given $x > y \geq y' > 0$, the number of confined paths from (x, y) to a point (x', y') for some x' is equal to the number of all possible lattice paths from (x, y) to $(y', y' - 1)$ minus the number of such paths that touch a diagonal point. Paths of the latter type are in one-to-one correspondence with lattice paths from (x, y) to $(y' - 1, y')$; the correspondence is obtained by interchanging x moves with y moves after the diagonal is first encountered. Hence the number of confined paths from (x, y) to points of the form (x', y'), given x, y, and y', is

$$\binom{x - y' + y - (y' - 1)}{x - y'} - \binom{x - (y' - 1) + y - y'}{y - y'};$$

and the total number of confined paths starting from (x, y) is

$$\sum_{y'=1}^{y} \left(\binom{x+y+1-2y'}{x-y'} - \binom{x+y+1-2y'}{y-y'} \right)$$

$$= \sum_{k=1}^{y} \left(\binom{x-y-1+2k}{k} - \binom{x-y-1+2k}{k-1} \right).$$

This is the quantity $V(x, y, 0)$. Notice that we have

$$V(n+1, n, 0) = \sum_{k=1}^{n} \left(\binom{2k}{k} - \binom{2k}{k-1} \right) = \sum_{k=1}^{n} \binom{2k}{k} \frac{1}{k+1} = \sum_{k=1}^{n} C_k,$$

the sum of the first n Catalan numbers.

Returning to the evaluation of $T(x, y, z)$, we can use the same approach, but we must add to $V(x, y, z)$ the values $T\big(t(a - 1, b, 0),$ $t(b - 1, 0, a), a\big)$ at every node of type $A(a, b)$, as well as the values $T\big(t(b - 1, 0, a), a, t(a - 1, b, 0)\big)$ at every node of type $B(a, b)$. Fortunately these additional amounts are mostly zero. Our knowledge about the values of $t(x, y, z)$ allows us to conclude that, when $a > b > 0$, we have

$$t(a - 1, b, 0) = a - 1; \qquad t(b - 1, 0, a) = \begin{cases} 0, & b = 1; \\ a, & b > 1. \end{cases}$$

Therefore $T\big(t(b - 1, 0, a), a, t(a - 1, b, 0)\big) = 0$; and $T\big(t(a - 1, b, 0),$ $t(b - 1, 0, a), a\big) = 0$ except when $b = 1$. Only the nodes of type $A(a, 1)$ acquire nonzero surcharges; at such nodes we should add $T(a - 1, 0, a)$.

The number of non-root nodes of type $A(a', 1)$ in a tree whose root is of type $A(a, b)$ or $B(a, b)$ is the number of nodes of type $A(a' + 1, 1)$ or $B(a' + 1, 1)$. And the number of such nodes is the number of confined lattice paths from (a, b) to $(a' + 1, 1)$, which is

$$\binom{a - (a' + 1) + b - 1}{b - 1} - \binom{a - 1 + b - (a' + 1)}{a - 1}$$

by André's reflection principle. Therefore

$$T(b, 0, a) = V(a, b, 0)$$
$$+ \sum_{a'=2}^{a-1} \left(\binom{a+b-a'-2}{b-1} - \binom{a+b-a'-2}{a-1} \right) T(a'-1, 0, a').$$

The same formula holds for $T(a, b, 0)$, except that we must add the quantity $T(a - 1, 0, a)$ when $b = 1$; a root node of type $A(a, 1)$ makes a contribution, but a root node of type $B(a, 1)$ does not. Putting these facts together yields the following recurrence for the numbers $T_n = T(n, 0, n + 1)$:

$$T_{n+1} = V(n + 2, n + 1, 0) + \sum_{k=0}^{n-1} \left(\binom{n+k}{n} - \binom{n+k}{n+1} \right) T_{n-k}.$$

Let $V_n = V(n + 1, n, 0)$; the first few values of these sequences are as follows:

$n =$	1	2	3	4	5	6	7	8	9
$V_n =$	1	3	8	22	64	196	625	2055	6917
$T_n =$	1	4	14	53	223	1034	5221	28437	165859

It is not difficult to deduce that the numbers T_n grow very rapidly, in fact faster than A^n for any constant A:

Lemma 2. *If $\epsilon > 0$, we have*

$$T_n > n^{(1-\epsilon)n}$$

for all sufficiently large n.

Proof. Choose k large enough so that $k/(k + 1) > 1 - \epsilon$. Looking only at the kth term of the recurrence for T_n tells us that, for all $n > k$, we have

$$T_{n+1} > \left(\binom{n+k}{n} - \binom{n+k}{n+1} \right) T_{n-k}$$

$$= \frac{(n + k)(n + k - 1) \dots (n + 2)(n + 1 - k)}{k!} T_{n-k}.$$

Thus

$$\ln T_{n+1} > \ln(n+k) + \cdots + \ln(n+2) + \ln(n+1-k) - \ln k! + \ln T_{n-k}.$$

Iterating this relation yields

$$\ln T_n > \frac{k}{k + 1} n \ln n + O(n).$$

and the result follows. (A similar but weaker result was obtained by Ilan Vardi [15], who used the fact that $T_{n+1} > n T_{n-1}$ to prove that $\ln T_n > \frac{1}{2} n \ln n + O(n)$.)   □

In fact, we can prove a stronger lower bound by observing that for all $n \geq 1$, we have $T_n \geq \varpi_n$, where ϖ_n is the Bell number defined by

$$\varpi_{n+1} = 1 + \sum_{k=0}^{n-1} \binom{n}{k} \varpi_{n-k} .$$

Each term in the recurrence for T_n is greater than or equal to the corresponding term in the recurrence for ϖ_n, by induction. It is known [1, (6.2.7)] that

$$\varpi_n > e^{n \ln n - n \ln \ln n - n}$$

for all sufficiently large n. Thus T_n grows faster than $\big(n/(e \ln n)\big)^n$.

On the other hand, we can prove the upper bound

$$T_n < 3n! .$$

This is clear for $n \leq 3$. Let $t_n = T_n/n!$, and rewrite the recurrence for T_n as follows:

$$t_{n+1} = \frac{V_{n+1}}{(n+1)!} + \frac{1}{n+1} \left(t_n + t_{n-1} + \frac{n+2}{2n} t_{n-2} + \right.$$

$$\left. + \frac{n+3}{3(n-1)} \frac{n+2}{2n} t_{n-3} + \frac{n+4}{4(n-2)} \frac{n+3}{3(n-1)} \frac{n+2}{2n} t_{n-4} + \cdots \right).$$

The coefficients inside the parentheses are all ≤ 1, so we have

$$t_{n+1} \leq \frac{V_{n+1}}{(n+1)!} + \frac{1}{n+1} (t_n + t_{n-1} + \cdots + t_1) < \frac{3n}{n+1} + \frac{V_{n+1}}{(n+1)!}$$

by induction. And it is easy to verify that $V_{n+1} < 3n!$ for $n \geq 3$, because $V_{n+1} \leq 4^n$. (The Catalan numbers C_n satisfy $C_{n+1} < 4C_n$; hence $V_{n+1} < C_1 + 4V_n$ and we have $V_{n+1} \leq 4V_n$.) We have proved

Theorem 2. *When the tarai recursion $t(x, y, z)$ is used in a memoryless manner to evaluate $t(n, 0, n+1)$, the recursive definition is expanded $1 + 4T(n, 0, n+1)$ times, where*

$$e^{n \ln n - n \ln \ln n - n} < T(n, 0, n+1) < e^{n \ln n - n + \ln n}$$

for all sufficiently large n.   □

On the other hand, only $O(n^2)$ evaluations are needed when previously computed results are remembered; thus memory is especially helpful here.

A more precise asymptotic formula for V_n can be obtained by using generating functions. We have

$$V(z) = \sum_{n \geq 1} V_n z^n = \frac{1}{1-z} \sum_{n \geq 1} C_n z^n = \frac{C(z) - 1}{1 - z},$$

where $C(z)$ is the well-known generating function for Catalan numbers [3, §5.4],

$$C(z) = \frac{1 - \sqrt{1 - 4z}}{2z}.$$

Darboux's lemma (see [5]) now shows that

$$\frac{V_n}{4^n} = [z^n] V\left(\frac{z}{4}\right) = -\frac{8}{3} \binom{n - 3/2}{n} + O(n^{-5/2}) = \frac{4n^{-3/2}}{3\sqrt{\pi}} + O(n^{-5/2}).$$

The generating function of the numbers T_n is much more complicated, but it does satisfy a remarkable functional equation. We have

$$T(z) = \sum_n T_n z^n$$

$$= \sum_n V_{n+1} z^{n+1} + \sum_{n,k} \left(\binom{n+k}{k} - \binom{n+k}{k-1} \right) T_{n-k} z^{n+1}$$

$$= \frac{C(z) - 1}{1 - z} + \sum_{n,k} \left(\binom{n+2k}{k} - \binom{n+2k}{k-1} \right) T_n z^{n+k+1}$$

$$= \frac{C(z) - 1}{1 - z} + \sum_n T_n z^{n+1} \frac{C(z)^n}{\sqrt{1 - 4z}} - \sum_n T_n z^{n+2} \frac{C(z)^{n+2}}{\sqrt{1 - 4z}}$$

$$= \frac{C(z) - 1}{1 - z} + \frac{z(2 - C(z))}{\sqrt{1 - 4z}} T(zC(z)),$$

because $zC(z)^2 = C(z) - 1$ and $\sum_k \binom{n+2k}{k} z^k = C(z)^n / \sqrt{1 - 4z}$.

Open Problem 2. Obtain further information about the asymptotic properties of the coefficients $T_1, T_2, \ldots$. □

The evaluation of $t(x, y, z)$ turns out to be much, much faster if we apply the technique of lazy evaluation or "call by need" when expanding the definition. (See Vuillemin [16][17].) Indeed, we can ignore the third argument $t(z-1, x, y)$ in the recursion, unless we have discovered that $t(x-1, y, z) > t(y-1, z, x)$; so the number of times the **else** clause needs to be expanded satisfies the recursion

$$K(x, y, z) = \textbf{if } x \leq y \textbf{ then } 0$$
$$\textbf{else } \big(1 + K(x-1, y, z) + K(y-1, z, x)$$
$$+ \textbf{ if } t(x-1, y, z) \leq t(y-1, z, x) \textbf{ then } 0$$
$$\textbf{else } \big(K(z-1, x, y)$$
$$+ K\big(t(x-1, y, z), t(y-1, z, x), t(z-1, x, y)\big)\big)\big).$$

And this recursion turns out to be quite simple. First, if $x > y \leq z$, we have

$$K(x, y, z) = 1 + K(x-1, y, z) = x - y$$

because $t(x-1, y, z) \leq z$ and $t(y-1, z, x) = z$. Second, if $x > y > z+1$, we have

$$K(x, y, z) = 1 + K(x-1, y, z) + K(y-1, z, x)$$
$$= 1 + K(x-1, y, z) + y - 1 - z = (x-y)(y-z),$$

because $t(x-1, y, z) = x - 1$ and $t(y-1, z, x) = x$. Finally, if $x > y = z+1$, we have $t(x-1, y, z) = x-1$, $t(y-1, z, x) = z$, and $t(z-1, x, y) = x$; hence

$$K(x, y, z) = 1 + K(x-1, y, z) + x - 1 - z = (x-y)(x-y+3)/2.$$

Incidentally, when $x > y > z+1$, the expansions of **else** clauses occur at the arguments (ξ, y, z) and (η, z, ξ) for $x \geq \xi > y$ and $y > \eta > z$; when $x > y = z+1$, they occur at (ξ, y, z) and (η, z, ξ) for $x \geq \xi > \eta \geq y$. Since these arguments are distinct, no additional savings over call-by-need would be obtained by remembering previously computed values, unless $t(x, y, z)$ is being evaluated at more than one point (x, y, z). The fact that the necessary arguments are limited underlies the simple mechanical proof of termination found by Moore [12].

3. False Takeuchi Functions

Vardi [15] has considered a general recursion scheme of the form

$$v_h(x, y, z) = \textbf{if } x \leq y \textbf{ then } h(x, y, z)$$
$$\textbf{else } v_h\big(v_h(x-1, y, z), v_h(y-1, z, x), v_h(z-1, x, y)\big).$$

If we set $h(x, y, z) = 0$, the function $v_h(x, y, z)$ will of course be identically zero; a LISP interpreter will deduce that its value is zero after expanding the definition exactly $1 + 4V(x, y, z)$ times, where $V(x, y, z)$ is the function considered in the previous section. This is clearly the minimum number of expansions necessary over all possible auxiliary functions $h(x, y, z)$, if we do not or cannot use call-by-need.

Richard Gabriel used a Takeuchi-like function in extensive benchmark tests of LISP compilers, but his function was slightly different from Takeuchi's original:

$$g(x, y, z) = \textbf{if } x \le y \textbf{ then } z$$
$$\textbf{else } g\big(g(x - 1, y, z),\ g(y - 1, z, x),\ g(z - 1, x, y)\big)\,.$$

(Notice that in this case call-by-need is inapplicable.) Gabriel explains the discrepancy as follows [2, pages 10–11]:

> When the Computer Science Department at Stanford University obtained the first two or three Xerox Dolphins, John McCarthy asked me to do a simple benchmark test with him. We sat down, and he tried to remember the Takeuchi function, which had had wide circulation. Because it was simple and because there were many results for it in the literature, he felt that it would be a good initial test. Of course, John misremembered the function. But we did not realize it until I had gathered a great many numbers for it.

Indeed, Gabriel's book [2] gives detailed timings for the computation of $g(18, 12, 6) = 7$ on 132 different configurations, and he lists four additional variants of g that provide further types of benchmark tests.

The seemingly trivial change from $t(x, y, z)$ to $g(x, y, z)$ actually makes $g(x, y, z)$ substantially easier to compute, if $t(x, y, z)$ is not evaluated with memory of previous results or with call-by-need. Vardi [15] has shown that the corresponding running time $G(n, 0, n + 1)$ is asymptotically less than $(3 + \sqrt{8}\,)^n$, although the exact order of growth is not known. Vardi has also observed that Gabriel's recursion defines the following curious pattern of values:

$$g(x, y, z) = \textbf{if } x \le y \textbf{ then } z$$
$$\textbf{else if } y \ge z \textbf{ then}$$
$$\textbf{if } y = z \textbf{ or } (x - y) \textbf{ odd then } y$$
$$\textbf{else } z + 1$$
$$\textbf{else if } z \le x + 1 \textbf{ and } (z \le x \textbf{ or } x > y + 1) \textbf{ then } y$$
$$\textbf{else if } (z - x) \textbf{ even then } x$$
$$\textbf{else } y + 1\,.$$

Here is another example of a generalized tarai recurrence whose solution exhibits odd-even behavior:

$$b(x, y, z) = \textbf{if } x \le y \textbf{ then if } x = y = z \textbf{ then } 0 \textbf{ else } 1$$
$$\textbf{else } b\big(b(x-1, y, z),\ b(y-1, z, x),\ b(z-1, x, y)\big).$$

This time the output of the function is boolean — always either 0 or 1 — although x, y, and z range over all integers. The computed values turn out to be

$$b(x, y, z) = \textbf{if } x \le y \textbf{ then if } x = y = z \textbf{ then } 0 \textbf{ else } 1$$
$$\textbf{else if } z > y + 1 \textbf{ then if } (x - z) \textbf{ odd then } 0 \textbf{ else } 1$$
$$\textbf{else if } y = z \textbf{ then if } (x - y) \textbf{ even then } 0 \textbf{ else } 1$$
$$\textbf{else if } (x - y) \textbf{ odd then } 0 \textbf{ else } 1.$$

The generalized recursion v_h does not always define a total function by repeated expansion. For example, consider the auxiliary function

$$e(x, y, z) = \textbf{if } x \textbf{ odd then } 0 \textbf{ else } 1;$$

then we get

$$v_e(1, 0, 0) = v_e\big(v_e(0, 0, 0),\ v_e(-1, 0, 1),\ v_e(-1, 1, 0)\big) = v_e(1, 0, 0)$$

and the recursion loops endlessly. There is a simple characterization of all cases where v_h is total in the boolean case:

Lemma 3. *Let $h(x, y, z)$ map arbitrary integers x, y, z into 0 or 1. Then the recursive equation for $v_h(x, y, z)$ defines a total function v_h except in the following three cases:*

(i) $h(0, 0, 0) = 1$ and $h(-1, 0, 1) = h(-1, 1, 0) = 0;$

(ii) $h(0, 0, 1) = h(0, 1, 0) = 1$ and $h(-1, 1, 1) = 0;$

(iii) $h(0, 0, 0) = h(0, 0, 1) = h(-1, 1, 0) = 1$ and
$h(-1, 0, 1) = h(-1, 1, 1) = 0.$

Proof. If $h(0, 0, 0) = 0$ or $h(-1, 0, 1) = 1$, we have the well-defined result

$$v_h(1, 0, 0) = h\big(h(0, 0, 0),\ h(-1, 0, 1),\ h(-1, 1, 0)\big);$$

otherwise we have

$$v_h(1, 0, 0) = v_h\big(1, 0, h(-1, 1, 0)\big),$$

which loops in case (i) but gives $v_h(1,0,0) = v_h(1,0,1)$ otherwise. Similarly, we find that $h(0,0,1) = 0$ or $h(-1,1,1) = 1$ implies

$$v_h(1,0,1) = h\big(h(0,0,1),\, h(-1,1,1),\, h(0,1,0)\big);$$

hence $v_h(1,0,1)$ is well defined whenever case (ii) does not hold, except in the case when it leads to $v_h(1,0,1) = v_h(1,0,0)$.

If neither case (i) nor case (ii) holds, then $v_h(x,y,z)$ is well defined for all boolean values x, y, z, except in case (iii). And when $v_h(x,y,z)$ is defined for all boolean x, y, z, we can evaluate $v_h(x,y,z)$ for all x, y, z in $O\big(V(x,y,z)\big)$ steps.   □

When the boolean function v_h of Lemma 3 isn't total, we can always complete it to a total function $v_h(x,y,z)$ that does satisfy the recurrence. We simply assign arbitrary boolean values to $v_h(1,0,0)$ and/or $v_h(1,0,1)$, whichever is undefined. For example, there are four total functions $v_e(x,y,z)$ that satisfy the recurrence arising from the auxiliary function $e(x,y,z)$ considered above:

$v_e^{00}(x,y,z) = $ **if** x odd **then** 0 **else** 1;

$v_e^{01}(x,y,z) = $ **if** $x \leq y$ **then if** x odd **then** 0 **else** 1
                    else if x even **then** 1
                    else if y odd **then** 0
                    else if z odd **then** 1 **else** 0;

$v_e^{10}(x,y,z) = $ **if** $x \leq y$ **then if** x odd **then** 0 **else** 1
                    else if x odd **then**
                               if y odd **or** z odd **then** 0 **else** 1
                    else if y odd **or** z odd **then** 1
                    else if $y \leq z \leq x$ **then** 1 **else** 0;

$v_e^{11}(x,y,z) = $ **if** $x \leq y$ **then if** x odd **then** 0 **else** 1
                    else if x even **then** 1
                    else if y odd **then** 0
                    else if $z \leq y$ **then** 1
                    else if z odd **then** 1 **else** 0.

However, the recurrence $v_h(x,y,z)$ cannot be completed to a total function for *arbitrary* auxiliary functions $h(x,y,z)$. Consider, for example, the (admittedly contrived) mapping

$$h(x,y,z) = 2xy - 4x + y + z - 1.$$

There is no total function v_h because we would otherwise have

$$v_h(2,1,4) = v_h\big(h(1,1,4),\, h(0,4,2),\, v_h\big(h(2,2,1),\, h(1,1,3),\, h(0,3,2)\big)\big)$$

$$= v_h\big(2, 5, v_h(2,1,4)\big) = 16 + v_h(2,1,4).$$

An incompletable function can even be constructed when we restrict ourselves to auxiliary functions that are limited by the condition

$$h(x, y, z) \leq \max(x, y, z).$$

For example, suppose we define

$$\begin{aligned}
h(x, y, z) = \ &\textbf{if } (x, y, z) = (1, 1, 4) \textbf{ then } 4 \\
&\textbf{else if } (x, y, z) = (3, 3, 3) \textbf{ then } 2 \\
&\textbf{else if } (x, y) = (2, 3) \textbf{ then } 1 \\
&\textbf{else if } \max(x, y, z) \geq 3 \textbf{ then } 3 \\
&\textbf{else } \max(x, y, z).
\end{aligned}$$

Then we have $v_h(x, y, 3) = 3$ whenever $3 > x \geq y$. For if $x = y$, clearly $v_h(y, y, 3) = h(y, y, 3) = 3$; otherwise

$$\begin{aligned}
v_h(x, y, 3) &= v_h\big(v_h(x - 1, y, 3),\, v_h(y - 1, 3, x),\, v_h(2, x, y)\big) \\
&= v_h(3, 3, \leq 2) = 3.
\end{aligned}$$

Therefore we have, for all $y < 3$,

$$\begin{aligned}
v_h(3, y, 3) &= v_h\big(v_h(2, y, 3),\, v_h(y - 1, 3, 3),\, v_h(2, 3, y)\big) \\
&= v_h(3, 3, 1) = 3.
\end{aligned}$$

It follows that

$$v_h(3, y, 3) \ = \ \textbf{if } y = 3 \textbf{ then } 2 \textbf{ else } 3.$$

But we also must have

$$\begin{aligned}
v_h(4, 3, 1) &= v_h\big(v_h(3, 3, 1),\, v_h(2, 1, 4),\, v_h(0, 4, 3)\big) \\
&= v_h\big(3,\, v_h\big(v_h(1, 1, 4),\, v_h(0, 4, 2),\, v_h(3, 2, 1)\big), 3\big) \\
&= v_h\big(3,\, v_h\big(4, 3, v_h\big(v_h(2, 2, 1),\, v_h(1, 1, 3),\, v_h(0, 3, 2)\big)\big), 3\big) \\
&= v_h\big(3,\, v_h\big(4, 3, v_h(2, 3, 3)\big), 3\big) \\
&= v_h\big(3,\, v_h(4, 3, 1),\, 3\big).
\end{aligned}$$

And there is no y such that $y = v_h(3, y, 3)$.

Open Problem 3. If we restrict $h(x, y, z)$ to be strictly less than $\max(x, y, z)$, is there always a total function $v_h(x, y, z)$ that satisfies the generalized tarai recurrence?   □

We have considered Takeuchi's special case $h(x, y, z) = y$ as well as Gabriel's special case $h(x, y, z) = z$, so it is natural to consider also the recurrence with $h(x, y, z) = x$. Let

$$k(x, y, z) = \text{if } x \leq y \text{ then } x$$
$$\text{else } k\big(k(x - 1, y, z),\ k(y - 1, z, x),\ k(z - 1, x, y)\big).$$

This recursive definition yields only a partial function because, for example, we have

$$k(x + 1, x, x) = k(x, x - 1, x - 1) = k(x - 1, x - 2, x - 2) = \cdots .$$

However, there are infinitely many ways to define a total function that does satisfy the k recurrence:

Theorem 3. *Let c be any integer. The function*

$$k_c(x, y, z) = \text{if } x \leq y \text{ then } x$$
$$\text{else if } y \leq z + 1 \text{ then } c \text{ else } \min(y, c)$$

satisfies the generalized tarai recurrence stated above for $k(x, y, z)$.

Proof.   Notice that we have the special values

$$k_c(x, c, z) = \min(x, c) \,;$$
$$\text{if } x > y \text{ then } k_c(x, y, c) = c \,.$$

The proof is now by induction on $x - y$.
   If $x = y + 1$ we have

$$k_c\big(k_c(x - 1, y, z),\ k_c(y - 1, z, x),\ k_c(z - 1, x, y)\big)$$
$$= k_c\big(y,\ k_c(y - 1, z, y + 1),\ k_c(z - 1, y + 1, y)\big) \,.$$

If $y \leq z + 1$, this reduces to

$$k_c(y, y - 1, z - 1 \text{ or } c) = c \,;$$

and if $y \geq z + 2$, it is

$$k_c\big(y,\ c,\ k_c(z - 1, y + 1, y)\big) = \min(y, c) \,.$$

Thus we obtain $k_c(x, y, z)$ when $x = y + 1$.

If $x \geq y + 2$ and $y \leq z + 1$ we have

$$k_c\big(k_c(x - 1, y, z),\ k_c(y - 1, z, x),\ k_c(z - 1, x, y)\big)$$
$$= k_c(c,\ y - 1,\ z - 1 \text{ or } c \text{ or } x),$$

which equals c since $y - 1 \leq z - 1 + 1$ and $y - 1 \leq x + 1$.

And finally if $x \geq y + 2$ and $y \geq z + 2$ the right side of the recurrence reduces to

$$k_c\big(\min(y, c), c, z - 1\big) = \min(y, c). \quad \square$$

Corollary. *The least fixed point of the recursive definition* $k(x, y, z)$ *is* **if** $x \leq y$ **then** x **else** ω.

Proof. Whenever $x > y$, we have $k_c(x, y, z) = y$ when $c = y$ but not when $c < y$. $\square$

4. The Tarai Recurrence in Higher Dimensions

If we define

$$t(w, x, y, z) = \textbf{if } w \leq x \textbf{ then } x$$
$$\textbf{else } t\big(t(w - 1, x, y, z),\ t(x - 1, y, z, w),$$
$$t(y - 1, z, w, x),\ t(z - 1, w, x, y)\big),$$

it turns out that the function reduces to the simple mapping

$$t(w, x, y, z) = \textbf{if } w \leq x \textbf{ then } x \textbf{ else if } x \leq y \textbf{ then } y$$
$$\textbf{else if } y \leq z \textbf{ then } z \textbf{ else } w.$$

Therefore it is natural to conjecture that the m-dimensional generalization

$$t(x_1, x_2, \ldots, x_m) = \textbf{if } x_1 \leq x_2 \textbf{ then } x_2$$
$$\textbf{else } t\big(t(x_1 - 1, x_2, \ldots, x_m),\ \ldots,$$
$$t(x_m - 1, x_1, \ldots, x_{m-1})\big)$$

is satisfied by the m-dimensional "first rise" function

$$u(x_1, x_2, \ldots, x_m) = \textbf{if } x_1 > \cdots > x_k \leq x_{k+1} \text{ for some } k \geq 1 \textbf{ then } x_{k+1}$$
$$\textbf{else } x_1.$$

But this is false, for all $m > 4$. Here, for example, is a 5-dimensional counterexample:

$$t(5,3,2,0,1) = t\big(t(4,3,2,0,1),\, 2,\, t(1,0,1,5,3),\, 1,\, 5\big)$$
$$= t\big(t(3,2,t(1,0,1,4,3),1,4),\, 2,\, t(0,1,\dots),\, 1,\, 5\big)$$
$$= t\big(t(3,2,t(0,1,\dots),1,4),\, 2,\, 1,\, 1,\, 5\big)$$
$$= t\big(t(3,2,1,1,4),\, 2,\, 1,\, 1,\, 5\big)$$
$$= t\big(t(2,1,1,4,3),\, 2,\, 1,\, 1,\, 5\big)$$
$$= t\big(t(1,1,4,3,2),\, 2,\, 1,\, 1,\, 5\big) = t(1,2,1,1,5) = 2\,,$$

while $u(5,3,2,0,1) = 1$.

The true general behavior is somewhat complicated, although (fortunately) the complications do not get worse and worse as the dimensionality m grows larger and larger. Let us define an auxiliary set of functions $g_j(x_1,\dots,x_j)$ for $j \geq 2$ as follows:

$$g_j(x_1,\dots,x_j) = \textbf{if } j = 2 \textbf{ then } x_2$$
$$\textbf{else if } x_1 > x_2 + 1 = x_3 + 2 \textbf{ then } \max(x_3, x_j)$$
$$\textbf{else } g_{j-1}(x_2,\dots,x_j)\,.$$

Theorem 4. *The function*

$$f(x_1,\dots,x_m) = \textbf{if } x_1 > \cdots > x_k \leq x_{k+1} \textit{ for some } k \geq 1$$
$$\textbf{then } g_{k+1}(x_1,\dots,x_{k+1}) \textbf{ else } x_1$$

satisfies the m-dimensional tarai recurrence.

Proof. Given $x_1,\dots,x_m$, with $x_1 > x_2$, let

$$y_j = f(x_j - 1, x_{j+1},\dots,x_m,x_1,\dots,x_{j-1})\,.$$

We want to show that $f(y_1,\dots,y_m) = f(x_1,\dots,x_m)$.

If $x_1 > \cdots > x_m$, we have $y_1 = x_1 - 1$. Also $y_2 = x_1$ or x_3; $\dots$; $y_{m-1} = x_1$ or x_m; and $y_m = x_1$. We cannot have $y_1 > \cdots > y_m$, because $y_m > y_1$. Hence there is a unique $k \geq 1$ such that $y_1 > \cdots > y_k \leq y_{k+1}$. And this can happen only if $y_{k+1} = x_1$; otherwise $y_{k+1} = x_{k+2} < y_k$. It follows that $f(y_1,\dots,y_m) = g_{k+1}(y_1,\dots,y_{k+1}) = x_1 = f(x_1,\dots,x_m)$.

Assume now that $x_1 > \cdots > x_k \leq x_{k+1}$, where $k \geq 2$, and let a be as large as possible such that $x_i = x_{i+1} + 1$ for $1 \leq i < a$.

Then $y_i = x_{i+1}$ for $1 \leq i < a$. If $a = k$, we have $y_k = x_{k+1}$ and it follows that $f(y_1, \ldots, y_m) = g_k(y_1, \ldots, y_k) = g_k(x_2, \ldots, x_{k+1}) = g_{k+1}(x_1, \ldots, x_{k+1}) = f(x_1, \ldots, x_m)$.

Assume therefore that $a < k$; hence $x_a > x_{a+1} + 1$. Let b be as large as possible such that $x_i > x_{i+1} + 1$ for $a \leq i < b$. If $b = k$, we have $y_i = x_{k+1}$ for $a \leq i \leq b$; hence $f(y_1, \ldots, y_m) = f(y_1, \ldots, y_{a+1}) = f(x_2, \ldots, x_a, x_{k+1}, x_{k+1}) = x_{k+1}$, and $x_{k+1} = g_{k+1}(x_1, \ldots, x_{k+1}) = f(x_1, \ldots, x_m)$.

Assume therefore that $b < k$; hence $x_b = x_{b+1} + 1$ and $y_b = x_{b+1}$. Let $z = \max(x_{b+1}, x_{k+1})$. We have $y_i = z$ for $a \leq i < b-1$. If $a > 1$ and $z \geq x_a$, we have $z = x_{k+1} = y_{b-1}$, hence $f(y_1, \ldots, y_m) = g_a(y_1, \ldots, y_a) = g_a(x_2, \ldots, x_a, z) = z = g_{k+1}(x_1, \ldots, x_{k+1}) = f(x_1, \ldots, x_m)$.

Assume therefore that $a = 1$ or $z < x_a$. If $x_{b-1} > x_b + 2$, then $y_{b-1} = z$; otherwise $y_{b-1} = x_l \geq x_{k+1}$ for some l in the range $b+1 < l \leq k + 1$. If $b > a + 2$, we have $f(y_1, \ldots, y_m) = g_{a+1}(y_1, \ldots, y_{a+1}) = g_{a+1}(x_2, \ldots, x_a, z, z) = z = g_{k+1}(x_1, \ldots, x_{k+1}) = f(x_1, \ldots, x_m)$. If $b = a + 2$, the same chain of equalities is valid unless $x_{b-1} = x_b + 2$ and $y_{b-1} = x_l$ and $x_l \neq z$. In the latter case we cannot have $z = x_{k+1}$, for that would imply $x_{k+1} \geq x_{b+1} \geq x_l$, hence $x_l = x_{k+1} = z$. It follows that $z = x_{b+1} > x_{k+1}$, and $x_l < z = y_b$. Then $f(y_1, \ldots, y_m) = g_{a+2}(y_1, \ldots, y_{a+2}) = g_{a+2}(x_2, \ldots, x_a, z, x_l, z) = z = f(x_1, \ldots, x_m)$.

Assume therefore that $b = a + 1$. If $z = x_{k+1}$ we have $x_{k+1} \geq x_i$ for $b < i \leq k$; hence $y_a = z$ and $y_i = x_{i+1}$ or z for $a < i \leq k$. The first appearance of z among $y_{a+1}, \ldots, y_{k+1}$ will show that $f(y_1, \ldots, y_m) = z = f(x_1, \ldots, x_m)$.

Assume therefore that $z = x_{b+1} > x_{k+1}$. If $x_a > x_b + 2$, then $y_a = y_b = z$; hence $f(y_1, \ldots, y_m) = g_b(x_2, \ldots, x_a, z, z) = z = f(x_1, \ldots, x_m)$.

Assume therefore (and finally) that $x_a = x_b + 2$, so that $y_a = x_l \geq x_{k+1}$, where $b + 1 < l \leq k + 1$. Then $x_l < x_{b+1} = y_b$, and $f(y_1, \ldots, y_m) = g_b(x_2, \ldots, x_a, x_l, x_{b+1}) = z = f(x_1, \ldots, x_m)$. We have proved that $f(y_1, \ldots, y_m) = f(x_1, \ldots, x_m)$ in all cases. $\square$

A machine-based proof of Theorem 4 would be very interesting, especially if it could cope with functions having a variable number of arguments. Indeed, the author has checked the proof by hand thrice, and he believes it to be correct, but he does not ever want to have to check it again! Therefore he hopes to see before long a solution to

Open Problem 4. Prove Theorem 4 by computer.

We cannot conclude from Theorem 4 that the m-dimensional tarai recursion $t(x_1, \ldots, x_m)$ actually defines a total function, when $m > 3$.

We have only shown that $f(x_1, \ldots, x_m)$ satisfies the recurrence. If the repeated expansion of $t(x_1, \ldots, x_m)$ actually terminates for some sequence of arguments $(x_1, \ldots, x_m)$, it must yield the value $f(x_1, \ldots, x_m)$; but we have not demonstrated that termination will occur, and there is apparently no obvious ordering on the integer m-tuples $(x_1, \ldots, x_m)$ that will yield such a proof. Therefore we come to a final question, which will perhaps prove to be the most interesting aspect of the present investigation, particularly if it has a negative answer:

Open Problem 5. Does the m-dimensional tarai recursion equation define a total function, for all $m \geq 3$, if it is expanded fully (without call-by-need)? Equivalently, does the recurrence

$$
\begin{aligned}
T(x_1, \ldots, x_m) = \ &\textbf{if } x_1 \leq x_2 \textbf{ then } 0 \\
&\textbf{else } 1 + T(x_1 - 1, x_2, \ldots, x_m) \\
&\quad + T(x_2 - 1, x_3, \ldots, x_m, x_1) + \cdots \\
&\quad + T(x_{m-1} - 1, x_m, x_1, \ldots, x_{m-2}) \\
&\quad + T(x_m - 1, x_1, \ldots, x_{m-1}) \\
&\quad + T\big(f(x_1 - 1, x_2, \ldots, x_m), \ldots, \\
&\qquad\quad f(x_m - 1, x_1, \ldots, x_{m-1})\big)
\end{aligned}
$$

define a total function on the integers $(x_1, \ldots, x_m)$, for all $m \geq 3$? (Here f is the function of Theorem 4.)   □

Close inspection of the proof of Theorem 4 implies that a call-by-need technique *will* always terminate when applied to the recursive equation for $t(x_1, \ldots, x_m)$. If $x_1 > x_2 > \cdots > x_k \leq x_{k+1}$, the values $y_i = t(x_i - 1, x_{i+1}, \ldots, x_{i-1})$ need be expanded only for $1 \leq i \leq k + 1$, and this will be sufficient to determine the value of $t(y_1, \ldots, y_m) = t(x_1, \ldots, x_m)$ in a finite number of steps. (The proof is by induction on k.) However, the possibility remains that an attempt to expand the "irrelevant" parameters $y_{k+2}, \ldots, y_m$ might loop forever. If so, the tarai recurrence would be an extremely interesting example to include in *all* textbooks about recursion.

Acknowledgments

Special thanks are due to Carolyn Talcott for her comments on the first draft, to Richard Manuck for discovering reference [14], and to Prof. Takayasu Ito for the story about "taraimawashi." The preparation of this paper was supported in part by the National Science Foundation.

References

[1] N. G. de Bruijn, *Asymptotic Methods in Analysis* (Amsterdam: North-Holland, 1961).

[2] Richard P. Gabriel, *Performance and Evaluation of Lisp Systems* (Cambridge, Massachusetts: MIT Press, 1985).

[3] Ronald L. Graham, Donald E. Knuth, and Oren Patashnik, *Concrete Mathematics: A Foundation for Computer Science* (Reading, Massachusetts: Addison–Wesley, 1989).

[4] Donald E. Knuth, *Fundamental Algorithms*, Volume 1 of *The Art of Computer Programming* (Reading, Massachusetts: Addison–Wesley, 1968).

[5] Donald E. Knuth and Herbert S. Wilf, "A short proof of Darboux's lemma," *Applied Mathematics Letters* **2** (1989), 139–140.

[6] Zohar Manna, *Mathematical Theory of Computation* (New York: McGraw–Hill, 1974).

[7] Zohar Manna and John McCarthy, "Properties of programs and partial function logic," *Machine Intelligence* **5** (1970), 27–37.

[8] Zohar Manna and Amir Pnueli, "The validity problem of the 91-function," Stanford Artificial Intelligence Project, Memo No. 68 (August 19, 1968), 20 pages.

[9] Zohar Manna and Amir Pnueli, "Formalization of properties of functional programs," *Journal of the Association for Computing Machinery* **17** (1970), 555–569.

[10] John McCarthy, "An interesting LISP function," unpublished notes (Autumn 1978), 3 pages.

[11] John McCarthy and Carolyn Talcott, *LISP: Programming and Proving*. Course notes, Computer Science Department, Stanford University (1980). "Under revision for publication as a book."

[12] J Strother Moore, "A mechanical proof of the termination of Takeuchi's function," *Information Processing Letters* **9** (1979), 176–181.

[13] I. Takeuchi, "On a recursive function that does almost recursion only," Memorandum, Musashino Electrical Communication Laboratory, Nippon Telephone and Telegraph Company (Tokyo: 1978).

[14] Ikuo Takeuchi, "Dai-Ni-Kai LISP Kontesuto [On the Second LISP Contest]," *Jōhō Shori* **20** (1979), 192–199.

[15] Ilan Vardi, "The running time of TAK," Chapter 9 of *Computational Recreations in Mathematica* (Redwood City, California: Addison–Wesley, 1991), 176–199.

[16] Jean Etienne Vuillemin, *Proof Techniques for Recursive Programs*, Ph.D. thesis, Stanford University (1973).

[17] Jean Vuillemin, "Correct and optimal implementations of recursion in a simple programming language," *Journal of Computer and System Sciences* **9** (1974), 332–354.

[18] Ben Wegbreit, "Mechanical program analysis," *Communications of the ACM* **18** (1975), 528–539.

Addendum

The "hard" half of Open Problem 1, namely the mechanical verification of Theorem 1, has been resolved by John R. Cowles using ACL2, a successor to the Boyer–Moore Theorem Prover developed by M. Kaufmann and J S. Moore ["Knuth's generalization of McCarthy's 91 function," in *Computer Aided Reasoning: ACL2 Case Studies* (Kluwer, 2000), 283–300].

Substantial progress has also been made on Open Problem 2: Thomas Prellberg has a heuristic argument and compelling numerical evidence to show that

$$T_n = C\varpi_n \exp\left(\frac{x^2}{2} - \frac{x(3+x)}{2(1+x)}e^{-x} + O(e^{-2x})\right), \qquad xe^x = n,$$

where $C \approx 2.239433104$ is a constant. ["On the asymptotics of the Takeuchi numbers," in *Symbolic Computation, Number Theory, Special Functions, Physics and Combinatorics* (Kluwer, 2001), 231–242.]

The author's original formulation of Theorem 4 was incorrect, but a correct definition of the function $g_j(x_1, \ldots, x_j)$ was found in May 2000 by Thomas A. Bailey as he was working with John R. Cowles on Open Problem 4. As of June 2000, ACL2 has verified the corrected version of Theorem 4 when $2 \leq m \leq 7$.

The answer to Open Problem 5 is, surprisingly, "No" — even when $m = 4$: Thomas A. Bailey, James Caldwell, and John R. Cowles discovered in January 2000 that $t(3, 2, 1, 5) = \cdots = t(2, 1, 5, 4) = \cdots = t(1, 5, 4, t(3, 2, 1, 5))$, hence $T(3, 2, 1, 5) > T(2, 1, 5, 4) > T(3, 2, 1, 5)$ and call-by-need wins big.

Chapter 23

An Exact Analysis of Stable Allocation

[Originally published in Journal of Algorithms **20** (1996), 431–442.]

Shapley and Scarf [8] introduced a notion of stable allocation between traders and indivisible goods, when each trader has rank-ordered each of the goods. The purpose of this note is to prove that the distribution of ranks after allocation is the same as the distribution of search distances in uniform hashing, when the rank-orderings are independent and uniformly random. Therefore the average sum of final ranks is just $(n+1)H_n - n$, and the standard deviation is $O(n)$. The proof involves a family of interesting one-to-one correspondences between permutations of a special kind.

0. Introduction

Suppose n traders have n indivisible goods to trade, and each trader k has ranked the goods of all traders (including himself or herself) as a permutation

$$p_k = p_{k1}\, p_{k2}\, \cdots\, p_{kn}$$

of $\{1, 2, \ldots, n\}$. If i precedes j in this list, we write "$i > j\ (k)$" and say that k prefers i to j. An allocation of goods to traders is a permutation $g_1 \ldots g_n$ of $\{1, \ldots, n\}$ such that trader k gets g_k. Shapley and Scarf [8] defined what they called a "core allocation" g, which is *stable* in the following sense: If C is any coalition of traders (any nonempty subset), and if h is any allocation of the goods of C to the members of C, then

$$h_k \geq g_k\ (k) \quad \text{for all } k \in C \quad \Longrightarrow \quad h_k = g_k \quad \text{for all } k \in C. \quad (*)$$

The hypothesis of this condition asserts that $h_k \in C$ whenever $k \in C$, but it does not assert that $g_k \in C$ whenever $k \in C$. An unstable allocation arises if the traders belonging to some coalition can improve the lot of at least one coalition member by trading among themselves, without harming anybody in the coalition.

415

For example, suppose $n = 3$ and the preference rankings are

$$p_1 = 2\,1\,3,$$
$$p_2 = 3\,1\,2,$$
$$p_3 = 2\,3\,1.$$

Then just three of the six possible allocations satisfy $(*)$ when C is the full set $\{1, 2, 3\}$, namely $2\,1\,3$, $2\,3\,1$, and $1\,3\,2$. But $2\,1\,3$ is unstable because traders 2 and 3 can both improve their lot by swapping goods between themselves. Similarly, $2\,3\,1$ is unstable, but it is not quite as bad: If the coalition $\{2, 3\}$ exchanges goods, trader 3 is happier than before, while 2 is no worse off. The remaining allocation, $1\,3\,2$, is stable.

It is not immediately obvious that a stable allocation always exists, for all $n!^n$ possible ranking sequences. But Shapley and Scarf presented an algorithm by David Gale that always finds one. In fact, there is always *exactly* one stable allocation. Gale's procedure is similar to the famous Gale–Shapley algorithm for stable marriage [2][4], but it incorporates a new twist.

Alan Frieze and Boris Pittel [1] recently analyzed Gale's algorithm and discovered some remarkable simplifications in the course of their study. One of the main purposes of the present note is to exhibit some underlying combinatorial structure that accounts for the surprising phenomena that they discovered. Frieze and Pittel proved, among other things, that the total sum of ranks in the stable allocation g (namely the sum $r_1 + \cdots + r_n$, where $g_k = p_{kr_k}$) lies between $(\frac{1}{2} - \epsilon)n \ln n$ and $(1 + \epsilon)n \ln n$ with high probability as $n \to \infty$, assuming that the preferences p_k are independent and uniformly random. We will deduce the exact distribution of $r_1 + \cdots + r_n$, showing in particular that its mean value is $(n+1)H_n - n$, and in fact we will see that the joint distribution of the multiset $\{r_1, \ldots, r_n\}$ has a particularly simple form.

1. Uniform Hashing

First let's consider a simpler problem, namely to find an allocation g that satisfies $(*)$ when C is the full set $\{1, \ldots, n\}$ but not necessarily when C is a smaller subset. Such an allocation is *locally optimal*, in the sense that no trader can improve a selection unless some other trader loses ground. It's easy to achieve such an allocation by simply letting g_k be the first item of list p_k that is not in $\{g_1, \ldots, g_{k-1}\}$, for $k = 1, \ldots, n$.

This trivial allocation algorithm, "first-come, first-served," is precisely the method of *uniform hashing* that arises in the study of information retrieval [5, §6.4], when the preference lists (called "hash sequences" in that context) are chosen randomly. The analysis of uniform hashing is particularly simple, and we will see below that stable allocation can be reduced to the same analysis.

A more general way to obtain a locally optimal allocation is to let π be any permutation of $\{1, \ldots, n\}$, and then to let $g_{\pi(k)}$ be the first item of $p_{\pi(k)}$ that is not in $\{g_{\pi(1)}, \ldots, g_{\pi(k-1)}\}$, for $k = 1, \ldots, n$. The permutation π gives top priority to trader $\pi(1)$, then to $\pi(2)$, and so on. Indeed, *every* allocation that satisfies $(*)$ for $C = \{1, \ldots, n\}$ will be found by this method, for some π. The reason is that we must have $g_k = p_{k1}$ for some k, in any locally optimum g; otherwise the mapping from p_{kr_k} to p_{k1} for all k would contain a cycle, and we could give everybody on that cycle their first choice. Let $\pi(1)$ be any value of k with $g_k = p_{k1}$. Remove k from all preference lists and apply the same reasoning recursively to the remaining $n - 1$ traders. This defines a permutation $\pi(1)\,\pi(2)\,\ldots\,\pi(n)$ such that $g_{\pi(k)}$ is the favorite of trader $\pi(k)$ in $\{1, \ldots, n\} \setminus \{g_{\pi(1)}, \ldots, g_{\pi(k-1)}\}$.

Since every locally optimum allocation is obtained in this way using some π, the stable allocation must itself result from some π. And when the preference lists are random, any π behaves like any other. Thus we might expect that stable allocation statistics are essentially identical to the statistics of uniform hashing. This, in fact, is true, but we must be careful to make the argument rigorous.

2. An Algorithm

Let's now consider a simple algorithm that computes the stable allocation, given any sequence of preference rankings $p_1 \ldots p_n$. The following procedure is a sequential variant of Gale's parallel method, analogous to the McVitie–Wilson version [7] of Gale and Shapley's original stable marriage algorithm. The basic idea is to look for cycles among the traders' best choices, and to put such cycles into the allocation whenever they are found.

A1. [Initialize.] Set $(q_1, \ldots, q_n) \leftarrow (-1, \ldots, -1)$, $(r_1, \ldots, r_n) \leftarrow (0, \ldots, 0)$, $(g_1, \ldots, g_n) \leftarrow (0, \ldots, 0)$, and $t \leftarrow 0$. (During this algorithm, t will be a trader who makes proposals to other traders, or zero when a new trader needs to enter the picture. Variable q_k will be the number of a trader who currently wants trader k's goods, or $q_k = 0$ if trader k has expressed interest in somebody else's wares but nobody has reciprocated; $q_k = -1$ if trader k has not yet entered. Variable r_k is the number of proposals made so far by trader k. Variable g_k is trader k's allocation, or 0 if no allocation has yet been made.)

A2. [Introduce a new trader.] (At this point $t = 0$, and $g_k = 0$ if and only if $q_k = -1$. The traders with $g_k > 0$ have been assigned a permutation of their goods.) If all g_k are nonzero, the algorithm terminates. Otherwise, set t to some k with $g_k = 0$, and set $q_t \leftarrow 0$.

A3. [Propose.] Increase r_t by 1, then set $s \leftarrow p_{tr_t}$. If $g_s > 0$, repeat this step. (Trader t has expressed interest in the best remaining choice of list t, namely s.)

A4. [Is s spoken for?] If $q_s \geq 0$, go to step A5. Otherwise set $q_s \leftarrow t$ and $t \leftarrow s$, then return to A3.

A5. [Remove a cycle.] (There is now a cycle $s = s_0 \rightarrow s_1 \rightarrow \cdots \rightarrow s_m = s$, where $m \geq 1$ and s_{j+1} is the best remaining choice of s_j for $0 \leq j < m$. This cycle must be part of any stable allocation, so we incorporate it into g.) Set $t \leftarrow q_s$; then repeatedly set $g_s \leftarrow p_{sr_s}$ and $s \leftarrow p_{sr_s}$ until finding $g_s > 0$. If $t = 0$, return to A2, otherwise go to A3. $\square$

In step A3 there is always a path

$$0 = t_0 \rightarrow t_1 \rightarrow t_2 \rightarrow \cdots \rightarrow t_m = t$$

connecting all traders k such that $g_k = 0$ and $q_k \geq 0$. Trader t_1 entered in step A2, and t_{j+1} is the best remaining choice of t_j, for $1 \leq j < m$; also $q_{t_j} = t_{j-1}$ for $1 \leq j \leq m$. These invariant relations justify the parenthesized assertions within the algorithm.

The final allocation $g_1 \ldots g_n$ is stable. For if C is a coalition such that (∗) fails, let $k \in C$ be such that $h_k > g_k$ (k), but $h_j = g_j$ for all $j \in C$ such that g_j was allocated earlier than g_k by the operation of the algorithm. Then $h_k = p_{kr}$ for some $r < r_k$, so h_k was rejected by the algorithm. Consequently h_k belongs to a cycle that was allocated before the cycle containing g_k, say $h_k = s(0) \rightarrow s(1) \rightarrow \cdots \rightarrow s(m) = h_k$, where $g_{s(j)} = s(j+1)$ for $0 \leq j < m$. And all elements of that cycle belong to C; indeed, $s(0) \in C$, and if $s(j) \in C$ we have $s(j+1) = g_{s(j)} = h_{s(j)}$ by the choice of k, hence $s(j+1) \in C$. But we cannot have $g_{s(m-1)} = h_{s(m-1)} = s(m) = h_k$ unless $k = s(m-1)$; contradiction.

Moreover, the stable allocation is unique. If g is assigned differently on any cycle that leads to step A5, that cycle will be a coalition violating (∗).

3. A Constructive Lemma

We have observed that the stable allocation will be found by a first-come-first-served algorithm equivalent to uniform hashing, if some appropriate permutation π is used to give priority to the traders. For example, in the introduction we considered a case where $n = 3$ and the stable allocation was $1\,3\,2$. Any π in which trader 3 has priority over trader 1 would find that allocation in the circumstances considered there.

We can also consider permutations of the preference lists. Let $\sigma = \sigma(1)\ldots\sigma(n)$ be a permutation of $\{1,\ldots,n\}$, and suppose that trader $\sigma(k)$ uses list $p'_{\sigma(k)} = p_k$. This will permute the locally optimum allocations, and it may also change the stable allocation. For example, if σ is $2\,1\,3$, so that

$$p'_2 = 2\,1\,3,$$
$$p'_1 = 3\,1\,2,$$
$$p'_3 = 2\,3\,1,$$

the stable allocation becomes $g'_2 g'_1 g'_3 = 2\,1\,3$, because g'_2 must be 2 and then g'_3 must be 3. Allocating goods in the order $2\,1\,3$ was the worst of the locally stable alternatives when σ was the identity permutation $1\,2\,3$, but it is best in the modified problem. Shuffling the preference lists corresponds to shuffling the goods that the traders started with.

We are now ready to prove a key fact about stable allocation. Let us say that the prioritization π is *consistent with* the shuffling σ, with respect to preferences $p = p_1 \ldots p_n$, if the locally optimum allocation $g_1 \ldots g_n$ obtained by uniform hashing with priorities π is the stable allocation $g'_{\sigma(1)} \ldots g'_{\sigma(n)}$ when $p'_{\sigma(k)} = p_k$. For example, $\pi(1)\,\pi(2)\,\pi(3) = 1\,3\,2$ produces the locally optimum $2\,1\,3$, so this permutation π is consistent with the shuffling $\sigma(1)\,\sigma(2)\,\sigma(3) = 2\,1\,3$ just considered.

Lemma. *Let p be any sequence of preference lists. There is a one-to-one correspondence between all permutations π of $\{1,\ldots,n\}$ and all permutations σ such that, if π corresponds to σ, the prioritization π is consistent with the shuffling σ.*

Proof. Given p and π, suppose uniform hashing with priorities π produces the locally optimum allocation $g_1 \ldots g_n$. Write the preference lists in rows, with each g_k circled in its list p_k. Delete all elements to the right of g_k.

We will construct a shuffling σ whose stable allocation agrees with g. The construction involves two dynamically growing sets X and Y, whose significance will become clear momentarily. Initially $X \leftarrow \emptyset$ and Y is the set of all k where $g_k = p_{k1}$ (namely all row numbers in which the circled element is all by itself). Set $m \leftarrow 0$; as the construction proceeds, we will have defined $\sigma(\pi(1)),\ldots,\sigma(\pi(m))$ as a permutation of $\{g_{\pi(1)},\ldots,g_{\pi(m)}\}$. We will also have $X \subseteq Y$ and $\pi(m+1) \in Y \setminus X$.

Find the minimum k in $m < k \leq n$ such that either $k = n$ or $\big(\pi(k+1) \in Y \setminus X$ and $\pi(k+1) > \pi(m+1)\big)$ or $\pi(k+1) \notin Y$. Define $\sigma\big(\pi(j)\big) = g_{\pi(j+1)}$ for $m < j < k$ and $\sigma\big(\pi(k)\big) = g_{\pi(m+1)}$. If $k = n$, the construction is complete. Otherwise, remove $\{g_{\pi(m+1)}, \ldots, g_{\pi(k)}\}$ from all preference lists where they aren't circled. If $\pi(k+1) \notin Y$, set $X \leftarrow Y$ and let Y be the set of all rows whose first elements are now circled. (Since π defines g by uniform hashing, $\pi(k+1)$ will be in the new Y.) Set $m \leftarrow k$ and repeat the instructions of this paragraph.

A worked example will help clarify this construction. Let

$$\pi(1) \ldots \pi(9) = 5\,3\,4\,9\,1\,8\,2\,7\,6.$$

Table 1 shows a sequence of preference lists for $n = 9$ in which π defines the locally optimum allocation indicated by circled elements. All elements to the right of the circled ones have been erased, since they are irrelevant for our present purposes.

1: ③	4: 1 ⑤	7: 5 3 ⑧
2: ④	5: ⑨	8: 9 ⑦
3: ①	6: ⑥	9: ②

TABLE 1. Preference lists and their stable allocation.

The stable allocation determined by these preference lists happens to coincide with the circled elements in Table 1, so in this case the priorities π produce the stable allocation; but our construction works for any π, whether or not its locally optimum allocation is stable. Initially $m = 0$, $X = \emptyset$, and $Y = \{1, 2, 3, 5, 6, 9\}$. According to the rules stated, we proceed to set $k = 2$, since $\pi(3) \notin Y$. So we define $\sigma(5) = g_3 = 1$ and $\sigma(3) = g_5 = 9$; then we delete 1 and 9 from lists 4 and 8, and we set $X \leftarrow \{1, 2, 3, 5, 6, 9\}$, $Y \leftarrow \{1, 2, 3, 4, 5, 6, 8, 9\}$, $m \leftarrow 2$. Next, $k = 5$ since $\pi(6) = 8 \in Y \setminus X$ and $8 > 4 = \pi(3)$. (The fact that $\pi(4)$ also exceeds $\pi(3)$ is irrelevant, because $\pi(4) = 9 \in X$.) This time $\sigma(4) = 2$, $\sigma(9) = 3$, $\sigma(1) = 5$. We delete 2, 3, and 5 where they are not circled. After setting $m \leftarrow 5$ we have $k = 7$, because $\pi(8) \notin Y$. (Notice that $7 \notin Y$, even though row 7 now contains only its circled element. The construction changes Y only in the case $\pi(k+1) \notin Y$.) This time $\sigma(8) = 4$, $\sigma(2) = 7$, $X \leftarrow \{1, 2, 3, 4, 5, 6, 8, 9\}$, $Y \leftarrow \{1, \ldots, 9\}$, $m \leftarrow 7$. On the final round we set $\sigma(7) = 6$ and $\sigma(6) = 8$; the shuffled preference lists are shown in Table 2. It is easy to verify that their stable allocation matches that of Table 1, using the algorithm given earlier.

5: ③   2: 1 ⑤   6: 5 3 ⑧

7: ④   1: ⑨   4: 9 ⑦

9: ①   8: ⑥   3: ②

TABLE 2. Shuffled precedence lists that have the same
stable allocation as those of Table 1.

The inverse construction is analogous. If σ is any shuffling, circle its
stable allocation and prepare an array like Table 2. Begin with $m \leftarrow 0$,
$X = \emptyset$, and Y as before. Then repeatedly consider all cycles

$$\sigma(a_1) \leftarrow \sigma(a_2) \leftarrow \cdots \leftarrow \sigma(a_t) \leftarrow \sigma(a_1)$$

formed by elements $\{a_1, \ldots, a_t\} \subseteq Y \setminus \{\pi(1), \ldots, \pi(m)\}$. Here $\sigma(a) \leftarrow$
$\sigma(b)$ means that $\sigma(a)$ is the (circled) element in list $\sigma(b)$; for example,
$\sigma(4) \leftarrow \sigma(9)$ in Table 2 because the circled element in list $\sigma(9) = 3$ is
$2 = \sigma(4)$. The properties of stable allocation guarantee that at least
one such cycle exists, and our inverse construction will guarantee that
each cycle will contain at least one $a_i \notin X$. Call the largest such a_i
the *cycle leader*, and renumber the subscripts so that a_1 is the cycle
leader. Take the cycle with smallest leader, and set $\pi(m+1) \leftarrow a_1, \ldots,$
$\pi(m+t) \leftarrow a_t$. Remove elements $\{\sigma(a_1), \ldots, \sigma(a_t)\}$ from the tableau
in places where they are not circled. Then set $m \leftarrow m + t$ and repeat
the same process until all cycles have been recorded in π. Then set
$X \leftarrow Y$ and let Y be the row numbers that now have but a single
element. Repetition of these steps will produce a priority permutation π
consistent with σ.

It is not difficult to verify that these constructions invert each
other. The reader will find easily, for example, that the permutation
$\sigma(1) \ldots \sigma(9) = 5\,7\,9\,2\,1\,8\,6\,4\,3$ in Table 2 leads back to $\pi(1) \ldots \pi(9) =$
$5\,3\,4\,9\,1\,8\,2\,7\,6$. $\square$

4. A Theorem

The lemma we have just proved makes it easy to establish the main result
of this note. We say that uniform hashing on $p_1 \ldots p_n$ with priorities π
produces ranks $r_1 \ldots r_n$ if $r_{\pi(k)}$ is minimum such that

$$p_{\pi(k)r_{\pi(k)}} \notin \{p_{\pi(1)r_{\pi(1)}}, \ldots, p_{\pi(k-1)r_{\pi(k-1)}}\}$$

for $1 \leq k \leq n$.

Theorem. *When preference lists $p_1 \ldots p_n$ are independent and uniformly random, the probability that the stable allocation $g_1 \ldots g_n = p_{1r_1} \ldots p_{nr_n}$ has a given value of the (unordered) multiset $\{r_1, \ldots, r_n\}$ is the same as the probability that uniform hashing yields $\{r_1, \ldots, r_n\}$.*

Proof. Let $\{r_1, \ldots, r_n\}$ be any given multiset. If $p = p_1 \ldots p_n$ is any sequence of preferences and if σ is any permutation of $\{1, \ldots, n\}$, let $s(\sigma, p) = 1$ if $\{r_1, \ldots, r_n\}$ is the multiset of ranks in the stable allocation when trader $\sigma(k)$ has preference list p_k; otherwise $s(\sigma, p) = 0$. Then the probability that stable allocation on random preferences has ranks $\{r_1, \ldots, r_n\}$ is

$$\frac{1}{n!^n} \sum_p s(\sigma, p)$$

for any fixed σ.

Similarly, if π is any permutation of $\{1, \ldots, n\}$, let $h(\pi, p) = 1$ if and only if $\{r_1, \ldots, r_n\}$ is the multiset of ranks produced by uniform hashing with priorities π. Then the probability that uniform hashing on random preferences has ranks $\{r_1, \ldots, r_n\}$ is

$$\frac{1}{n!^n} \sum_p h(\pi, p)$$

for any fixed π.

We want to show that these sums are equal. This is now obvious, because the lemma implies that

$$\sum_\sigma \sum_p s(\sigma, p) = \sum_p \sum_\sigma s(\sigma, p) = \sum_p \sum_\pi h(\pi, p) = \sum_\pi \sum_p h(\pi, p)$$

and we simply divide by $n!^{n+1}$. □

Notice that this proof of the theorem remains valid even when the preference lists $p_1 \ldots p_n$ are not uniformly random. All we are assuming is a symmetry condition, that shuffled preference lists $p_{\sigma(1)} \ldots p_{\sigma(n)}$ have the same distribution for all σ.

5. Corollaries

The analysis of uniform hashing is quite simple, so our theorem immediately characterizes many properties of the ranks in random stable allocations. For example, let us find the expected value of

$$(z + r_1)(z + r_2) \ldots (z + r_n) ;$$

since this polynomial is a function of the multiset $\{r_1, \ldots, r_n\}$, we can analyze it by considering its behavior with respect to uniform hashing.

Let q_{kj} be the probability that $r_k > j$ in uniform hashing. This is the probability that $p_{k1}, \ldots, p_{kj} \in \{p_{1r_1}, \ldots, p_{(k-1)r_{k-1}}\}$, so

$$q_{kj} = \left(\frac{k-1}{n}\right)\left(\frac{k-2}{n-1}\right)\cdots\left(\frac{k-j}{n-j+1}\right) = \binom{k-1}{j}\Big/\binom{n}{j}. \qquad (1)$$

Standard binomial coefficient summation techniques [3] show that

$$\sum_{j=0}^{\infty} \binom{j}{m} q_{kj} = \frac{n+1}{n+m+2-k}\binom{k-1}{m}\Big/\binom{n+m+1-k}{m}. \qquad (2)$$

The expected value of $(z + r_1)\ldots(z + r_n)$ is therefore

$$\sum_{r_1,\ldots,r_n} \prod_{k=1}^{n} \left(q_{k(r_k-1)} - q_{kr_k}\right)(z + r_k)$$

$$= \prod_{k=1}^{n} \sum_{r=1}^{\infty} \left(q_{k(r-1)} - q_{kr}\right)(z + r)$$

$$= \prod_{k=1}^{n} \left(z + \sum_{j=0}^{\infty} q_{kj}\right)$$

$$= \prod_{k=1}^{n} \left(z + \frac{n+1}{n+2-k}\right) = \frac{1}{(n+1)!} \prod_{k=2}^{n+1} (kz + n + 1). \qquad (3)$$

In particular, the expected value of $r_1 + \cdots + r_n$, which is the coefficient of z^{n-1}, is

$$\sum_{k=1}^{n} \frac{n+1}{n+2-k} = (n+1)(H_{n+1} - 1) = (n+1)H_n - n. \qquad (4)$$

The other coefficients can be expressed in terms of Stirling cycle numbers if we note that the expected value of $(z + r_1)\ldots(z + r_n)(z + n + 1)$ is

$$\frac{1}{(n+1)!} \prod_{k=1}^{n+1} (kz + n + 1) = \sum_{k=0}^{n+1} \begin{bmatrix} n+2 \\ k+1 \end{bmatrix} \frac{(n+1)^k}{(n+1)!} z^{n+1-k}. \qquad (5)$$

For example, the coefficient of z^{n-2} in $\mathrm{E}(z+r_1)\ldots(z+r_n)$ is

$$\begin{bmatrix} n+2 \\ 3 \end{bmatrix}\frac{(n+1)^2}{(n+1)!} - (n+1)\begin{bmatrix} n+2 \\ 2 \end{bmatrix}\frac{(n+1)}{(n+1)!} + (n+1)^2\begin{bmatrix} n+2 \\ 1 \end{bmatrix}\frac{1}{(n+1)!}$$

$$= (n+1)^2\Big(\frac{H_{n+1}^2 - H_{n+1}^{(2)}}{2} - H_{n+1} + 1\Big)$$

$$= \frac{(n+1)^2}{2}\big(H_n^2 - H_n^{(2)}\big) - n(n+1)(H_n - 1)\,; \tag{6}$$

see [3, exercise 6.33].

So far we have used only the case $m = 0$ of (2). A similar argument, using $m = 1$, shows that

$$\mathrm{E}(z+r_1^2)\ldots(z+r_n^2) = \prod_{k=1}^{n}\Big(z + \frac{(n+1)(n+1+k)}{(n+2-k)(n+3-k)}\Big). \tag{7}$$

In particular,

$$\mathrm{E}(r_1^2+\cdots r_n^2) = \sum_{k=1}^{n}\frac{(n+1)(n+1+k)}{(n+2-k)(n+3-k)}$$

$$= (n+1)\sum_{k=1}^{n}\Big(\frac{2n+4}{(n+2-k)(n+3-k)} - \frac{1}{n+2-k}\Big)$$

$$= (n+1)(n - H_{n+1} + 1) = (n+1)(n - H_n) + n\,. \tag{8}$$

Hence, by (6) and (8),

$$\mathrm{E}\big((r_1+\cdots+r_n)^2\big) = \mathrm{E}(r_1^2+\cdots+r_n^2) + 2\,[z^{n-2}]\,\mathrm{E}(z+r_1)\ldots(z+r_n)$$

$$= (n+1)^2\big(H_n^2 - H_n^{(2)}\big) - (n+1)(2n+1)H_n$$
$$+ n(3n+4)\,. \tag{9}$$

The expected value of the variance of the ranks is therefore

$$\mathrm{E}\Big(\frac{r_1^2+\cdots+r_n^2}{n}\Big) - \mathrm{E}\Big(\Big(\frac{r_1+\cdots+r_n}{n}\Big)^2\Big) = n + O(\log n)^2 \tag{10}$$

while the variance of the rank sum is

$$\mathrm{E}\big((r_1\cdots+r_n)^2\big) - \big(\mathrm{E}(r_1+\cdots+r_n)\big)^2$$

$$= 2n(n+2) - (n+1)^2 H_n^{(2)} - (n+1)H_n$$

$$= \Big(2 - \frac{\pi^2}{6}\Big)n^2 + O(n\log n)\,. \tag{11}$$

The final rank r_n in uniform hashing is uniformly distributed in $\{1,\ldots,n\}$. Therefore the probability is $\geq \frac{1}{2}$ that at least one trader in a random stable allocation will be stuck with a piece of goods ranked in the lower half of his or her preference list. Indeed, the probability that $\max(r_1,\ldots,r_n) \leq \frac{1}{2}n$ is exactly

$$(1 - q_{1m})(1 - q_{2m})\ldots(1 - q_{nm}),$$

where $m = \lfloor \frac{1}{2}n \rfloor$; this is asymptotically

$$(1 - \tfrac{1}{2})(1 - \tfrac{1}{4})(1 - \tfrac{1}{8})(1 - \tfrac{1}{16})\ldots \approx .288788. \tag{12}$$

6. Conclusions and Conjectures

The running time of the simple algorithm we have presented for stable allocation is essentially proportional to the sum of ranks in the unique allocation, $r_1 + \cdots + r_n$. We have proved that the statistical properties of any symmetric function of $(r_1 \ldots r_n)$ are identical to the corresponding statistics for uniform hashing, provided only that the distribution of preference lists $p_1 \ldots p_n$ is invariant under shuffling. When the preferences are uniformly random, the expected value of $r_1 + \cdots + r_n$ is exactly $(n + 1)H_n - n$, and the standard deviation is $O(n)$.

Uniform hashing is equivalent to the classical stable marriage problem when all the girls have the same preference list. (See [6, Lecture 5].) A tantalizing research problem about stable marriages, stated in the author's lectures of 1975 [6], has still not been resolved: If the girls have any fixed set of preferences and the boys propose at random, does it follow that the expected rank sum $r_1 + \cdots + r_n$ of the male-optimum stable marriage is always $\geq (n + 1)H_n - n$? In other words, does the case of equal preferences for the girls (uniform hashing) give the greatest lower bound for $E(r_1 + \cdots + r_n)$? If so, the average would be tightly bounded, because the upper bound $(n - 1)H_n + 1$ is easy to prove [6, Lecture 3].

In fact, computer experiments for small n suggest a further conjecture: The maximum value of $E(r_1 + \cdots + r_n)$, when the girls have a fixed set of preferences and the boys propose independently at random, appears to be obtained if and only if the girls' preferences are cyclic, in the sense that we could rename boys and girls so that girl j's kth choice is congruent to $j + k \pmod{n}$.

Both conjectures about $\min E(r_1 + \cdots + r_n)$ and $\max E(r_1 + \cdots + r_n)$ have been verified by exhaustive enumeration when $n \leq 4$, and in several hundred random experiments when $n = 5$. Presumably there is a (simple?) reason for the empirical observation that, in some sense, the more the girls agree in their ranking, the less the men will have to propose, on the average.

Is there a simple expression for $E(r_1 + \cdots + r_n)$ when the girls' preferences are cyclic? For $n = 3, 4, 5$ the values are respectively $306/3!^3$, $884224/4!^4$, $104035560000/5!^5$. When $n = 4$, the worst seven preference matrices for the girls are

1 2 3 4	1 2 3 4	1 2 3 4	1 2 3 4	1 2 3 4	1 2 3 4	1 2 3 4
2 3 4 1	2 3 1 4	2 3 1 4	2 3 4 1	2 3 1 4	2 3 1 4	1 2 3 4
3 4 1 2	3 4 1 2	3 4 2 1	3 1 4 2	3 4 1 2	3 4 1 2	3 4 1 2
4 1 2 3	4 1 2 3	4 1 2 3	4 1 2 3	4 1 3 2	4 2 1 3	4 2 3 1

with respective total rank sums

884224,   879488,   875264,   875072,   874752,   874624,   872192.

All preference matrices not isomorphic to these seven, under renumbering of boys and girls, have smaller total rank sum, considered over all $4!^4$ preference matrices for the boys.

Acknowledgment

I want to thank Boris Pittel for introducing me to this problem and for patiently correcting my original misunderstanding of the definitions.

References

[1] Alan Frieze and Boris G. Pittel, "Probabilistic analysis of an algorithm in the theory of markets in indivisible goods," *Annals of Applied Probability* **5** (1995), 768–808.

[2] D. Gale and L. S. Shapley, "College admissions and the stability of marriage," *American Mathematical Monthly* **69** (1962), 9–15.

[3] Ronald L. Graham, Donald E. Knuth, and Oren Patashnik, *Concrete Mathematics: A Foundation for Computer Science* (Reading, Massachusetts: Addison–Wesley, 1989).

[4] Dan Gusfield and Robert W. Irving, *The Stable Marriage Problem* (Cambridge, Massachusetts: MIT Press, 1989).

[5] Donald E. Knuth, *Sorting and Searching*, Volume 3 of *The Art of Computer Programming* (Reading, Massachusetts: Addison–Wesley, 1973).

[6] Donald E. Knuth, *Mariages Stables* (Montréal: Les Presses de l'Université de Montréal, 1976). English translation by Martin Goldstein, *Stable Marriage and its Relation to Other Combinatorial Problems* (Providence, Rhode Island: American Mathematical Society, 1997).

[7] D. G. McVitie and L. B. Wilson, "The stable marriage problem," *Communications of the ACM* **14** (1971), 486–492.

[8] Lloyd Shapley and Herbert Scarf, "On cores and indivisibility," *Journal of Mathematical Economics* **1** (1974), 23–38.

Chapter 24

Stable Husbands

[Written with Rajeev Motwani and Boris Pittel. Originally published in Random Structures & Algorithms **1** *(1990), 1–14.]*

Suppose n boys and n girls rank each other at random. We show that any particular girl has at least $(.5 - \epsilon) \ln n$ *and at most* $(1 + \epsilon) \ln n$ *different husbands in the set of all Gale/Shapley stable matchings defined by these rankings, with probability approaching 1 as* $n \to \infty$*, if* ϵ *is any positive constant. The proof emphasizes general methods that appear to be useful for the analysis of many other combinatorial algorithms.*

1. Introduction

This is a tale of n girls and n boys who play a game called "stable matching," invented by Gale and Shapley [4]. Each player ranks each player of the opposite sex according to preference; thus, there are n permutations of the set of boys, representing the preferences of the individual girls, and there are n permutations of the set of girls, representing the preferences of the individual boys. The object of the game is for the boys and girls to match up so as to obtain n marriages that are *stable*, in the sense that no girl and boy prefer each other to their current partners.

For example, suppose Alice, Brigitte, Cindy, and Debra play with Wilfred, Xavier, Yuri, and Zeke; and suppose their preference rankings are as follows, from favorite to least desired:

Alice likes	$Y > X > Z > W$	Wilfred likes	$A > B > D > C$
Brigitte likes	$X > W > Y > Z$	Xavier likes	$C > A > D > B$
Cindy likes	$W > Y > X > Z$	Yuri likes	$B > D > A > C$
Debra likes	$X > W > Z > Y$	Zeke likes	$B > A > C > D$

The matching (AW, BX, CY, DZ) is unstable because, for example, A prefers Z to W and at the same time Z prefers A to D. But the matching (AZ, BW, CX, DY) is stable; most of the players are matched with a person other than their first choice, but the objects of their affections don't want to change. The given preferences also admit another stable matching, namely (AY, BW, CX, DZ). In this example only two matchings are stable.

The *stable husbands* of a girl are the boys she can be married to in at least one stable matching. Thus, Alice's stable husbands in the example are Yuri and Zeke. Brigitte has only one stable husband, namely Wilfred; she likes Xavier better, but he can't stand her.

2. An Algorithm

Gale and Shapley [4] gave a procedure to find a stable matching, given any set of preferences; McVitie and Wilson [11] extended the method so that all stable matchings would be found. More recently, Gusfield [6] exploited the interesting lattice structure of stable matchings to construct an elegant algorithm that simultaneously determines the stable husbands of all girls in $O(n^2)$ steps. For our purposes in the present paper it suffices to consider a simplified variant of these procedures, which finds the stable husbands of just one given girl G.

The basic idea is to maintain partial matchings in which each boy who currently has a partner is paired with his best possible choice among all stable matchings of a certain class. One of the boys who doesn't have a current partner is temporarily called P; he will *propose* to one of the girls, and she will then decide whether to accept or to reject his proposal (at least for the time being). The role of P passes from boy to boy according to the following simple rules:

A0. Initially all boys and girls are unpaired.

A1. If at least one boy has no current partner, let P be one such boy. Otherwise all boys and girls are already paired, and we have a stable matching; output G's partner S as one of her stable husbands, then remove the pair GS from the current matching and let $P = S$. (Henceforth we will consider only stable matchings in which G is not married to S.)

A2. If P has already proposed to all the girls, terminate the algorithm. Otherwise let H be the girl P likes best among all those he hasn't approached so far; P now proposes to H.

A3. If girl H has already been proposed to by a boy she prefers to P, she rejects P's proposal. Otherwise, she accepts P, and they become paired in the current matching; her previous partner (if any) now assumes the role of P. If she had no previous partner, the algorithm continues at step A1, otherwise it continues at A2. ☺

For example, suppose we run this algorithm on the preference rankings given in the introduction, always choosing the alphabetically least boy when there is a choice in step A1. Let the special girl G be Alice. Then the following events occur:

Step	Current matching	P	H	Actions
A1		W		
A2		W	A	A accepts W
A1	AW	X		
A2	AW	X	C	C accepts X
A1	AW, CX	Y		
A2	AW, CX	Y	B	B accepts Y
A1	AW, BY, CX	Z		
A2	AW, BY, CX	Z	B	B rejects Z
A2	AW, BY, CX	Z	A	A accepts Z
A2	AZ, BY, CX	W	B	B accepts W
A2	AZ, BW, CX	Y	D	D accepts Y
A1	AZ, BW, CX, DY	Z		output Z
A2	$(AZ), BW, CX, DY$	Z	C	C rejects Z
A2	$(AZ), BW, CX, DY$	Z	D	D accepts Z
A2	$(AZ), BW, CX, DZ$	Y	A	A accepts Y
A1	AY, BW, CX, DZ	Y		output Y
A2	$(AY), BW, CX, DZ$	Y	C	C accepts Y
A2	$(AY), BW, CY, DZ$	X	A	A rejects X
A2	$(AY), BW, CY, DZ$	X	D	D accepts X
A2	$(AY), BW, CY, DX$	Z		terminate.

Each girl is paired with the boy who has made her the best offer so far, except that the special girl Alice never has a partner in step A2 after the first stable matching has been found. The notation '(AZ)' in this chart means that Alice has no current partner, but that her best proposal so far has come from Zeke. In one place where '(AY)' appears, A rejects X even though she is currently unattached, because she prefers Y to X and she will not lower her previous standards.

To prove that this algorithm finds all stable husbands of G, let us suppose for convenience that exactly one proposal is made per unit of time, so that the tth execution of step A2 takes place at time t. Denote by M_t the set of all stable matchings such that G is not married to any of the S's already output before time t. Then M_0 is the set of all stable matchings, and $t \leq t'$ implies that $M_t \supseteq M_{t'}$. The correctness of the algorithm relies on the following crucial fact:

> If girl H rejects a suitor R between time t and $t+1$,
> then the pair HR is not part of any stable matching in M_{t+1}.   (∗)

The proof is by induction on t. If (∗) fails for the first time at t, suppose H rejects R in step A3 because she prefers Q. (Either $Q = P$ and R is her previous best partner, or $R = P$ and Q is her previous best.) Then we are assuming that HR is part of a stable matching in M_{t+1}, and in this matching the stability condition tells us that boy Q must be paired with some girl J he prefers to H. But Quentin must then have proposed to Jane before he proposed to Helen, so he must have been rejected by J at some time $t' < t$. Therefore, by (∗) and induction, JQ is not part of a stable matching from $M_{t'}$, contradicting the fact that $M_{t'} \supseteq M_{t+1}$. Rejection of R by H must therefore have occurred not in step A3 but in step A1; in other words, we must have $H = G$ and $R = S$, a stable husband. But then M_{t+1} does not include GS, by definition. Therefore (∗) must be true.

The matchings found in step A1 must be stable. For if some girl H prefers boy U to her current partner, she has not yet been proposed to by U; hence he prefers his current mate. In fact, (∗) tells us that the stable matchings found in A1 are characterized by the property that each boy has his best choice among all matchings in M_t. Thus, *when the algorithm outputs S, each boy has his best choice among all stable matchings such that G is paired with S.*

The algorithm terminates when some boy has been rejected by all the girls. According to (∗), this happens at some time t when $M_t = \emptyset$, namely when all the stable husbands S of G have been output.

3. A Random Model

We wish to show that the algorithm just stated will produce at least $c \ln n$ outputs with probability approaching 1, if c is any given constant less than $1/2$, assuming that the $n!^{2n}$ possible preference sequences are selected uniformly at random.

The basic idea will be to use the principle of *late binding*, which also has been called the principle of "conservation of ignorance" or "deferred decisions" — *le principe d'ajournement des décisions* in [8]. Instead of fixing the preference sequences in advance, we simply let them unfold to whatever extent the algorithm needs them as it runs. Thus, whenever a boy is asked to propose, he proposes to a random girl chosen uniformly from among the girls he hasn't tried yet. Whenever a girl receives her kth proposal, she accepts it with probability $1/k$. A stochastic process with these characteristics is equivalent to the original algorithm running on random preference sequences, because it has the same transition probabilities between states.

We can also simplify the algorithm further by assuming that each proposal is uniformly random, as if each boy has "amnesia" [8] and cannot remember any of the girls he has previously asked. If it turns out that he has just repeated himself, we will say that he has just made a *redundant proposal*; such proposals are always rejected. The algorithm now reduces to a fairly simple stochastic process, which uses the following data structures:

l = the number of boys who have played the role of proposer.
p = the boy who is currently proposing.
h = the girl who is currently being proposed to.
$x_1, \ldots, x_n$ = the boys who made the best offer so far to girls 1 to n, or zero if the relevant girl has received no offer.
$k_1, \ldots, k_n$ = the number of proposals received by girls 1 to n.
$A_1, \ldots, A_n$ = the sets of girls proposed to so far by boys 1 to n.

B0. Set $A_j \leftarrow \emptyset$, $x_j \leftarrow 0$, and $k_j \leftarrow 0$, for $1 \leq j \leq n$; also set $l \leftarrow 0$.

B1. If $l < n$, increase l by 1 and set $p \leftarrow l$. Otherwise output x_g, where g is the number of the special girl G; and set $p \leftarrow x_g$.

B2. Let h be a random number, uniformly chosen between 1 and n. (We say that boy p has proposed to girl h.) If $h \in A_p$ (that is, if p's proposal is redundant), repeat this step. Otherwise replace A_p by $A_p \cup \{h\}$ and go on to step B3.

B3. Increase k_h by one. With probability $1 - 1/k_h$, return to B2 (we say that girl h rejects the proposal). Otherwise interchange $p \leftrightarrow x_h$ (she accepts the proposal and her former partner will have to propose to somebody else). If the new value of p is zero, or if $h = g$ and at least one output has already occurred, go back to step B1; otherwise continue with step B2.   ☺

Algorithm B faithfully models the previous Algorithm A on random input, except for the redundant proposals. Notice that the new algorithm never terminates; step A2 stops when P has nobody left to propose to, but step B2 keeps making redundant proposals ad infinitum when $A_p = \{1, \ldots, n\}$. The details of Algorithm B aren't extremely simple, but we will see that certain aspects of its probable behavior are fairly easy to analyze, in part because it never terminates.

4. Probabilistic Preliminaries

Algorithm B can be regarded as a branching process, an infinite tree with nodes at levels $t = 1, 2, 3, \ldots$ corresponding to the tth time step B2 is performed. Every node α in this tree corresponds to a unique path from the root, representing one of the possible behaviors of the algorithm up to time t. This path determines the values of the data structures $(l, p_1, h, x_1, \ldots, x_n, k_1, \ldots, k_n, A_1, \ldots, A_n)$ at node α.

Every node α has $2n$ children $\alpha_1^a, \alpha_1^r, \ldots, \alpha_n^a, \alpha_n^r$, where α_h^a and α_h^r represent the nodes following a proposal that has been accepted or rejected by h. If $h \in A_p$, the transition probability from α to α_h^a is 0 and the transition probability from α to α_h^r is $1/n$; this case corresponds to a redundant proposal, which is always rejected. If $h \notin A_p$, the transition probability from α to α_h^a is $1/(k_h + 1)n$ and the transition probability from α to α_h^r is $k_h/(k_h + 1)n$, where k_h is the data value that becomes $k_h + 1$ in step B3.

The probability $\Pr(\alpha)$ of node α is the product of the transition probabilities on the path from the root to α; this is the probability that Algorithm B will take the computational path represented by α. Since the transition probabilities from each node to its children sum to 1, the sum of $\Pr(\alpha)$ for all nodes α on a given level t is 1.

We say that an event occurs at node α with *local probability* ρ if ρ is the conditional probability of the event given that the algorithm reaches α. Thus, for example, the local probability that a proposal is accepted at α is

$$\frac{1}{n} \sum_{h \notin A_p} \frac{1}{k_h + 1},$$

the sum of the transition probabilities in which the event occurs.

An event at α that depends only on the transition probabilities from α to its children will be called an *immediate event*. More general events may involve a sequence of node transitions in the subtree below node α; all such events have local probabilities at α as defined above. For example, we might speak of the local probability that at most five consecutive rejections immediately follow node α. Local probabilities at α are equivalent to unconditional probabilities in the branching process represented by the subtree whose root is α.

Our proofs will often be based on a technique of probability estimation that can conveniently be called the *principle of negligible perturbation*. The idea will be to change the transition probabilities between certain nodes, obtaining a "perturbed" probability distribution $\Pr'$ on which it is relatively easy to compute the probability of some given event.

Let t be a level of the tree, and let E be the set of all nodes at level t such that the given event is true. Let C be the set of all nodes α at level t whose probability has been perturbed somewhere along the path from the root to α; thus, $\Pr(\alpha) = \Pr'(\alpha)$ for all $\alpha \notin C$. Summing over all $\alpha \notin C$ and taking complements tells us that $\Pr(C) = \Pr'(C)$. If $\Pr(C)$ is small, then the perturbation will have a negligible effect on the probability of E, because

$$|\Pr(E) - \Pr'(E)| = \left| \sum_{\alpha \in E} \Pr(\alpha) - \sum_{\alpha \in E} \Pr'(\alpha) \right|$$

$$= \left| \sum_{\alpha \in E \cap C} (\Pr(\alpha) - \Pr'(\alpha)) \right|$$

$$\leq \sum_{\alpha \in C} |\Pr(\alpha) - \Pr'(\alpha)|$$

$$\leq \sum_{\alpha \in C} |\Pr(\alpha)| + \sum_{\alpha \in C} |\Pr'(\alpha)| = 2\Pr(C).$$

Expected values can be estimated in a similar way.

(The principle of negligible perturbation seems almost absurdly simple, but we will see that it simplifies our analyses in surprisingly nontrivial ways. The idea is similar in spirit to Laplace's method [10] of asymptotic analysis, where integrals are estimated by changing the integrand in unimportant portions of the domain. Another kindred method is Wilkinson's well-known technique of "backward error analysis" [13], in which numerical errors are conveniently studied by assuming that exact answers have been obtained from approximate data; the actual situation, in which approximate answers are calculated from exact data, is more difficult to handle directly.)

Many of the proofs below are based on estimates of the tails of probability distributions, using the following fundamental inequalities that we shall call the *tail inequalities*: Let

$$P(z) = p_0 + p_1 z + p_2 z^2 + \cdots = \mathrm{E}(z^X)$$

be the probability generating function (pgf) for a random variable X that takes nonnegative integer values. Then

$$\Pr(X \leq r) \leq x^{-r} P(x) \qquad \text{for } 0 < x \leq 1;$$
$$\Pr(X \geq r) \leq x^{-r} P(x) \qquad \text{for } x \geq 1.$$

The proof is easy, since we have $p_k \leq x^{-r} p_k x^k$ when $0 < x \leq 1$ and $k \leq r$, and also when $x \geq 1$ and $k \geq r$. In spite of this easy proof, the tail inequalities lead to quite effective bounds because we can often choose x to make $x^{-r} P(x)$ small.

(The history of these elementary inequalities takes us back to the early days of probability theory. Bienaymé [1] and Chebyshev [2] observed that $\Pr\big((X - \mu)^2 \geq r\big) \leq \mathrm{E}\big((X - \mu)^2\big)/r$ for all $r > 0$. Kolmogorov [9] went further and remarked that $\Pr(X \geq r) \leq \mathrm{E}\big(f(X)\big)/s$ for any nonnegative function $f(X)$, provided that $\mathrm{E}\big(f(X)\big)$ exists and $f(x) \geq s > 0$ for all $x \geq r$. In particular [9, equation 4.3.2], we get the second tail inequality when $f(x) = e^{cx}$ and $c \geq 0$. Chernoff [3] pointed out the wide applicability of such estimates.)

5. Probabilistic Lemmas

Consider the behavior of Algorithm B as $n \to \infty$. We will say that an event occurs *almost surely*, or 'a.s.', if the probability that it doesn't happen is $o(1)$, i.e., if the probability of nonoccurrence approaches zero as $n \to \infty$. We will also say that an event occurs *quite surely*, or 'q.s.', if the probability that it doesn't happen is superpolynomially small, i.e., $O(n^{-K})$ for all fixed K. If $p(n)$ is any polynomial function, the sum of $O\big(p(n)\big)$ superpolynomially small probabilities is superpolynomially small; hence if $m = O\big(p(n)\big)$ and if the events $E_1, \ldots, E_m$ individually happen q.s., the combined event 'E_1 and ... and E_m' also happens q.s.

Let $N = \lfloor n^{1+\delta} \rfloor$, where δ is a constant in the range $0 < \delta < \frac{1}{2}$. Throughout this section we shall consider only the first N proposals made by Algorithm B. Thus, probabilities of events are measured by summing $\Pr(\alpha)$ over all nodes α at time $N + 1$ such that the event occurs as the algorithm follows the path to α.

Lemma 1. *Each girl q.s. receives at least $\frac{1}{2} n^{\delta}$ proposals and at most $2n^{\delta}$ proposals (including redundant ones).*

The statement of this lemma and those below is deliberately somewhat ambiguous. One interpretation is that, if g is any particular girl, she q.s. receives the stated number of proposals. Another interpretation is that q.s. all n of the girls receive the stated number. The second statement is a corollary of the first, because of the nature of 'q.s.'; therefore we can prove each lemma using the first (weak) interpretation, but we can apply each lemma by using the second (strong) interpretation.

Proof. Let g be one of the girls, and let E_k be the event that the kth proposal is to g. This immediate event has local probability $\frac{1}{n}$, because each proposal in step B2 is uniformly random. Therefore proposals to g are like Bernoulli trials with parameter $\frac{1}{n}$, and the pgf for the total number of proposals received by girl g in the first N levels is simply

$$P(z) = \left(\frac{n-1+z}{n}\right)^N .$$

Let $r = \frac{1}{2}n^\delta$. By the first tail inequality, the probability that g receives at most r proposals is at most

$$\left(\frac{1}{2}\right)^{-r} P\left(\frac{1}{2}\right) = 2^r \left(1 - \frac{1}{2n}\right)^{\lfloor 2nr \rfloor} \le 2^r \left(1 - \frac{1}{2n}\right)^{2nr-1} \le 2^{r+1} e^{-r}$$

since $1 - x \le e^{-x}$, and this is superpolynomially small.

Similarly, if $r = 2n^\delta$, the second tail inequality tells us that g receives r or more proposals with probability at most

$$2^{-r} P(2) = 2^{-r} \left(1 + \frac{1}{n}\right)^{\lfloor \frac{1}{2} nr \rfloor} \le 2^{-r} \left(1 + \frac{1}{n}\right)^{\frac{1}{2} nr} \le 2^{-r} e^{\frac{1}{2} r}$$

since $1 + x \le e^x$, again superpolynomially small. ☺

Let us say that a boy begins a *run of proposals* when he becomes the proposer p in step B1 or B3; his run ends when one of his subsequent proposals is first accepted in step B3. In terms of the branching process, a run continues when a transition is from node α to a "rejected" node of the form α_h^r, and it ends at a transition from α to an "accepted" node of the form α_h^a.

Lemma 2. *Each boy q.s. begins at most $2n^\delta$ runs of proposals.*

Proof. Let b be one of the boys. His first run of proposals begins just after variable l increases to b in step B1; his subsequent runs occur just after variable p is set to $x_g = b$ in step B1 or to $x_h = b$ in step B3. Thus, at most two of his runs begin immediately after p becomes b in step B1.

The other runs occur when p becomes $b = x_h$ in step B3; and this can happen only if h is the girl who accepted b at the end of his previous run. Let E_t be the immediate event that the proposal at time t is to the girl who has most recently accepted b, or to girl 1 if b has never yet been accepted. Then the number of runs begun by b is at most 2 plus the number of occurrences of E_t; in other words, b can begin r or more runs only if E_t occurs $r - 2$ or more times. But the local probability of E_t is clearly $\frac{1}{n}$, so again we have the binomial pgf

$$P(z) = \left(\frac{n-1+z}{n}\right)^N$$

for the distribution of occurrences of E_t.

We now complete the proof as in Lemma 1, by setting $r = 2n^\delta$; the probability of r or more runs is at most $x^{2-r}P(x)$ for all $x > 1$. And we have seen that this bound is superpolynomially small when $x = 2$. ☺

Lemma 3. *Each run q.s. contains at most $n^\delta(\log n)^2$ nonredundant proposals.*

Proof. We will prove that for any fixed time t, $1 \le t \le N$, a run starting at t q.s. has the stated property. Let α be any node at level t, and let $P(\alpha, m, t)$ be the local probability that the proposals immediately following α will include at least m rejected nonredundant proposals before reaching time $N+1$ or before the first acceptance, whichever comes first. Then we have the recursive formulas

$$P(\alpha, m, t) = \begin{cases} 1, & \text{if } m = 0; \\ 0, & \text{if } m > 0 \text{ and } t = N + 1; \\ \displaystyle\sum_{h \in A_p} \frac{P(\alpha_h, m, t+1)}{n} + \sum_{h \notin A_p} \frac{k_h P(\alpha_h^r, m-1, t+1)}{(k_h + 1)n}, \\ & \text{otherwise.} \end{cases}$$

According to Lemma 1, we may assume that the upper bounds $k_h \le 2n^\delta$ hold for $1 \le h \le n$. (The validity of this assumption is discussed below.) Then it follows by induction on $N + 1 - t$ that

$$P(\alpha, m, t) \le \left(\frac{2n^\delta}{2n^\delta + 1}\right)^m.$$

If we now choose $m = \lfloor n^\delta(\log n)^2 \rfloor$, the local probability that there are more than m nonredundant proposals in a run starting at α is at most

$$\exp\left(\frac{-m}{(2n^\delta + 1)}\right) = \exp\left(-\frac{1}{2}(\log n)^2 + o(1)\right).$$

Multiplying by $\Pr(\alpha)$ and summing over all α on level t gives a total probability of at most $\exp\left(-\frac{1}{2}(\log n)^2 + o(1)\right)$, which is superpolynomially small. ☺

The previous proof uses a convenient simplification, indicated by the words "According to Lemma 1, we may assume that ...". The assumption we are making holds q.s., but it is not always true; moreover, it is a probabilistic assertion about time $N + 1$. So we should be careful that we are not fallaciously using the future to influence probability calculations in the past. A rigorous justification can be made by appealing to the principle of negligible perturbation: We simply recompute the transition probabilities when the assumption $k_h \leq 2n^\delta$ is invalid.

More precisely, if α is any node in the branching process, we let the perturbed transition probabilities from α to α_h^a and α_h^r be $1/(k_h' + 1)n$ and $k_h'/(k_h' + 1)n$, respectively, where

$$k_h' = \min(k_h, 2n^\delta).$$

The proof of Lemma 3 is valid for the perturbed branching process, using k_h' in place of k_h in the formula for $P(\alpha, m, t)$. Thus, the proof establishes that each run in the perturbed branching process q.s. contains at most $n^\delta (\log n)^2$ nonredundant proposals. And this same conclusion also holds q.s. in the unperturbed branching process, because the probability of its falsity can increase by at most $2\Pr(C)$, where C is the condition that some transition probability has been perturbed between the root and level $N + 1$. Lemma 1 tells us that $\Pr(C)$ is superpolynomially small, because the path to a node α at level $N + 1$ involves a perturbed transition probability only if some girl in the state represented by α has received more than $2n^\delta$ proposals before time $N + 1$.

Lemma 4. *Each boy q.s. proposes to at most $2n^{2\delta}(\log n)^2$ girls.*

Proof. Multiply the results of Lemmas 2 and 3. ☺

Lemma 5. *Each run q.s. contains at most $n^\delta (\log n)^2$ proposals.*

Proof. Let t be a fixed time, $1 \leq t \leq N$, and let α be any node at level t. A proposal is rejected with local probability $\sum_{h \in A_p} 1/n + \sum_{h \notin A_p} k_h/(k_h + 1)n$.

By the previous lemmas and the principle of negligible perturbation, we can assume that $\|A_p\| \leq 2n^{2\delta}(\log n)^2$ and $k_h \leq 2n^\delta$. Let $\rho = \|A_p\|/n$. Then the local probability of a run continuing one more step is at most

$$\rho + (1 - \rho)\frac{2n^\delta}{2n^\delta + 1} = \frac{2n^\delta + \rho}{2n^\delta + 1} \leq \frac{2n^\delta + 2n^{2\delta-1}(\log n)^2}{2n^\delta + 1} = \rho'.$$

(If the assumptions fail and the local probability is actually greater than this number ρ', we can perturb it by artificially decreasing the probability of rejection and increasing the probability of acceptance. For example, we can define the transition probabilities from α to α_h^a and α_h^r to be respectively $(1 - \rho')/n$ and ρ'/n, for $1 \leq h \leq n$. The perturbed algorithm need not behave at all like the original algorithm does; for example, a boy's redundant proposals might be accepted with positive probability. The principle of negligible perturbations requires only that the nodes of the tree remain the same and that the transition probabilities be consistent with all assumptions of the proof.)

Since $\delta < \frac{1}{2}$, the local probability of m consecutive redundant or rejected proposals is at most

$$(\rho')^m < \left(1 - \frac{1}{3n^\delta}\right)^m$$

for sufficiently large n. Consequently we can complete the proof as in Lemma 3. ☺

Notice that the principle of negligible perturbations has permitted us, in this proof, to estimate probabilities of events that start at time t by using assumptions that might fail at some future time $> t$. (Thus, $\|A_p\|$ might be $\leq 2n^{2\delta}(\log n)^2$ at the beginning of a run but not at the end.) Arguments based on a weaker principle, which would require only that the assumptions hold at time t, would be more complicated; we would have to argue that $\|A_p\|$ cannot grow by more than 1 at each time step, and our upper bound would be $\left(\rho' + m/\left(n(2n^\delta + 1)\right)\right)^m$ instead of $(\rho')^m$.

Lemma 6. *Each boy q.s. makes at most $2n^{2\delta}(\log n)^2$ proposals.*

Proof. Multiply the results of Lemmas 2 and 5. ☺

Lemma 7. *Each boy q.s. proposes to a given girl at most $\log n$ times.*

Proof. Let b be one of the boys and let j be one of the girls. Perturb the process so that after b makes n proposals, none of his subsequent proposals has positive probability of being made to j. This perturbation is negligible, because b q.s. makes fewer than n proposals (Lemma 6).

Furthermore, if b hasn't made n proposals by time $N + 1$, pretend that he continues proposing until he has done it n times. This can only increase the number of proposals he makes to j.

The pgf for the total number of proposals by b to j is then

$$P(z) = \left(\frac{n - 1 + z}{n}\right)^n ,$$

because b has amnesia; each of his n proposals is uniform among the girls. The probability that he has made more than $\log n$ of them to j is therefore at most

$$(\ln n)^{-\log n} \left(\frac{n - 1 + \ln n}{n} \right)^n = \exp\bigl(-(\log n)(\ln \ln n) + O(\ln n)\bigr),$$

and this is superpolynomially small. ☺

Incidentally, we have adopted here the convention of [5, Section 9.2] that 'log' is used for logarithms in contexts where the base is immaterial, while 'ln' denotes the special case of natural logs.

Lemma 8. *Each girl q.s. receives at least $\frac{1}{2} n^{\delta} / \log n$ nonredundant proposals.*

Proof. A girl q.s. receives $\frac{1}{2} n^{\delta}$ proposals by Lemma 1, but at most $\log n$ from any one boy by Lemma 7. ☺

6. The Main Theorem

We are almost ready to show that Algorithm B a.s. produces $\Theta(\log n)$ outputs. (This final result will be "almost sure" but not "quite sure.") First we need to analyze the time of the first output, because steps B1 and B3 change their behavior at that time.

The first output occurs as soon as each of the n girls has received at least one proposal. We can prove that this q.s. happens long before time $N = \lfloor n^{1+\delta} \rfloor$:

Lemma 9. *Let $N_0 = \lfloor n \ln n \ln \ln n \rfloor$. Each girl q.s. receives at least one proposal and at most $\ln n \, (\ln \ln n)^2$ proposals during the first N_0 steps.*

Proof. The pgf for proposals to g satisfies

$$P(x) = \left(\frac{n - 1 + x}{n} \right)^{N_0} \leq \exp\bigl((x - 1) \ln n \ln \ln n + o(1)\bigr)$$

for all real x. The probability that g receives no proposal is $P(0) \leq \exp\bigl(-\ln n \ln \ln n + o(1)\bigr)$; on the other hand the probability that she receives $\ln n \, (\ln \ln n)^2$ or more is at most

$$2^{-\ln n \, (\ln \ln n)^2} P(2) \leq \exp\bigl(-(\ln 2)(\ln n)(\ln \ln n)^2 + \ln n \ln \ln n + o(1)\bigr).$$

Both of these bounds are superpolynomially small. ☺

Lemma 10. *Let ϵ be a positive constant. A girl who has received m nonredundant proposals will accept at least $(1 - \epsilon) \ln m$ of them, with probability $1 - O(m^{-\epsilon^2/2})$ as $m \to \infty$. She will accept at most $(1 + \epsilon) \ln m$ of them with probability $1 - O(m^{-\epsilon^2/2+\epsilon^3/6})$ as $m \to \infty$. Moreover, she will accept at most $m/(\ln m)^3$ of them with probability $1 - O\left(\exp(-m/(\ln m)^2 + 7m \, (\ln \ln m)/(\ln m)^3)\right)$ as $m \to \infty$.*

Proof. She accepts the kth with probability $1/k$, so the pgf for the total number of acceptances is

$$P(z) = \frac{z}{1} \frac{1+z}{2} \cdots \frac{m-1+z}{m} = \binom{m-1+z}{m} = \frac{1}{\Gamma(z)m^{\underline{1-z}}}.$$

(The notation $z^{\underline{w}} = z!/(z-w)!$ for factorial powers is discussed in [5, Section 5.5].) The probability that she accepts fewer than $(1 - \epsilon) \ln m$ is at most

$$(1-\epsilon)^{-(1-\epsilon)\ln m} P(1-\epsilon) = \frac{m^{-(1-\epsilon)\ln(1-\epsilon)}}{\Gamma(1-\epsilon)\,m^{\underline{\epsilon}}} \leq \frac{m^{\epsilon-\epsilon^2/2}}{\Gamma(1-\epsilon)\,m^{\underline{\epsilon}}},$$

and this is $O(m^{-\epsilon^2/2})$ because $m^{\underline{\epsilon}} = m^\epsilon + O(m^{\epsilon-1})$. (See the answer to exercise 9.44 in [5].) Similarly, she accepts more than $(1 + \epsilon) \ln n$ with probability at most

$$(1+\epsilon)^{-(1+\epsilon)\ln m} P(1+\epsilon) \leq \frac{m^{-\epsilon-\epsilon^2/2+\epsilon^3/6}}{\Gamma(1+\epsilon)\,m^{\underline{-\epsilon}}} = O(m^{-\epsilon^2/2+\epsilon^3/6}).$$

The probability that she accepts more than $m_0 = m/(\ln m)^3$ of them is at most

$$m_0^{-m_0} P(m_0) = \exp\left(-m_0 \ln m_0 + \ln \Gamma(m+m_0) - \ln \Gamma(m_0) - \ln m!\right)$$

$$= \exp\left(-m_0(\ln m - 6 \ln \ln m + O(1))\right)$$

by Stirling's approximation. ☺

Theorem. *Assume that n girls and n boys have independent random preference rankings, and let G be one of the girls. Let c be a constant $< \frac{1}{2}$ and let C be a constant > 1. Then G a.s. has at least $c \ln n$ and at most $C \ln n$ stable husbands.*

Proof. The stable husbands of G are output by Algorithm A, which is equivalent to Algorithm B. The number of outputs is the number of times g accepts a proposal in Algorithm B, minus the number of times she accepts a proposal before the first output.

We have shown in Lemma 8 that g will q.s. receive at least $\frac{1}{2}n^\delta/\log n$ nonredundant proposals, among the first $n^{1+\delta}$ proposals made by Algorithm B, if δ is any constant between 0 and $\frac{1}{2}$. Therefore, by the first estimate of Lemma 10, she will a.s. accept at least $(1-\epsilon)\delta\ln n - O(\log\log n)$ proposals.

On the other hand, g receives at most n nonredundant proposals altogether. Therefore, by the second estimate of Lemma 10, she will a.s. accept at most $(1+\epsilon)\ln n$ of them.

Furthermore, by Lemma 9, the first output q.s. occurs before she has received $m = \ln n\,(\ln\ln n)^2$ nonredundant proposals. Therefore (by the third estimate of Lemma 10) she will accept at most

$$\frac{m}{(\ln m)^3} = \frac{\ln n}{\ln\ln n}\left(1 + O\left(\frac{\log\log\log n}{\log\log n}\right)\right) = o(\log n)$$

proposals before the first output, with probability

$$1 - O\left(\exp\left(-\ln n + O\left(\frac{\log n\log\log\log n}{\log\log n}\right)\right)\right) = 1 - \frac{1}{n^{1+o(1)}}\,.$$

So the number of outputs will a.s. exceed $c\ln n$ and be less than $C\ln n$ for all large n, if we choose δ and ϵ so that $(1-\epsilon)\delta > c$ and $1+\epsilon < C$.   ☺

7. Remarks

Inspection of the proof of the theorem shows that the conclusion holds with probability $1 - O(n^{-\gamma})$, where γ is any constant less than both $(1-2c)^2/2$ and $(C-1)^2/2 - (C-1)^3/6$. We cannot improve this estimate to $1 - O(n^{-1})$, because there is probability $\sqrt{\ln n}/n$ that the first proposal to G will come from one of her $\sqrt{\ln n}$ favorite boys. In such a case she can have at most $\sqrt{\ln n}$ stable husbands, because the first stable marriage found by Algorithm A gives every girl her *least* preferred stable husband.

Our theorem proves that random preferences a.s. guarantee an unbounded number of stable matchings, since every stable husband is part of at least one stable matching. Can it be shown that the a.s. lower bound of stable matchings grows faster than this, say as $\Omega(\log n)^2$? Pittel [12] has proved that the *expected* number of stable matchings is asymptotically $e^{-1}n \ln n$. However, Pittel's theorem does not prove that a large number of matchings will almost surely occur; constructions are known [7] where certain preference matrices give rise to at least 2^{n-1} stable matchings, and such examples may be common enough to account for the relatively high expected value.

This research was supported in part by the National Science Foundation and in part by the Office of Naval Research.

References

[1] J. Bienaymé, "Considérations à l'appui de la découverte de Laplace sur la loi de probabilité dans la méthode des moindres carrés," *Comptes Rendus hebdomadaires des séances de l'Académie des Sciences* **37** (Paris: 1853), 309–324.

[2] P. L. Chebyshev, "О средних величинах," *Matematicheskiĭ Sbornik'* **2** (1867), 1–9; reprinted in his *Polnoe Sobranie Sochineniĭ*, volume 2, 431–437. French translation, "Des valeurs moyennes," *Journal de Mathématiques pures et appliquées* (2) **12** (1867), 177–184; reprinted in *Œuvres de P.-L. Tchébyshef* **1** (1899), 685–694.

[3] Herman Chernoff, "A measure of asymptotic efficiency for tests of a hypothesis based on the sum of observations," *Annals of Mathematical Statistics* **23** (1952), 493–507.

[4] D. Gale and L. S. Shapley, "College admissions and the stability of marriage," *American Mathematical Monthly* **69** (1962), 9–15.

[5] Ronald L. Graham, Donald E. Knuth, and Oren Patashnik, *Concrete Mathematics: A Foundation for Computer Science* (Reading, Massachusetts: Addison–Wesley, 1989).

[6] Dan Gusfield, "Three fast algorithms for four problems in stable marriage," *SIAM Journal on Computing* **16** (1987), 111–128.

[7] Robert W. Irving and Paul Leather, "The complexity of counting stable marriages," *SIAM Journal on Computing* **15** (1986), 655–667.

[8] Donald E. Knuth, *Mariages Stables* (Montréal: Les Presses de l'Université de Montréal, 1976). English translation by Martin Goldstein, *Stable Marriage and its Relation to Other Combinatorial Problems* (Providence, Rhode Island: American Mathematical Society, 1997).

[9] A. Kolmogoroff, *Grundbegriffe der Wahrscheinlichkeitsrechnung* (Berlin: Springer, 1933). English translation by Nathan Morrison, *Foundations of the Theory of Probability* (Chelsea, 1950).

[10] P. S. La Place, "Mémoire sur les approximations des formules qui sont fonctions de très grands nombres," *Mémoires de l'Academie royale des Sciences de Paris* (1782), 1–88. Reprinted in his *Œuvres Complètes* **10**, 207–291.

[11] D. G. McVitie and L. B. Wilson, "The stable marriage problem," *Communications of the ACM* **14** (1971), 486–492.

[12] Boris Pittel, "The average number of stable matchings," *SIAM Journal on Discrete Mathematics* **2** (1989), 530–549.

[13] J. H. Wilkinson, *Rounding Errors in Algebraic Processes* (Englewood Cliffs, New Jersey: Prentice–Hall, 1963).

Chapter 25

Shellsort With Three Increments

*[Written with Svante Janson. Originally published in Random Structures & Algorithms **10** (1997), 125–142.]*

A perturbation technique can be used to simplify and sharpen A. C. Yao's theorems about the behavior of shellsort with increments $(h, g, 1)$. In particular, when $h = \Theta(n^{7/15})$ and $g = \Theta(h^{1/5})$, the average running time is $O(n^{23/15})$. The proof involves interesting properties of the inversions in random permutations that have been h-sorted and g-sorted.

Shellsort [10], also known as the "diminishing increment sort" [6, Algorithm 5.2.1D], puts the elements of an array $(X_0, \ldots, X_{n-1})$ into order by successively performing a straight insertion sort on larger and larger subarrays of equally spaced elements. The algorithm consists of t passes defined by increments $(h_{t-1}, \ldots, h_1, h_0)$, where $h_0 = 1$; the jth pass makes $X_k \le X_l$ whenever $l - k = h_{t-j}$.

A. C. Yao [11] has analyzed the average behavior of shellsort in the general three-pass case when the increments are $(h, g, 1)$. The most interesting part of his analysis dealt with the third pass, where the running time is $O(n)$ plus a term proportional to the average number of inversions that remain after a random permutation has been h-sorted and g-sorted. Yao proved that if g and h are relatively prime, the average number of inversions remaining is

$$\psi(h, g)n + \widehat{O}(n^{2/3}), \tag{0.1}$$

where the constant implied by $\widehat{O}$ depends on g and h. He gave a complicated triple sum for $\psi(h, g)$, which is too difficult to explain here; we will show that

$$\psi(h, g) = \frac{1}{2} \sum_{d=1}^{g-1} \sum_{r} \binom{h-1}{r} \left(\frac{d}{g}\right)^r \left(1 - \frac{d}{g}\right)^{h-1-r} \left| r - \left\lfloor \frac{hd}{g} \right\rfloor \right|. \tag{0.2}$$

447

Moreover, we will prove that the average number of inversions after such h-sorting and g-sorting is

$$\psi(h,g)n + O(g^3 h^2), \tag{0.3}$$

where the constant implied by O is independent of g, h, and n.

The main technique used in proving (0.3) is to consider a stochastic algorithm $\mathcal{A}$ whose output has the same distribution as the inversions of the third pass of shellsort. Then by slightly perturbing the probabilities that define $\mathcal{A}$, we will obtain an algorithm $\mathcal{A}^*$ whose output has the expected value $\psi(h,g)n$ exactly. Finally we will prove that the perturbations cause the expected value to change by at most $O(g^3 h^2)$.

Section 1 introduces basic techniques for inversion counting, and Section 2 adapts those techniques to a random input model. Section 3 proves that the crucial random variables needed for inversion counting are nearly uniform; then Section 4 shows that the leading term $\psi(h,g)n$ in (0.3) would be exact if those variables were perfectly uniform. Section 5 explains how to perturb them so that they are indeed uniform, and Section 6 shows how this perturbation yields the error term $O(g^3 h^2)$ of (0.3).

The asymptotic value of $\psi(h,g)$ is shown to be $(\pi h/128)^{1/2}g$ in Section 7. The cost of the third pass in $(ch, cg, 1)$-shellsort for $c > 1$ is analyzed in Section 8. This makes it possible to bound the total running time for all three passes, as shown in Section 9, leading to an $O(n^{23/15})$ average running time when h and g are suitably chosen.

The bound $O(g^3 h^2)$ in (0.3) may not be best possible. Section 10 discusses a conjectured improvement, consistent with computational experiments, which would reduce the average cost to $O(n^{3/2})$ if it could be proved.

The tantalizing prospect of extending the techniques of this paper to more than three increments is explored briefly in Section 11.

1. Counting Inversions

We shall assume throughout this paper that g and h are relatively prime. To fix the ideas, suppose $h = 5$, $g = 3$, $n = 20$, and suppose we are sorting the 2-digit numbers

$$(X_0, X_1, \ldots, X_{n-1}) = (03, 14, 15, 92, 65, 35, 89, 79, 32, 38,$$
$$46, 26, 43, 37, 31, 78, 50, 28, 84, 19).$$

The first pass of shellsort, h-sorting, replaces this array by

$$(X'_0, X'_1, \ldots, X'_{n-1}) = (03, 14, 15, 32, 19, 35, 26, 28, 37, 31,$$
$$46, 50, 43, 84, 38, 78, 89, 79, 92, 65).$$

The second pass, g-sorting, replaces it by

$$(X_0'', X_1'', \ldots, X_{n-1}'') = (03, 14, 15, 26, 19, 35, 31, 28, 37, 32,$$
$$46, 38, 43, 65, 50, 78, 84, 79, 92, 89).$$

Our task is to study the inversions of this list, namely the pairs (k, l) for which $k < l$ and $X_k'' > X_l''$.

The result of g-sorting is the creation of g ordered lists $X_j'' < X_{j+g}'' < X_{j+2g}'' < \cdots$ for $0 \le j < g$, each of which contains no inversions within itself. So the inversions remaining are inversions between different sublists. For example, the 20 numbers sorted above lead to

$$\text{list } 0 = (03, 26, 31, 32, 43, 78, 92),$$
$$\text{list } 1 = (14, 19, 28, 46, 65, 84, 89),$$
$$\text{list } 2 = (15, 35, 37, 38, 50, 79);$$

the inversions between list 0 and list 1 are the inversions of

$$(03, 14, 26, 19, 31, 28, 32, 46, 43, 65, 78, 84, 92, 89).$$

It is well known [6, §5.2.1] that two interleaved ordered lists of length m have $\sum_{r=0}^{m-1} |r - s_r|$ inversions, where s_r of the elements of the second list are less than the $(r + 1)$st element of the first list; for example, $(03, 14, 26, 19, 31, 28, 32, 46, 43, 65, 78, 84, 92, 89)$ has

$$|0 - 0| + |1 - 2| + |2 - 3| + |3 - 3| + |4 - 3| + |5 - 5| + |6 - 7| = 4$$

inversions. If $r \ge s_r$, the $(r + 1)$st element of the first list is inverted by $r - s_r$ elements of the second; otherwise it inverts $s_r - r$ of those elements. (We assume that the list elements are distinct.) The same formula holds for interleaved ordered lists of lengths m and $m - 1$, because we can imagine an infinite element at the end of the second list.

Let Y_{kl} be the number of elements $X_{k'}$ such that $k' \equiv k \pmod{h}$ and $X_{k'} < X_l$. The n numbers Y_{ll} for $0 \le l < n$ clearly characterize the permutation performed by h-sorting; and it is not hard to see that the full set of hn numbers Y_{kl} for $0 \le k < h$ and $0 \le l < n$ is enough to determine the relative order of all the X's.

There is a convenient way to enumerate the inversions that remain after g-sorting, using the numbers Y_{kl}. Indeed, let

$$J_{kl} = (k \bmod h + hY_{kl}) \bmod g. \tag{1.1}$$

Then X_l will appear in list $j = J_{ll}$ after g-sorting. Let S_{jl} be the number of elements $X_{k'}$ such that $X_{k'} < X_l$ and $X_{k'}$ is in list j. The inversions between lists j and j' depend on the difference $|S_{jl} - S_{j'l}|$ when X_l goes into list j.

Given any values of j and j' with $0 \le j < j' < g$, let

$$j_s = (j + hs) \bmod g,$$

and let d be minimum with $j_d = j'$. Thus, d is the distance from j to j' if we count by steps of h modulo g. Let

$$H = \{j_1, j_2, \ldots, j_d\} \tag{1.2}$$

be the h numbers between j and j' in this counting process, and let Q_l be the number of indices k such that $0 \le k < h$ and $J_{kl} \in H$. Then we can prove the following basic fact:

Lemma 1. *Using the notation above, we have*

$$S_{jl} - S_{j'l} = Q_l - \lfloor hd/g \rfloor \tag{1.3}$$

for all j, j', and l with $0 \le j < j' < g$ and $0 \le l < n$.

Proof. Since the X's are distinct, there is a permutation $(l_0, l_1, \ldots, l_{n-1})$ of $\{0, 1, \ldots, n-1\}$ such that $X_{l_0} < X_{l_1} < \cdots < X_{l_{n-1}}$. We will prove (1.3) for $l = l_t$ by induction on t.

Suppose first that $l = l_0$, so that X_l is the smallest element being sorted. Then $Y_{kl} = 0$ for all k; hence $J_{kl} = k \bmod g$ for $0 \le k < h$. Also $S_{jl} = S_{j'l} = 0$. Therefore (1.3) is equivalent in this case to the assertion that *precisely $\lfloor hd/g \rfloor$ elements of the multiset*

$$\{0 \bmod g, \ 1 \bmod g, \ \ldots, \ (h-1) \bmod g\}$$

belong to H.

A clever proof of that assertion surely exists, but what is it? We can at any rate use brute force by assuming first that $j = 0$. Then the number of solutions to $x \equiv hd \pmod{g}$ and $0 \le x < h$ is the number of integers in the interval $[-hd/g \mathinner{.\,.} - h(d-1)/g)$, namely

$$\lceil -h(d-1)/g \rceil - \lceil -hd/g \rceil = \lfloor hd/g \rfloor - \lfloor h(d-1)/g \rfloor.$$

Therefore the assertion for $j = 0$ follows by induction on d. And once we've proved it for some pair $j < j'$, we can prove it for $j+1 < j'+1$, assuming that $j'+1 < g$: The value of d stays the same, and the values of $j_1, j_2, \ldots, j_d$ increase by 1 (mod g). So we lose one solution if $j_s \equiv h - 1$ (mod g) for some s with $1 \leq s \leq d$; we gain one solution if $j_s \equiv -1$ (mod g) for some s. Since $j_s \equiv h - 1 \iff j_{s-1} \equiv -1$, the net change is zero unless $j_1 \equiv h - 1$ (but then $j = g - 1$) or $j_d \equiv -1$ (but then $j' = g - 1$). This completes the proof by brute force when $l = l_0$.

Suppose (1.3) holds for $l = l_t$; we want to show that it also holds when l is replaced by $l' = l_{t+1}$. The numbers Y_{kl} and $Y_{kl'}$ are identical for all but one value of k, since

$$Y_{kl'} = Y_{kl} + [l \equiv k \,(\mathrm{mod}\, h)].$$

Thus, the values of J_{kl} and $J_{kl'}$ are the same except that J_{kl} increases by h (mod g) when $k \equiv l$ (mod h). It follows that

$$Q_{l'} = Q_l + [J_{ll} = j] - [J_{ll} = j'].$$

This completes the proof by induction on t, since $S_{jl'} = S_{jl} + [J_{ll} = j]$ for all j. $\square$

Corollary. *Using the notations above, the total number of inversions between lists j and j' is*

$$\sum_{l=0}^{n-1} \left| Q_l - \lfloor hd/g \rfloor \right| [J_{ll} = j]. \tag{1.4}$$

Proof. This is $|S_{jl} - S_{j'l}| = |r - s_r|$ summed over all r such that X_l is the $(r+1)$st element of list j. $\square$

In the example of $n = 20$ two-digit numbers given earlier, with $h = 5$, $g = 3$, $j = 0$, and $j' = 1$, we have $d = 2$, $H = \{2, 1\}$,

$l =$	0	1	2	3	4	5	6	7	8	9	10	11	12	13	14	15	16	17	18	19
$X_l =$	03	14	15	92	65	35	89	79	32	38	46	26	43	37	31	78	50	28	84	19
$Y_{0l} =$	0	1	1	4	3	1	4	4	1	2	2	1	2	2	1	3	3	1	4	1
$Y_{1l} =$	0	0	1	4	3	2	3	3	2	2	2	1	2	2	2	3	2	2	3	1
$Y_{2l} =$	0	0	0	4	3	2	4	3	2	2	3	1	2	2	2	3	3	1	4	1
$Y_{3l} =$	0	0	0	3	2	1	3	2	0	2	2	0	2	1	0	2	2	0	2	0
$Y_{4l} =$	0	0	0	4	3	2	4	4	2	2	3	1	3	2	1	4	3	1	4	0
$J_{0l} =$	0	2	2	2	0	2	2	2	2	1	1	2	1	1	2	0	0	2	2	2
$J_{1l} =$	1	1	0	0	1	2	1	1	2	2	2	0	2	2	2	1	2	2	1	0
$J_{2l} =$	2	2	2	1	2	0	1	2	0	0	2	1	0	0	0	2	2	1	1	1
$J_{3l} =$	0	0	0	0	1	2	0	1	0	1	1	0	1	2	0	1	1	0	1	0
$J_{4l} =$	1	1	1	0	1	2	0	0	2	2	1	0	1	2	0	0	1	0	0	1
$Q_l =$	3	4	3	2	4	4	3	4	3	4	5	2	4	4	2	3	4	3	4	3

and the underlined values J_{ll} are zero for $l = 0, 3, 8, 11, 12, 14, 15$ (accounting for the seven elements in list 0). The inversions between lists 0 and 1 are therefore

$$|3 - 3| + |2 - 3| + |3 - 3| + |2 - 3| + |4 - 3| + |2 - 3| + |3 - 3| = 4$$

according to (1.4).

2. Random Structures

We obtain a random run of shellsort if we assume that the input array $(X_0, X_1, \ldots, X_{n-1})$ is a random point in the n-dimensional unit cube. For each integer l in the range $0 \le l < n$ and for each "time" t in the range $0 \le t \le 1$, we will consider the contribution made by X_l to the total number of inversions if $X_l = t$.

Thus, instead of the quantities Y_{kl} and J_{kl} defined in the previous section, we define

$$Y_{kl}(t) = \sum_{\substack{k' \equiv k \pmod{h} \\ 0 \le k' < n}} [X_{k'} < t], \tag{2.1}$$

$$J_{kl}(t) = \big(k \bmod h + h Y_{kl}(t)\big) \bmod g. \tag{2.2}$$

These equations are almost, but not quite, independent of l, because we assume that $X_l = t$ while all other X's are uniformly and independently random.

For each pair of indices j and j' with $0 \le j < j' < g$, we define H as in (1.2), and we let

$$Q_l(t) = \sum_{k=0}^{h-1} [J_{kl}(t) \in H][k \ne l \bmod h]. \tag{2.3}$$

This definition is slightly different from our original definition of Q_l, because we have excluded the term for $k = l \bmod h$. However, formula (1.4) remains valid because $j \notin H$; when $J_{ll} = j$, the excluded term is therefore zero.

Notice that, for fixed l, the random variables $Y_{kl}(t)$ for $0 \le k < h$ are independent. Therefore the random variables $J_{kl}(t)$ are independent; and $Q_l(t)$ is independent of $J_{ll}(t)$. The average contribution of X_l to the inversions between lists j and j' when $X_l = t$ is therefore

$$W_{jj'l}(t) = \Pr[J_{ll}(t) = j] \, \mathrm{E} \, \big|Q_l(t) - \lfloor hd/g \rfloor\big| \tag{2.4}$$

by (1.4), where probabilities and expectations are computed with respect to $(X_0, \ldots, X_{l-1}, X_{l+1}, \ldots, X_{n-1})$. The average total contribution of X_l is obtained by integrating over all values of t:

Lemma 2. *Let*

$$W_{jj'l} = \int_0^1 W_{jj'l}(t)\, dt\,. \tag{2.5}$$

Then the average grand total number of inversions in the third pass of shellsort is

$$\sum_{\substack{0 \le j < j' < g \\ 0 \le l < n}} W_{jj'l}\,. \quad \square \tag{2.6}$$

Our goal is to find the asymptotic value of this sum, by proving that it agrees with the estimate (0.3) stated in the introduction.

3. Near Uniformity

The complicated formulas of the previous section become vastly simpler when we notice that each random variable $J_{kl}(t)$ is almost uniformly distributed: The probability that $J_{kl}(t) = j$ is very close to $1/g$, for each j, as long as t is not too close to 0 or 1. To prove this statement, it suffices to show that $Y_{kl}(t) \bmod g$ is approximately uniform, because h is relatively prime to g. Notice that $Y_{kl}(t)$ has a binomial distribution, because it is the sum of approximately n/h independent random 0–1 variables that take the value 1 with probability t.

Lemma 3. *If Y has the binomial distribution with parameters (m, t), then*

$$\left| \Pr[Y \bmod g = j] - \frac{1}{g} \right| < \frac{1}{g}\, \phi_{gm}(t) \tag{3.1}$$

for $0 \le j < g$, where

$$\phi_{gm}(t) = 2 \sum_{k=1}^{\infty} e^{-8t(1-t)k^2 m/g^2}\,. \tag{3.2}$$

Proof. Let $y_j = \Pr[Y \bmod g = j]$, and consider the discrete Fourier transform

$$\hat{y}_k = \sum_{j=0}^{g-1} \omega^{kj} y_j = \mathrm{E}\, \omega^{kY},$$

where $\omega = e^{2\pi i/g}$. We have

$$\hat{y}_k = \sum_{l=0}^{m} \binom{m}{l} t^l (1-t)^{m-l} \omega^{kl} = (\omega^k t + 1 - t)^m\,, \tag{3.3}$$

and

$$|\omega^k t + 1 - t|^2 = t^2 + (1-t)^2 + t(1-t)(\omega^k + \omega^{-k})$$
$$= 1 - 2t(1-t)\big(1 - \cos(2\pi k/g)\big)$$
$$= 1 - 4t(1-t)\sin^2(\pi k/g). \tag{3.4}$$

If $0 \le x \le \pi/2$ we have $\sin x \ge 2x/\pi$; hence, if $0 \le k \le \frac{1}{2}g$,

$$|\omega^k t + 1 - t|^2 \le 1 - 16t(1-t)k^2/g^2 < e^{-16t(1-t)k^2/g^2}.$$

And if $\frac{1}{2}g < k < g$ we have $|\hat{y}_k| = |\hat{y}_{g-k}|$. Therefore

$$\sum_{k=1}^{g-1} |\hat{y}_k| \le 2 \sum_{k=1}^{g/2} e^{-8t(1-t)k^2 m/g^2} < \phi_{gm}(t). \tag{3.5}$$

The desired result follows since

$$y_j = \frac{1}{g} \sum_{k=0}^{g-1} \omega^{-kj} \hat{y}_k$$

and thus

$$\left| y_j - \frac{1}{g} \right| = \left| \frac{1}{g} \sum_{k=1}^{g-1} \omega^{-kj} \hat{y}_k \right| \le \frac{1}{g} \sum_{k=1}^{g-1} |\hat{y}_k|. \quad \square$$

Corollary. *We have*

$$\left| \Pr[J_{kl}(t) = j] - \frac{1}{g} \right| < \frac{1}{g} \phi(t) \tag{3.6}$$

for $0 \le k < h$, where

$$\phi(t) = \begin{cases} 2 \sum_{k=1}^{\infty} e^{-4t(1-t)k^2 n/g^2 h}, & \text{if } n \ge 4h; \\ g, & \text{if } n < 4h. \end{cases} \tag{3.7}$$

Proof. Each variable $Y_{kl}(t)$ in (2.1) for $0 \le k < h$ has the binomial distribution with parameters (m, t), where if $n \ge 4h$

$$m = \lceil (n-k)/h \rceil - [k = l \bmod h] \ge \frac{n}{h} - 2 \ge \frac{n}{2h}.$$

Now $J_{kl}(t) = j$ if and only if $Y_{kl}(t)$ has a certain value mod g. The case $n < 4h$ is trivial. $\square$

4. Uniformity

Let's assume now that, for given l and t, the random variables $J_{kl}(t)$ have a perfectly uniform distribution. Since the variables $J_{kl}(t)$ are independent for $0 \leq k < h$, this means that

$$\Pr[J_{0l}(t) = j_0, J_{1l}(t) = j_1, \ldots, J_{(h-1)l}(t) = j_{h-1}] = \frac{1}{g^h} \qquad (4.1)$$

for all h-tuples $(j_0, j_1, \ldots, j_{h-1})$.

In such a case the random variable $Q_l(t)$ defined in (2.3) is the sum of $h-1$ independent indicator variables, each equal to 1 with probability d/g because H has d elements. Hence $Q_l(t)$ has the binomial distribution with parameters $(h-1, d/g)$, and it is equal to r with probability

$$\binom{h-1}{r} \left(\frac{d}{g}\right)^r \left(1 - \frac{d}{g}\right)^{h-1-r}. \qquad (4.2)$$

Let $W^*_{jj'l}(t)$ be the value of $W_{jj'l}(t)$ under the assumption of uniformity (see (2.4)). This quantity $W^*_{jj'l}(t)$ is independent of t, and we let $W^*_{jj'l} = W^*_{jj'l}(t)$ in accordance with (2.5). Then

$$W^*_{jj'l} = \frac{1}{g} \sum_{r=0}^{h-1} \binom{h-1}{r} \left(\frac{d}{g}\right)^r \left(1 - \frac{d}{g}\right)^{h-1-r} \left| r - \left\lfloor \frac{hd}{g} \right\rfloor \right|. \qquad (4.3)$$

For given values of d and j, the index $j' = (j + hd) \bmod g$ is at distance d from j. Suppose that $a(d)$ of these pairs (j, j') have $j < j'$. Then $g - a(d)$ of them have $j > j'$, and $a(g - d) = g - a(d)$ since j is at distance $g - d$ from j'. The sum of (4.3) over all $j < j'$ is therefore independent of $a(d)$:

$$\sum_{0 \leq j < j' < g} W^*_{jj'l} = \sum_{d=1}^{g-1} \frac{a(d)}{g} \sum_{r=0}^{h-1} \binom{h-1}{r} \left(\frac{d}{g}\right)^r \left(1 - \frac{d}{g}\right)^{h-1-r} \left| r - \left\lfloor \frac{hd}{g} \right\rfloor \right|$$

$$= \sum_{d=1}^{g-1} \frac{a(g-d)}{g} \sum_{r=0}^{h-1} \binom{h-1}{h-1-r} \left(\frac{g-d}{g}\right)^{h-1-r} \left(1 - \frac{g-d}{g}\right)^r$$

$$\times \left| h - 1 - r - \left\lfloor \frac{h(g-d)}{g} \right\rfloor \right|$$

$$= \frac{1}{2} \sum_{d=1}^{g-1} \sum_{r=0}^{h-1} \binom{h-1}{r} \left(\frac{d}{g}\right)^r \left(1 - \frac{d}{g}\right)^{h-1-r} \left| r - \left\lfloor \frac{hd}{g} \right\rfloor \right|.$$

(We have used the fact that $\lfloor h(g - d)/g \rfloor = h - 1 - \lfloor hd/g \rfloor$ when hd/g is not an integer.) But this is just the quantity $\psi(h, g)$ in (0.2), for each value of l. We have proved

Lemma 4. *If we assume that the variables $J_{kl}(t)$ have exactly the uniform distribution, the quantity (2.6) is exactly $\psi(h,g)n$.* ☐

5. Perturbation

To complete the proof of (0.3), we use a general technique applicable to the analysis of many algorithms: If a given complicated algorithm $\mathcal{A}$ almost always has the same performance characteristics as a simpler algorithm $\mathcal{A}^*$, then the expected performance of $\mathcal{A}$ is the same as the performance of $\mathcal{A}^*$ plus an error term based on the cases where $\mathcal{A}$ and $\mathcal{A}^*$ differ. (See, for example, the analysis in [7], where this "principle of negligible perturbation" is applied to a nontrivial branching process.)

In the present situation we retain the $(n-1)$-dimensional probability space $(X_0, \ldots, X_{l-1}, t, X_{l+1}, \ldots, X_{n-1})$ on which the random variables $J_{kl}(t)$ were defined in (2.2), and we define a new set of random variables $J_{kl}^*(t)$ on the same space, where $J_{kl}^*(t)$ has exactly a uniform distribution on $\{0, 1, \ldots, g-1\}$. This can be done in such a way that $J_{kl}(t) = J_{kl}^*(t)$ with high probability.

More precisely, when l and t are given, $J_{kl}(t)$ depends only on the variables $X_{k'}$ with $k' \equiv k \pmod{h}$ and $k' \neq l$. The unit cube on those variables is partitioned into g parts $P_0, P_1, \ldots, P_{g-1}$ such that $J_{kl}(t) = j$ when the variables lie in P_j; the volume of P_j is $\Pr[J_{kl}(t) = j]$. We will divide each P_j into g sets $P'_{j0}, P'_{j1}, \ldots, P'_{j(g-1)}$, and define $J_{kl}^*(t) = i$ on P'_{ji}. This subdivision, performed separately for each k, will yield independent random variables $J_{0l}^*(t), J_{1l}^*(t), \ldots, J_{(h-1)l}^*(t)$. We will show that the subdivision can be done in such a way that

$$\Pr[J_{kl}^*(t) = j] = 1/g, \tag{5.1}$$

$$\Pr[J_{kl}^*(t) \neq J_{kl}(t)] < \phi(t), \tag{5.2}$$

for $0 \leq j < g$ and $0 \leq k < h$. Thus, we will have perturbed the values of $J_{kl}(t)$ with low probability when $\phi(t)$ is small.

The following construction does what we need, and more:

Lemma 5. *Let $p_1, \ldots, p_m$ and $p_1^*, \ldots, p_m^*$ be nonnegative real numbers with $p_1 + \cdots + p_m = p_1^* + \cdots + p_m^* = 1$. Then there are nonnegative reals p'_{ij} for $1 \leq i, j \leq m$ such that*

$$p_i = \sum_{j=1}^{m} p'_{ij}, \tag{5.3}$$

$$p_j^* = \sum_{i=1}^{m} p'_{ij}, \tag{5.4}$$

and

$$\sum_{i \neq j} p'_{ij} = 1 - \sum_j p'_{jj} = \frac{1}{2} \sum_j |p_j - p^*_j|. \tag{5.5}$$

Proof. This is a special case of "maximal coupling" in probability theory [5][8, §III.14]; it can be proved as follows.

Let $p'_{jj} = \min(p_j, p^*_j)$, and observe that

$$\sum_j p'_{jj} = \sum_j \min(p_j, p^*_j) = \sum_j \frac{(p_j + p^*_j - |p_j - p^*_j|)}{2} = 1 - \sum_j \frac{|p_j - p^*_j|}{2}.$$

The existence of nonnegative p'_{ij}, $i \neq j$, such that (5.3) and (5.4) hold follows from the max-flow/min-cut theorem [4]: Consider a network with a source s, a sink t, and $2m$ nodes $v_1, \ldots, v_m, v^*_1, \ldots, v^*_m$; the edges are $s \mathrel{-\!\!-} v_j$ with capacity $p_j - p'_{jj}$, $v^*_j \mathrel{-\!\!-} t$ with capacity $p^*_j - p'_{jj}$, and $v_i \mathrel{-\!\!-} v^*_j$ with infinite capacity. $\square$

6. The Effect of Perturbation

When independent random variables $J^*_{kl}(t)$ have been defined satisfying (5.1) and (5.2), we can use them to define $Q^*_l(t)$ as in (2.3) and $W^*_{jj'l}(t)$ as in (2.4). This value $W^*_{jj'l}(t)$ has already been evaluated in (4.3); we want now to use the idea of perturbation to see how much $W_{jj'l}(t)$ can differ from $W^*_{jj'l}(t)$.

Since $Q_l(t) = O(h)$ and

$$|Q_l(t) - Q^*_l(t)| \leq \sum_{k=0}^{h-1} [J_{kl}(t) \neq J^*_{kl}(t)], \tag{6.1}$$

the difference $|W_{jj'l}(t) - W^*_{jj'l}(t)|$ is

$$\left| (\Pr[J_{ll}(t) = j] - \Pr[J^*_{ll}(t) = j]) \operatorname{E} |Q_l(t) - \lfloor hd/g \rfloor| \right.$$

$$\left. + \Pr[J^*_{ll}(t) = j] (\operatorname{E} |Q_l(t) - \lfloor hd/g \rfloor| - \operatorname{E} |Q^*_{kl}(t) - \lfloor hd/g \rfloor|) \right|$$

$$< \frac{1}{g} \phi(t) O(h) + \frac{1}{g} \sum_{k=0}^{h-1} \Pr[J_{kl}(t) \neq J^*_{kl}(t)]$$

$$= O\left(\frac{h}{g}\right) \phi(t). \tag{6.2}$$

(We assume that $J^*_{kl}(t) = J^*_{(k \bmod h)l}(t)$ when $k \geq h$.) To complete our estimate, we need to integrate this difference over all t.

Lemma 6. $\int_0^1 \phi(t)\, dt = O(g^2 h/n)$.

Proof.   The case $n < 4h$ is trivial. Otherwise we have

$$\int_0^1 \phi(t)\, dt = 2 \int_0^{1/2} \phi(t)\, dt$$

$$< 4 \int_0^{1/2} \sum_{k=1}^{\infty} e^{-2tk^2 n/g^2 h}\, dt$$

$$< 4 \int_0^{\infty} \sum_{k=1}^{\infty} e^{-2tk^2 n/g^2 h}\, dt$$

$$= 4 \sum_{k=1}^{\infty} \frac{g^2 h}{2k^2 n} = \frac{\pi^2}{3} \frac{g^2 h}{n}. \quad \square$$

Theorem 1. *The average number of inversions remaining after h-sorting and then g-sorting a random permutation of n elements, when h is relatively prime to g, is $\psi(h,g)n + O(g^3 h^2)$, where $\psi(h,g)$ is given by (0.2).*

Proof.   By (6.2) and Lemmas 2, 4, and 6, the average is $\psi(h,g)n$ plus

$$\sum_{\substack{0 \le j < j' < g \\ 0 \le l < n}} \int_0^1 \left(W_{jj'l}(t) - W^*_{jj'l}(t) \right) dt = O(g^2 n) O(h/g) \int_0^1 \phi(t)\, dt$$

$$= O(g^3 h^2). \quad \square$$

Notice that the proof of this theorem implicitly uses Lemma 5 for each choice of l and t, without requiring any sort of continuity between the values of $J^*_{kl}(t)$ as t varies. We could have defined $J^*_{kl}(t)$ in a continuous fashion; indeed, the random variables $[X_k < t]$ partition the $(n-1)$-cube into 2^{n-1} subrectangles in each of which $J_{kl}(t)$ has a constant value, so we could define $J^*_{kl}(t)$ over $(n-1)$-dimensional rectangular prisms with smooth transitions as a function of t. But such complicated refinements are not necessary for the validity of the perturbation argument.

7. Asymptotics

Our next goal is to estimate $\psi(h,g)$ when h and g are large. Notice that

$$\psi(h,g) = \frac{1}{2} \sum_{d=1}^{g-1} \mathrm{E} \left| Z\left(h-1, \frac{d}{g}\right) - \left\lfloor \frac{hd}{g} \right\rfloor \right|, \tag{7.1}$$

where $Z(m, p)$ has the binomial distribution with parameters m and p. The mean of $Z(h - 1, d/g)$ is $(h - 1)d/g = \lfloor hd/g \rfloor + O(1)$, and the variance is $(h - 1)d(g - d)/g^2$. If we replace Z by a normally distributed random variable with this same mean and variance, the expected value of $|Z - \lfloor hd/g \rfloor|$ is approximately $(2\pi)^{-1/2} \int_{-\infty}^{\infty} |t| e^{-t^2/2} \, dt = 2/\sqrt{2\pi}$ times the standard deviation, so (7.1) will be approximately

$$\frac{1}{g} \sqrt{\frac{h}{2\pi}} \sum_{d=1}^{g-1} \sqrt{d(g - d)} \, . \tag{7.2}$$

The detailed calculations in the remainder of this section justify this approximation and provide a rigorous error bound.

Lemma 7. *If Z has the binomial distribution with parameters (m, p), and $\lfloor mp \rfloor \le a \le \lceil mp \rceil$, then*

$$\mathrm{E} \, |Z - a| = \sqrt{\frac{2p(1 - p)m}{\pi}} + O\left(\frac{1}{\sqrt{mp(1 - p)}}\right) . \tag{7.3}$$

Proof. Consider first the case $a = mp$. By a formula of de Moivre [1, page 101] and Poincaré [9, pages 56–60], see Diaconis and Zabell [2],

$$\mathrm{E} \, |Z - mp| = 2\lceil mp \rceil \binom{m}{\lceil mp \rceil} p^{\lceil mp \rceil} (1 - p)^{m + 1 - \lceil mp \rceil} . \tag{7.4}$$

In order to prove (7.3) in this case we may assume that $p \le 1/2$, since $|Z - mp| = |m - Z - m(1 - p)|$. Moreover, we may assume that $mp > 1$ since (7.3) otherwise is trivial. Then a routine application of Stirling's approximation shows that

$$\mathrm{E} \, |Z - mp| = \sqrt{\frac{2p(1 - p)m}{\pi}} \exp\left(O\left(\frac{1}{mp}\right)\right) . \tag{7.5}$$

Next observe that if $\lfloor mp \rfloor \le a \le \lceil mp \rceil$, we have

$$\mathrm{E} \, |Z - a| = \mathrm{E} \, |Z - mp| + (mp - a)\big(1 - 2\Pr[Z \le mp]\big) . \tag{7.6}$$

Since $\Pr[Z \le mp] = \frac{1}{2} + O\big((mp(1 - p))^{-1/2}\big)$, for example by the Berry–Esseen estimate of the error in the central limit theorem [3, §XVI.5], the result follows. $\square$

Corollary. *The asymptotic value of $\psi(h, g)$ is*

$$\psi(h, g) = \sqrt{\frac{\pi h}{128}}\, g + O(g^{-1/2}h^{1/2}) + O(gh^{-1/2}). \qquad (7.7)$$

Proof. Since $\lfloor hd/g \rfloor \le \lfloor (h+1)d/g \rfloor \le \lfloor (hd + g - 1)/g \rfloor = \lceil hd/g \rceil$, Lemma 7 yields

$$\psi(h+1, g) = \frac{1}{2}\sum_{d=1}^{g-1} \text{E}\left| Z\left(h, \frac{d}{g}\right) - \left\lfloor \frac{(h+1)d}{g} \right\rfloor \right|$$

$$= \sum_{d=1}^{g-1}\left(\sqrt{\frac{h}{2\pi}\frac{d}{g}\left(1 - \frac{d}{g}\right)} + O\left(\left(h\frac{d}{g}\left(1 - \frac{d}{g}\right)\right)^{-1/2}\right)\right)$$

$$= \sqrt{\frac{h}{2\pi}}\sum_{d=1}^{g-1}\sqrt{\frac{d}{g}\left(1 - \frac{d}{g}\right)} + O(gh^{-1/2}).$$

And Euler's summation formula with $f(x) = \sqrt{(x/g)(1 - x/g)}$ tells us that

$$\sum_{d=1}^{g-1} f(d) = \int_1^{g-1} f(x)\, dx + \frac{f(1)}{2} + \frac{f(g-1)}{2} + \frac{f'(g-1)}{12} - \frac{f'(1)}{12} - R$$

$$= g\int_0^1 \sqrt{t(1-t)}\, dt + O(g^{-1/2}) = \frac{\pi g}{8} + O(g^{-1/2})$$

because

$$|R| = \left| \int_1^{g-1} \frac{B_2(x \bmod 1)}{2} f''(x)\, dx \right|$$

$$\le \frac{1}{12}\int_1^{g-1} |f''(x)|\, dx = \frac{1}{12}f'(1) - \frac{1}{12}f'(g-1). \quad \square$$

The error term is thus $O(g^{1/2})$ when $h = g^2 + 1$; for example, we have

h	g	$\psi(h, g)$	$\sqrt{\pi h/128}\, g$	difference$/\sqrt{g}$
901	30	140.018	141.076	0.1933
1601	40	249.539	250.741	0.1900
2501	50	390.412	391.739	0.1877

8. Common Factors

Now let's consider the behavior of shellsort with increments $(ch, cg, 1)$, where c is an integer > 1. It is easy to see that the first two passes are equivalent to the first two passes of $(h, g, 1)$ shellsort on c independent subarrays $(X_a, X_{a+c}, X_{a+2c}, \ldots)$ of size $\lceil (n-a)/c \rceil$ for $0 \le a < c$. The inversions that remain are the $\psi(h, g)n + O(g^3 h^2 c)$ inversions within these subarrays, plus "cross-inversions" between $\binom{c}{2}$ pairs of subarrays.

Yao [11, Theorem 2] proved that the average number of cross-inversions is $\frac{1}{8}\sqrt{\pi c}\,(1 - c^{-1})n^{3/2} + O(cghn)$. The following lemma improves his error term slightly.

Lemma 8. *The average number of cross-inversions after ch-sorting and cg-sorting is*

$$\frac{1}{8}\sqrt{\pi c}\,(1 - c^{-1})n^{3/2} + O(cgh^{1/2}n) + O(c^2 g^3 h^2). \tag{8.1}$$

Proof. Let's consider first the process of h-sorting and g-sorting two independent arrays $(X_0, X_1, \ldots, X_{n-1})$ and $(\widehat{X}_0, \widehat{X}_1, \ldots, \widehat{X}_{n-1})$, then interleaving the results to obtain $(X_0'', \widehat{X}_0'', X_1'', \widehat{X}_1'', \ldots, X_{n-1}'', \widehat{X}_{n-1}'')$. The cross inversions are then the pairs $\{X_l'', \widehat{X}_{l'}''\}$ where either $X_l'' > \widehat{X}_{l'}''$ and $l \le l'$ or $X_l'' < \widehat{X}_{l'}''$ and $l > l'$.

Recasting this process in the model of Section 2 above, we assume that $X_l = t$, while the other $2n - 1$ variables $(X_0, \ldots, X_{l-1}, \ldots, X_{n-1}, \widehat{X}_0, \ldots, \widehat{X}_{n-1})$ are independent and uniformly distributed between 0 and 1. We define

$$Y_{kl}(t) = \sum_{\substack{k' \equiv k \,(\mathrm{mod}\ h) \\ 0 \le k' < n}} [X_{k'} < t], \quad \widehat{Y}_{kl}(t) = \sum_{\substack{k' \equiv k \,(\mathrm{mod}\ h) \\ 0 \le k' < n}} [\widehat{X}_{k'} < t] \tag{8.2}$$

as in (2.1). The elements of each array are divided into h subarrays by h-sorting, and the elements $< t$ have $Y_{kl}(t)$ and $\widehat{Y}_{kl}(t)$ elements in the kth subarrays. Then g-sorting will form g lists, with

$$L_{jl}(t) = \sum_{k=0}^{h-1} \left\lceil \frac{Y_{kl}(t) - a_{kj}}{g} \right\rceil \tag{8.3}$$

elements $< t$ in the jth list of the first array, where $a_{kj} \in \{0, 1, \ldots, g-1\}$ is given by $k + a_{kj}h \equiv j \pmod g$. Similarly, there will be

$$\widehat{L}_{jl}(t) = \sum_{k=0}^{h-1} \left\lceil \frac{\widehat{Y}_{kl}(t) - a_{kj}}{g} \right\rceil \tag{8.4}$$

elements $< t$ in the jth list of the second. Element $X_l = t$ of the first array will go into list $j = J_{ll}(t)$ as before, where $J_{kl}(t)$ is defined in (2.2). The number of cross-inversions between this element and the elements of the second array will then be

$$V_l(t) = \sum_{j'=0}^{g-1} \left| \widehat{L}_{j'l}(t) - L_{jl}(t) - [j' < j] \right|. \tag{8.5}$$

The average total number of cross-inversions is the sum of $\mathrm{E}\, V_l(t)$ over all l, integrated for $0 \le t \le 1$.

We know from Lemma 3 that the numbers $Y_{kl}(t) \bmod g$ have approximately a uniform distribution. Therefore

$$\left\lceil \frac{Y_{kl}(t) - a_{kj}}{g} \right\rceil = \frac{Y_{kl}(t) - a_{kj} + R_{jkl}(t)}{g}$$

where $R_{jkl}(t)$ is approximately uniform on $\{0, 1, \ldots, g - 1\}$. It follows that

$$L_{jl}(t) = \frac{Z_l(t)}{g} + \sum_{k=0}^{h-1} \left(\frac{R_{jkl}(t) - a_{kj}}{g} \right), \tag{8.6}$$

where

$$Z_l(t) = \sum_{k=0}^{h-1} Y_{kl}(t)$$

is the total number of elements in the first array that are $< t$.

Since $R_{jkl}(t)$ depends on $Y_{kl}(t) \bmod g$ only, or equivalently on $J_{kl}(t)$, we may use the perturbed truly uniform random variables $J^*_{kl}(t)$ in Section 5 (or repeat the argument there with $R_{jkl}(t)$) and construct random variables $R^*_{jkl}(t)$ that are uniform on $\{0, 1, \ldots, g - 1\}$ and satisfy $\Pr[R^*_{jkl}(t) \ne R_{jkl}(t)] < \phi(t)$; moreover, the variables $R^*_{jkl}(t)$ are independent for $0 \le k < h$ and fixed j and l. Consequently

$$\mathrm{E}\, |R^*_{jkl}(t) - R_{jkl}(t)| \le g \Pr[R^*_{jkl}(t) \ne R_{jkl}(t)] < g\phi(t). \tag{8.7}$$

By independence and the fact that $\mathrm{E}\, R^*_{jkl}(t) = (g - 1)/2$,

$$\mathrm{E}\left(\sum_{k=0}^{h-1} R^*_{jkl}(t) - h(g-1)/2 \right)^2 = \sum_{k=0}^{h-1} \mathrm{E}\left(R^*_{jkl}(t) - (g-1)/2 \right)^2 < hg^2,$$

which by the Cauchy–Schwarz inequality yields

$$\mathrm{E}\left|\sum_{k=0}^{h-1} R_{jkl}^*(t) - h(g-1)/2\right| < \sqrt{hg}. \tag{8.8}$$

Let $W_{jl} = \frac{1}{g}\left(\sum_{k=0}^{h-1} R_{jkl}(t) - h(g-1)/2\right)$ and $b_j = \frac{1}{g}\left(h(g-1)/2 - \sum_{k=0}^{h-1} a_{kj}\right)$; then

$$L_{jl}(t) = \frac{Z_l(t)}{g} + W_{jl} + b_j, \tag{8.9}$$

where by (8.7) and (8.8)

$$\mathrm{E}\,|W_{jl}(t)| < \sqrt{h} + h\phi(t).$$

A similar argument shows that

$$\widehat{L}_{jl}(t) = \frac{\widehat{Z}_l(t)}{g} + \widehat{W}_{jl} + b_j.$$

Hence

$$V_l(t) = \sum_{j'=0}^{g-1} \left(\frac{|\widehat{Z}_l(t) - Z_l(t)|}{g} + O(|W_{j'l}| + |\widehat{W}_{j'l}| + 1)\right)$$

and

$$\mathrm{E}\,V_l(t) = \mathrm{E}\,|\widehat{Z}_l(t) - Z_l(t)| + O(g\sqrt{h}) + O(gh)\phi(t). \tag{8.10}$$

The quantity $|\widehat{Z}_l(t) - Z_l(t)|$ is just what we would get if we were counting the cross-inversions between two fully sorted arrays that have been interleaved. Therefore

$$\int_0^1 \sum_{l=0}^{n-1} \mathrm{E}\,|\widehat{Z}_l(t) - Z_l(t)|\,dt$$

must be the average number of inversions of a random 2-ordered permutation of $2n$ elements; this, according to Douglas H. Hunt in 1967, is exactly $n2^{2n-2}/\binom{2n}{n}$ [6, exercise 5.2.1–14]. Since $\binom{2n}{n}$ is asymptotically $(1 + O(1/n))4^n/\sqrt{\pi n}$, we obtain the desired total

$$\int_0^1 \mathrm{E}\sum_{l=0}^{n-1} V_l(t)\,dt = \frac{\sqrt{\pi}\,n^{3/2}}{4} + O(gh^{1/2}n) + O(g^3h^2) \tag{8.11}$$

by Lemma 6. Similarly, the same result holds for two arrays of different sizes $n + O(1)$.

Lemma 8 follows if we replace n by $n/c + O(1)$ in (8.11) and multiply by $\binom{c}{2}$. □

9. The Total Cost

So far we have been considering only the number of inversions removed during the third pass of a three-pass shellsort. But the first two passes can be analyzed as in Yao's paper [11]:

Theorem 2. *Let the positive integers g and h be relatively prime and let c be a positive integer. The average number of inversions removed when $(ch, cg, 1)$-shellsort is applied to a random n-element array is*

$$\frac{n^2}{4ch} + O(n) \tag{9.1}$$

on the first pass,

$$\frac{1}{8g}\sqrt{\frac{\pi}{ch}}\,(h-1)n^{3/2} + O(hn) \tag{9.2}$$

on the second, and

$$\psi(h,g)n + \frac{1}{8}\sqrt{\frac{\pi}{c}}\,(c-1)n^{3/2} + O((c-1)gh^{1/2}n) + O(c^2g^3h^2) \tag{9.3}$$

on the third.

Proof. The first pass removes an average of $\frac{1}{4}(n/ch+O(1))^2$ inversions from ch subarrays of size $\lfloor n/ch\rfloor$ or $\lceil n/ch\rceil$; this proves (9.1). The second pass is equivalent to the second pass of $(h,g,1)$-shellsort on c independent subarrays of sizes $\lfloor n/c\rfloor$ or $\lceil n/c\rceil$. Equation (9.3) is Lemma 8. So the theorem will follow if we can prove (9.2) in the case $c=1$. And that case follows from [11, equation (32)], with the $O(n)$ term replaced by $O(n/kh)$ in the notation of that paper. (See also [6, second edition, exercise 5.2.1–40].) □

Corollary. *If $h = \Theta(n^{7/15})$, $g = \Theta(n^{1/5})$, and $\gcd(g,h) = 1$, the running time of $(h,g,1)$-shellsort is $O(n^{23/15})$.*

Proof. The first pass takes time $O(n^{2-7/15})$, by (9.1); the second takes $O(n^{3/2+7/30-1/5}) + O(n^{1+7/15})$, by (9.2); and the third takes $O(n^{1+1/5+7/30}) + O(n^{3/5+14/15})$ by (7.6) and (9.3). □

10. Two Conjectures

Our estimate $O(g^3h^2)$ for the difference between $\psi(h,g)n$ and the average number of third-pass inversions may not be the best possible. In fact, the authors conjecture that the difference is at most $O(g^3h^{3/2})$. This sharper bound may perhaps follow from methods analogous to those in the proof of Lemma 8.

g	inversions	$\psi(h,g)n$	g	inversions/10^5	$\psi(h,g)n/10^5$
1	0 ± 0	0	17	$36.6 \pm 2.36/32$	37.3
2	$7.12 \pm 2.09/100$	7.5	18	$51.7 \pm 3.35/32$	52.6
3	$94.4 \pm 13.6/100$	98.3	19	$71.5 \pm 4.81/32$	72.9
4	$563 \pm 59.1/100$	581	20	$97.3 \pm 6.14/10$	99.2
5	$2210 \pm 195/100$	2280	21	$130 \pm 8.93/10$	133
6	$6740 \pm 560/100$	6910	22	$174 \pm 12.3/10$	176
7	$17200 \pm 1300/100$	17600	23	$226 \pm 14.0/10$	230
8	$38600 \pm 2820/100$	39500	24	$291 \pm 16.8/10$	297
9	$78900 \pm 5670/100$	80600	25	$368 \pm 23.7/10$	380
10	$149000 \pm 10600/100$	152000	26	$475 \pm 29.1/10$	480
11	$265000 \pm 17200/32$	271000	27	$595 \pm 39.0/10$	603
12	$447000 \pm 30300/32$	458000	28	$735 \pm 44.9/10$	750
13	$727000 \pm 49300/32$	742000	29	$922 \pm 52.1/10$	926
14	$1140000 \pm 75400/32$	1160000	30	$1110 \pm 74.0/10$	1140
15	$1730000 \pm 116000/32$	1760000	31	$1370 \pm 97.9/10$	1380
16	$2530000 \pm 166000/32$	2590000	32	$1650 \pm 101/10$	1670

TABLE 1. Empirical results when $h \approx g^2$ and $n \approx g^4$.

If such a conjecture is valid, the running time of $(h, g, 1)$-shellsort will be $O(n^{3/2})$ when $h \approx n^{1/2}$ and $g \approx n^{1/4}$. A computer program was written to test this hypothesis by applying $(h, g, 1)$-shellsort to random arrays of n elements with $h = g^2+1$ and $n = g^2h = g^4+g^2$. Table 1 shows the results, to three significant figures. (The empirical inversion counts appear in the form $\mu \pm \sigma/\sqrt{r}$, where μ and σ are the empirical mean and standard derivation in r independent trials; 10000 trials were made when $g \leq 10$, but only 100 trials were made when $g \geq 20$.) Both mean and standard derivation seem to grow proportionately to $g^6 \approx n^{3/2}$, with $\sigma \approx \mu/15$ for $g \geq 10$.

These data suggest also another conjecture, that the average number of inversions is $\leq \psi(h,g)n$ when h and g are relatively prime. Indeed, the deviations from uniformity between $\mathcal{A}$ and $\mathcal{A}^*$ should tend to cause fewer inversions, because $\mathcal{A}$ forces the balance condition $Y_{kl}(1) = n/h + O(1)$ for all k and l. This second conjecture obviously implies running time $\Theta(n^{3/2})$ when $h = \Theta(n^{1/2})$ and $g = \Theta(n^{1/4})$.

11. More Than Three Increments?

It may be possible to extend this analysis to $(h, g, f, 1)$-shellsort, by analyzing the following stochastic algorithm. "Initialize two sets of counters $(I_0, I_1, \ldots, I_{g-1})$ and $(J_0, J_1, \ldots, J_{h-1})$ by setting $I_j \leftarrow j \bmod f$ and $J_k = k \bmod g$ for all j and k. Then execute the following procedure n times: Choose a random k in the range $0 \leq k < h$. Set $j \leftarrow J_k$ and $i \leftarrow I_j$; then set $J_k \leftarrow (J_k + h) \bmod g$ and $I_j \leftarrow (I_j + g) \bmod f$."

Consider the transition from $l = l_t$ to $l' = l_{t+1}$ in the proof of Lemma 1. When elements enter the array in increasing order, the choice of k represents the subarray that will contain a new element X during the h-sort; then X goes into list j during the g-sort, and into list i during the f-sort. We can therefore obtain the contribution of X to the inversions between lists i and i' for $i < i' < f$, by considering a state P_l obtained from the I table just as Q_l was obtained from the J table in Lemma 1.

References

[1] Abraham de Moivre, *Miscellanea Analytica de Seriebus et Quadraturis* (London: J. Tonson and J. Watts, 1730).

[2] Persi Diaconis and Sandy Zabell, "Closed form summation for classical distributions: Variations on a theme of De Moivre," *Statistical Science* **6** (1991), 284–302.

[3] William Feller, *An Introduction to Probability Theory and Its Applications* **2** (New York: Wiley, 1966).

[4] L. R. Ford, Jr., and D. R. Fulkerson, "Maximal flow through a network," *Canadian Journal of Mathematics* **8** (1956), 399–404.

[5] Sheldon Goldstein, "Maximal coupling," *Zeitschrift für Wahrscheinlichkeitstheorie und verwandte Gebiete* **46** (1979), 193–204.

[6] Donald E. Knuth, *Sorting and Searching*, Volume 3 of *The Art of Computer Programming* (Reading, Massachusetts: Addison–Wesley, 1973). Second edition, 1998.

[7] Donald E. Knuth, Rajeev Motwani, and Boris Pittel, "Stable husbands," *Random Structures & Algorithms* **1** (1990), 1–14. [Reprinted as Chapter 24 of the present volume.]

[8] Torgny Lindvall, *Lectures on the Coupling Method* (New York: Wiley, 1992).

[9] Henri Poincaré, *Calcul des Probabilités* (Paris: Carré, 1896).

[10] D. L. Shell, "A high-speed sorting procedure," *Communications of the ACM* **2**, 7 (July 1959), 30–32.

[11] Andrew Chi-Chih Yao, "An analysis of $(h, k, 1)$-Shellsort," *Journal of Algorithms* **1** (1980), 14–50.

Addendum

Tao Jiang, Ming Li, and Paul Vitányi, "A lower bound on the average-case complexity of Shellsort," *Journal of the Association for Computing Machinery* **47** (2000), 905–911, have applied Kolmogorov complexity theory to show that t-pass shellsort always removes an average of at least $\Omega(tn^{1+1/t})$ inversions, given any sequence of increments, $1 \leq t \leq n$.

Chapter 26

The Average Time for Carry Propagation

[To Professor N. G. de Bruijn on his 60th birthday, 9 July 1978. Originally published in Indagationes Mathematicæ 40 (1978), 238–242.]

1. Introduction

Given two integers $x = (\ldots x_2 x_1 x_0)_b$ and $y = (\ldots y_2 y_1 y_0)_b$ expressed in radix-b notation, one way to form their sum is to compute the two integers $s_{xy} = (\ldots s_2 s_1 s_0)_b$ and $c_{xy} = (\ldots c_2 c_1 c_0)_b$, where $c_0 = 0$ and

$$0 \leq s_i = x_i + y_i - b c_{i+1} < b \quad \text{for} \quad i \geq 0.$$

Here c_{xy} represents the so-called "carry" digits. If we let

$$\Sigma x = x_0 + x_1 + x_2 + \cdots$$

denote the sum of the digits in x, it follows immediately that

$$x + y = s_{xy} + c_{xy},$$
$$\Sigma x + \Sigma y = \Sigma s_{xy} + \Sigma c_{xy} + (b-1)\Sigma c_{xy}.$$

We obtain the sum $x + y$ by repeating the iteration

$$(x, y) \leftarrow (s_{xy}, c_{xy}) \quad \text{until} \quad y = 0;$$

the final value of x will be the original value of $x + y$, because each iteration preserves the value of $x+y$, and the process will terminate after finitely many steps because each iteration except the last one decreases the value of $\Sigma x + \Sigma y$.

It is natural to ask how many iterations will be required to add "typical" numbers x and y by this scheme. Let $t(x,y)$ be the number of iterations required, so that

$$t(x,0) = 0,$$
$$t(x,y) = 1 + t(s_{xy}, c_{xy}) \quad \text{if} \quad y > 0.$$

467

The *average carry propagation time* to add n-place numbers may then be defined as

$$t_n = \frac{1}{b^{2n}} \sum_{0 \le x,\, y < b^n} t(x, y).$$

John von Neumann first raised the question of estimating t_n when $b = 2$, in his 1946 notes on computer design [3], and he proved that

$$t_n < l(n) + n/2^{l(n)} \le \lg n + 2,$$

where $l(n) = \lceil \lg n \rceil$ is the least integer greater than or equal to $\lg n$. A lower bound on t_n was obtained in 1973 by V. Claus [1], who showed that

$$t_n > l(n) - 1$$

and gave a table of values indicating that t_n is approximately $\log_2 n + \frac{1}{3}$.

The purpose of this note is to show that the asymptotic behavior of t_n can be deduced by using a technique suggested by N. G. de Bruijn in connection with another problem. In particular, for any fixed b we shall derive the formula

$$t_n = \log_b n + \frac{\gamma}{\ln b} + \frac{1}{2} + \log_b \left(\frac{b-1}{2} \right) - \delta(n) + O\left(\frac{(\log n)^4}{n} \right),$$

where $\delta(n)$ is a periodic function of $\log n$ having "average" value zero. (When $b = 2$, the average value of $t_n - \log_2 n$ is therefore not $\frac{1}{3}$ but $\gamma/\ln 2 - \frac{1}{2} = .33275$.) The method we shall use could be extended to obtain further terms of the expansion, with the help of a computer.

2. Preliminary Formulas

Let p_{nk} be the probability that more than k iterations are required, namely the probability that $t(x, y) > k$ when x and y are independent random integers, uniformly distributed in the range $0 \le x, y < b^n$. Then

$$p_{n0} = 1 - b^{-n};$$

and for $k \ge 1$ it is not difficult to prove that

$$p_{nk} = a_{nk}/b^{2n}$$

where a_{nk} is the number of pairs of integers

$$x = (x_{n-1} \ldots x_1 x_0)_b, \quad y = (y_{n-1} \ldots y_1 y_0)_b$$

such that

$$x_j + y_j \geq b \quad \text{and} \quad x_i + y_i = b - 1 \quad \text{for} \quad j < i < j + k$$

for some j in the range $0 \leq j \leq n - k$. Now $a_{nk} = 0$ when $k > n$, and we have

$$a_{nk} = b^2 a_{(n-1)k} + b^{k-1} \binom{b}{2} (b^{2n-2k} - a_{(n-k)k}), \quad \text{for} \quad 1 \leq k \leq n,$$

by considering separately those pairs that satisfy the stated condition for some $j < n - k - 1$ and those that satisfy it only for $j = n - k - 1$.

It follows that the generating function

$$P_k(z) = \sum_{n \geq 0} p_{nk} z^n$$

has the rather simple form

$$P_k(z) = \frac{1}{1-z} - \frac{1}{Q_k(z)},$$

where

$$Q_0(z) = 1 - \frac{z}{b};$$

$$Q_k(z) = 1 - z + \frac{b-1}{2} \left(\frac{z}{b}\right)^k, \quad \text{for} \quad k \geq 1.$$

Let $k \geq 1$. As z traverses the circle $|z| = 2$ in the complex plane, the value of $Q_k(z)$ winds around the origin exactly once, hence the polynomial Q_k has exactly one root in $|z| \leq 2$. Calling this root $1 + \varepsilon_k$, we have

$$\varepsilon_k = \frac{b-1}{2} \left(\frac{1+\varepsilon_k}{b}\right)^k,$$

and it follows that

$$\varepsilon_k = \frac{b-1}{2b^k} (1 + O(kb^{-k})) \quad \text{as} \quad k \to \infty.$$

(The proof is by "bootstrapping," first observing that $Q_k(1 + 1/k)$ is negative for large k, hence $\varepsilon_k = O(1/k)$; then using the first observation to prove that $\ln \varepsilon_k = \ln((b-1)/2b^k) + O(1)$; then using the second observation to prove that $\ln \varepsilon_k = \ln((b-1)/2b^k) + O(k/b^k)$.)

3. Analysis

Our goal is to find the asymptotic behavior of

$$t_n = p_{n0} + p_{n1} + \cdots + p_{nn},$$

and for this purpose we need an estimate of p_{nk}. By the residue theorem,

$$\left| 1 - p_{nk} + \frac{1}{(1+\varepsilon_k)^{n+1} Q'_k(1+\varepsilon_k)} \right| = \left| \frac{1}{2\pi i} \oint_{|z|=2} \frac{dz}{z^{n+1} Q_k(z)} \right|$$

$$\leq \frac{2^{-n-1}}{2\pi} \oint_{|z|=2} \frac{dz}{|Q_k(z)|}$$

$$\leq 2^{-n-1} b$$

for all $k \geq 1$, since $|Q_k(z)| \geq 1 - ((b-1)/2)(2/b)^k \geq b^{-1}$ when $|z| = 2$. Using the fact that

$$Q'_k(1+\varepsilon_k) = -1 + \frac{k\varepsilon_k}{1+\varepsilon_k},$$

we obtain

$$p_{nk} = 1 - \frac{1}{(1+\varepsilon_k)^n (1 - (k-1)\varepsilon_k)} + O(2^{-n})$$

uniformly in k.

Let us consider replacing p_{nk} by the simpler expression

$$q_{nk} = 1 - \exp(-(b-1)n/(2b^k)).$$

When k is relatively small, say $b^k \leq (b-1)n/(4\ln n)$, our estimate for ε_k shows that both p_{nk} and q_{nk} are $1 - O(n^{-2})$. Similarly, when k is somewhat larger, say $b^k \geq (b-1)n^3/2$, we find that both p_{nk} and q_{nk} are $O(n^{-2})$. Between these two values of k we have

$$(1+\varepsilon_k)^{-n} = \exp\left(-n \left(\frac{b-1}{2b^k} + O\left(\frac{k}{b^{2k}} \right) \right) \right)$$

$$= \exp(-(b-1)n/(2b^k)) \left(1 + O\left(\frac{nk}{b^{2k}} \right) \right),$$

hence $p_{nk} = q_{nk} + O((\log n)^3/n)$. It follows that only $O(\log n)$ terms contribute significantly to the error of approximation, and

$$t_n = \sum_{k \geq 0} q_{nk} + O\left(\frac{(\log n)^4}{n}\right),$$

since the sum of q_{nk} for $k > n$ is exponentially small.

The remaining task is to find the asymptotic value of

$$t_n = \sum_{k \geq 0} q_{nk},$$

and this can be done by arguing as suggested by N. G. de Bruijn in [2, equations 5.2.2–(38) through 5.2.2–(48)]. In fact, the necessary formula has essentially already appeared in connection with the analysis of "trie search" [2, exercise 6.3–19], if we substitute $b(b-1)n/2$ for n and b for m in the formulas obtained there for $V_{n+1}/(n+1)$. The result is

$$t_n = \log_b n + \frac{\gamma}{\ln b} + \frac{1}{2} + \log_b\left(\frac{b-1}{2}\right) - \delta(n) + O(n^{-1}),$$

where

$$\delta(n) = \frac{2}{\ln b} \sum_{k \geq 1} \Re\left(\Gamma\left(\frac{-2\pi i k}{\ln b}\right) \exp\left(2\pi i k \log_b \frac{(b-1)n}{2}\right)\right).$$

This completes the proof of the result stated in the introduction. Note that $\delta(nb) = \delta(n)$, and that the "average" value of each term of $\delta(n)$ is zero if we assume that $\log_b n$ is uniformly distributed. In practice, $\delta(n)$ is negligible, since it is bounded by

$$\frac{2}{\ln b} \sum_{k \geq 1} \left|\Gamma\left(\frac{-2\pi i k}{\ln b}\right)\right| = \frac{2}{\ln b} \sum_{k \geq 1} \left(\frac{\ln b}{2k \sinh(2\pi^2 k/\ln b)}\right)^{\frac{1}{2}};$$

for example, when $b = 2$ or $b = 10$ we have

$$|\delta(n)| < .000001574 \quad \text{or} \quad |\delta(n)| < .01831,$$

respectively.

References

[1] Volker Claus, "Die mittlere Additionsdauer eines Paralleladdier-werks," *Acta Informatica* **2** (1973), 283–291.

[2] Donald E. Knuth, *Sorting and Searching*, Volume 3 of *The Art of Computer Programming* (Reading, Massachusetts: Addison–Wesley, 1973).

[3] John von Neumann, *Collected Works* **5** (New York: Pergamon, 1963), 45–46.

Chapter 27

Linear Probing and Graphs

*[Dedicated to Philippe Patrick Michel Flajolet. Originally published in Algorithmica **22** (1998), 561–568.]*

Mallows and Riordan showed in 1968 that labeled trees with a small number of inversions are related to labeled graphs that are connected and sparse. Wright enumerated sparse connected graphs in 1977, and Kreweras related the inversions of trees to the so-called "parking problem" in 1980. A combination of these three results leads to a surprisingly simple analysis of the behavior of hashing by linear probing, including higher moments of the cost of successful search.

The well-known algorithm of *linear probing* for n items in $m > n$ cells can be described as follows: Begin with all cells $(0, 1, \ldots, m - 1)$ empty; then, for $1 \leq k \leq n$, insert the kth item into the first nonempty cell in the sequence h_k, $(h_k + 1) \bmod m$, $(h_k + 2) \bmod m$, $\ldots$, where h_k is a random integer in the range $0 \leq h_k < m$. (See, for example, [7, Algorithm 6.4L].)

The purpose of this note is to exhibit a surprisingly simple solution to a problem that appears in a recent book by Sedgewick and Flajolet [12]:

> **Exercise 8.39** Use the symbolic method to derive the exponential generating function of the number of probes required by linear probing in a successful search, for fixed M.

The authors admitted that they did not know how to solve the problem, in spite of the fact that a "symbolic method" was the key to the analysis of all the other algorithms in their book. Indeed, the second moment of the distribution of successful search by linear probing was unknown when [12] was published in 1996.

If the kth item is inserted into position q_k, the quantity $d = \sum_{k=1}^{n}(q_k - h_k) \bmod m$ is the *total displacement* of the items from their

473

hash addresses. The average number of probes needed in a successful search is then $1 + d/n$. Our goal in the following is to study the probability distribution of d as a function of the table size m and the number of items n.

1. Generating Functions

Let $D_{mn}(x) = \sum x^d$, summed over all m^n possible hash sequences $h_1 \ldots h_n$, and let $F_{mn}(x)$ be the same sum restricted to hash functions that are *confined*, in the sense that linear probing with $h_1 \ldots h_n$ will leave cell 0 unoccupied.

Given $h_1 \ldots h_n$, the m hash sequences

$$\big((h_1 + j) \bmod m \ \ldots \ (h_n + j) \bmod m\big) \qquad \text{for } 0 \le j < m$$

all lead to the same total displacement d. And exactly $(m-n)/m$ of them will be confined, in the sense above. Therefore $D_{mn}(x) = \frac{m}{m-n} F_{mn}(x)$, and the probability generating function for d is

$$\frac{D_{mn}(x)}{D_{mn}(1)} = \frac{F_{mn}(x)}{F_{mn}(1)} . \tag{1.1}$$

The quantity $F_{mn}(x)$ is easier to deal with than $D_{mn}(x)$, since linear probing does not "wrap around" when the hash sequence is confined. We obviously have $0 < h_k \le q_k < m$ in a confined sequence; therefore remainders mod m are not actually taken and the behavior is simpler.

The special case of confined linear probing in which $m = n + 1$ has been called the *parking problem* [8], because we can think of n cars that try to park in n consecutive spaces, where the kth car starts its search in position h_k. The number of sequences $h_1 \ldots h_n$ such that all cars are successfully parked is the number of confined hash sequences, namely $\frac{m-n}{m} m^n = (n+1)^{n-1}$, when $m = n + 1$. We will write

$$F_n(x) = F_{n+1,n}(x) \tag{1.2}$$

for the generating function of total displacement in the parking problem.

The general case is clearly related to the special case $m = n + 1$ by

$$F_{n+r,n}(x) = \sum_{n_1 + n_2 + \cdots + n_r = n} \frac{n!}{n_1! \, n_2! \, \ldots \, n_r!} F_{n_1}(x) \, F_{n_2}(x) \, \ldots \, F_{n_r}(x) , \tag{1.3}$$

because every confined hash sequence leaves r cells

$$\{0, n_1 + 1, n_1 + n_2 + 2, \ldots, n_1 + \cdots + n_{r-1} + r - 1\}$$

empty, and defines parking sequences on blocks of sizes $n_1 + 1$, $n_2 + 1$, ..., $n_r + 1$ for some nonnegative integers $n_1, n_2, \ldots, n_r$. The number of ways to fit such subsequences into $h_1 \ldots h_n$ is the multinomial coefficient $n!/n_1! \, n_2! \ldots n_r!$.

Let

$$F(x, z) = \sum_{n \geq 0} F_n(x) \frac{z^n}{n!} \tag{1.4}$$

generate the displacements of successfully parked cars. Equation (1.3) tells us that

$$\frac{F_{mn}(x)}{n!} = [z^n] \, F(x, z)^{m-n} \, ; \tag{1.5}$$

hence the bivariate generating function $F(x, z)$ is the key to the distribution of total displacement.

2. Solution to the Parking Problem

Suppose $h_1 \ldots h_n$ is a confined hash sequence for the special case $m = n+1$, with $n \geq 1$. This holds if and only if $h_n \geq 1$ and $h_1 \ldots h_{n-1}$ leaves cells 0 and k empty for some k in the range $h_n \leq k \leq n$. The sequence $h_1 \ldots h_{n-1}$ then decomposes into parking subsequences for $k - 1$ and $n - k$ cars.

Therefore, by arguing as in (1.3) above, we see that the polynomials $F_n(x)$ satisfy the recurrence

$$F_n(x) = \sum_{k=1}^{n} \binom{n-1}{k-1} (1 + x + \cdots + x^{k-1}) \, F_{k-1}(x) \, F_{n-k}(x) \, . \tag{2.1}$$

(The factor $1 + x + \cdots + x^{k-1}$ corresponds to the displacement of the nth car, while $\binom{n-1}{k-1}$ is the number of ways to mix the two subsequences.) The first few values are

$$F_0(x) = 1 \, ;$$
$$F_1(x) = 1 \, ;$$
$$F_2(x) = 2 + x \, ;$$
$$F_3(x) = 6 + 6x + 3x^2 + x^3 \, . \tag{2.2}$$

Recurrence (2.1) can be put into a more user-friendly form if we write

$$A_n(x) = (x-1)^n F_n(x).\tag{2.3}$$

Then $A_0(x) = 1$, and for $n > 0$ we have

$$A_n(x) = \sum_{k=1}^{n} \binom{n-1}{k-1}(x^k - 1)A_{k-1}(x)A_{n-k}(x).\tag{2.4}$$

For fixed x, this recurrence can be analyzed by using the exponential generating functions

$$A(z) = \sum_{n=0}^{\infty} A_n(x)\,\frac{z^n}{n!},\tag{2.5}$$

$$B(z) = \sum_{n=1}^{\infty} B_n(x)\,\frac{z^n}{n!},\tag{2.6}$$

where

$$B_n(x) = (x^n - 1)A_{n-1}(x),\tag{2.7}$$

because (2.4) is then equivalent to

$$A(z) = e^{B(z)},\tag{2.8}$$

by Euler's well-known formula for power series exponentiation (see, for example, [6, exercise 4.7–4]).

Now (2.6) and (2.7) tell us that

$$B(z) = C(xz) - C(z),\tag{2.9}$$

where

$$C(z) = \sum_{n=1}^{\infty} C_n(x)\,\frac{z^n}{n!},\tag{2.10}$$

$$C_n(x) = A_{n-1}(x);\tag{2.11}$$

and we have

$$C'(z) = \sum_{n=1}^{\infty} C_n(x)\,\frac{z^{n-1}}{(n-1)!} = \sum_{n=0}^{\infty} A_n(x)\,\frac{z^n}{n!} = A(z).\tag{2.12}$$

In other words $C'(z) = e^{C(xz)-C(z)}$; and if we set

$$G(z) = e^{C(z)} \tag{2.13}$$

we find

$$G'(z) = C'(z)G(z) = e^{C(xz)} = G(xz). \tag{2.14}$$

But this functional relation is easy to solve, for if we set

$$G(z) = \sum G_n(x) \frac{z^n}{n!} \tag{2.15}$$

the relation $G(xz) = G'(z)$ says simply that $x^n G_n(x) = G_{n+1}(x)$. Therefore

$$G(z) = \sum_{n=0}^{\infty} x^{n(n-1)/2} \frac{z^n}{n!}, \tag{2.16}$$

and we have deduced that

$$\sum_{n=1}^{\infty} (x-1)^{n-1} F_{n-1}(x) \frac{z^n}{n!} = C(z) = \ln \sum_{n=0}^{\infty} x^{n(n-1)/2} \frac{z^n}{n!}. \tag{2.17}$$

3. Connected Graphs

We are interested in the behavior of $F_n(x)$ near $x = 1$, so it is convenient to write $x = 1 + w$. Then (2.17) becomes

$$\sum_{n=1}^{\infty} w^{n-1} F_{n-1}(1+w) \frac{z^n}{n!} = \ln \sum_{n=0}^{\infty} (1+w)^{n(n-1)/2} \frac{z^n}{n!}. \tag{3.1}$$

Aha — the right side of this equation is well known as the exponential generating function for labeled connected graphs [11]. Thus we have

$$w^{n-1} F_{n-1}(1+w) = C_n(1+w) = \sum w^{\text{edges}(G)}, \tag{3.2}$$

where the sum is over all connected graphs on n labeled vertices. From this interpretation of $C_n(w)$, we see that

$$F_n(1+w) = C_{n,n+1} + w \, C_{n+1,n+1} + w^2 \, C_{n+2,n+1} + \cdots, \tag{3.3}$$

where $C_{m,n}$ is the number of connected labeled graphs on n vertices and m edges. In particular, $C_{n,n+1}$ is $(n+1)^{n-1}$, the number of labeled trees on $n+1$ vertices; this checks with the value of $F_n(1)$ that we already knew.

4. Sparse Connected Graphs

Let

$$W_k(z) = \sum_{n=1}^{\infty} C_{n-1+k,n} \frac{z^n}{n!} \tag{4.1}$$

be the generating function for k-cyclic components of a labeled graph; thus $W_0(z)$ generates unrooted trees, $W_1(z)$ generates connected components that have exactly one cycle, $W_2(z)$ generates bicyclic components, and in general $W_k(z)$ generates connected graphs that have $k-1$ more edges than vertices. From (3.3) and (1.4) we have

$$F(1+w, z) = W_0'(z) + wW_1'(z) + w^2 W_2'(z) + \cdots . \tag{4.2}$$

E. M. Wright [14] showed how to compute the W's systematically, and proved that they are all expressible in terms of the *tree function*

$$T(z) = \sum_{n=1}^{\infty} n^{n-1} \frac{z^n}{n!}, \tag{4.3}$$

which generates rooted trees. (See [4] for simplifications and extensions of Wright's results. In that paper, $W_0(z)$, $W_1(z)$, and $W_2(z)$ are called respectively $\widehat{U}(z)$, $\widehat{V}(z)$, and $\widehat{W}(z)$.)

The known results about $W_k(z)$ for small k show that we have

$$F(1+w, z) = \frac{T(z)}{z} f(w, T(z)), \tag{4.4}$$

where $f(w, t)$ has the following leading terms:

$$
\begin{aligned}
f(w, t) = 1 + w\,&\frac{t^2}{2(1-t)^2} \\
+ w^2 \bigg(&\frac{5}{24} \frac{t^4}{(1-t)^5} (5 - 2t) + \frac{1}{4} \frac{t^3}{(1-t)^4} (4 - 2t) \bigg) \\
+ w^3 \bigg(&\frac{5}{16} \frac{t^7}{(1-t)^8} (8 - 2t) + \frac{55}{48} \frac{t^6}{(1-t)^7} (7 - 2t) \\
&+ \frac{73}{48} \frac{t^5}{(1-t)^6} (6 - 2t) + \frac{3}{4} \frac{t^4}{(1-t)^5} (5 - 2t) \\
&+ \frac{1}{24} \frac{t^3}{(1-t)^4} (4 - 2t) \bigg) \\
+ w^4 \bigg(&\frac{1105}{1152} \frac{t^{10}}{(1-t)^{11}} (11 - 2t) + \cdots \bigg) \\
+ \cdots . &
\end{aligned}
\tag{4.5}
$$

(See formula (8.13) in [4], and use the fact that $zT'(z)$ is equal to $T(z)/\big(1 - T(z)\big)$.)

5. Application to Linear Probing

We can now put everything together and calculate factorial moments of the distribution of total displacement when n items are inserted into m cells by linear probing. The tree function has a wonderful property that leads to considerable simplification, thanks to Lagrange's inversion formula and the identity $T(z) = ze^{T(z)}$:

$$
\begin{aligned}
[z^n]\, F(1 + w, z)^{m-n} &= [z^n]\, \frac{T(z)^{m-n}\, f\big(w, T(z)\big)^{m-n}}{z^{m-n}} \\
&= [z^m]\, T(z)^{m-n}\, f\big(w, T(z)\big)^{m-n} \\
&= [t^n]\, e^{mt}(1 - t)\, f(w, t)^{m-n}.
\end{aligned}
\tag{5.1}
$$

(See [6, exercise 4.7–16], for a simple algorithmic proof of Lagrange's formula.)

We will need to use the hypergeometric functions

$$
Q_r(m, n) = \binom{r}{0} + \binom{r+1}{1}\frac{n}{m} + \binom{r+2}{2}\frac{n(n-1)}{m^2} + \cdots
$$

$$
= {}_2F_0(r+1, -n\,;\,;-1/m),
\tag{5.2}
$$

which are known to appear in the analysis of linear probing (see Theorem 6.4K of [7]); they have the simple generating function

$$
\sum_{n=0}^{\infty} Q_r(m, n)\,\frac{t^n}{n!} = \frac{e^t}{(1 - t/m)^{r+1}}.
\tag{5.3}
$$

The formulas above now allow us to compute the expected total displacement as follows, using (5.3) and (4.5):

$$
\begin{aligned}
\frac{[wz^n]\, F(1 + w, z)^{m-n}}{[z^n]\, F(1, z)^{m-n}} &= \frac{[t^n]\, e^{mt}(1 - t)(m - n)\, t^2/\big(2(1 - t)^2\big)}{[t^n]\, e^{mt}(1 - t)} \\
&= \frac{\frac{1}{2}(m - n)\,[t^n]\, e^{mt} t\big(1/(1 - t) - 1\big)}{m^n/n! - m^{n-1}/(n - 1)!} \\
&= \frac{\frac{1}{2}(m - n)\, m^{n-1}\big(Q_0(m, n - 1) - 1\big)/(n - 1)!}{(m - n)\, m^{n-1}/n!} \\
&= \frac{n}{2}\big(Q_0(m, n - 1) - 1\big).
\end{aligned}
\tag{5.4}
$$

This agrees with the known result that a successful search requires $\frac{1}{2}\big(Q_0(m, n-1) + 1\big)$ probes, on the average [7, Theorem 6.4K].

Moreover, a similar calculation gives

$$\frac{[w^2 z^n]\, F(1+w, z)^{m-n}}{[z^n]\, F(1, z)^{m-n}} = \frac{n(n-1)(n-2)}{24m^2}\,\big(15Q_3(m, n-3)$$
$$+ (4 + 3m - 3n)Q_2(m, n-3)$$
$$+ (5 - 3m + 3n)Q_1(m, n-3)\big).\quad (5.5)$$

This is the expected value of $\binom{d}{2}$, from which of course we obtain the expected value of d^2 by doubling and adding (5.4). All moments can in principle be obtained in this way, although the expressions get more and more complicated.

Formulas such as (5.5) can be rewritten in many ways using the identities

$$rQ_r(m, n) = mQ_{r-2}(m, n) - (m - n - r)Q_{r-1}(m, n);\quad (5.6)$$
$$rQ_r(m, n) = mQ_{r-1}(m, n+1) - mQ_{r-1}(m, n);\quad (5.7)$$
$$nQ_r(m, n-1) = mQ_r(m, n) - mQ_{r-1}(m, n).\quad (5.8)$$

However, none of these transformations seems to convert (5.5) into a substantially simpler formula.

6. Related Work

Germain Kreweras [9] discussed the polynomials $F_n(x)$ at length, showing that they are the generating functions for "suites majeures," which are equivalent to parking sequences with displacements enumerated. He also showed that $F_n(-1)$ is the number of "up-down" permutations, and that $F_n(x)$ is the generating function for inversions in a labeled tree of $n + 1$ nodes. The concept of inversions in trees was first defined by Colin Mallows and John Riordan [10], who established their relation to connected graphs. Thus, all of the main ideas of Sections 2–4 above were already in the literature, waiting to be applied to the analysis of linear probing.

A one-to-one correspondence that maps labeled trees on $\{0, 1, \ldots, n\}$ with k inversions to parking sequences on $\{1, \ldots, n\}$ with k displacements appears in [7, answer to exercise 6.4–31]. A beautiful construction that uses depth-first search to establish (3.2), by relating each n-node tree with k inversions to 2^k connected graphs having $w^n(1 + w)^k$ edges, was found by Ira Gessel and Da-Lun Wang [3]. Therefore the relation between linear probing and graphs can be made quite explicit, although there is apparently no really simple connection.

Ira Gessel and Bruce Sagan had, in fact, found relations between the generating functions for linear probing and the polynomials of Kreweras. Section 7 of their paper [2] obtains the expected value of d.

The expected value of d^2 was first obtained by Alfredo Viola and Patricio Poblete [13], who discovered a formula equivalent to (5.5) about one week before the author had independently carried out the calculations above. Their starting point was equivalent to the symmetry-breaking strategy of Section 1; their other methods provide an interesting alternative to those of the present note. In subsequent work with Philippe Flajolet [1], they proved that when $m = n + 1$ the distribution of $d/n^{3/2}$ converges to the distribution of a random Brownian excursion, and they found connections between linear probing and many other areas of mathematics.

7. Personal Remarks

The problem of linear probing is near and dear to my heart, because I found it immensely satisfying to deduce (5.4) when I first studied the problem in 1962 (see [5]). Linear probing was the first algorithm that I was able to analyze successfully, and the experience had a significant effect on my future career as a computer scientist. None of the methods available in 1962 were powerful enough to deduce the expected square displacement, much less the higher moments, so it is an even greater pleasure to be able to derive such results today from other work that has enriched the field of combinatorial mathematics during a period of 35 years.

It is also gratifying to know that the field of algorithmic analysis has matured to the point where researchers in different parts of the world are now able to resolve such difficult problems working independently.

The reader will note that Sedgewick and Flajolet's exercise 8.39 has not truly been solved, strictly speaking, because we have not found the exponential generating function

$$\sum_{n=0}^{m-1} F_{mn}(x) \frac{z^n}{n!}$$

as requested. However, Sedgewick and Flajolet should be happy with any analysis of linear probing that uses symbolic methods associated with generating functions in an informative way.

I thank the referees for their perceptive remarks and extremely valuable suggestions.

Finally, I wish to pay tribute to my secretary of more than twenty-five years, Phyllis Astrid Benson Winkler, who is retiring this year. The present paper is the last of more than one hundred that she has typed and typeset beautifully for me at Stanford.

References

[1] P. Flajolet, P. Poblete, and A. Viola, "On the analysis of linear probing hashing," *Algorithmica* **22** (1998), 490–515.

[2] Ira Gessel and Bruce E. Sagan, "The Tutte polynomial of a graph, depth-first search, and simplicial complex partitions," *Electronic Journal of Combinatorics* **3** (2) (1996), #R9.

[3] Ira Gessel and Da-Lun Wang, "Depth-first search as a combinatorial correspondence," *Journal of Combinatorial Theory* (A) **26** (1979), 308–313.

[4] Svante Janson, Donald E. Knuth, Tomasz Łuczak, and Boris Pittel, "The birth of the giant component," *Random Structures & Algorithms* **4** (1993), 233–358.

[5] Donald E. Knuth, "Notes on 'open' addressing," typewritten manuscript (27 July 1963); see `http://pauillac.inria.fr/algo/AofA/Research/11-97.html`.

[6] Donald E. Knuth, *Seminumerical Algorithms*, Volume 2 of *The Art of Computer Programming*, third edition (Reading, Massachusetts: Addison–Wesley, 1997).

[7] Donald E. Knuth, *Sorting and Searching*, Volume 3 of *The Art of Computer Programming*, second edition (Reading, Massachusetts: Addison–Wesley, 1998).

[8] Alan G. Konheim and Benjamin Weiss, "An occupancy discipline and applications," *SIAM Journal on Applied Mathematics* **14** (1966), 1266–1274.

[9] G. Kreweras, "Une famille de polynômes ayant plusieurs propriétés énumératives," *Periodica Mathematica Hungarica* **11** (1980), 309–320.

[10] C. L. Mallows and John Riordan, "The inversion enumerator for labelled trees," *Bulletin of the American Mathematical Society* **74** (1968), 92–94.

[11] Robert James Riddell Jr., *Contributions to the Theory of Condensation* (Ann Arbor: University of Michigan, 1951). The main results

of this dissertation were published as R. J. Riddell, Jr., and G. E. Uhlenbeck, "On the theory of the virial development of the equation of the state of monoatomic gases," *Journal of Chemical Physics* **21** (1953), 2056–2064.

[12] Robert Sedgewick and Philippe Flajolet, *An Introduction to the Analysis of Algorithms* (Reading, Massachusetts: Addison–Wesley, 1996).

[13] Alfredo Viola and Patricio V. Poblete, "Analysis of the total displacement in linear probing hashing," presented at the third Dagstuhl Seminar in Analysis of Algorithms (9 July 1997).

[14] E. M. Wright, "The number of connected sparsely edged graphs," *Journal of Graph Theory* **1** (1977), 317–330.

Addendum

Svante Janson, in a letter dated 15 February 1999, observed that (1.5) is equivalent to the identity

$$\sum_{m,n} F_{mn}(x)\, t^m\, \frac{z^n}{n!} = \frac{1}{1 - tF(x, tz)} \, .$$

Therefore we can in fact claim to have found the exponential generating function desired by Sedgewick and Flajolet.

Janson also pointed out an interesting combinatorial interpretation of the coefficients of $F_{mn}(1+w)$, valid for all m and n: $[w^k]\, F_{mn}(1+w)$ is the number of graphs on labeled vertices $\{1, \ldots, m\}$ having $n + k$ edges and $m - n$ components, such that vertices $n + 1, \ldots, m$ belong to different components. (Equation (3.3) is the special case $m = n + 1$.)

Chapter 28

A Terminological Proposal

*[Originally published in SIGACT News **6**, 1 (January 1974), 12–18.]*

While preparing a book on combinatorial algorithms, I felt a strong need for a new technical term, a word that is essentially a one-sided version of 'polynomial complete'. A great many problems of practical interest have the property that they are at least as difficult to solve in polynomial time as those of the Cook–Karp class NP. I needed an adjective to convey such a degree of difficulty, both formally and informally; and since the range of practical applications is so broad, I concluded that such a term should be established as soon as possible.

The goal is to find an adjective x that sounds good in sentences like this:

The covering problem is x.

It is x to decide whether a given graph has a Hamiltonian circuit.

It is unknown whether or not primality testing is an x problem.

We also probably need the associated noun 'x-ness' or 'x-hood' as appropriate. Here x is not supposed to imply that a problem is necessarily in NP, merely that everything in NP can be reduced to such a problem.

For example, let's imagine the situation a few months ago before Pratt showed that primality testing is in NP. The third sentence above does not raise the issue of primality testing belonging to NP; but if I say, "It's unknown whether or not primality testing is polynomial complete," I imply that there is uncertainty either about primality in NP or about NP reducing to primality.

In my lectures at Oslo last year I used $x =$ 'hard'. But this turned out to be unsatisfactory because the word 'hard' is so common; people couldn't distinguish when it was being used in a technical sense. I also thought of 'tough', because 'tough' is informal enough that we can be pretty sure when technical usage is intended; however, it conflicts with some graph-theoretic terminology and doesn't sound quite right. When non-specialists talk about difficult computational problems, they unfortunately call them 'combinatorial', which of course is a completely unwelcome usage.

I think many people are interested in how terminology gets started. New terms often seem to evolve by accident, with the originators having no idea that they are fixing a name for all time. That certainly was the case with me when I defined the term 'LR(k)'; I had no idea that anyone else would ever use it. And I imagine that misleading terms like 'statement' (in programming languages), or 'context-free language', or 'AVL tree', etc., were never considered very seriously for their appropriateness when they were first proposed.

In this case I wanted to try to do something better, to get a large number of qualified people helping to decide on a name before the first publication. So I did two things: (1) I got out my copy of Roget and my unabridged dictionary, and found a set of candidates for x. (2) I wrote to about 30 people asking them to vote on these choices. [My sincere apologies to all readers whom I forgot to include in the balloting.]

The three choices I listed were 'Herculean', 'formidable', and 'arduous'. I asked all voters to assign a real number between 0 and 1 to each term, indicating the degree to which they approved of it. (Thus, 0 meant complete disagreement, 1 meant complete agreement, and 1/2 or more meant "would use if it became standard.") I also left space for write-in votes.

After mailing the ballots, I personally came to the conclusion that *Herculean* would be best; I tried using it for a week, and found that it felt comfortable in all the necessary contexts, and in fact I began to like it. Then a week later the returns began to come in, and I was reminded of the fact that nobody but me has my tastes; I had forgotten that everybody else in the world is hopeless when it comes to terminology (and that they think the same about me). The first week's returns were comparatively few, but there was a strong preference for *formidable* and only very weak responses for *Herculean*. I had favored *Herculean* partly because it translates immediately into all the prominent languages, but I found that even my foreign-speaking correspondents didn't like it. That night I met Dick Karp socially, and we decided to start saying *formidable*. This worked well in conversation and seemed to be a good solution. I went home and replaced *Herculean* by *formidable* in my files.

The next week, many more ballots arrived, and I found to my chagrin that *formidable* was losing its early popularity. I began to wonder how chemists ever got any of their horrible terms adopted, especially their names for the four constituents of DNA code. And I also began to wonder whether my task of assessing the results of votes was going to be Herculean, formidable, or merely arduous.

The final results are shown on the histograms below, showing the distributions by which the 31 respondents assigned numbers in various ranges for each word. [I've multiplied the range by 10, so that the number of x's above digit n indicates the number of votes in the range $n/10 \leq v < (n+1)/10$. It wasn't trivial to make these charts, since Mike Harrison used $(\sqrt{5}-1)/2$ as one choice, and Al Aho used ϵ and ϵ^2. I presume Al meant ϵ to be a small positive real, not a large ordinal.]

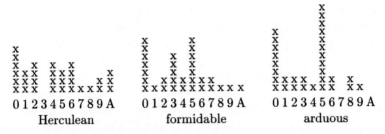

```
                                                              x
                                                              x
                                                              x
                                   x        x          x      x
                                   x        x          x      x
         x                         x    x   x          x      x
         x                         x    x   x          x      x
         x    x   x                x    x   x          x      x
        xxx  xxx                   x    x   x          x      x
        xxx  xxx       x x         x  xxxxxxx         xxxx  xx    x
        xxx  xxxxxxx  xx x         xxxxxxxxxxx xx x   xxxxxx  xx
        0 1 2 3 4 5 6 7 8 9 A      0 1 2 3 4 5 6 7 8 9 A      0 1 2 3 4 5 6 7 8 9 A
           Herculean                   formidable                 arduous
```

The distributions are remarkably different, *Herculean* being rather uniform and *arduous* very peaked. But one thing was perfectly clear: All three words fared rather badly. Only *arduous* was able to get $\geq .5$ from a majority of the voters, and this majority (16 votes to 15) was hardly conclusive.

Then I applied a secret weighting factor to all the ballots, based on approximately how many papers related to this subject I felt each particular voter would be writing, in the next few years, and how much influence on computer science students they have, etc. [Naturally I had assigned the weights before looking at the ballots.] It's preposterous to do such a thing in a democracy, but I did it. The resulting weighted average scores were

Herculean	.369
formidable	.373
arduous	.353

In other words, very low. [I'll bet that the term *polynomial complete* would have fared even worse in the early days; but I'm just trying to heal my wounded feelings when I say this.]

Fortunately, there was a ray of hope remaining, namely the space for write-in votes. I received very many ingenious suggestions; indeed, the write-ins proved conclusively that creative research workers are as full of ideas for new terminology as they are empty of enthusiasm for adopting it.

The write-in votes were so interesting, I'd like to discuss them here at some length. First, several other English words were suggested:

impractical	prodigious	obdurate
bad	difficult	obstinate
heavy	intractable	exorbitant
tricky	costly	interminable
intricate		

Also, Ken Steiglitz suggested 'hard-boiled', in honor of Cook who originated this subject. Al Meyer tried 'hard-ass' (hard as satisfiability). [You can see what I mean about creative researchers.]

Bob Floyd suggested *Sisyphean* instead of *Herculean*, since the problem of Sisyphus was time-consuming while Hercules needed great strength. The difficult NP problems seem to be more time-consuming than energy-spending, so this may be a better term. On the other hand, Sisyphus never finished his task, so we could use this more appropriately for unsolvable problems. A similar remark applies to *Tithonian*. I prefer *Ulyssean* to these, because Ulysses was noted for his persistence and he also finished. Incidentally, Al Aho said he lauds my intent in "trying to clean the theory of computing of its Augean terminology." Thus we find classicists amongst us.

The next group of suggestions was based on acronyms. Shen Lin thought of calling them PET problems, as he likes to work on the traveling salesman problem and similar tasks in spite of their difficulty. He points out that PET stands for "probably exponential time." But if this gets proved, PET stands for "provably exponential time." And if the proof goes the other way, it stands for "previously exponential time."

There's also another Al Meyerism, to let x = 'GNP' (greater than or equal to NP in difficulty, with the possibility of costing more than the GNP to resolve). Or, x = 'XS' (seeming to demand an e̲x̲haustive s̲earch, which requires an excess of time).

The most tantalizing suggestions I received were based on newly-coined words, taken from appropriate classical roots. This, after all, is the way biologists and their colleagues get nearly all of their highfaluting terms. Mike Paterson contributed two nice ones:

exparent   (literally, seeming outside; also joc.
           fr. exponential + apparent);

perarduous   (since 'per' means "through, in space or time"
           and/or "completely, extremely").

Al Meyer tried also 'supersat', meaning greater than or equal to satisfiability. Another excellent one comes from Ed Reingold and his classicist friend Howard Jacobson:

> *polychronious.*

This pleasant word curiously appears in Webster's 2nd unabridged, but not in the 3rd or in the Oxford English or apparently any other dictionary. The definition given in Webster's is quite appropriate: "enduringly long; chronic (rare)." However, to my ears the word polychronious actually implies polynomial time rather than the contrary.

I can see many words in the list above that I wouldn't mind using, but none that I can see becoming standard. There was, however, one further class of write-in votes, based on hyphenated compound words that clearly dominate what we now are saying, although they also relate strongly to the presently entrenched terminology. Since these words were proposed as write-in candidates by quite a few people, apparently acting independently of each other, I believe that the solution to the problem lies here.

The "winning" write-in vote is the term *NP-hard*, which was put forward mainly by several people at Bell Labs, after what I understand was considerable discussion. Similar if not identical proposals were made by Steve Cook, by Ron Rivest, and in earlier publications by Sartaj Sahni. This term is intended for use together with another new one, *NP-complete*, which abbreviates 'polynomial complete' and is at the same time more exact.

Motivation for these terms is easy to describe to a novice, once the concept of NP is understood, namely

> *NP-hard* means as hard as the most difficult problem in NP.
> *NP-complete* means representative of the complete class NP
> with respect to difficulty.

In recent weeks, Karp and I have tried this terminology, and it seems to stand up well in practice. As Jeff Ullman remarked in his letter, "The natural thing to do is substitute *hard* or some other word for *complete* so that 'blah hard' means 'blah complete or worse'."

The strength of support for this write-in vote makes it reasonable to propose it for immediate adoption by all workers in the field. I will conclude this note by examining such a proposal critically and concluding that it survives all the attacks I can muster.

First, are the terms well-defined? Answer: Well, not by the discussion above, but we can make them so. One of the things I learned from the letters received was that Cook's original definition of polynomial reducibility is not known to be the same as the one Karp used to relate so many combinatorial problems to each other. Since the latter is simpler to deal with and supports all the constructions that I believe are of interest to real-world programmers, I propose to make the following explicit definitions (following Karp):

A *problem* L is a subset of the strings on some finite alphabet; in other words, a problem is a language.

A *polynomial-bounded transduction* f is a function $\Sigma^* \to \Sigma'^*$, where Σ and Σ' are finite alphabets, such that, for some integer k, the output $f(x)$ is computable in at most $(|x| + 2)^k$ steps for all x, on (say) a one-tape Turing machine.

If L and L' are problems, we say L *reduces to* L' if there is a polynomial-bounded transduction f such that $x \in L$ if and only if $f(x) \in L'$.

The *satisfiability problem* S is the set of all strings α in (say) the context-free language A over the alphabet $\{(,),\wedge,\vee,\neg,x,'\}$ defined by the syntax and integer-valued semantics

$$
\begin{array}{ll}
A \to (C) & m(A) = m(C) \\
A_1 \to A_2 \wedge (C) & m(A_1) = m(A_2)m(C) \\
C \to L & m(C) = m(L) \\
C_1 \to C_2 \vee L & m(C_1) = m(C_2) + m(L) \\
L \to V & m(L) = f(m(V)) \\
L \to \neg V & m(L) = 1 - f(m(V)) \\
V \to x & m(V) = 1 \\
V_1 \to V_2' & m(V_1) = m(V_2) + 1
\end{array}
$$

such that there exists a function $f\colon N \to \{0,1\}$ for which $m(A) > 0$.

A problem L is *NP-hard* if and only if S reduces to L. It is *in NP* if and only if L reduces to S. It is *NP-complete* if and only if both conditions hold.

Thus, there exists a way to define the terminology precisely. Note that the definition relies on Cook's theorem to relate NP to nondeterministic polynomial time, so that *S-hard* and *S-complete* look like better terms in the sense of a satisfiability-based definition.

A more general definition would say that, for any class C of problems, we define C-hard to mean "L' reduces to L for all $L' \in C$." Also, C-complete is C-hard plus "L reduces to L' for some $L' \in C$." We get immediate metatheorems from the fact that "reduces to" is transitive and reflexive; for example,

If L is C-hard and L reduces to M then M is C-hard.

If L is C-complete then L reduces to M if and only if M is C-hard.

The class C of context-sensitive languages is just one interesting example.

Cook's definition of reducibility was different; he said that L reduces to L' if and only if L is accepted in polynomial time by a Turing machine extended with the capability of deciding membership in L' in one step. This definition corresponds of course to similar definitions with respect to recursive functions and unsolvable problems. We might call this *Turing-reducibility* or *Cook-reducibility*. However, I must admit that I don't see a critical distinction here. Unless I'm mistaken, it is possible to prove the following theorem, by extending Cook's original construction slightly:

If L reduces to S and L' Cook-reduces to L on a nondeterministic Turing machine, then L' reduces to S.

(The clauses generated for those instants of time when L problems are to be solved are replaced by clauses corresponding to the reduction of L to S.) If we set $L = S$ we get "Cook-reducibility to S implies nondeterministic Cook-reducibility to S implies reducibility to S." But reducibility obviously implies Cook-reducibility, so the three concepts are the same at this level of the hierarchy unless I've missed something.

Even if my supposed proof of the above theorem breaks down when I get around to writing the details, I would argue that it is best to use the simpler definitions in connection with notions that will be used by non-automata-theorists. There is an enormous literature on combinatorial algorithms applied to practical problems, and a large body of practical people who get excited about them but not about the technical details of what can happen in weird cases on curious abstract machines. For more technical discussions, the terminology issue is comparatively unimportant, even though the concepts are likely to be important in the total theory, since fewer people are involved; but NP-hard problems hit lots of people, and that's why I began searching for a special term.

In other words, I don't consider it a major goal to invent completely descriptive terminology for every conceivably interesting question of the type considered here. The major goal is to have a good term to use for the masses, in the one case that experience shows is almost omnipresent. To say *NP-hard* actually smacks of being a little too technical for a mass audience, but it's not so bad as to be unusable; fortunately the term does easily generalize to a lot of other cases considered by automata theorists, so it appears to be an excellent compromise. When more technicalities are introduced, there is less need for a universally accepted term or notation. Although things like log-space reductions are quite interesting, I don't think it's necessary to come up with a special short name for them.

John Hopcroft's suggestion was 'NP-time' instead of 'NP-hard', with the corresponding 'NP-space' (which equals P-space). I considered this seriously but decided that it was not satisfactory (mostly because *time* and *space* are nouns). The words 'NP-long' or 'NP-big' might be OK; but really, as I have said, the practical problems of mass interest are all associated with one case, and terminology should be optimized for that case.

NP-hard meets Mike Fischer's objection to my original words, which gave an absolute meaning to a relative quantity; he said that calling some problems formidable is as bad as deciding to say that 'big' means "greater than 17." [I don't agree here; after all, the word 'positive' has merit, and NP-hard problems are just those above the 0th level of difficulty.] Mike was afraid of running out of terms; he said that problems of double exponential difficulty might be called 'hopeless', and triple exponential 'disastrous', but then he was at a loss for words.

One final criticism (which applies to all the terms suggested) was stated nicely by Vaughan Pratt: "If the Martians know that P = NP for Turing Machines and they kidnap me, I would lose face calling these problems *formidable*." Yes; if P = NP, there's no need for any term at all. But I'm willing to risk such an embarrassment, and in fact I'm willing to give a prize of one live turkey to the first person who proves that P = NP.

Chapter 29

Postscript About NP-Hard Problems

*[Originally published in SIGACT News **6**, 2 (April 1974), 15–16.]*

The proposal to call a problem *NP-hard* if every problem in NP reduces to it, as discussed in the January SIGACT newsletter, seems to have gotten widespread support. (For example, I have had favorable reactions from Steve Cook, Dick Karp, Albert Meyer, and several others, and no unfavorable reactions so far.) However, these people have convinced me that I should use reducibility in Cook's sense as opposed to Karp's in the definition of NP-hard. The main reason is that we naturally think of the complement of a problem being just as "hard" as the problem itself, when using actual computers.

This led me to ponder the terminology a little more, and I think I have found a decent way to avoid the dilemma between Cook's "Turing reducibility" and Karp's "many-one reducibility." The former has a standard meaning in recursive function theory, which is different from the meaning we now intend; and the latter appears to be a simple transformation of the data. Hence I propose to use different words for the two concepts.

If L_1 and L_2 are problems, let us say

$$L_1 \ transforms \ to \ L_2$$

if there is a polynomial-time transformation

$$f : \mathrm{domain}(L_1) \to \mathrm{domain}(L_2)$$

such that $x \in L_1 \iff f(x) \in L_2$. Let us say

$$L_1 \ reduces \ to \ L_2$$

if there is a way to solve L_1 by a deterministic polynomial-time program when that program is allowed to use the operation of computing the characteristic function of L_2 in unit time.

493

The advantage of these definitions in lectures (where we have to speak what we mean instead of simply writing it) is obvious. There doesn't seem to be any problem in mentally confusing reducibility with transformability either, since transforming is done by a data transformation, while reducing is done by any construction that makes the efficient solution of one problem reduce to the efficient solution of another.

The terminology "L is NP-hard" means that any problem in NP reduces to L. If we wish to state the stronger condition that any problem in NP *transforms* to L, we may use stronger language and say "L is NP-hard by transformation."

This terminology has further advantages in that it extends easily to other relations; for example, "L_1 linearly transforms to L_2" might mean that the transformation increases the length of input by at most a constant factor. The statement "L_1 transforms to L_2 in linear time" has an obvious meaning, given a particular computational model, as does the statement "L_1 reduces to L_2 in linear time." It seems wisest to single out polynomial time for the words *transform* and *reduce* when they are used without qualification, because this makes them independent of the common models of computation.

I proposed this to Meyer and he used it in five lectures at Stanford in January; the terminology consistently worked well.

P.P.S. I have of course found a fatal error in my supposed proof that reducibility often implies transformability, so please ignore that part of my January note.

Addendum

The term 'NP-complete' became widespread in 1974, thanks primarily to *The Design and Analysis of Computer Algorithms* by Alfred V. Aho, John E. Hopcroft, and Jeffrey D. Ullman. The term 'NP-hard' was also adopted quickly.

Unfortunately, however, the exact meaning of 'NP-hard' has not converged. David S. Johnson uses Cook reducibility, as recommended in the present chapter, in his survey paper "A catalog of complexity classes," *Handbook of Theoretical Computer Science*, Volume A: *Algorithms and Complexity* (Amsterdam: Elsevier, and Cambridge, Massachusetts: MIT Press, 1990), 67–161, §2.3. But Thomas H. Cormen, Charles E. Leiserson, and Ronald L. Rivest use Karp reducibility (that is, transformability), as recommended in the previous chapter, in their widely used textbook *Introduction to Algorithms* (Cambridge, Massachusetts: MIT Press, 1990), §36.3. Neither alternative clearly dominates the other.

Chapter 30

An Experiment in Optimal Sorting

[Written with E. B. Kaehler. Originally published in Information Processing Letters 1 (1972), 173–176.]

Since Ford and Johnson published their "merge-insertion" method of sorting in 1959 [1], nobody has been able to discover a sorting algorithm that uses fewer comparisons in its worst case. Their method has been proved optimal when at most 12 elements are being sorted, yet we can reasonably conjecture that a better algorithm exists for 13 or 14 elements. The possibilities are so enormous, however, that an exhaustive computer search appears to be out of the question. The purpose of this note is to report the results of an unsuccessful attempt to improve on merge insertion when $n = 13$ or 14, in the hope that our experiments might suggest a new approach to the problem.

The maximum number of comparisons needed by merge insertion is known [2] to be

$$F(n) = \sum_{k=1}^{n} \left\lceil \lg \frac{3}{4} n \right\rceil.$$

Since $F(n) - F(n-1) = \lceil \lg n \rceil$ when $12 \le n \le 16$, or when $24 \le n \le 32$, or $48 \le n \le 64$, etc., the Ford–Johnson procedure is no better in its worst case than simply sorting $n-1$ elements with $F(n-1)$ comparisons, then inserting the nth element by binary insertion, for all such n. Surely there must be a better way than this!

Mark Wells proved [4] that there is no better way when $n = 12$. An independent confirmation of his proof (see [3], Section 5.3.1) reveals a particularly efficient line of attack with respect to 9 elements. By combining this line with efficient constructions for 4 or 5 elements, the authors hoped to come up with improved sorting procedures for 13 or 14 elements.

Suppose that the elements to be sorted are $\{K_1, \ldots, K_n\}$, and that they are distinct. Let the relation "$i \prec j$" mean that K_i has been compared to K_j and that $K_i < K_j$. Let S be a set of such relations, and let $P(S)$ be the number of permutations $K_1 K_2 \ldots K_n$ of the set $\{1, 2, \ldots, n\}$ such that the relations of S are valid. For example, if $n = 4$ and $S = \{1 \prec 2, 3 \prec 4, 2 \prec 4\}$ then $P(S) = 3$, since there are only three permutations $K_1 K_2 K_3 K_4$ of $\{1, 2, 3, 4\}$ such that $K_1 < K_2 < K_4$ and $K_3 < K_4$, namely 1234, 1324, and 2314.

When $P(S) = 1$, the sorting has been completed. When $P(S) > 1$, we need to make another comparison, say between K_i and K_j, after which the two cases $S_1 = S \cup \{i \prec j\}$ and $S_2 = S \cup \{j \prec i\}$ must both be dealt with. Notice that $P(S_1) + P(S_2) = P(S)$. When $P(S) \geq 2^k$, we must have either $P(S_1) \geq 2^{k-1}$ or $P(S_2) \geq 2^{k-1}$ (or both); hence at least k more comparisons must be made in some branch of the algorithm before the sorting is complete. Intuitively it seems best to choose i and j so that $P(S_1)$ and $P(S_2)$ are each approximately half of $P(S)$.

Suppose 8 elements are to be sorted, and suppose that the first four comparisons are $K_1 : K_2$, $K_3 : K_4$, $K_5 : K_6$, $K_7 : K_8$. By renaming the elements if necessary, we may assume without loss of generality that the results are $1 \prec 2$, $3 \prec 4$, $5 \prec 6$, $7 \prec 8$. Then we may compare $K_1 : K_3$ and $K_5 : K_7$, and assume by symmetry that $1 \prec 3$ and $5 \prec 7$. And then we may compare $K_4 : K_8$ and assume that $4 \prec 8$. All of these comparisons split the number of possibilities perfectly into two equal parts; hence if $S^{(7)}$ is the set of seven relations known so far we have $P(S^{(7)}) = 8!/2^7 = 315$.

If we now compare $K_4 : K_6$, we find 157 cases with $4 \prec 6$ and 158 cases with $6 \prec 4$. Let's work on the latter possibility, since it is probably a little harder. If we compare $K_1 : K_5$ it turns out that $1 \prec 5$ occurs 77 times but $5 \prec 1$ occurs 81 times, and again we focus attention on the latter case. Introducing a new element K_9, it may be in any of 9 relative positions with respect to the original 8 elements, hence there are $9 \times 81 = 729$ cases to consider. In 372 of these, $7 \prec 9$, while $9 \prec 7$ in the remaining 357. The 372 cases can be broken into 192 with $4 \prec 9$ and 180 with $9 \prec 4$.

Let's look at those 192 cases in detail. The eleven relations $S^{(11)} = \{1 \prec 2, 3 \prec 4, 5 \prec 6, 7 \prec 8, 1 \prec 3, 5 \prec 7, 4 \prec 8, 6 \prec 4, 5 \prec 1, 7 \prec 9, 4 \prec 9\}$ can be diagrammed as follows:

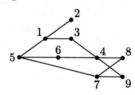

The symmetry between 8 and 9 implies that we can assume $8 \prec 9$ without loss of generality; this leads to $S^{(12)} = S^{(11)} \cup \{8 \prec 9\}$, with 96 possibilities. Curiously a perfect split occurs if we now compare K_2 with K_4. There are 48 possibilities with $2 \prec 4$, namely with

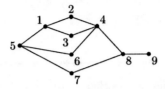

By symmetry we may assume $2 \prec 3$, and then 6 can be inserted into its proper place relative to $\{1, 2, 3\}$ in two more comparisons; and now we may compare K_7 with the middle element of $\{K_1, K_2, K_3, K_4, K_6\}$. The result will leave us with one of the two configurations

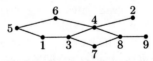

or

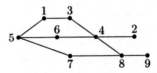

each of which has 3 remaining possibilities.

In the other branch, the 48 possibilities in $S^{(12)} \cup \{4 \prec 2\}$ can also be reduced to $48/16 = 3$ in four more comparisons. Starting with

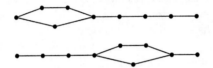

we compare K_3 with K_7. If $3 \prec 7$ we obtain the diagram

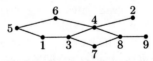

which has left/right symmetry if we remove the least element, 5; consequently we obtain a perfect split by comparing the two "middle" elements, $K_4 : K_7$. After three more comparisons we obtain either

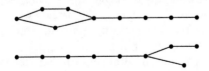

or

On the other hand if $7 \prec 3$, there is symmetry between 7 and 1, and again the reduction is straightforward.

We have now worked out the "hardest" lines of a partial sorting procedure; in each case considered, we discovered a way to reduce the 9! initial possibilities to only 3, after a grand total of 17 comparisons. This is remarkably efficient, since

$$\frac{9!}{2^{17}} = \frac{945}{1024} \cdot 3$$

is only slightly less than 3; in other words, each of the comparisons has split the possibilities very nearly in half.

Let us therefore assume that a 17-step procedure exists for 9 items such that each of the sets $S^{(17)}$ that occurs has at most 3 corresponding permutations. (We haven't proved this, but we have grounds to suspect it is true since the lines not yet considered have fewer possibilities and comparatively more freedom.) It is plausible to suspect that this fact could be used to discover a sorting procedure for 14 items. If we add five more elements $K_{10}, \ldots, K_{14}$ and sort them using seven comparisons, we obtain configurations $S^{(24)}$ such as

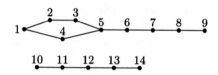

after 24 comparisons have been made. This configuration represents $3\binom{14}{5} = 6006$ possibilities; and since the number 6006 is comfortably less than $2^{13} = 8192$, it appears likely that this $S^{(24)}$ can be sorted with 13 further comparisons, for a total of $24 + 13 = 37 < 38 = F(14)$.

Therefore an exhaustive search was programmed, based on the configuration above. The matrix in Table 1 shows, for each i and j, the value of $P(S^{(24)} \cup \{i \prec j\})$. The two median elements, K_5 and K_{12}, can be compared, giving a perfect 3003 to 3003 split. The next best choice is to compare K_7 to K_{13}, giving 3276 to 2730. Each of the 13 possible comparisons such that both numbers are ≤ 4096 was pursued further in the exhaustive search.

The program was designed so that if, for example, the "large" 3276 branch could be sorted, the "small" 2730 branch was tried too. The two branches were often found to be isomorphic, in which case only one was pursued. However, we discovered to our chagrin that it was impossible to complete any of the "large" branches further than 9 levels; thus, the

0	6006	6006	6006	6006	6006	6006	6006	6006	**3861**	5346	5841	5976	6003
0	0	6006	**4004**	6006	6006	6006	6006	6006	**2046**	**3996**	5220	5788	5973
0	0	0	**2002**	6006	6006	6006	6006	6006	966	**2604**	4228	5348	5873
0	**2002**	**4004**	0	6006	6006	6006	6006	6006	1506	**3300**	4724	5568	5923
0	0	0	0	0	6006	6006	6006	6006	378	1428	**3003**	4578	5628
0	0	0	0	0	0	6006	6006	6006	168	798	**2058**	**3738**	5250
0	0	0	0	0	0	0	6006	6006	63	378	1218	**2730**	4620
0	0	0	0	0	0	0	0	6006	18	138	570	1650	**3630**
0	0	0	0	0	0	0	0	0	3	30	165	660	**2145**
2145	**3960**	5040	4500	5628	5838	5943	5988	6003	0	6006	6006	6006	6006
660	**2010**	**3402**	**2706**	4578	5208	5628	5868	5976	0	0	6006	6006	6006
165	786	1778	1282	**3003**	**3948**	4788	5436	5841	0	0	0	6006	6006
30	218	658	438	1428	**2268**	**3276**	4356	5346	0	0	0	0	6006
3	33	133	83	378	756	1386	**2376**	**3861**	0	0	0	0	0

TABLE 1. Permutations remaining after $24 + 1$ comparisons.

isomorphism test (designed to simplify the solution we thought would be found) was never actually useful.

The program was written in IBM Assembler language and carefully tested on smaller cases. In the 6006-case example above, 14×14 matrices were generated a total of 1235 times, and the computation took about 23.6 minutes on a 360/67.

A similar experiment was tried on the 13-element configurations

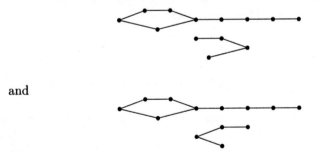

and

each of which represents 6435 permutations. But neither of these could be sorted with 13 comparisons. Hence merge insertion still is the champion.

This research was supported in part by the National Science Foundation and the Office of Naval Research.

References

[1] Lester R. Ford, Jr., and Selmer M. Johnson, "A tournament problem," *American Mathematical Monthly* **66** (1959), 387–389.

[2] A. Hadian, *Optimality Properties of Various Procedures for Ranking n Different Numbers Using Only Binary Comparisons* (Ph.D. thesis, University of Minnesota, 1969), 38–42.

[3] Donald E. Knuth, *Sorting and Searching*, Volume 3 of *The Art of Computer Programming* (Reading, Massachusetts: Addison–Wesley, 1973).

[4] Mark B. Wells, "Applications of a language for computing in combinatorics," *Proceedings of IFIP Congress 65* (1965), 497–498. [His book *Elements of Combinatorial Computing* (Oxford: Pergamon, 1971) gives further details on pages 206–215.]

Addendum

Glenn K. Manacher discovered that the Ford–Johnson method can be beaten for infinitely many values of n beginning with $n = 189$ ["The Ford–Johnson sorting algorithm is not optimal," *Journal of the ACM* **26** (1979), 441–456], and Jürgen Schulte Mönting subsequently found infinitely many cases beginning with $n = 47$ ["Merging of 4 or 5 elements with n elements," *Theoretical Computer Science* **14** (1981), 19–37].

Marcin Peczarski [*Lecture Notes in Computer Science* **2461** (2002), 785–794] has extended Wells's method to prove that merge insertion is actually unbeatable when $n = 13$. But the optimum procedure for sorting 14, 15, or 16 elements remains unknown.

Chapter 31

Duality in Addition Chains

[Written with Christos H. Papadimitriou. Originally published in Bulletin of the European Assocation for Theoretical Computer Science (EATCS) 13 (February 1981), 2–4.]

Let $N = [n_{ij}]$ be an $m \times p$ matrix of nonnegative integers such that no row or column of N is entirely 0. We define an *addition chain for N* to be a sequence

$$C = \langle c_{-m+1}, c_{-m+2}, \ldots, c_0, c_1, \ldots, c_k, c_{k+1}, \ldots, c_{k+p} \rangle$$

of $m \times 1$ vectors, such that the following conditions hold.

a) The vectors $c_{-m+1}, \ldots, c_0$ are the m possible unit $m \times 1$ vectors, in their natural order.

b) For each j, $1 \leq j \leq p$, the vector c_{k+j} equals the jth column of N.

c) For each i, $1 \leq i \leq k + p$, there is an integer $r(i) \geq 1$, and a sequence of $r(i)$ integers $j(i, 1), \ldots, j(i, r(i)) \leq \min(i - 1, k)$, such that $c_i = \sum_{q=1}^{r(i)} c_{j(i,q)}$.

The *length* of C is defined to be $l(C) = \sum_{i=1}^{k+p}(r(i) - 1)$. We denote by $l(N)$ the smallest integer l such that there exists an addition chain C for N with $l(C) = l$.

The classical addition chain problem for integers [1][6][2][3] is the special case of this formulation with $m = p = 1$. The problem of addition chains for vectors [7] corresponds to the case $p = 1$, whereas addition chains for sets of integers [8] correspond to the case $m = 1$. The general problem was studied by Pippenger [5], who derived tight upper and lower bounds for $l(N)$ as a function of m, p, and the largest integer appearing in N. Notice that our definition differs from the usual one in that we allow more than two addends in each "step" of the addition chain. Naturally, such a step with r addends is counted as $r - 1$

additions. In this way we disregard differences between addition chains of the traditional type that are equivalent by the commutativity and associativity of vector addition; and we allow the case $r = 1$.

In this note we use a graph-theoretic formulation of the problem — first employed by Pippenger [5] — in order to give a simple proof of a rather unexpected *duality* property of addition chains. Specifically, we prove the following:

Theorem. *Let N be as above. Then $l(N) - m = l(N^T) - p$.*

Proof. The case $m = 1$ of this theorem was first proved by Olivos [4], using an interesting but rather complicated argument.

Given any addition chain $C = \langle c_{-m+1}, \ldots, c_{k+p} \rangle$ for N, we define a directed acyclic graph $G_C = (V_C, E_C)$, possibly with multiple edges. The vertices $V_C = \{v_{-m+1}, \ldots, v_{k+p}\}$ correspond to the vectors in C. The set E_C of directed edges is defined as follows: $(v_j, v_i) \in E_C$ if and only if $j = j(i, q)$ for some $q \leq r(i)$. For example, the addition chain

$$C = \left\langle \begin{bmatrix} 1 \\ 0 \end{bmatrix}, \begin{bmatrix} 0 \\ 1 \end{bmatrix}, \begin{bmatrix} 1 \\ 1 \end{bmatrix}, \begin{bmatrix} 1 \\ 2 \end{bmatrix}, \begin{bmatrix} 3 \\ 3 \end{bmatrix}, \begin{bmatrix} 3 \\ 4 \end{bmatrix}, \begin{bmatrix} 1 \\ 2 \end{bmatrix} \right\rangle$$

for the matrix

$$N = \begin{bmatrix} 3 & 3 & 1 \\ 3 & 4 & 2 \end{bmatrix}$$

corresponds to the following digraph G_C:

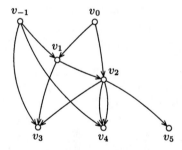

It is very easy to prove (by induction on j) that G_C has the following property: For any i and j such that $1 \leq i \leq m$ and $1 \leq j \leq k + p$, the number of distinct paths from v_{-m+i} to v_j equals the ith component of the vector c_j. As a consequence, for any i and j such that $1 \leq i \leq m$ and $1 \leq j \leq p$, there are exactly n_{ij} paths from v_{-m+i} to v_{k+j}.

Conversely, consider any directed acyclic graph $G = (V, E)$ with m sources and p sinks. Following the previous discussion we can associate with G an addition chain $C(G)$ for the $m \times p$ matrix $N = [n_{ij}]$, where n_{ij} is the number of distinct paths from the ith source to the jth sink. It is important to notice that the length of $C(G)$ is the sum of the in-degree, minus one, over all nodes except the sources. This adds up to $|E| - |V| + m$.

Now, for the duality result, simply notice that the graph $G_C^- = (V_C, E_C^-)$, which results from G_C by reversing the directions of all the arcs, has p sources, m sinks, and exactly n_{ji} arcs from the jth source to the ith sink. Therefore $C(G_C^-)$ is an addition chain for N^T; and its length is $|E_C^-| - |V_C| + p = l(C) + p - m$. Consequently,

$$l(N^T) - p \leq l(N) - m.$$

We obtain the reverse inequality by symmetry. $\quad \square$

Addition chain duality is interesting even when $m = p = 1$. Of course, the theorem then reduces to a trivial equation $l(n) = l(n)$. Still, the graph-theoretic model suggests an intriguing duality among addition chains for the same integer. For example, for each integer n there are two "standard" addition chains. The first corresponds to the following *iterative* algorithm to compute n:

First compute 1, 2, 4, ..., $2^{\lfloor \lg n \rfloor}$, by repeatedly adding the latest integer to itself.

Then add together those powers of 2 that correspond to 1s in the binary representation of n.

The second standard addition chain is the following *recursive* scheme to compute n:

If $n = 1$, do nothing.

Otherwise, if n is odd then compute $n - 1$ and add 1 to it.

Otherwise compute $n/2$ and add it to itself.

These two addition chains for n are easily seen to be dual.

References

[1] H. Dellac, "Question 49," L'*Intermédiaire des Mathématiciens* **1** (1894), 20.

[2] P. Erdös, "Remarks on number theory III: On addition chains," *Acta Arithmetica* **6** (1960), 77–81.

[3] Donald E. Knuth, *Seminumerical Algorithms*, Volume 2 of *The Art of Computer Programming* (Reading, Massachusetts: Addison–Wesley, 1969).

[4] Jorge Olivos, "On vectorial addition chains," *Journal of Algorithms* **2** (1981), 13–21.

[5] Nicholas Pippenger, "On the evaluation of powers and monomials," *SIAM Journal on Computing* **9** (1980), 230–250.

[6] Arnold Scholz, "Aufgabe 253," *Jahresbericht der deutschen Mathematiker-Vereinigung*, II. Abteilung, **47** (1937), 41–42.

[7] E. G. Straus, "Addition chains of vectors," *American Mathematical Monthly* **71** (1964), 806–808. (Partial solution to a problem posed by Richard Bellman.)

[8] Andrew Chi-Chih Yao, "On the evaluation of powers," *SIAM Journal on Computing* **5** (1976), 100–103.

Addendum

Strictly speaking, an addition chain should specify the sets of integers $\{j(i,q) \mid 1 \le q \le r(i)\}$ as well as the sequence of vectors C, because the latter does not uniquely define the former.

Chapter 32

Complexity Results for Bandwidth Minimization

[Written with M. R. Garey, R. L. Graham, and D. S. Johnson. Originally published in SIAM Journal on Applied Mathematics **34** *(1978), 477–495.]*

We present a linear-time algorithm for sparse symmetric matrices, which converts a matrix into pentadiagonal form ("bandwidth 2") whenever there is a way to do so using simultaneous row and column permutations. On the other hand when an arbitrary integer k and graph G are given, we show that it is NP-complete to determine whether or not there exists an ordering of the vertices such that the adjacency matrix has bandwidth ≤ k, even when G is restricted to the class of free trees with all vertices of degree ≤ 3. Related problems for acyclic directed graphs (upper triangular matrices) are also discussed.

1. Introduction

Let G be a graph on the set of vertices V, where $\|V\| = n$. We shall write $u - v$ if vertex u is adjacent to vertex v in G, and $u \,+\!\!\!\!/\, v$ if they are not adjacent. A *layout* of G is a one-to-one mapping f that takes V into the positive integers; equivalently, a layout can be regarded as a string of vertices and "blanks," with each vertex of V appearing exactly once, for instance $b\_c\_\_da$. The correspondence between these two definitions is simply that $f(v) = k$ if and only if v is the kth element of the string; thus $b\_c\_\_da$ corresponds to $f(a) = 7$, $f(b) = 1$, $f(c) = 3$, and $f(d) = 6$, where $V = \{a, b, c, d\}$.

Telecommunications engineers have a concept called "bandwidth" that refers to an interval of frequencies; computer hardware designers have a concept called "bandwidth" that refers to the number of bits processed per second. But numerical analysts and graph theorists use the term "bandwidth" in yet a third sense, which will be our concern in the present paper. The *bandwidth* of a layout f is defined to be

$$bandwidth(f) = \max\{|f(u) - f(v)| \mid u \!\!-\!\! v\},$$

the greatest distance between G-adjacent vertices in the string corresponding to f. The bandwidth of graph G is then

$$Bandwidth(G) = \min\{bandwidth(f) \mid f \text{ is layout of } G\}.$$

It is clear that

$$Bandwidth(G) = \max\{Bandwidth(G') \mid$$
$$G' \text{ is a connected component of } G\};$$

for if f is any layout there is another layout f', having the same bandwidth, in which the connected components of G appear "unmixed" as substrings. (We can let $f'(v) = f(v) + Nc(v)$, for example, where $c(v)$ is the number of the component containing v, and where N is sufficiently large.)

Perhaps the most important application of the bandwidth notion arises in connection with sparse matrices. Given a sparse $n \times n$ matrix $A = (a_{ij})$, let G be the graph on vertices $\{v_1, \ldots, v_n\}$ where $v_i \!\!-\!\! v_j$ for $i \neq j$ if and only if $a_{ij} \neq 0$ or $a_{ji} \neq 0$. Then $Bandwidth(G) \leq k$ if and only if there is a permutation matrix P such that all nonzero elements of $P^T A P$ lie on the diagonal or on one of the first k superdiagonals or the first k subdiagonals. This is easily proved by observing that blanks may be removed from a layout without increasing the bandwidth.

When G has no edges, its bandwidth is trivially $-\infty$. Otherwise the bandwidth will be as low as 1 if and only if each component of G is an isolated point or a *path*, namely a subgraph of the form $v_1 \!\!-\!\! v_2 \!\!-\!\! \cdots \!\!-\!\! v_n$, where $v_i \!\!-\!\! v_j$ if and only if $|i - j| = 1$. It is easy to determine whether or not $Bandwidth(G) = 1$, even when G is not known to be connected, in linear time; in other words, there is an algorithm that decides in $O(n)$ steps whether or not a sparse matrix can be converted to tridiagonal form by simultaneous row and column permutations. (See [13].) The simplicity of this algorithm suggests naturally that the next harder case might not be too difficult, and indeed we shall see below that the condition $Bandwidth(G) = 2$ can also be tested in linear time. However, the algorithm that achieves this is quite intricate, and there appears to be no elegant way to characterize graphs of bandwidth 2.

The authors have been unable to construct a polynomial-time algorithm that decides whether or not $Bandwidth(G) = 3$. The case of bandwidth 2 indicates some of the difficulties that must be surmounted. Section 8 below shows that the general problem of deciding whether or not $Bandwidth(G)$ is k or less, given k and G, is NP-complete, even if G is a free tree with all vertices of degree ≤ 3. This restriction to trees is of special interest because the analogous problem of minimizing $\sum |f(u) - f(v)|$ instead of $\max |f(u) - f(v)|$ over all layouts can be done in polynomial time when the graph is a free tree [31], yet it is NP-complete for general graphs [17].

Section 9 considers the analogous problems that arise when acyclic directed graphs replace undirected graphs. Several open problems conclude the paper.

2. Preliminaries for the Algorithm

In this section we shall begin to develop an algorithm that tests whether or not $Bandwidth(G) = 2$. We shall assume that G is connected and that it has at least one vertex of degree ≥ 3. (If all vertices are of degree ≤ 2, it is easy to see that $Bandwidth(G) \leq 2$, since such a graph is a collection of isolated points, paths, and cycles.) The connectedness assumption implies that G has at least $n - 1$ edges, and on the other hand we may assume that G has at most $2n - 3$ edges since a graph of bandwidth k cannot have more than $(n-1)+(n-2)+\cdots+(n-k)$ pairs of adjacent vertices. Therefore our algorithm will take $O(n)$ steps if its running time is bounded by a constant times the number of edges in G.

The best way to get into the right frame of mind for this problem is to construct a bandwidth-2 layout for a typical case such as the graph in Figure 1. Like all graphs of bandwidth 2, this one is rather "skinny"; a breadth-first search will not involve many unexplored nodes at any time. The puzzle that the reader is now asked to try is simply this: *Arrange the 27 vertices of Figure 1 into a straight line so that all pairs of directly linked vertices are separated by at most one other vertex.*

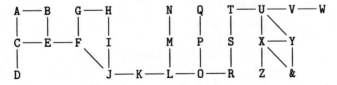

FIGURE 1. An example graph, which the reader is urged to arrange into a bandwidth-2 layout before proceeding further.

(This puzzle is not quite so easy as it looks. The algorithm we shall develop is supposed to work in linear time, essentially without backing up, but no such restriction is being imposed on the reader.)

Perhaps the most important notion that arises in connection with graphs of bandwidth 2 is the concept of *chains* within G. We say that v begins a chain of length k if there are vertices $v = v_1, \ldots, v_k$ such that

$$v_1 - v_2 - \cdots - v_k$$

in G, and each of $v_1, \ldots, v_{k-1}$ has degree 2; furthermore v_k must be of degree 1, an endpoint.

Let us define $l(v) = 1$ if $\deg(v) = 1$, and $l(v) = k + 1$ if $\deg(v) = 2$ and $v - w$ where $l(w) = k$; otherwise $l(v) = \infty$. This function is well-defined since $Bandwidth(G) > 1$; and we can readily compute $l(v)$, for all v, in $O(n)$ steps. Therefore our algorithm will assume that this precomputation has been carried out. The values of l for the example graph in Figure 1 are shown in Figure 2. Note that vertex v is part of a chain if and only if $l(v) < \infty$.

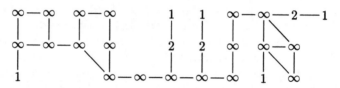

FIGURE 2. The l function for the example graph in Figure 1; there are three chains of length 2.

We shall say that a layout f is *chain-stretched* if $|f(v_i) - f(v_{i+1})| = 2$ whenever v_i and v_{i+1} are consecutive vertices of a chain. This terminology is justified because of the following observation.

Lemma. *Every graph of bandwidth ≤ 2 has a chain-stretched layout of bandwidth ≤ 2.*

Proof. Let f be a layout for the graph G, where $Bandwidth(G) \leq 2$; we may assume that G is connected. Furthermore we shall choose f to have the maximum "range span" over all bandwidth-2 layouts for G; that is, $\left(\max_{v \in V} f(v)\right) - \left(\min_{v \in V} f(v)\right)$ is to be maximum over all f with $bandwidth(f) \leq 2$. (The maximum range span is finite, at most $2n - 2$, since G is connected.) We shall prove that f is chain-stretched.

If not, the string φ corresponding to f contains the substring uv, where u and v are consecutive vertices of a chain. By definition, $\deg(u)$ and $\deg(v)$ are at most 2, and $u - v$, hence u and v are each adjacent to at most one other vertex. By maximality of f's range span, the strings obtained from φ by replacing uv by u_-v and v_-u are not layouts of bandwidth ≤ 2. It follows that φ contains the substring $uvab$ or $abuv$, where $a - u - v - b$; by left-right symmetry we may assume that φ contains $abuv$. Then v must be the rightmost nonblank element of φ. If $l(u) > l(v) = k$, graph G contains the chain $v_k - v_{k-1} - \cdots - v_1$ where $v = v_k$ and $b = v_{k-1}$; but then φ must end with $v_1u_2\ldots u_{k-1}v_{k-1}u_kv_k$ and it can be lengthened by replacing this substring by $_-u_2-\ldots-u_{k-1}-u_k-v_k-v_{k-1}-\ldots-v_1$. On the other hand if $l(v) > l(u) = k$, a similar argument shows that φ ends with $u_1v_1u_2\ldots u_{k-1}v_{k-1}u_kv_k$ where $u = u_k$ and $a = u_{k-1}$, and this substring can be replaced by $_-v_1-\ldots-v_k-u_k-u_{k-1}-\ldots-u_1$. In both cases the maximality of range span has been contradicted. $\square$

The algorithm we shall develop below is based on a subalgorithm that solves the following problem: "Given a connected graph G and two vertices a and b, decide whether or not there exists a layout f of bandwidth ≤ 2 such that $f(a) = 1$ and $f(b) = 2$." If such a layout beginning with ab exists, the algorithm will construct one; and in all cases the algorithm will terminate after $O(n)$ steps. The idea is to build the layout step by step, working with *partial layouts*, namely with one-to-one functions f that are defined only on a subset of the vertices. All partial layouts we shall deal with will satisfy the bandwidth 2 condition, in the sense that $|f(u) - f(v)| \leq 2$ whenever $f(u)$, $f(v)$ are both defined and $u - v$. Furthermore we know by the lemma that it suffices to restrict attention to chain-stretched partial layouts.

If f is a partial layout defined on the set of vertices U, the *active* vertices of f are those elements $u \in U$ such that $u - v$ for some $v \notin U$. If f_1 is a partial layout defined on V_1 and f_2 is a partial layout defined on $V_2 \supseteq V_1$, we say that f_2 is an *extension* of f_1 if $f_2(v) = f_1(v)$ for all $v \in V_1$. We also say that f_2 is a *complete* layout if $V_2 = V$ and $bandwidth(f_2) \leq 2$. Thus the task of our subalgorithm will be to decide whether or not the partial layout f defined by the string ab (namely the layout $f(a) = 1$ and $f(b) = 2$) can be extended to a complete layout.

The subalgorithm actually does more, since its initial task leads to a family of similar subtasks of three types:

Type A. Given a partial layout defined by the string αab, where at most a and b are active, can it be extended to a complete layout?

Type B. Given two partial layouts defined by the respective strings $\alpha a_m b_m \ldots a_1 b_1$ and $\alpha b_m a_m \ldots b_1 a_1$, for some $m \geq 1$, where at most a_1 and b_1 are active, can at least one of these be extended to a complete layout?

Type C. Given a partial layout defined by a string of the form $\varphi = \alpha_- a_m - \cdots - a_1$ for some $m \geq 1$, where at most a_1 is active, can it be extended to a complete layout?

In each case α is a (possibly empty) initial string that has no important influence on the algorithm, since it represents inactive vertices and blanks that have already been permanently placed. The string α in tasks of Type C will have length ≥ 2, and its final two elements will be nonblank. The two strings in tasks of Type B will be denoted by $\varphi = \alpha \langle a_m b_m \rangle \ldots \langle a_1 b_1 \rangle$.

The idea of the subalgorithm is quite simple, namely to "keep doing something useful." Let f be a partial layout of one of the three types, defined on the vertices U. (Actually f represents *two* partial layouts if it is of Type B, but we can safely ignore this fine distinction in our informal discussion.) By looking at how the active vertices of f interact with vertices $\notin U$, we might conclude that f obviously cannot be completed. Otherwise the subalgorithm will find a sufficiently general extension of f, namely an extension layout f' that can be completed whenever f can be; and f' will have one of the three basic types. If any suitable extension is found, the string φ corresponding to f will be replaced by the string φ' corresponding to f', and the process will continue until either reaching an impasse or a complete layout. The running time for each extension step will be bounded, except in one case where the running time can be "charged" to subsequent extension steps; hence the total time will be $O(n)$.

In Section 7 we shall show how the subalgorithm can be used to construct an algorithm that solves the general bandwidth 2 problem (without any given partial layout), in linear time.

3. The Subalgorithm for Types A and B

We shall present the subalgorithm informally, with proofs of the validity of each extension intermixed with specifications of the actual operations to be carried out. The actions will be of three kinds: (a) Terminate successfully because φ is complete; (b) terminate unsuccessfully because φ cannot be completed; (c) set φ' to a sufficiently general extension of φ, after which φ should be replaced by φ'. This manner of presenting the procedure is intended to make it reasonably easy to understand and reasonably enjoyable to read. Several examples of the subalgorithm in operation appear in Section 6 below.

The following notation will be used for convenience:

$$U = \text{set of vertices appearing in } \varphi$$
$$= \text{domain of current partial layout } f;$$
$$S(u) = \{v \mid u \text{---} v \text{ and } v \notin U\} = \text{``successors'' of vertex } u;$$
$$n(u) = \|S(u)\| = \text{number of ``successors'' of } u;$$
$$l(u) = \text{chain level of } u \text{ (defined earlier)}.$$

It is clearly possible to build and maintain data structures so that references to $S(u)$, $n(u)$, and $l(u)$ take a bounded amount of time. The subalgorithm consists of a long but exhaustive list of cases covering which actions are appropriate under various circumstances that can arise.

First let us consider Type A, recalling that tasks of this type are specified by the string $\varphi = \alpha ab$, where at most a and b are active.

Case A1. $n(a) > 1$ or $n(b) > 2$. Failure.

Case A2. $n(a) = 1$. Set $\varphi' = \alpha abc$ where $S(a) = \{c\}$.

Case A3. $n(a) = 0$ and $n(b) = 2$. Set φ' equal to $\alpha ab\langle cd\rangle$ where $S(b) = \{c, d\}$.

Case A4. $n(a) = 0$ and $n(b) = 1$. Set $\varphi' = \alpha ab\_c$ where $S(b) = \{c\}$.

Case A5. $n(a) = 0$ and $n(b) = 0$. Success.

Note that Cases A2, A3, A4 lead to new problems of Type A, B, C respectively; the proofs of validity in each case are trivial.

Next we consider tasks of Type B, which are specified by the string $\varphi = \alpha\langle a_m b_m\rangle \ldots \langle a_1 b_1\rangle$ for some $m \geq 1$, where at most a_1 and b_1 are active. Actually φ represents a potential choice between two partial layouts, $\alpha a_m b_m \ldots a_1 b_1$ and $\alpha b_m a_m \ldots b_1 a_1$. For convenience we shall write $a = a_1$, $b = b_1$; we may assume by symmetry that $n(a) \leq n(b)$.

Case B1. $\|S(a) \cup S(b)\| > 2$ or $n(a) = n(b) = 2$. Failure.

Case B2. $n(a) = 1$ and $n(b) = 2$. Set $\varphi' = \alpha a_m b_m \ldots a_1 b_1 cd$ where $S(a) = \{c\}$ and $S(b) = \{c, d\}$.

Case B3. $n(a) = 0$ and $n(b) = 2$. Set $\varphi' = \alpha a_m b_m \ldots a_1 b_1 \langle cd\rangle$ where $S(b) = \{c, d\}$.

Case B4. $n(a) = 1$, $n(b) = 1$, and $S(a) = S(b)$. Set φ' equal to $\alpha a_m b_m \ldots a_1 b_1 c$ where $S(a) = \{c\}$.

Case B5. $n(a) = 1$, $n(b) = 1$, and $S(a) \neq S(b)$. Set φ' equal to $\alpha\langle a_m b_m\rangle \ldots \langle a_1 b_1\rangle\langle cd\rangle$ where $S(a) = \{c\}$, $S(b) = \{d\}$.

Case B6. $n(a) = 0$ and $n(b) = 1$. Set $\varphi' = \alpha a_m b_m \ldots a_1 b_1\_c$ where $S(b) = \{c\}$.

Case B7. $n(a) = 0$ and $n(b) = 0$. Success.

Again the proofs in each case are trivial; we shall discuss only Case B6 here: Any completion of φ must be of the forms $\alpha a_m b_m \ldots a_1 b_1 x c\,\omega$ (where x is a vertex or a blank), $\alpha a_m b_m \ldots a_1 b_1 c\,\omega$, or $\alpha b_m a_m \ldots b_1 a_1 c\,\omega$. The first of these is an extension of φ'; and the second or third imply that $\alpha a_m b_m \ldots a_1 b_1 {\scriptscriptstyle\_} c\,\omega$ is also a complete extension.

4. The Subalgorithm for Type C

Recall that tasks of Type C are specified by the string $\varphi = \alpha {\scriptscriptstyle\_} a_m \ldots {\scriptscriptstyle\_} a_1$, for some $m \geq 1$, where at most a_1 is active and α contains no usable blanks. This type of partial layout allows considerably more flexibility than Types A and B do, since it may be possible to make good use of the m blanks. Let us write a as a shorthand for a_1. Furthermore we shall write $U' = U \cup S(a)$, with $S'(u)$ and $n'(u)$ defined correspondingly.

    Case C1. $n(a) > 3$. Failure.

    Case C2. $S(a) = \{b, c, d\}$.

In this case the final neighborhood of a in a complete extension must be *bacd*, *badc*, *cabd*, *cadb*, *dabc*, or *dacb*. The possibilities can be narrowed down by considering various subcases. Symmetry between b, c, d is used in order to reduce the number of alternatives; in other words, there is always a way to rename the elements of $S(a)$ so that some subcase applies. We shall say that a vertex u in $S(a)$ is *feasible* if it can conceivably fit to the left of a_1. More precisely, u is feasible if $S'(u) = \{v\}$ where $l(v) < m$, or if $n'(u) = 0$. In the former case we say that u is $l(v)$-feasible; in the latter case we say that u is 0-feasible.

    Case C2.1. $b {\,\relbar\,} c$, $b {\,\relbar\,} d$, $c {\,\relbar\,} d$. Failure.

    Case C2.2. $b {\,+\,} c$, $b {\,\relbar\,} d$, $c {\,\relbar\,} d$.

In this case we must decide between *badc* and *cadb*.

    Case C2.2.1. Neither b nor c is feasible. Failure.

    Case C2.2.2. b is feasible but not c. Set $\varphi' = \alpha[ba]dc$.

Here and in the sequel we shall use the following notation: $[ba] = {\scriptscriptstyle\_} a_m \ldots {\scriptscriptstyle\_} a_{k+2} b_k a_{k+1} \ldots b_0 a_1$ if $b = b_0$ is k-feasible and $b_1 {\,\relbar\,} \cdots {\,\relbar\,} b_k$ is the corresponding chain of length k. In other words, $[ba]$ stands for the string ${\scriptscriptstyle\_} a_m \ldots {\scriptscriptstyle\_} a_1$ with b and its successors inserted into the appropriate blank spaces.

    Case C2.2.3. b is k-feasible and c is l-feasible where $k \geq l$. Set
$$\varphi' = \alpha[ba]dc.$$
To justify this step, we shall prove that

$$\alpha[ba]dc \geq \alpha[ca]db,$$

where we say that partial layout φ_1 *dominates* φ_2 (written $\varphi_1 \geq \varphi_2$) if every completion of φ_2 implies the existence of a completion of φ_1.

In our case any chain-stretched completion of φ that is not an extension of φ' must be an extension of $\alpha[ca]db$, so it must have the form $\varphi'' = \alpha[ca]d_0b_0d_1b_1\ldots d_kb_k\omega$. Let $c_0 - c_1 - \cdots - c_l$ be the chain adjacent to $c = c_0$ and let c_j be blank if $l < j \leq k$. Then we may interchange $c_0, \ldots, c_k$ with $b_0, \ldots, b_k$ in φ'', obtaining a valid completion of φ that extends φ'.

The reader should pause to understand the justification of step C2.2.3 at this point before proceeding further. Although the argument is very simple, we shall be using it repeatedly in the sequel, with various refinements and extensions as the cases get more complex.

Case C2.3. $b - c$, $b + d$, $c + d$.

In this case we must decide between *bacd*, *cabd*, *dabc*, and *dacb*.

> *Case* C2.3.1. Neither b nor c is feasible. Failure, unless d is feasible.
> In the latter case, set $\varphi' = \alpha[da]\langle bc\rangle$.

> *Case* C2.3.2. b is feasible but not c; say b is k-feasible. If d is l-feasible where $l \geq k$, set $\varphi' = \alpha[da]bc$, otherwise set $\varphi' = \alpha[ba]cd$.

To justify this step, note that $\alpha[ba]cd$ is forced unless d is feasible. In the latter case $\alpha[da]cb$ cannot be better than $\alpha[da]bc$, since $b = b_0$ must be followed by $b_1, \ldots, b_k$, with b_{i+1} following two positions after b_i; any completion of $\alpha[da]cb$ can clearly be converted into a completion that extends $\alpha[da]bc$. Thus we must simply distinguish between *bacd* and *dabc*, and the argument is similar to Case C2.2.3.

> *Case* C2.3.3. b is k-feasible and c is l-feasible, where $k \geq l$. Set $\varphi' = \alpha[ba]cd$.

The argument is like Case C2.2.3 again; if d is feasible too, we will soon be successful, regardless of which alternative is chosen.

Case C2.4. $b + c$, $b + d$, $c + d$.

All six possibilities of Case C2 still remain, but we can make use of the symmetry.

> *Case* C2.4.1. None of b, c, d is feasible. Failure.

> *Case* C2.4.2. b is feasible but c and d are not. Set $\varphi' = \alpha[ba]\langle cd\rangle$.

> *Case* C2.4.3. b is k-feasible and c is l-feasible, where $l \leq k$, but d is infeasible. Set $\varphi' = \alpha[ba]cd$.

In this case $\alpha[ba]cd \geq \alpha[ba]dc$ and $\alpha[ca]bd \geq \alpha[ca]db$ as in Case C2.3.2, while $\alpha[ba]cd \geq \alpha[ca]bd$ as in Case C2.2.3.

> *Case* C2.4.4. All of b, c, d are feasible. Set $\varphi' = \alpha[ba]cd$.

Success is imminent.

Case C3. $S(a) = \{b, c\}$. See Section 5 below.

This is by far the hardest case to handle, and we shall postpone it for a moment since the remaining cases are very simple.

Case C4. $S(a) = \{b\}$. Set $\varphi' = \alpha_- a_m \ldots_- a_1 {}_- b$.
This clearly dominates $\alpha_- a_m \ldots_- a_2 b a_1$ and $\alpha_- a_m \ldots_- a_1 b$.
   Case C5. $n(a) = 0$. Success.

5. The Subalgorithm for Type C, Case C3

Now we must face up to Case C3; as above we have $\varphi = \alpha_- a_m \ldots_- a_1$
and $a = a_1$ and $S(a) = \{b, c\}$. We should replace the substring $_- a$ at the
right of φ by either $_- abc$, $_- acb$, bac, $ba_- c$, cab, or $ca_- b$, where the dashes
may or may not get filled in later. Fortunately we can rule out two of
these possibilities immediately, since bac is never better than $_- abc$ and
cab is (similarly) never better than $_- acb$: The complete layout $\alpha[ba]c\,\omega$
that extends $\alpha_- a_m \ldots_- a_2 bac$ can always be converted to a complete
layout $\alpha[b_1 a]bc\,\omega$ that extends $\alpha_- a_m \ldots_- abc$.
   Case C3.1. $b \text{---} c$.
In this case we have to distinguish between $_- abc$ and $_- acb$. Let us say
that b is k-*lucky* if $S'(b)$ contains a vertex b_1 with $l(b_1) = k$ and $k \le m$.
(If there are two or more such vertices b_1, choose one with maximum k.)
Similarly c might be lucky; we can use the blanks left of a for one of the
successors of a lucky vertex.
   Case C3.1.1. Neither b nor c is lucky. Set $\varphi' = \alpha_- a_m \ldots_- a_1 \langle bc \rangle$.
   Case C3.1.2. b is k-lucky and c is either (i) unlucky or (ii) l-lucky
          where $l < k$, or (iii) k-lucky and $n'(b) \le n'(c)$. Set
          $\varphi' = \alpha[b_1 a]bc$.
To justify this step, we first argue (as in Case C2.2.3) that the layout
$\alpha_- a_m \ldots_- a_1 bcb_1$ has no advantage over φ'. Therefore the only competing possibility is $\alpha_- a_m \ldots_- a_1 cb$. The two ways to place b_1 in the
latter string give us two possible types of completion to consider, say
$\varphi'' = \alpha[c_1 a]cbx_1 b_1 \ldots x_k b_k \omega$ and $\varphi''' = \alpha[c_1 a]cbb_1 x_1 \ldots x_{k-1} b_k \omega$, since
b_1 has degree ≤ 2 and is part of a stretched chain. (Here c_1 is blank if c
is unlucky or if we do not choose to make use of c's luckiness.) We can
always replace φ'' by $\alpha[b_1 a]bcx_1 c_1 \ldots x_k c_k \omega$, an extension of φ'; similarly, φ''' can always be replaced by $\alpha[b_1 a]bcx_1 c_1 \ldots x_{k-1} c_{k-1} \omega$ unless c
is k-lucky. But in the latter case we have $n'(b) \le n'(c) = 1$ by hypothe-
sis, so the x_i are all blank and ω is empty; φ''' can therefore be replaced
by $\alpha[b_1 a]bc_- c_1 \ldots_- c_k$.
   Case C3.2. $b + c$ and $n'(b) > 3$. Failure.
   Case C3.3. $b + c$ and $n'(b) = 3$. If $S'(b) \cap S'(c) = \{d\}$ and either
          $S'(c) = \{d\}$ or $S'(c) = \{c_1, d\}$ where $l(c_1) < m$, set
          $\varphi' = \alpha[ca]db$. If $S'(b) \cap S'(c) = \emptyset$ and either $S'(c) = \emptyset$
          or $S'(c) = \{c_1\}$ where $l(c_1) < m$, set $\varphi' = \alpha[ca]_- b$.
          Otherwise failure.

Case C3.4. $b + c$ and $\max(n'(b), n'(c)) = 2$.

Case C3.4.1. $S'(b) = S'(c)$. Failure.

Case C3.4.2. $S'(b) \cap S'(c) = \{d\}$. If $n'(b) = 2$, let $S'(b) = \{b_1, d\}$; if $n'(c) = 2$ let $S'(c) = \{c_1, d\}$.

In this case we say that b is k-lucky if $l(b_1) = k$ and $k \leq m$; b is 0-lucky if $n'(b) = 1$; otherwise b is unlucky. Similarly c can be lucky or unlucky. There are four viable alternatives to decide between, namely $\alpha[ba]dc$, $\alpha[b_1 a]bcd$, $\alpha[ca]db$, and $\alpha[c_1 a]cbd$.

Case C3.4.2.1. Neither b nor c is lucky. Failure.

Case C3.4.2.2. b is k-lucky and c is unlucky. If $k \neq m$, set
$$\varphi' = \alpha_{-}a_m \ldots {}_{-}a_{k+2}\langle b_k a_{k+1}\rangle \ldots \langle ba_1\rangle\langle dc\rangle.$$
Otherwise set $\varphi' = \alpha[b_1 a]bcd$.

This is the neatest part of the entire algorithm, since the two viable alternatives $\alpha[ba]dc$ and $\alpha[b_1 a]bcd$ turn out to be essentially a Type B situation. (On the other hand it may also be considered the sloppiest part of the algorithm, since an abuse of notation is involved here: If the Type B specification is ultimately completed to a string of the form $\alpha_{-}a_m \ldots {}_{-}a_{k+2}a_{k+1}b_k \ldots a_1 bcd\omega$, a blank should actually be inserted just before a_{k+1}.)

Case C3.4.2.3. b is k-lucky and c is l-lucky, where $k \geq l$. Set
$$\varphi' = \alpha[b_1 a]bcd.$$

It is easy to check that φ' dominates the other three alternatives, using arguments like those in Section 4.

Case C3.4.3. $S'(b) \cap S'(c) = \emptyset$ and $n'(b) = n'(c) = 2$. Let $S'(b) = \{b_1, b_1'\}$ and $S'(c) = \{c_1, c_1'\}$, where $l(b_1) \leq l(b_1')$ and $l(c_1) \leq l(c_1')$.

The only possibilities are $\alpha[ba]b_1' cc_1 c_1'$ and $\alpha[ca]c_1' bb_1 b_1'$, perhaps interchanging b_1 with b_1' and/or c_1 with c_1'.

Case C3.4.3.1. $l(b_1) \geq m$. If $l(c_1) \geq m$, failure; otherwise if $l(c_1') \geq m$, set $\varphi' = \alpha[ca]c_1' b$; otherwise set $\varphi' = \alpha[c'a]c_1 b$, where "$[c'a]$" means that the blanks are to be filled by c and the chain containing c_1'.

These actions are forced unless $l(c_1) = l(c_1') = 1$, for if c_1 and c_1' both have finite level we must have $l(c_1) = 1$ or failure will be imminent.

Case C3.4.3.2. $l(b_1) < m \leq l(b_1')$, $l(c_1) < m \leq l(c_1')$, and $n'(b_1') \leq n'(c_1')$. If $S'(b_1') \neq \{c_1'\}$, failure; otherwise set $\varphi' = \alpha[ba]b_1' c$.

In this case it is impossible to complete φ with $\alpha[ba]b_1' cc_1 c_1'$, since $l(b_1') > 1$; the only viable alternatives are $\alpha[ba]b_1' cc_1' c_1$ and $\alpha[ca]c_1' bb_1' b_1$, and we must have $b_1' - c_1'$. Now if $S'(c_1') \neq \{b_1'\}$, the stated value of φ' is forced, otherwise success is imminent.

Case C3.4.3.3. $l(b_1) < m \le l(b_1')$ and $l(c_1') < m$. Set $\varphi' = \alpha[c'a]c_1b$. This is essentially forced, since $\alpha[ba]b_1'c\langle c_1 c_1'\rangle$ implies $l(b_1') = 1$ when c_1 and c_1' have finite level.

Case C3.4.3.4. $l(b_1') < m$, $l(c_1') < m$, and $l(b_1) \le l(c_1)$. Set $\varphi' = \alpha[b'a]b_1c$.

As in Case C3.4.3.1 we see that failure will occur unless $l(b_1) = 1$.

Case C3.4.4. $S'(b) \cap S'(c) = \emptyset$, $n'(b) = 2$, and $n'(c) \le 1$. Let $S'(b) = \{b_1, b_1'\}$, where $l(b_1) \le l(b_1')$; and if $n'(c) = 1$, let $S'(c) = \{c_1\}$, otherwise let c_1 be blank and $l(c_1) = 0$.

There are many possible arrangements to choose from, and the subcases require careful analysis.

Case C3.4.4.1. $l(b_1) > m$. If $l(c_1) > m$, set $\varphi' = \alpha_- a_m \ldots {}_- a_2 cac_1 b$. If $l(c_1) = m$, set $\varphi' = \alpha[c_1a]cb$. Otherwise set $\varphi' = \alpha[ca]_- b$.

Case C3.4.4.2. $l(b_1) \le m$ and $l(c_1) \le m$. If $l(c_1) = m$ or $l(b_1') < \infty$, set $\varphi' = \alpha[c_1a]cb$. Otherwise if $l(c_1) < l(b_1) - 2$, set $\varphi' = \alpha[b_1a]bc$; otherwise set $\varphi' = \alpha[ca]b_1b$.

If $l(b_1') < \infty$, success is imminent, so we may assume that $l(b_1') = \infty$. Then $\alpha[b_1a]bcb_1' \ge \alpha[ba]b_1'c$; and we have $\alpha[ca]_- b \ge \alpha[c_1a]cb \ge \alpha_- a_m \ldots {}_- a_2 cac_1 b$, unless $l(c_1) = m$ when $\alpha[ca]_- b$ is inapplicable. If $l(c_1) = m$, it is clear that $\alpha[c_1a]cb \ge \alpha[b_1a]bcb_1'$; otherwise we need to compare $\alpha[b_1a]bcb_1'$ with $\alpha[ca]_- b$, and the best place for b_1 in the latter string is $\alpha[ca]b_1 b_- b_1'$. The stretched chains in these two alternatives now fill respectively $l(c_1)$ and $l(b_1) - 2$ positions to the right of b_1', and it is best to minimize this quantity.

Case C3.4.4.3. $l(b_1) \le m$ and $l(c_1) > m$. If $l(b_1) = m$, set φ' equal to $\alpha[b_1a]bcb_1'c_1$. Otherwise if $l(b_1') = m$, set φ' equal to $\alpha[b_1'a]bcb_1c_1$. Otherwise if $l(b_1') < m$, set $\varphi' = \alpha[b'a]b_1c$. Otherwise let $k = l(b_1)$; set $\varphi' = \alpha_- a_m \ldots {}_- a_{k+2}\langle b_k a_{k+1}\rangle \ldots \langle b_1 a_2\rangle\langle ba_1\rangle\langle b_1'c\rangle$.

As in Case C3.4.2.2, this is a slight abuse of notation.

Case C3.5. $b + c$ and $S'(b) = S'(c) = \{d\}$. Set $\varphi' = \varphi bc$.

Case C3.6. $b + c$, $S'(b) \cap S'(c) = \emptyset$, and $\max(n'(b), n'(c)) \le 1$. If $n'(b) = 1$, let $S'(b) = \{b_1\}$; otherwise let b_1 be blank and set $l(b_1) = 0$. Define c_1 similarly.

Case C3.6.1. $l(b_1) \le m$ and $l(c_1) \le m$. Set $\varphi' = \varphi bc$.

Success is imminent.

Case C3.6.2. $l(b_1) \le m$ and $l(c_1) > m$. If $l(b_1) = m$, set $\varphi' = \alpha[b_1a]bc$, otherwise set $\varphi' = \alpha[ba]_- c$.

Case C3.6.3. $l(b_1) > m$ and $l(c_1) > m$.

In this final case we must "look ahead" before deciding what to do.

For $k \geq 1$ if b_k has degree 2, let b_{k+1} be the vertex adjacent to b_k that has not yet been given a name; continue until having found the sequence $b \!-\! b_1 \!-\! \cdots \!-\! b_k$ where $\deg(b_k) \neq 2$. Similarly, find the sequence $c \!-\! c_1 \!-\! \cdots \!-\! c_l$ where $\deg(c_l) \neq 2$.

(This process must terminate, since G is not a cycle.)

Case C3.6.3.1. $b_k = c_l = a$ or $\deg(b_k) = \deg(c_l) = 1$. Set $\varphi' = \varphi bc$. Success is imminent.

Case C3.6.3.2. $\deg(b_k) = 1$ and $\deg(c_l) > 2$. Set φ' equal to $\alpha_- a_m \ldots - a_2 bab_1 c$.

Case C3.6.3.3. $\deg(b_k) > 2$, $\deg(c_l) > 2$, and $k \leq l$.

In this case we must decide among four layouts $\_abcb_1 c_1 \ldots b_{k-1} c_{k-1} b_k$, $\_acbc_1 b_1 \ldots c_{k-1} b_{k-1} c_k$, $bab_1 cb_2 c_1 \ldots b_k c_{k-1}$, and $cac_1 bc_2 b_1 \ldots c_k b_{k-1}$; by acquiring a little more information about b_k, c_l, k, and l we will learn which of these dominates:

Case C3.6.3.3.1. $b_k = c_l$. If $k = l$, set $\varphi' = \varphi bcb_1 c_1$; otherwise set $\varphi' = \alpha_- a_m \ldots - a_2 ca_1 c_1 b$.

Case C3.6.3.3.2. $b_k \!-\! c_l$. If $k = l$, set $\varphi' = \varphi \langle bc \rangle \langle b_1 c_1 \rangle$; otherwise set $\varphi' = \alpha_- a_m \ldots - a_2 \langle ac \rangle \langle bc_1 \rangle$.

Case C3.6.3.3.3. $b_k \neq c_l$, $b_k \!+\! c_l$. Failure.

Note that the "lookahead time" required to find k and l in Case C3.6.3 is $O(k+l)$, not $O(1)$; but Case C3.6.3 cannot occur again until elements $b_1, \ldots, b_{k-1}, c_1, \ldots, c_{l-1}$ have all been included in the string φ. Thus the lookahead time can be distributed among the subsequent steps, and the subalgorithm runs in linear time.

We have now exhausted all possible cases, and the subalgorithm is complete.

6. Examples

Here is how the subalgorithm would proceed to search for a layout for the graph of Figure 1, beginning with DC:

Case	φ
	DC
A3	DC$\langle$AE$\rangle$
B2	DCAEBF
A3	DCAEBF$\langle$GJ$\rangle$
B1	Failure.

On the other hand, if we begin with DA, the algorithm succeeds:

A2	DA
A2	DAC
A2	DACB
A4	DACBE
C3.4.4.1(i)	DACBE_F
A2	DACBEGFHJ
A2	DACBEGFHJI
A4	DACBEGFHJIK
C3.4.4.1(ii)	DACBEGFHJIK_L
A3	DACBEGFHJIKNLMO
B5	DACBEGFHJIKNLMO⟨PR⟩
B6	DACBEGFHJIKNLMO⟨PR⟩⟨QS⟩
C4	DACBEGFHJIKNLMOPRQS_T
C2.3.1(ii)	DACBEGFHJIKNLMOPRQS_T_U
B2	DACBEGFHJIKNLMOPRQSWTVU⟨XY⟩
A5	DACBEGFHJIKNLMOPRQSWTVUYX&Z
	Success.

And here is how the algorithm would construct the same solution with left and right reversed, starting with Z&:

A2	Z&
A2	Z&X
A2	Z&XY
A3	Z&XYU
B5	Z&XYU⟨TV⟩
B6	Z&XYU⟨TV⟩⟨SW⟩
C4	Z&XYUVTWS_R
C3.4.4.2(iii)	Z&XYUVTWS_R_O
A2	Z&XYUVTWSQRPOML
A2	Z&XYUVTWSQRPOMLN
A4	Z&XYUVTWSQRPOMLNK
C3.4.4.1(i)	Z&XYUVTWSQRPOMLNK_J
A2	Z&XYUVTWSQRPOMLNKIJHF
A2	Z&XYUVTWSQRPOMLNKIJHFG
A3	Z&XYUVTWSQRPOMLNKIJHFGE
B2	Z&XYUVTWSQRPOMLNKIJHFGE⟨BC⟩
A5	Z&XYUVTWSQRPOMLNKIJHFGEBCAD
	Success.

If the algorithm had chosen the somewhat tempting alternative layout Z&XYUVTWSNRMOLPK at step C3.4.4.2 in this example, failure would have followed soon after.

Suppose Figure 1 were changed so that F — J became F — $*$ — J. Then the algorithm would invoke further cases:

C3.6.3.3.1(ii)	`Z&XYUVTWSQRPOMLNK_J`
A2	`Z&XYUVTWSQRPOMLNKIJH*`
A2	`Z&XYUVTWSQRPOMLNKIJH*G`
A4	`Z&XYUVTWSQRPOMLNKIJH*GF`
C3.4.2.3	`Z&XYUVTWSQRPOMLNKIJH*GF_E`
A5	`Z&XYUVTWSQRPOMLNKIJH*GFDECBA`
	Success.

7. Applications of the Subalgorithm

The subalgorithm determines in $O(n)$ steps whether or not G has a bandwidth-2 layout beginning with ab; by trying all possible a and b we have an $O(n^3)$ algorithm for deciding whether or not $Bandwidth(G) \leq 2$. This can be improved to an $O(n^2)$ algorithm, by using the subalgorithm to decide whether or not G has a complete layout that extends xy_a, for some vertex a and some (nonexistent) dummy vertices x and y. However, we really want an $O(n)$ algorithm, so it is necessary to be a little more careful.

We observed at the beginning of Section 2 that G may be assumed to contain a vertex v of degree ≥ 3; suppose v — a, v — b, and v — c. Then any layout for G must contain one of the six substrings

$$vab, \quad vba, \quad vac, \quad vca, \quad vbc, \quad vcb,$$

or their left-right reflections, since two of $\{a, b, c\}$ must appear on the same side of v. To test $Bandwidth(G) \leq 2$ in linear time, it therefore suffices to have a linear-time algorithm that determines whether or not a complete layout exists containing a given substring of three vertices. (Recall that a "complete layout" always has bandwidth 2 according to the definition in Section 2.)

Let us first develop an algorithm that decides in $O(n)$ steps whether or not there is a complete layout for a given connected graph G, containing a given substring $abcd$ of length 4:

A1. [Sanity check.] Stop with failure if a — d.

A2. [Safety check.] Let G_0 be the graph obtained from G by deleting all edges among $\{a, b, c, d\}$. If there is a path in G_0 from a or b to c or d, stop with failure. (This path cannot possibly be incorporated into a complete layout containing $abcd$, since it cannot get to the right of b.)

A3. [Divide and conquer.] Let the vertices of $V \backslash \{a, b, c, d\}$ be partitioned into two subsets

$$V_1 = \{v \mid \text{a path exists in } G_0 \text{ from } v \text{ to } a \text{ or } b\},$$
$$V_2 = \{v \mid \text{a path exists in } G_0 \text{ from } v \text{ to } c \text{ or } d\}.$$

(By step A2, V_1 and V_2 are disjoint. Furthermore we have $V = \{a, b, c, d\} \cup V_1 \cup V_2$, since G was connected.) Let G_1 be G_0 restricted to $V_1 \cup \{a, b\}$, and let G_2 be G_0 restricted to $V_2 \cup \{c, d\}$. Use the subalgorithm to find a layout φ_1 for G_1 beginning with ba, and also to find a layout φ_2 for G_2 beginning with cd. If either attempt fails, stop with failure; otherwise stop with success, since $\varphi_1^R \varphi_2$ is a complete layout for G as required. $\square$

Now to solve the similar problem given a substring abc of length 3, we consider two cases:

i) There is at least one vertex $d \notin \{a, c\}$ such that $b \,\text{—}\, d$. Then the complete layout must contain either $abcd$ or $dabc$, and we use the previous algorithm to try both cases.

ii) There is no such vertex. Then we can use an algorithm analogous to the one above: Let G_0 be G minus all edges among $\{a, b, c\}$ and stop if there is a path from a to c in G_0. Otherwise partition $V \backslash \{a, b, c\}$ into disjoint sets V_1 and V_2, where V_1 contains the vertices reachable from a and V_2 those reachable from c. Any complete layout containing the substring abc must be composed of a complete layout for G_1 ending with ab and a complete layout for G_2 beginning with bc.

It is also possible to construct a linear-time algorithm that decides whether or not a complete layout exists containing a given substring ab of length 2; details are left to the reader.

8. Tree Bandwidth is NP-complete

In this section we will shift gears and prove that the general problem of determining the bandwidth of a graph is NP-complete. That is, we shall prove that any problem in the large class NP can be transformed into the problem of determining whether or not the bandwidth of some graph is less than some integer k, with at most a polynomial increase in the size of the problem specification. (See [25] and [2, Chapter 10] for surveys of NP-complete problems.) This particular result was first obtained by Christos H. Papadimitriou [28]; we shall prove it in a sharper form, by severely restricting the form of G.

Theorem. *The following problem is NP-complete: Given an integer k, and given a graph G that is a free tree with no vertices of degree > 3, is Bandwidth$(G) \leq k$?*

Proof. The problem of determining whether or not Bandwidth$(G) \leq k$, given k and an *arbitrary* graph G, is clearly in NP. We shall complete the proof by showing that the "3-partition problem," which is known to be NP-complete [16, page 120], can be polynomially transformed into the restricted bandwidth problem stated in the theorem.

Given a sequence of $3n$ integers $\langle a_1, a_2, \ldots, a_{3n} \rangle$, where $a_1 + a_2 + \cdots + a_{3n} = nA$ and $A/4 < a_j < A/2$ for each j, the 3-partition problem asks whether or not there is a way to partition the integers $\{1, 2, \ldots, 3n\}$ into disjoint triples $T_1, \ldots, T_n$ so that $\sum \{a_j \mid j \in T_i\} = A$ for $1 \leq i \leq n$. In other words it is a special bin-packing problem, where we are to take $3n$ objects of integer sizes $a_1, a_2, \ldots, a_{3n}$ and pack them into n boxes of size A whenever possible. The condition $A/4 < a_j < A/2$ means that each box in any such packing must contain exactly three objects.

Given the specification of a 3-partition problem, our job is to construct an integer k and a free tree G whose vertices all have degree ≤ 3, such that there is a 3-partition if and only if Bandwidth$(G) \leq k$. From the proof in [14] it suffices to do this with a tree whose size is at most a polynomial in n and A, since the 3-partition problem is NP-complete even when the magnitudes of all $3n$ numbers are bounded above by a (suitably large) polynomial function of n. (See [15] for a discussion of this "strong NP-completeness" property.)

The free trees we shall construct bear more resemblance to pelagic hydrozoa of the order Siphonophora than to actual trees, so we shall find it convenient to use terms from marine biology rather than botany. Our construction involves parameters $m_1, \ldots, m_{3n}$, d, and k that we will specify later after the properties we need for the proof have been explained.

The graphs of interest to us all have the general structure shown in Figure 3. There is a long *stem*, a path in which every dth vertex has a special name; the respective names of these special stem vertices are

$$b_0 \; h_1 \; b_1 \; p_1 \; b_2 \; f_1 \; b_3 \; p_2 \; b_4 \; f_2 \ldots p_n \; b_{2n} \; f_n \; b_{2n+1} \; h_2 \; b_{2n+2} \; h_3 \; b_{2n+3}$$

from left to right. It follows that the stem contains $4dn + 6d + 1$ vertices in all. There are also $3n$ long *tentacles* attached to special vertices t_1, $\ldots$, t_{3n}; the ith tentacle consists of a long *filament* followed by $2m_i$ *nematocysts* as shown in Figure 4. If we break off each tentacle just below the node t_i, and if we remove the boundary nodes $b_0, b_1, \ldots, b_{2n+3}$,

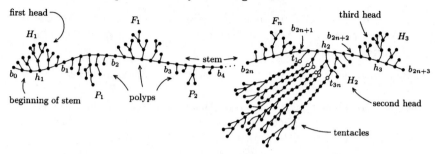

FIGURE 3. Schematic view of a siphonophore graph.

the remaining graph consists of $2n + 3$ connected pieces called *polyps*, named respectively

$$H_1 \ P_1 \ F_1 \ P_2 \ F_2 \ldots P_n \ F_n \ H_2 \ H_3$$

from left to right. The vertices t_1, ..., t_{3n} all belong to the polyp called H_2, the animal's "second head."

We have noted that the special stem vertices b_0, h_1, b_1, ..., b_{2n+3} are separated by distance d; our construction will also have the property that every node of a polyp H_i, P_i, or F_i is at distance $\leq d$ from its "central" node h_i, p_i, or f_i.

Now we shall impose further constraints on the construction, so that it will not be easy to make layouts of bandwidth k. In the first place, we will require each of the heads H_i to contain exactly $2dk - 1$ vertices. This means that there are exactly $2dk$ vertices $\neq h_i$ at distance $\leq d$ from h_i (since each head touches two boundary nodes b_j), so it is necessary to lay these vertices out in such a way that the dk nearest locations on each side of h_i are occupied by precisely those elements at distance d or less in the graph. In particular, consider the layout of H_1, and assume without loss of generality that vertex b_1 occurs to the right of h_1; then all of the other polyps must appear to the right of H_1 in the layout, since there is no way for any of their vertices to get to the left of h_1 without making the bandwidth exceed k. A similar argument applies to the third head H_3, which therefore must appear (together somehow with b_{2n+3}) at the extreme right of the layout. All of the other polyps, and all of the tentacles, must appear between H_1 and H_3.

We shall arrange things so that the total number of vertices in the graph is exactly $(2n + 3)(2dk) + 1$. This means that the situation will be very "tight": There are $(2n + 1)(2dk) - 1$ vertices that must appear in the layout between b_1 and b_{2n+2}, but vertices b_1 and b_{2n+2} are at

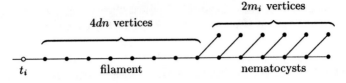

FIGURE 4. General form of the ith tentacle.

distance $(2n+1)(2d)$ from each other in the graph, so we must conclude that *the stem between b_1 and b_{2n+2} is stretched tightly*. In other words, two adjacent nodes in this portion of the stem must be placed k positions apart. (It does not follow that the stem from b_0 to h_1 or from h_3 to b_{2n+3} is stretched; b_0 might even appear to the right of h_1. But all we are using H_1 and H_3 for is to confine the other nodes and therefore to assign a rigid structure to the interior parts of the layout.)

Since the stem is stretched tightly, and since the polyps contain no nodes at distance $> d$ from their central node, the layout must now appear as a sequence of regions that we may represent as follows:

$$H_1' \ b_1 \ P_1' \ b_2 \ F_1' \ b_3 \ P_2' \ b_4 \ F_2' \ldots P_n' \ b_{2n} \ F_n' \ b_{2n+1} \ H_2' \ b_{2n+2} \ H_3'.$$

Here H_1' is a layout of $H_1 \cup \{b_0\}$, H_2' is a layout of H_2, H_3' is a layout of $H_3 \cup \{b_{2n+3}\}$, and (P_i', F_i') are respectively layouts of (P_i, F_i) plus portions of the tentacles that just manage to fit. Each of the regions P_i' and F_i' includes exactly $2dk - 1$ vertices of the layout. The reader should stop at this point to review the construction before going on.

If we choose the sizes of P_i and F_i carefully, the tentacles will be difficult to place. Let us say that

$\quad F_i$ contains exactly $2dk - 1 - 6di$ vertices,

and

$\quad P_i$ contains exactly $2dk - 1 - c - 18di + 12d$ vertices,

so that

$\quad F_i'$ contains exactly $6di$ tentacle vertices,

and

$\quad P_i'$ contains exactly $c + 18di - 12d$ tentacle vertices,

where c is a constant to be determined later. Since the tentacles are all connected to H_2, they must emanate from near the right end of the layout, passing through F_i' before coming to P_i'. If $P_1', \ldots, P_i'$ together contain portions of at least r_i different tentacles then F_i' must contain at least $2dr_i$ vertices of these tentacles, since a path cannot cross F_i' without using up at least $2d$ positions; hence $2dr_i \leq 6di$, that is,

$$r_i \leq 3i.$$

Furthermore if $r_i = 3i$ each tentacle must use exactly $2d$ positions of F'_i, so there can be no nematocysts in F'_i in such a case.

By choosing the values of $c, m_1, \ldots, m_{3n}$ we will be able to guarantee that exactly $3i$ tentacles come through F'_i. Consider first P'_1, which must contain $c + 6d$ tentacle vertices; these must come from at most three different tentacles because of the constraint on r_1. If we choose each m_i as a function of the given numbers a_i so that the number of nodes in two tentacles is always less than $c + 6d$, then P'_1 must contain vertices from exactly three different tentacles, and it must include all of their nematocysts too because of the constraint on F'_1. Furthermore we will be able to argue in the same way that P'_2 must now include all the nematocysts of three other tentacles because of the constraint on F'_2, and so on.

In order to make this argument go through properly we will want to define things so that the three tentacles whose nematocysts appear in P'_i have their filaments "pulled completely through" the succeeding regions, with exactly $2d$ vertices of their filaments appearing in each of $F'_i, P'_{i+1}, \ldots, P'_n, F'_n$. It turns out that we can do this by making each m_i a multiple of $6dn$, and requiring that $a_i + a_j + a_l = A$ if and only if $2(m_i + m_j + m_l) = c$. Let us set

$$m_i = 6dna_i, \qquad c = 12dnA;$$

we shall prove that a layout of bandwidth k implies the existence of a 3-partition:

Lemma. *For $1 \leq i \leq n$, region P'_i contains all of the nematocysts from exactly three tentacles, namely the tentacles connected to t_j where j is in some triple T_i, and $\sum\{a_j \mid j \in T_i\} = A$. Furthermore P'_i also contains as much as possible of the filaments from these tentacles; that is, each tentacle in T_i has only $2d$ vertices in each of $F'_i, P'_{i+1}, \ldots, P'_n, F'_n$.*

Proof. By induction on i, we know that F'_i and P'_i each contain exactly $3(i-1)(2d)$ filament nodes from tentacles whose nematocysts appear in $P'_1, \ldots, P'_{i-1}$. That leaves $6d$ empty positions in F'_i and $12dnA + 12di - 6d$ in P'_i. Now P'_i must contain vertices from at least three tentacles, since two tentacles have at most $8dn + 2(m_j + m_l) = 8dn + 12dn(a_j + a_l) \leq 8dn + 12dn(A - 1) = 12dnA - 4dn$ vertices altogether. Hence P'_i has vertices from exactly three tentacles, defined by some triple $T_i \subseteq \{1, 2, \ldots, 3n\}$, and it includes all of their nematocysts because F'_i has room for only $6d$ more vertices from all three tentacles. Let $\alpha = \sum\{a_j \mid j \in T_i\}$; then the $12dnA + 12di - 6d$ available positions in P'_i, are taken up by $12dn\alpha$ nematocysts and somewhere between 0 and $3(4dn - (2n - 2i + 1)(2d)) = 12di - 6d$ filament nodes. It follows that $\alpha = A$ and exactly $12di - 6d$ filament nodes are present.   □

The lemma proves that a bandwidth-k layout for a graph of this kind necessarily leads to a valid 3-partition. To complete the proof of the theorem, we must define the graphs so that existence of a 3-partition is sufficient to imply the existence of a layout with bandwidth k. This means in particular that we will have to choose d and k appropriately. Furthermore the graphs must be constructible by an algorithm whose running time is bounded by a polynomial in n and A.

In the first place we want to choose k large enough that P_n contains at least $2d - 1$ vertices, hence we require

$$k \geq 6nA + 9n - 5.$$

For convenience we let k be the smallest power of 2 satisfying this condition, and we write

$$k = 2^l.$$

Finally we choose

$$d = lk.$$

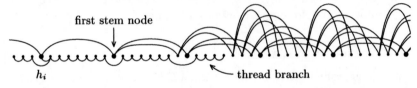

first stem node

h_i thread branch

FIGURE 5. Layout of a head polyp H_i in the immediate vicinity of its center node h_i.

From these parameters k and d we can construct G by explaining how to construct each polyp. The head polyps H_i are formed by the bandwidth-2^l layout indicated in Figure 5 for $l = 3$ (although l will never be this small). A periodic pattern begins to repeat after the lth stem node to the right of h_i: The jth node preceding a stem node branches to the $(2j)$th and $(2j + 1)$st nodes preceding the next stem nodes, for $0 \leq j < 2^{l-1}$. Before this pattern is established, we have $(1, 2, 4, \ldots, 2^{l-2})$ as the respective limits on j. An additional "thread branch" goes out of h_i to fill up the remaining

$$(2^l - 1) + (2^l - 2) + \cdots + (2^l - 2^{l-1}) = lk - 2^l + 1 = d - k + 1$$

holes near the center. To the left of h_i we use essentially the same idea in mirror image; thus it is clear that no vertex is at distance greater than d from the center node. The special nodes $t_1, \ldots, t_{3n}$ in H_2 are taken to be the leftmost $3n$ nodes in its layout.

A similar procedure is used to construct the other polyps P_i and F_i. In each case we wish to remove $2dx$ nodes from a full head polyp, for some integer x, and we do this by removing x nodes between each pair of adjacent stem nodes. The x nodes immediately to the right of each stem node in Figure 5 are simply deleted from the graph, together with all edges touching them, and the "thread branch" is reconnected for the remaining nodes; again the mirror image of this pattern is used to the left of the center vertex, and we clearly have a tree. It is easy to see that the resulting polyp has a layout of length $2dk - 1$ in which the x positions just to the *left* of each stem node are empty. (Simply shift all nonstem vertices that lie to the right of the center vertex exactly x places to the left.) These x slots form x parallel "channels" through which filaments can pass.

Now it is not difficult to see how to embed the tentacles into these polyp layouts whenever a 3-partition is given. For example, we can place filaments for the three tentacles specified by T_1 into the rightmost three channels of $F_1, P_2, F_2, \ldots, P_n, F_n$. Now it is easy to make the remaining nematocyst and filament nodes fit into the remaining spaces in P_1 without exceeding bandwidth k; further details are left to the reader. It is possible to link up any channel in F_n with any t_i, since $k \geq 6n$. $\square$

9. Directed Bandwidth

Analogous problems can be studied when G is an acyclic *directed* graph, where we require its layout to be a topological sorting of the vertices; in other words, we stipulate that $f(u) < f(v)$ whenever $u \to v$ in the graph, and we ask for the minimum bandwidth subject to this constraint.

The algorithm in Sections 2 through 7 above can readily be modified to test for "directed bandwidth 2." In fact, the situation becomes so much simpler that it is tempting to try for directed bandwidth 3 in polynomial time.

The NP-completeness construction in Section 8 can be modified in a straightforward way to obtain an analogous result.

Theorem. *The following problem is NP-complete: Given an integer k, and given a directed graph that is an oriented tree having no vertices of in-degree > 2, is its directed bandwidth $\leq k$?*

(Each vertex of an oriented tree has out-degree ≤ 1, and there are no oriented cycles.)

The analogous problem of minimizing $\sum(f(v) - f(u))$ over all topological sortings of a general acyclic directed graph has recently been proved NP-complete by E. L. Lawler [26]; on the other hand Adolphson and Hu [1] have resolved this problem in polynomial time when the directed graph is an oriented tree, even when the arcs have been assigned arbitrary weights. Thus the bandwidth problem is somewhat harder than this optimal ordering problem, in the directed as well as the undirected case.

10. Some Open Problems

The following related questions are still waiting for an answer:

a) Is the problem "*Bandwidth*$(G) \leq 3$" NP-complete, given an arbitrary graph (or perhaps a tree) G?

b) Is there a polynomial time algorithm to enumerate the number of distinct bandwidth-2 layouts of a given connected graph G?

c) For which exponents p is the problem "Some layout of G satisfies $\sum\{|f(u) - f(v)|^p \mid u \longrightarrow v \text{ in } G\} \leq k$" NP-complete, when G is a free tree?

d) What is the expected bandwidth, for random graphs on n vertices and m edges, as n and $m \to \infty$?

Question (b) is of potential interest because there seems to be a vague connection between efficient algorithms for enumeration and efficient algorithms for testing existence. For example, there is a determinant formula for evaluating the number of spanning trees of a graph, and there are efficient algorithms for testing connectedness. The problems of enumerating the number of Hamiltonian paths of a graph, or the number of ways to satisfy a given set of clauses, etc., do not seem to be in NP; there most likely are polynomial-time reducibilities between such problems, but such transformations remain to be investigated. In the case of bandwidth-2 layouts for a graph, there is a linear time algorithm for existence, yet no apparently "nice" characterization. So this is a candidate problem in which enumeration might be definitely more difficult than existence.

Question (c) is suggested by the fact that Yossi Shiloach [31] has shown how to solve the stated problem in polynomial time for $p = 1$, but as p increases the best layouts are eventually those with minimum bandwidth.

All four problems can be considered also for the case of directed bandwidth.

Another interesting question is to discover how far from optimum the various heuristic methods for bandwidth reduction can be; see the references below for several approaches that have been proposed.

The preparation of this paper was supported in part by the National Science Foundation and the Office of Naval Research.

References

[1] D. Adolphson and T. C. Hu, "Optimal linear ordering," *SIAM Journal of Applied Mathematics* **25** (1973), 403–423.

[2] A. V. Aho, J. E. Hopcroft, and J. D. Ullman, *The Design and Analysis of Computer Algorithms* (Reading, Massachusetts: Addison–Wesley, 1974).

[3] F. A. Akyuz and Senol Tuku, "An automatic node-relabeling scheme for bandwidth minimization of stiffness matrices," *American Institute of Aeronautics and Astronautics [AIAA] Journal* **6** (1968), 728–730.

[4] G. G. Alway and D. W. Martin, "An algorithm for reducing the bandwidth of a matrix of symmetrical configuration," *The Computer Journal* **8** (1965), 264–272.

[5] Ilona Arany, Lajos Szoda, and W. F. Smyth, "An improved method for reducing the bandwidth of sparse symmetric matrices," *Proceedings of IFIP Congress 71* (Amsterdam: North-Holland, 1972), 1246–1250.

[6] J. H. Bolstad, G. K. Leaf, A. J. Lindeman, and H. G. Kaper, "An empirical investigation of reordering and data management for finite element systems of equations," Technical Report ANL8056 (Argonne National Laboratories, 1973).

[7] Kuo Young Cheng, "Note on minimizing the bandwidth of sparse, symmetric matrices," *Computing* **11** (1973), 27–30; "Minimizing the bandwidth of sparse symmetric matrices," *Computing* **11** (1973), 103–110.

[8] Václav Chvátal, "A remark on a problem of Harary," *Czechoslovak Mathematical Journal* **20** (1970), 109–111.

[9] Jarmila Chvátalová, "Optimal labelling of a product of two paths," *Discrete Mathematics* **11** (1975), 249–253.

[10] P. Z. Chinn, J. Chvátalová, A. K. Dewdney, and N. E. Gibbs, "The bandwidth problem for graphs and matrices — a survey," *Journal of Graph Theory* **6** (1982), 223–254.

[11] E. Cuthill and J. McKee, "Reducing the bandwidth of sparse symmetric matrices," *Proceedings of the ACM National Conference* **24** (1969), 157–172.

[12] Richard A. DeMillo, Stanley C. Eisenstat, and Richard J. Lipton, "Preserving average proximity in arrays," *Communications of the ACM* **21** (1978), 228–231.

[13] D. R. Fulkerson and O. A. Gross, "Incidence matrices and interval graphs," *Pacific Journal of Mathematics* **15** (1965), 835–855. [Generalized bandwidth-1 problem for hypergraphs.]

[14] M. R. Garey and D. S. Johnson, "Complexity results for multiprocessor scheduling under resource constraints," *SIAM Journal on Computing* **4** (1975), 397–411.

[15] M. R. Garey and D. S. Johnson, " 'Strong' NP-completeness results: Motivation, examples and implications," *Journal of the Association for Computing Machinery* **25** (1978), 499–508.

[16] M. R. Garey, D. S. Johnson, and Ravi Sethi, "The complexity of flowshop and jobshop scheduling," *Mathematics of Operations Research* **1** (1976), 117–129.

[17] M. R. Garey, D. S. Johnson, and L. Stockmeyer, "Some simplified *NP*-complete graph problems," *Theoretical Computer Science* **1** (1976), 237–267.

[18] J. Alan George, *Computer Implementation of the Finite Element Method*, Computer Science Technical Report STAN-CS-71-208 (Ph.D. thesis, Stanford University, 1971).

[19] Norman E. Gibbs and William G. Poole Jr., "Tridiagonalization by permutations," *Communications of the ACM* **20** (1974), 20–24.

[20] R. L. Graham, "On primitive graphs and optimal vertex assignments," *Annals of the New York Academy of Sciences* **175** (1970), 170–186.

[21] Henry R. Grooms, "Algorithm for matrix bandwidth reduction," *Journal of the Structural Division, Proceedings of the American Society of Civil Engineers* **98** (1972), 203–214.

[22] L. H. Harper, "Optimal assignments of numbers to vertices," *Journal of the Society for Industrial and Applied Mathematics* **12** (1964), 131–135.

[23] L. H. Harper, "Optimal numberings and isoperimetric problems on graphs," *Journal of Combinatorial Theory* **1** (1966), 385–393.

[24] L. H. Harper, "A necessary condition on minimal cube numberings," *Journal of Applied Probability* **4** (1967), 397–401.

[25] Richard M. Karp, "Reducibility among combinatorial problems," in *Complexity of Computer Computations*, edited by Raymond E. Miller and J. W. Thatcher (New York: Plenum, 1972), 85–104.

[26] E. L. Lawler, "Sequencing jobs to minimize total weighted completion time subject to precedence constraints," *Annals of Discrete Mathematics* **2** (1978), 75–90.

[27] R. J. Lipton, S. C. Eisenstat, and R. A. DeMillo, "Space and time hierarchies for classes of control structures and data structures," *Journal of the Association for Computing Machinery* **23** (1976), 720–732. [Generalized bandwidth problem of embedding one graph in another.]

[28] Ch. H. Papadimitriou, "The *NP*-completeness of the bandwidth minimization problem," *Computing* **16** (1976), 263–270.

[29] Richard Rosen, "Matrix bandwidth minimization," *Proceedings of the ACM National Conference* **23** (1968), 585–595.

[30] Arnold L. Rosenberg, "Preserving proximity in arrays," *SIAM Journal on Computing* **4** (1975), 443–460.

[31] Yossi Shiloach, "A minimum linear arrangement algorithm for undirected trees," *SIAM Journal on Computing* **8** (1979), 15–32.

[32] Paul Tiing Renn Wang, *Bandwidth Minimization, Reducibility Decomposition, and Triangularization of Sparse Matrices*, Computer and Information Science Research Center Report OSU-CISRC-TR-73-5 (Ph.D. thesis, Ohio State University, 1973).

Addendum

Substantial progress has been made on the research problems that were posed at the end of this paper. James B. Saxe ["Dynamic-programming algorithms for recognizing small-bandwidth graphs in polynomial time," *SIAM Journal on Algebraic and Discrete Methods* **1** (1980), 363–369] found an elegant algorithm to test if $Bandwidth(G) \leq k$ and to enumerate all such layouts in polynomial time. Refinements of his algorithm by Eitan M. Gurari and Ivan Hal Sudborough ["Improved dynamic programming algorithms for bandwidth minimization and the MinCut linear arrangement problem," *Journal of Algorithms* **5** (1984), 531–546] lead to a worst-case running time of $O(2^k k^{k+1} n^k)$.

Efficient algorithms are known for exact bandwidth computation in a few special classes of graphs. For example, the bandwidth of an *interval graph*, in which the vertices correspond to intervals of the real line and $u — v$ means that intervals u and v overlap, can be compared to a given threshold k in $O(n \log n)$ steps. [See Daniel J. Kleitman and Rakesh V. Vohra, "Computing the bandwidth of interval graphs," *SIAM Journal on Discrete Mathematics* **3** (1990), 373–375; Alan P. Sprague, "An $O(n \log n)$ algorithm for bandwidth of interval graphs," *SIAM Journal on Discrete Mathematics* **7** (1994), 213–220.] The bandwidth of a *theta graph*, which consists of a set of paths joining two endpoints and having only those endpoints in common, can be computed directly from the lengths of the paths [G. W. Peck and Aditya Shastri, "Bandwidth of theta graphs with short paths," *Discrete Mathematics* **103** (1992), 177–187]. The bandwidth of a *chain graph*, which is a bipartite graph on vertices $\{x_1, \ldots, x_p\}$ and $\{y_1, \ldots, y_q\}$ such that x_i —— y_j implies x_{i+1} —— y_j for $1 \le i < p$, can be computed in $O(n^2 \log n)$ steps, where $n = p + q$ [Ton Kloks, Dieter Kratsch, and Haiko Müller, "Bandwidth of chain graphs," *Information Processing Letters* **68** (1998), 313–315]. A graph in which all vertices of degree > 1 belong to a sequence of cliques on vertices $(Q_1, \ldots, Q_m)$, where $\|Q_i \cap Q_{i+1}\| = 1$ for $1 \le i < m$ but $\|Q_i \cap Q_j\| = 0$ when $|i - j| > 1$, has a bandwidth that can be found in linear time because an obvious lower bound is achievable [Le Tu Quoc Hung, Maciej M. Sysło, Margaret L. Weaver, and Douglas B. West, "Bandwidth and density for block graphs," *Discrete Mathematics* **189** (1998), 163–176].

A *generalized caterpillar* is a very special case of a free tree obtained by starting with a stem and attaching any number of short paths called "hairs" to the stem vertices. If all the hairs have length 1 or 2, and if each stem vertex has fewer than h hairs, the bandwidth can be computed in $O(n \log h)$ steps. [S. F. Assmann, G. W. Peck, M. M. Sysło, and J. Zak, "The bandwidth of caterpillars with hairs of length 1 and 2," *SIAM Journal on Algebraic and Discrete Methods* **2** (1981), 387–393.] But Burkhard Monien showed, surprisingly, that the problem becomes NP-complete if all hairs have length 1 or 3, even if only one stem vertex is allowed to have hairs of length 3. ["The bandwidth minimization problem for caterpillars with hair length 3 is NP-complete," *SIAM Journal on Algebraic and Discrete Methods* **7** (1986), 505–512.] Monien also proved that the problem is NP-complete for generalized caterpillars of degree 3; in such graphs the hair length is unbounded, but each stem vertex is allowed to have at most one hair. This gives a sharper form of the theorem in Section 8.

Algorithms that are often able to compute the bandwidth of graphs on, say, 100 vertices in a reasonable amount of time have been described by G. M. Del Corso and G. Manzini, "Finding exact solutions to the bandwidth minimization problem," *Computing* **62** (1999), 189–203.

It is, of course, natural to turn from exact methods to approximate methods when we are faced with an NP-hard problem. An important study of the classical approaches to bandwidth minimization was carried out by Jonathan S. Turner, "On the probable performance of heuristics for bandwidth minimization," *SIAM Journal on Computing* **15** (1986), 561–580.

A significant new approach was developed by Uriel Feige, who constructed a randomized polynomial-time algorithm that finds a graph layout whose bandwidth is at most $O(\log n)^{9/2}$ times the optimum, more than half of the time. ["Approximating the bandwidth via volume respecting embeddings," *Journal of Computer and System Sciences* **60** (2000), 510–539.] His algorithm is not practical in its present form — for example, even when $n = 10^9$ we have $(\lg n)^{9/2} \approx 4 \cdot 10^6$ — but it is the first algorithm known to approximate the bandwidth of general graphs (or even of trees) within a factor that is polynomial in $\log n$, hence it suggests that better approximation schemes may well be possible.

Ton Kloks, Dieter Kratsch, and Haiko Müller have found efficient ways to approximate the bandwidth within a factor of 2 on a general class of graphs that includes *permutation graphs*, whose edges correspond to inversions of a permutation. ["Approximating the bandwidth for asteroidal triple-free graphs," *Journal of Algorithms* **32** (1999), 41–57.]

On the other hand, there is a definite limit to the degree of approximation that is possible. Walter Unger has proved the following theorem: *Let F be any positive integer. If there is a polynomial time algorithm to approximate the bandwidth of any given graph within a multiplicative factor of F, then* P = NP. In fact, his theorem holds even when the given graph is required to be a generalized caterpillar of degree 3. ["The complexity of the approximation of the bandwidth problem (Extended abstract)," *Proceedings of the 39th Annual Symposium on Foundations of Computer Science* (1998), 82–91.]

Open problem (d) has also been resolved in many cases. For example, Y. Kuang and C. McDiarmid have proved that if $u \text{—} v$ holds with probability p, independently for all pairs of vertices u and v of a random graph on n vertices, the bandwidth will be

$$n - \frac{(2 + \sqrt{2}) \ln n + O(\log \log n)}{\ln(1/(1 - p))}$$

with probability $\to 1$ as $n \to \infty$. This result holds not only for fixed p but also when p varies with n in such a way that $\omega(1/\log n) \le p \le 1 - e^{-|o(\log n)|}$. Such random graphs have more than order $n^2/\log n$ edges, so it is not surprising that their bandwidth is large; at the other extreme, almost all random graphs with $\Theta(n^{(2k+1)/(2k+2)})$ edges have bandwidth equal to k. ["On the bandwidth of a random graph," *Ars Combinatoria* **20A** (1985), 29–36.] The bandwidth of random graphs with $\lfloor cn \rfloor$ edges is known to be $\Omega(n)$ when $c > 1$; see W. Fernández de la Vega, "On the bandwidth of random graphs," *Annals of Discrete Mathematics* **17** (1983), 633–638. The average bandwidth of a random free tree, when all n^{n-2} free trees on n labeled vertices are equally likely, is $\Omega(\sqrt{n})$ and $O(\sqrt{n \log n})$; see Andrew M. Odlyzko and Herbert S. Wilf, "Bandwidths and profiles of trees," *Journal of Combinatorial Theory* (B) **42** (1987), 348–370.

In spite of all this progress, problem (c) remains open, even in the special case of minimizing $\sum\{(f(u) - f(v))^2 \mid u \!-\! v\}$ over all layouts f.

Chapter 33

The Problem of
Compatible Representatives

[Written with Arvind Raghunathan. Originally published in SIAM Journal on Discrete Mathematics **5** *(1992), 422–427.]*

The purpose of this note is to attach a name to a natural class of combinatorial problems and to point out that this class includes many important special cases. We also show that a simple problem of placing nonoverlapping labels on a rectangular map is NP-complete.

1. Introduction

Many combinatorial tasks can be formulated in the following way: Is there a sequence $(x_1, x_2, \ldots, x_n)$ such that $x_j \in A_j$ for all j, and x_j is compatible with x_k for all $j < k$? Here A_1, A_2, $\ldots$, A_n are given sets, and "compatibility" is a given relation on $A_1 \cup A_2 \cup \cdots \cup A_n$.

Such a problem is NP-hard in general. For example, if all sets A_j are the same, and if compatibility is a symmetric, irreflexive relation, a sequence of compatible representatives is nothing but an n-clique in the compatibility graph.

The problem of coloring a graph G with c colors is another NP-hard special case of the general compatibility question. Let A_j be the set of pairs $\{(j, 1), \ldots, (j, c)\}$, and say that (j, a) is compatible with (k, b) if either $a \neq b$ or v_j is not adjacent to v_k in G, where the vertices of G are $\{v_1, \ldots, v_n\}$. Then a sequence of compatible representatives is essentially a c-coloring of G. Therefore the problem is NP-hard for all $c \geq 3$.

On the other hand, the compatibility problem also has important special cases that are efficiently solvable. If the compatibility relation is '$\neq$', then a solution sequence $(x_1, \ldots, x_n)$ is traditionally called a system of distinct representatives [4] [3, Chapter 5], and the problem of finding such systems is well known to be equivalent to bipartite matching. Indeed, if the compatibility relation is the complement of any equivalence relation, a sequence $(x_1, x_2, \ldots, x_n)$ of compatible representatives exists if and only if there is a matching of cardinality n in a bipartite graph on the vertices $\{v_1, \ldots, v_n, c_1, \ldots, c_m\}$, where $\{c_1, \ldots, c_m\}$ are the equivalence classes and we have the adjacency relation $v_j \,\text{---}\, c_k$ if and only if A_j contains an element of class c_k.

Another nice special case is equivalent to identifying increasing subsequences of a permutation. Let $\pi_1 \ldots \pi_m$ be a permutation of $\{1, \ldots, m\}$, and let A_j be the set of pairs $\{(j, 1), \ldots, (j, m)\}$. Say that (j, a) is compatible with (k, b) if and only if $j < k$ and $\pi_a < \pi_b$. Then a compatible sequence $\big((1, a_1), \ldots, (n, a_n)\big)$ is equivalent to an increasing subsequence $(\pi_{a_1}, \ldots, \pi_{a_n})$ of $\pi_1 \ldots \pi_m$.

The example in the prevous paragraph illustrates that compatibility need not be a symmetric relation. But when the sets A_j are pairwise disjoint, as in that case, we could just as well assume that compatibility is symmetric and reflexive, since our definition of compatible representatives makes it immaterial whether elements x_j of A_j and x_k of A_k are compatible unless we have $j < k$.

There are, however, important special cases in which compatibility is asymmetric. Consider, for example, a scheduling problem in which A_j is a set of tasks that can be done at time j, and where x_j is compatible with x_k only when task x_j does not require the prior completion of x_k.

Cartographers face an interesting case of the general compatibility problem when they attach alphabetic labels to dots on a map. Let A_j represent the possible ways to place the name of city j, and let x_j be compatible with x_k when positions x_j and x_k do not overlap each other or otherwise mislead a potential reader. Then a good map should be a solution to the problem of compatible representatives.

Notice that the cartographic problem makes sense even if the sets A_j are infinite. The task of placing disjoint labels is a fairly natural question of combinatorial geometry that does not appear to be a special case of any other well-known problem.

In light of this discussion, it seems worthwhile to add the problem of compatible representatives to the class of "combinatorial problems that deserve a name," and to investigate heuristics and additional special cases that turn out to have efficient solutions.

2. Simple Special Cases

We have noted that the compatibility problem is equivalent to bipartite matching when incompatibility is an equivalence relation. The problem also has a polynomial-time solution when compatibility is transitive. Let $B_1 = A_1$, and for $j > 1$ let

$$B_j = \{ y \in A_j \mid \exists x \in B_{j-1} \ (x \text{ compatible with } y) \} .$$

Then the transitive compatibility problem has a solution if and only if B_n is nonempty. We can decide this in at most $\sum_{j=2}^{n} \|A_{j-1}\| \, \|A_j\|$ steps.

Another noteworthy special case occurs when each set A_j contains at most two elements. Then the compatibility problem is equivalent to an instance of 2SAT: We can assume that $A_j = \{v_j, \bar{v}_j\}$; the clauses are $(\bar{\sigma}_j \vee \bar{\sigma}_k)$ for every pair of literals such that $j < k$ and σ_j is incompatible with σ_k.

In general, if each $\|A_j\| \leq k$ and $k \geq 2$, the problem reduces directly to an instance of kSAT in which each literal occurs positively just once. The literals are (j, a) for $a \in A_j$, and the clauses are

$$\bigvee_{n \in A_j} (j, a), \qquad \text{for } 1 \leq j \leq n;$$

$$\overline{(j, a)} \vee \overline{(k, b)}, \qquad \text{for } 1 \leq j < k \leq n \text{ and } a \text{ incompatible with } b.$$

Conversely, any instance of kSAT with m clauses reduces to the compatibility problem of finding representatives $(x_1, \ldots, x_m)$, with x_j a member of the jth clause and with two literals compatible if and only if they aren't negatives of each other.

The general compatibility problem with finite sets A_j can also be reduced to an independent set problem in a natural way. Consider the graph G with vertices (j, a) for $a \in A_j$, having edges

$$(j, a) \!-\!\!\!-\! (j, b), \qquad \text{if } a \neq b;$$
$$(j, a) \!-\!\!\!-\! (k, b), \qquad \text{if } j < k \text{ and } a \text{ is incompatible with } b.$$

Then G has an independent set of size n if and only if the compatibility problem has a solution.

Therefore we obtain simple solutions of the compatibility problem when there is a simple solution to the corresponding independent set problem. One such case occurs when compatibility is a symmetric relation that satisfies the following condition: If $i < j < k$ and the elements x_i, x_j, x_k are mutually compatible, then (1) every element of A_i is compatible with either x_j or x_k; (2) every element of A_j is compatible with either x_i or x_k; (3) every element of A_k is compatible with either x_i or x_j; and (4) every element not in $A_i \cup A_j \cup A_k$ is compatible with either x_i, x_j, or x_k. In such a case the graph G is claw-free, and we can use Minty's algorithm [7] to find a maximum independent set.

Grötschel, Lovász, and Schrijver [2, Chapter 9] have compiled a survey of cases where the independent set problem is known to have a simple solution.

3. Another Hard Case

A very special case of the general mapmaker's problem, alluded to in the introduction, proves to be NP-complete.

Consider a set of integer points $p_1, \ldots, p_n$ on the plane. We wish to find integer points $x_1, \ldots, x_n$ with the following properties for all $j \neq k$:

$$|x_j - p_j| = 1; \qquad |x_j - p_k| > 1; \qquad |x_j - x_k| \geq 2.$$

(Motivation: Each x_j is the center of a 2×2 square in which a "label" for point p_j can be placed. The label at x_j should be closer to p_j than to any other point; distinct labels should not overlap.) We will call this the MFL problem, for "METAFONT labeling," because it arises in connection with the task of attaching labels to points in diagrams drawn by METAFONT [5, page 328].

Solutions to the MFL problem can conveniently be represented by showing each point p_j as a heavy dot and drawing an arrow from p_j to x_j for each j; at most four possibilities exist from each of the given points. For example, it is easy to see that a cluster of four adjacent points can be labeled in only two ways:

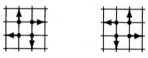

There is no way to attach a label to the middle point in a configuration like

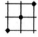

because each of the four positions adjacent to that point is too close to one of the other given points. The MFL problem provides an amusing pastime for people who are sitting in a boring meeting and who happen to have a tablet of graph paper to doodle on.

The general MFL problem is clearly in NP. In order to show that it is NP-complete, we observe first that there are only two solutions to the

problem

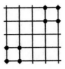

namely the two solutions for four-point clusters given earlier, using the same orientation in each cluster. Thus we can construct large chainlike tree networks of four-point clusters, for example,

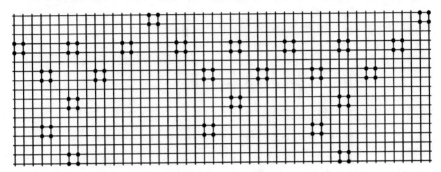

in which there are only two solutions, "positive" and "negative." This construction provides a way to represent the values of boolean variables in a satisfiability problem.

We can now use Lichtenstein's theorem that planar **3SAT** is NP-complete [6]. An instance of planar **3SAT** is a set of variables $v_1, \ldots, v_n$ arranged in a straight line, together with a set of three-legged clauses above and below them, where the clauses are properly nested so that none of the legs between clauses and variables cross each other. We can always put the clauses into a rectilinear configuration such as

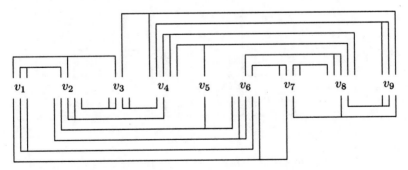

which corresponds to Lichtenstein's "crossover box" [6, Figure 5].

We construct an instance of MFL from a given instance of planar 3SAT by representing the vertical legs for each variable as chains of four-point clusters; this guarantees that each variable will have one of two values, corresponding to the common orientation of all its clusters. We can easily stretch out the diagram so that there is no interference between the variables except at places where three legs of a clause come together in a horizontal segment.

It remains to specify the representation of the clauses. By symmetry we need only describe the representation that appears above the variables. Each horizontal section of a comb-like clause in the upper portion will be represented by a configuration of the form

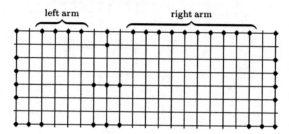

with $6l + 4$ dots in the left arm and $6m + 4$ dots in the right arm, for some l and m. (The three triples at the bottom will connect to clusters that represent variables, as explained below. Those clusters will occur at positions that are congruent mod 6; the arms of a comb stretch out so that they reach the variables appropriate to the clause.)

In each group of three dots at the bottom of this construction, the arrow for the middle dot must go either up or down. All three middle arrows cannot go up, because that would force

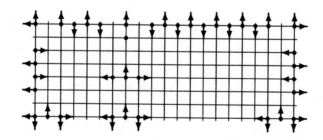

and there is no way to attach an arrow to the middle dot in the second row.

However, there are solutions in which any one of the middle arrows goes down. For example, we can choose

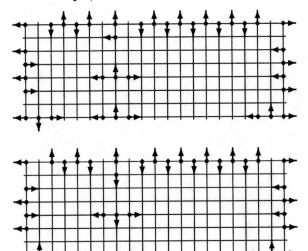

or

and there is a third solution that is essentially a mirror image of the first.

We can place four-point clusters below a row of three dots in such a way that a downward arrow on the top middle dot forces an orientation on the clusters, but an upward arrow on the top middle dot forces nothing:

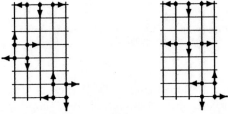

By choosing one of these junction configurations for each variable in the clause, depending on whether the variable is negated or not, we obtain an instance of MFL that has a solution if and only if the given planar clauses are satisfiable.

4. Backtracking

We have now proved that MFL is NP-hard. However, in practice a solution or proof of nonexistence can often be found quickly by backtracking, using the idea of "preclusion" introduced by Golomb and Baumert [1]. When a trial value x_j is selected from A_j, it precludes all selections of other x_k that are incompatible with it; precluded values can be (temporarily) removed from A_k. The problem of compatible representatives is precisely the abstract general setting that supports this notion of preclusion.

Golomb and Baumert suggest choosing x_j at each stage from a currently smallest set A_j whose representative has not yet been chosen. If we are simply looking for a solution, instead of enumerating all solutions, it would also be worthwhile to select elements that preclude as few others as possible.

For example, if an element of A_j doesn't preclude any others, we can set x_j equal to that element without loss of generality. If $x \in A_j$ precludes only one element $y \in A_k$ and no others, and if we find no solution when $x_j = x$, then we can set $x_k = y$ without loss of generality.

5. Further Work

A recent paper by Simon [8] considers the assignment of channels to transmitters in a radio communication system. This is another case of a compatibility problem, rather like the mapmaker's problem because nearby transmitters must not broadcast on the same channel. Simon presents a polynomial-time approximation scheme that is guaranteed to find at least a fixed fraction of the optimum number of compatible channels. This suggests that many useful approximation schemes for other instances of the general compatibility problem might remain to be found.

This research was supported in part by the National Science Foundation and in part by Semiconductor Research Corporation.

References

[1] Solomon Golomb and Leonard D. Baumert, "Backtrack programming," *Journal of the Association for Computing Machinery* **12** (1965), 516–524.

[2] Martin Grötschel, László Lovász, and Alexander Schrijver, *Geometric Algorithms and Combinatorial Optimization* (Berlin: Springer-Verlag, 1987).

[3] Marshall Hall, Jr., *Combinatorial Theory* (Waltham, Massachusetts: Blaisdell, 1967).

[4] P. Hall, "On representatives of subsets," *Journal of the London Mathematical Society* **10** (1935), 26–30.

[5] Donald E. Knuth, *The METAFONTbook*, Volume C of *Computers & Typesetting* (Reading, Massachusetts: Addison–Wesley and American Mathematical Society, 1986).

[6] David Lichtenstein, "Planar formulæ and their uses," *SIAM Journal on Computing* **11** (1982), 329–343.

[7] G. Minty, "On maximal independent sets of vertices in claw-free graphs," *Journal of Combinatorial Theory* (B) **28** (1980), 284–304.

[8] Hans Ulrich Simon, "Approximation algorithms for channel assignment in cellular radio networks," *Lecture Notes in Computer Science* **380** (1989), 405–415.

Addendum

The problem of compatible representatives was in fact defined and named by J. L. Carter in his Ph.D. dissertation, *On the Existence of a Projective Plane of Order Ten* (Berkeley, California: Mathematics Department, University of California, 1974). It is also known as the problem of *constraint satisfaction with unary and binary predicates*; see Alan K. Mackworth, "Consistency in networks of relations," *Artificial Intelligence* **8** (1977), 99–118. This special case of the general constraint satisfaction problem was also called the *satisficing assignment problem* by John Gaschnig, "Experimental case studies of backtrack vs. Waltz-type vs. new algorithms for satisficing assignment problems," *Proceedings of the Second National Conference of the Canadian Society for Computational Studies of Intelligence* (Toronto: 1978), 268–277.

Chapter 34

The Complexity of Nonuniform Random Number Generation

[Written with Andrew C. Yao. Originally published in Algorithms and Complexity, edited by J. F. Traub (New York: Academic Press, 1976), 357–428.]

The purpose of this paper is to introduce a type of complexity theory that is relevant to the problem of generating random numbers with nonuniform distributions, given a source of uniform random bits. We shall examine procedures that minimize the average number of bits required to generate random numbers from arbitrary numeric distributions in arbitrary systems of notation.

Section 1 presents some informal examples of the algorithms we shall be considering, and previews some of the theorems that will follow. Optimum algorithms for generating samples from a discrete distribution are developed in Section 2. The concept of a general representation system for real numbers is defined in Section 3, then Section 4 constructs an optimum generation procedure for any distribution in any representation. The quantitative aspects of this construction are analyzed in Section 5.

Section 6 applies some of the theory to a problem unrelated to random number generation: It is shown that any monotone function from $[0 . . 1]$ into $[0 . . 1]$ can be computed in such a way that the first k bits of the output require a knowledge of fewer than the first $k + 4$ bits of the input, when averaged over all inputs in $[0 . . 1]$.

Algorithms for random number generation that are optimum under the unrestricted model of Sections 1–6 are usually unwieldy in practice, so Section 7 discusses the important special case of finite state algorithms. A model somewhat stronger than a finite state device is used to generate the exponential distribution in Section 8.

The authors have tried to keep this paper self-contained, since it introduces a new topic. Section 9 discusses some possible directions for further research into this type of complexity theory.

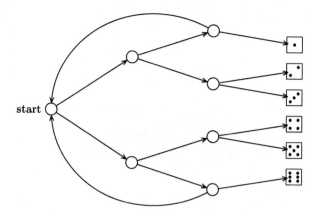

FIGURE 1. Simulating one die with three flips of a coin.

1. Introductory Examples

Suppose you want to play a dice game, but there are no dice on hand; all you have is a single coin that you can flip, to get a "random bit." Your coin is perfectly unbiased, so that each flip yields "heads" or "tails" with exactly equal probability; furthermore each toss of the coin is independent of the results of other tosses. The problem is to generate a result equivalent to rolling two true dice and taking the sum of their pips; thus, the values $(2, 3, \ldots, 6, 7, 8, \ldots, 12)$ are to occur with the respective probabilities $(\frac{1}{36}, \frac{2}{36}, \ldots, \frac{5}{36}, \frac{6}{36}, \frac{5}{36}, \ldots, \frac{1}{36})$.

For brevity, let's encode "heads" as 1 and "tails" as 0, so the result of a sequence of tosses can be represented as a string of 0s and 1s. One way to solve the stated problem is to flip the coin three times in order to simulate the rolling of one die: The results $(001, 010, 011, 100, 101, 110)$ can be interpreted as binary numbers, representing the respective rolls $(1, 2, 3, 4, 5, 6)$. If the sequence of flips produces three identical results 000 or 111, simply repeat the process until a sequence of three non-identical flips is obtained. Then simulate the roll of a second die in the same way.

This three-flip procedure to simulate a single die can be represented schematically as shown in Figure 1. Each circle denotes a single flip of the coin, which has two outcomes shown to the right of that circle; each square denotes a "terminal node," a value assigned to the simulated die.

The average number of flips in the procedure specified by Figure 1 is easily seen to be exactly 4, since it satisfies the equation $T = 3 + \frac{2}{8}T$. We can also derive this average number in a less special way that will apply to other problems discussed later: Let p_m be the probability that there will be exactly m flips, and let $q_m = p_{m+1} + p_{m+2} + \cdots$ be the probability that there will be more than m. Then the average value is

$$\sum_{m \geq 1} m p_m = \sum_{m \geq 1} \sum_{j=0}^{m-1} p_m = \sum_{j \geq 0} \sum_{m > j} p_m = \sum_{j \geq 0} q_j. \tag{1.1}$$

(The interchange of summation is justified since each p_m is nonnegative.) In Figure 1 we see therefore that the average number of flips is

$$\frac{1}{1} + \frac{2}{2} + \frac{4}{4} + \frac{2}{8} + \frac{4}{16} + \frac{8}{32} + \frac{4}{64} + \frac{8}{128} + \frac{16}{256} + \cdots,$$

and this infinite series sums to 4. In general, it is easy to see that *every* coin-flipping algorithm will satisfy

$$q_m = \frac{l(m)}{2^m} \tag{1.2}$$

for some integer $l(m) \geq 0$; indeed, $l(m)$ is the number of "live" (not terminated) branches of the algorithm after m flips have been made. We can imagine expanding Figure 1 into an infinite binary tree, with the starting node at level 0 and with $l(m)$ branch nodes at level m.

Notice that it is possible to go on forever in Figure 1, without ever coming to a terminal node. This must be true for any procedure that correctly simulates a true die with a true coin, since 6 is never a divisor of 2^m for any m. If there are no infinite paths in a binary tree, the infinity lemma (see [5, Section 2.3.4.3]) implies that there is some m with $q_m = 0$; hence the probability of each outcome in such a tree would be a multiple of $1/2^m$. An analysis of the complexity of coin-flipping algorithms had therefore better not be based simply on the worst case running time. Fortunately the chance of a long sequence of flips in Figure 1 is exceedingly small; the probability is only $\left(\frac{2}{8}\right)^m$ that we will need more than $3m$. Thus for all practical purposes the procedure always terminates, except perhaps in books or plays [10]. In this paper we shall use the word "algorithm" for such possibly infinite procedures, although strictly speaking we should be calling them "computational methods" since algorithms are traditionally supposed to be finite in their worst case.

The reader may have noticed a source of inefficiency in Figure 1: When three equal values are obtained, we could have used this common

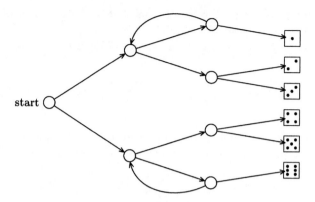

FIGURE 2. A more efficient way to simulate one die.

result as the value of the next flip, since 000 and 111 are equally probable. Thus we get the procedure sketched in Figure 2, requiring only $3\frac{2}{3}$ flips on the average.

If we use Figure 2 to simulate each of two rolls of a die, we will need $7\frac{1}{3}$ flips, on the average. Actually it is possible to do considerably better than this, since we do not require complete information about the individual simulated dice. All we need to know is the sum of the pips; it doesn't matter whether 7 occurs as $\boxed{\cdot\,}$ + $\boxed{\because}$ or as $\boxed{::}$ + $\boxed{\cdot\,}$. The procedure of Figure 3 can be shown to yield the correct probabilities, and it requires an average of only $4\frac{7}{18}$ flips.

The general question of generating samples from any discrete distribution, when any given finite or countably infinite set of quantities is to be generated with specified rational or irrational probabilities, is investigated in Section 2. We will see that Figure 3 is an optimum algorithm for simulating the sum of two random dice, among all algorithms based on flipping a coin, where "optimum" is meant in a very strong sense: Let q_m be the probability that the procedure of Figure 3 flips the coin more than m times, and let Q_m be the corresponding probability in any valid algorithm for this problem; then $Q_m \geq q_m$. In particular, the algorithm of Figure 3 minimizes every term in the sum (1.1), so it has the minimum average time among all valid algorithms.

If we want to simulate rolling a single die, Figure 2 turns out to be an optimum procedure. But if we wish to record the complete information from two successive rolls, with each of the 36 possibilities equally likely, there is a *better* way to do this than to apply Figure 2 twice! The results of Section 2 will imply that two rolls of a die can be simulated with an

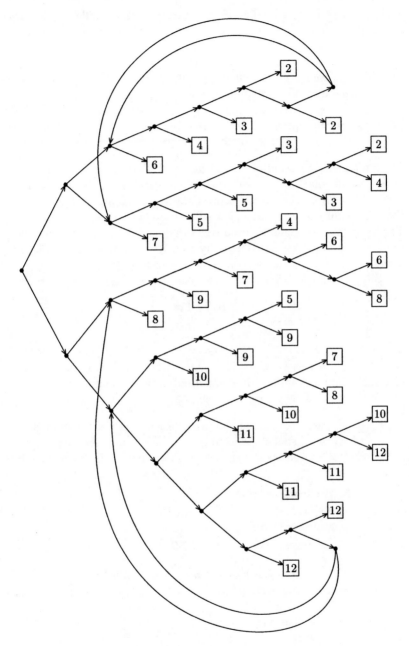

FIGURE 3. An optimum way to simulate the sum of two dice.

average of $6\frac{2}{3}$ flips of a coin. Furthermore we can simulate a sequence of k rolls with an average of fewer than $2 + k \lg 6$ flips of the coin; for $k = 3$ the optimum average number is $8\frac{35}{57}$.

Let us turn now to another problem, which seems to be quite different although we shall see that it actually is strongly related: Instead of dealing with discrete probabilities like $1/6$ or $1/36$, let us consider the continuous case, where we wish to generate a random *real number* X having a specified probability distribution

$$F(x) = \Pr(X \le x), \qquad -\infty < x < \infty. \tag{1.3}$$

We can't generate infinitely many digits of X in finite time on a computer, so we shall be content with algorithms that generate as many successive bits of the binary representation of X as needed; if we let the algorithm run long enough it will supply arbitrarily high precision. The problem is to generate such random deviates using only a source of uniform random bits — that is, only by flipping a true coin sufficiently many times.

Suppose, for example, that we wish to generate X with the distribution

$$F(x) = \begin{cases} 0, & \text{if } x < 0; \\ x^2, & \text{if } 0 \le x \le 1; \\ 1, & \text{if } x > 1. \end{cases} \tag{1.4}$$

One way to do this is to set $X \leftarrow \sqrt{U}$, where U is a uniform deviate (a random number uniformly distributed between 0 and 1); then

$$\Pr(X \le x) = \Pr(\sqrt{U} \le x) = \Pr(U \le x^2) = x^2,$$

for $0 \le x \le 1$, as desired. The following procedure, written in an ad hoc dialect of ALGOL, spells out exactly how this could be done, using an adaptation of the classical pencil-and-paper algorithm for square root extraction:

```
A:   begin integer n, r;
         n ← r ← 0;
         while true do
             begin r ← 4 × r + 2 × flip + flip;  n ← 2 × n;
             if r > n then
                 begin r ← r − n − 1;  n ← n + 2;
                 output(1)
             end
             else output(0);
         end;
     end;
```

Here *flip* denotes a random input bit, either 0 or 1, and *output* produces the next bit for the desired representation of X as a binary fraction. The validity of this algorithm is a consequence of the following relations connecting the input and output with n and r at the beginning of the **while** loop:

If the first $2k$ bits input to the algorithm are the 0s and 1s that define the integer m in binary notation, then the output is the binary string of length k that defines the integer $\lfloor \sqrt{m} \rfloor$; furthermore

$$n = \lfloor \sqrt{m} \rfloor \quad \text{and} \quad r = m - n^2/4.$$

As an example of this algorithm, suppose the first ten flips are 1 0 1 0 0 1 1 1 0 0; then the first five bits output are 1 1 0 0 1, and indeed the square root of $(.1010011100\ldots)_2$ is $(.11001\ldots)_2$. Notice that Algorithm A consumes two input bits for every output bit it produces.

Students of random number generation know that there is an alternative to taking the square root of a uniform deviate: We can equivalently take the maximum of two independent deviates U and V, since

$$\Pr(\max(U,V) \leq x) = \Pr(U \leq x \text{ and } V \leq x) = x^2, \quad \text{for } 0 \leq x \leq 1.$$

This enables us to get by with fewer than two input bits per output bit in many cases; once we have seen enough bits of U and V to conclude that $U \neq V$, we need only look at the remaining bits of the larger number in order to compute the maximum. Thus, we may use the following algorithm.

B: **begin integer** u, v;
        $u \leftarrow v \leftarrow 0$;
        while $u = v$ **do**
           begin $u \leftarrow$ *flip*; $v \leftarrow$ *flip*;
            output $(\max(u,v))$;
          end;
        while *true* **do** *output* $(flip)$;
    end;

The average number of input bits needed to produce k output bits with this algorithm satisfies

$$T_k = 2 + \frac{1}{2}T_{k-1} + \frac{1}{2}(k-1), \quad k \geq 1; \qquad T_0 = 0;$$

and this recurrence implies that $T_k = k + 2 - 2^{1-k}$.

Closer study reveals that we can improve on Algorithm B if we let the first of the two *flips* tell us whether or not $u = v$; if $u \neq v$ then the second flip is redundant. We obtain a simpler algorithm:

C: **begin integer** u;
  $u \leftarrow 0$;
  while $u = 0$ **do**
   begin $u \leftarrow$ *flip*;
    if $u = 1$ **then** *output*(1) **else** *output*(*flip*);
   end;
  while *true* **do** *output*(*flip*);
 end;

The average number of flips to produce k outputs by this procedure is the solution to

$$T_k = \frac{1}{2}k + \frac{1}{2}(2 + T_{k-1}), \quad k \geq 1; \qquad T_0 = 0;$$

namely

$$T_k = k + 1 - 2^{-k}. \tag{1.5}$$

We shall prove below that Algorithm C is an optimum way to generate X with distribution (1.4). In fact, the method is optimum in a very strong sense: For all integers k and m, Algorithm C minimizes the probability that m or more flips need to be made before k bits have been output, over all valid algorithms for this distribution. Furthermore we shall prove constructively that optimum algorithms in this strong sense exist for *any* given distribution $F(x)$.

The problem of simulating k tosses of a die, for $k = 1, 2, 3, \ldots$, can be regarded as the problem of generating a random real number between 0 and 1 in the radix-6 number system, given a sequence of random bits. There is in fact a general framework that includes both types of problems as special cases: We shall discuss the idea of a general *representation system* for real numbers in Section 3, using a general model that includes binary as well as other possibly mixed-radix systems, and even signed-magnitude floating point representations and continued fraction representations as special cases. The general nonuniform random number generation problem now becomes one of generating random variables X with a given distribution $F(x)$ and in a given representation system; and we shall construct optimum methods for all cases of this general problem. The discrete probability distributions of Section 2 correspond simply to determining the most significant digit of the representation of an appropriate random variable.

Before we return to take a closer look at the discrete case, let us remark that Ahrens [1, Section 2d] has presented a somewhat different method for generating X with distribution (1.4). In our notation, his so-called "bit scrambling" method is

D: **begin integer** i, j;
      $j \leftarrow 0$;
      while *flip* $= 0$ **do** $j \leftarrow j + 1$;
      for $i \leftarrow 1$ **step** 1 **until** j **do** *output* (*flip*);
      output (1);
      while *true* **do** *output* (*flip*);
   end;

This procedure is rather like Algorithm C, except that it delays the first j outputs; the resulting average number of flips to produce k outputs comes to

$$k + 1 + 2^{-k}, \tag{1.6}$$

slightly more than (1.5). Thus, Ahrens's method is not optimal by our standards. However, from a practical standpoint it turns out that j is usually very small, k is usually 10 or more, and Algorithm D can usually be implemented very efficiently using the shift operations on a binary computer. Therefore Algorithm D is actually more useful in practice than the optimum Algorithm C!

As always, we must be careful not to read too much into our theoretical results about complexity of algorithms. The theory is very helpful for locating bottlenecks, for discovering new algorithms, and for gaining a high level understanding of a problem domain; it also has mathematical elegance and beauty. But we should never forget that the models of computation we deal with are only simplified idealizations of reality. (See [7] for further discussion about the abuse of theory.)

2. Generating Discrete Random Variables

Suppose X is to be assigned the distinct values x_1, x_2, ..., x_n with the respective nonnegative probabilities p_1, p_2, ..., p_n, where

$$p_1 + p_2 + \cdots + p_n = 1. \tag{2.1}$$

We shall allow n to be infinite. Without loss of generality the number of possible values x_i is at most countably infinite, since (2.1) implies that there are at most N values of i such that $p_i > 1/N$, hence only countably many p_i are nonzero. We shall study the class of all algorithms that generate X with this distribution by flipping coins as discussed in Section 1. Every such algorithm can be represented as a (usually infinite) binary tree, containing nodes of two types:

i) Branch nodes, which have two children, and which mean "flip a coin and go to the left or right child node according as the result is 0 or 1."

ii) Terminal nodes, which have no children; these are marked with one of the desired output values x_i, and the meaning is "output x_i and terminate the algorithm."

The diagrams in Figures 1–3 fit this framework if they are expanded into infinite trees in the obvious manner. In such a binary tree we say that the root is at level 0, and the children of nodes on level m are at level $m + 1$. Terminal nodes are conventionally given a square shape. If $t_i(m)$ is the number of square nodes on level m that are marked x_i we must have

$$\sum_{m \geq 0} \frac{t_i(m)}{2^m} = p_i \qquad (2.2)$$

for each i. When these conditions are satisfied we shall say that we have a *DDG-tree* (discrete distribution generating tree), and the corresponding algorithms will be called DDG-tree algorithms. Our goal in this section is to study the DDG-trees that define the fastest algorithms.

Let

$$t(m) = t_1(m) + t_2(m) + \cdots + t_n(m) \qquad (2.3)$$

be the total number of terminal nodes on level m of a DDG-tree. Equations (2.1), (2.2), and (2.3) imply that

$$\sum_{m \geq 0} \frac{t(m)}{2^m} = 1, \qquad (2.4)$$

hence the DDG-tree algorithm terminates with probability 1.

Recall from Section 1 that the average running time of such an algorithm is

$$\sum_{m \geq 0} q_m = \sum_{m \geq 0} \frac{l(m)}{2^m} \qquad (2.5)$$

flips of the coin, where q_m is the probability that more than m flips will occur and $l(m)$ is the number of branch nodes on level m. We shall find a lower bound for the average running time by finding a lower bound for each $l(m)$.

The derivation is quite simple. In the first place we have

$$l(m) + t(m) = \begin{cases} 1, & \text{if } m = 0, \\ 2l(m-1), & \text{if } m > 0, \end{cases} \tag{2.6}$$

since each branch node on level $m - 1$ has two children. Furthermore

$$l(m) = \sum_{\mu > m} \frac{t(\mu)}{2^{\mu - m}}, \tag{2.7}$$

since this relation holds for $m = 0$ by (2.4) and it follows for $m > 1$ by induction using (2.6). For each index i we have

$$\sum_{\mu > m} \frac{t_i(\mu)}{2^\mu} = p_i - \sum_{\mu = 0}^{m} \frac{t_i(\mu)}{2^\mu} \geq \frac{\{2^m p_i\}}{2^m}, \tag{2.8}$$

where $\{x\}$ denotes the fractional part of x, namely $x - \lfloor x \rfloor = x \bmod 1$, since the left-hand sum is nonnegative and the sum for $\mu \leq m$ is an integer multiple of 2^{-m}. The combination of (2.7) and (2.8) now yields

$$l(m) \geq \{2^m p_1\} + \{2^m p_2\} + \cdots + \{2^m p_n\}. \tag{2.9}$$

This is the desired lower bound. Combining it with (2.5) shows that the average running time of any DDG-tree algorithm is at least

$$\nu(p_1) + \nu(p_2) + \cdots + \nu(p_n), \tag{2.10}$$

in terms of a "new" function defined by the relation

$$\nu(x) = \sum_{m \geq 0} \frac{\{2^m x\}}{2^m}, \qquad \text{for } 0 \leq x \leq 1. \tag{2.11}$$

When $n = \infty$, the lower bound (2.10) might be infinite (as we shall see below), and in such cases all DDG-trees must have infinite average running time.

If the lower bound is finite, a DDG-tree will attain it if and only if equality holds in (2.8) for all i and m; this means that

$$\sum_{\mu = 0}^{m} t_i(\mu) 2^{m - \mu} = \lfloor 2^m p_i \rfloor. \tag{2.12}$$

But equation (2.12) for $m = 0, 1, 2, \ldots$ says simply that $t_i(m)$ is the mth bit to the right of the binary point in the representation of p_i.

Since we will be referring frequently to binary expansions, we shall use the family of functions

$$\varepsilon_m(x) = \lfloor 2^m x \rfloor \bmod 2, \qquad (2.13)$$

which specify the coefficient of 2^{-m} in the standard binary representation of x; thus, the identity

$$x = \sum_m \frac{\varepsilon_m(x)}{2^m} \qquad (2.14)$$

holds for all nonnegative x, if we sum over all integer values of m. Our discussion leads us to conclude that a DDG-tree algorithm has the minimum average running time (2.10) if and only if

$$t_i(m) = \varepsilon_m(p_i) \qquad (2.15)$$

for all i and m.

Conversely we must show that DDG-trees satisfying (2.15) exist, for all probability distributions $(p_1, p_2, \ldots, p_n)$ satisfying (2.1). Let $t_i(m)$ and $t(m)$ be defined by (2.15) and (2.3), so that (2.2) and (2.4) hold. Clearly a DDG-tree with this $t_i(m)$ specification exists if and only if the integers $l(m)$ defined by (2.6) are nonnegative. But (2.4) and (2.6) imply (2.7); hence $l(m) \geq 0$ and optimal DDG-trees satisfying (2.15) exist.

As an example of this construction, consider the probability distribution defined by the irrational probabilities

$$
\begin{aligned}
p_1 &= 1/\pi & &= (0.010100010111110\ldots)_2, \\
p_2 &= 1/e & &= (0.010111100010110\ldots)_2, \qquad (2.16) \\
p_3 &= 1 - p_1 - p_2 & &= (0.010100000101010\ldots)_2.
\end{aligned}
$$

One of the optimum DDG-trees for this distribution is shown in Figure 4. This particular tree is inherently infinite; it could not be obtained by expanding a finite state diagram such as those in Figures 1–3. It is clear that finite state algorithms are possible if and only if the probabilities are all rational. On the other hand an algorithm for optimum generation of any discrete distribution is easy to construct as a function of the (infinite) binary representations of the given probabilities.

The following theorem summarizes what we have learned so far about generating discrete distributions.

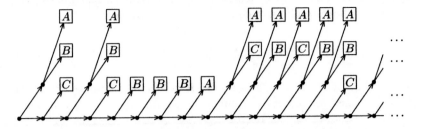

FIGURE 4. An optimum DDG-tree to generate (A, B, C)
with the respective probabilities in (2.16).

Theorem 2.1. Let $(p_1, p_2, \ldots, p_n)$ specify a discrete probability distribution, where n may be infinite, and let $\mathcal{A}$ be a DDG-tree algorithm for this distribution. Then the average running time $T(\mathcal{A})$ (that is, the expected number of random bits input by $\mathcal{A}$) satisfies

$$T(\mathcal{A}) \geq \nu(p_1) + \nu(p_2) + \cdots + \nu(p_n), \qquad (2.17)$$

where $\nu(x)$ is defined in (2.11). The following statements are equivalent:

i) For all $m \geq 0$, Algorithm $\mathcal{A}$ minimizes the probability that more than m random bits will be input, over all DDG-tree algorithms for this distribution.

ii) For all $m \geq 0$ and $1 \leq i \leq n$, the DDG-tree for $\mathcal{A}$ has exactly $\varepsilon_m(p_i)$ terminal nodes marked x_i on level m, where $\varepsilon_m(x)$ denotes the coefficient of 2^{-m} in the binary representation of x.

Furthermore, if $T(\mathcal{A})$ is finite, the following statement is also equivalent to (i) and (ii):

iii) $T(\mathcal{A}) = \nu(p_1) + \nu(p_2) + \cdots + \nu(p_n)$. $\square$

Let us now study the function $\nu(x)$ that appears in the formula for the optimum average running time. We have

$$\nu(x) = \sum_{m \geq 0} \frac{1}{2^m} \sum_{\mu > m} \frac{\varepsilon_\mu(x)}{2^{\mu - m}}$$

$$= \sum_{\mu \geq 0} \sum_{m=0}^{\mu-1} \frac{\varepsilon_\mu(x)}{2^\mu}$$

$$= \sum_{\mu \geq 0} \mu \frac{\varepsilon_\mu(x)}{2^\mu}, \qquad \text{for } 0 \leq x \leq 1. \qquad (2.18)$$

It will prove convenient to define $\nu(x)$ for arbitrary real positive x by extending this formula; consequently we shall write

$$\nu(x) = \sum_m m\frac{\varepsilon_m(x)}{2^m}, \qquad \text{for } x \geq 0, \qquad (2.19)$$

where the sum is over all integers m between $-\infty$ and ∞. This sum is well defined for any fixed x, since $\varepsilon_m(x)$ will be 0 for all sufficiently negative values of m. For example, $\nu(7) = (-2)2^2 + (-1)2^1 = -10$.

When x is a power of 2 we have $\nu(x) = H(x)$, where $H(x)$ is the entropy function,

$$H(x) = x\lg(1/x), \quad \text{for } x > 0; \qquad H(0) = 0. \qquad (2.20)$$

Furthermore it is easy to see that

$$\nu(x/2^n) = nx/2^n + \nu(x)/2^n, \qquad (2.21)$$

an identity also satisfied by $H(x)$. Thus we are led to suspect that $\nu(x)$ is approximately equal to $H(x)$, and indeed it is:

Theorem 2.2. $H(x) \leq \nu(x) < H(x) + 2x$ for all $x \geq 0$, and these bounds are best possible.

Proof. Clearly $\nu(0) = H(0)$. When $x > 0$, let $2^{-m} \leq x < 2^{1-m}$; then

$$\nu(x) = \sum_{\mu \geq m} \mu\frac{\varepsilon_\mu(x)}{2^\mu} \geq \sum_{\mu \geq m} \lg(1/x)\frac{\varepsilon_\mu(x)}{2^\mu} = H(x).$$

Also

$$H(x) + 2x - \nu(x) = \sum_{\mu \geq m} \left(\lg(1/x) + 2 - \mu\right)\frac{\varepsilon_\mu(x)}{2^\mu}$$

$$> \sum_{\mu \geq m} (m + 1 - \mu)\frac{\varepsilon_\mu(x)}{2^\mu}$$

$$= 2^{-m} - \sum_{\mu \geq m+2} (\mu - m - 1)\frac{\varepsilon_\mu(x)}{2^\mu}$$

$$> 2^{-m} - \sum_{\mu \geq 1} \frac{\mu}{2^{\mu+m+1}} = 0$$

since $\varepsilon_m(x) = 1$.

The fact that these limits are best possible comes by considering the values $x = 2^{-m}$ and $x = 2^{1-m} - 2^{1-m-n}$. $\quad\square$

Corollary. *Let* $H(p_1, p_2, \ldots, p_n) = H(p_1) + H(p_2) + \cdots + H(p_n)$ *be the entropy of the probability distribution* $(p_1, p_2, \ldots, p_n)$. *The average running time of an optimum DDG-tree algorithm for this distribution lies between* $H(p_1, p_2, \ldots, p_n)$ *and* $H(p_1, p_2, \ldots, p_n) + 2$. □

Perhaps the most famous property of $H(x)$ is the fundamental inequality

$$H(x) + H(y) \le H(x + y) + x + y, \tag{2.22}$$

with equality if and only if $x = y$. The function $\nu(x)$ does not satisfy this relation (consider, for example, the case $x = 1/3$, $y = 2/3$, $\nu(x) = 8/9$, $\nu(y) = 10/9$, $\nu(x+y) = 0$); but $\nu(x)$ actually satisfies a related *equality*,

$$\nu(x) + \nu(y) = \nu(x + y) + (x \wedge y) \tag{2.23}$$

where '$x \wedge y$' is the binary number that has 1s exactly where the *carries* occur when adding x to y:

$$x \wedge y = \sum_m \frac{(\varepsilon_m(x + y) + \varepsilon_m(x) + \varepsilon_m(y)) \bmod 2}{2^m}. \tag{2.24}$$

Equation (2.23) follows from the observation that we reduce ν by 2^{-m} when carrying into position m, since $(m + 1)/2^{m+1} + (m + 1)/2^{m+1} = m/2^m + 1/2^m$. Note that

$$x \wedge y \le 2(x + y), \tag{2.25}$$

for if $2^m \le x+y < 2^{m+1}$ we have $x \wedge y \le 2^m + 2^{m-1} + 2^{m-2} + \cdots = 2^{m+1}$.

One of the most important discrete distributions is, of course, the uniform distribution, when $p_1 = \cdots = p_n = 1/n$. (Rolling k dice is equivalent to taking $n = 6^k$.) In this case the average running time of an optimal algorithm is $n\nu(1/n)$; one can show without difficulty that

$$\lceil \lg n \rceil \le n\nu(1/n) < \lceil \lg n \rceil + 1, \tag{2.26}$$

with equality if and only if n is a power of 2. If n is odd and if l is the smallest positive integer such that $2^l \equiv 1 \pmod{n}$, we have

$$n\nu(1/n) = \frac{2^l l}{2^l - 1} + \frac{\nu(a)}{a}, \qquad a = \frac{2^l - 1}{n}, \tag{2.27}$$

because $1/n = a/2^l + a/2^{2l} + a/2^{3l} + \cdots$.

Let us conclude this section by finding the extreme values of the optimum average running time.

Theorem 2.3. *Let* $\nu(p_1, p_2, \ldots, p_n) = \nu(p_1) + \nu(p_2) + \cdots + \nu(p_n)$ *be the "new entropy" of the probability distribution* $(p_1, p_2, \ldots, p_n)$. *Then*

$$\nu(p_1, p_2, \ldots, p_n) \leq \lceil \lg n \rceil + (n-1)/2^{\lceil \lg n \rceil - 1}. \qquad (2.28)$$

Furthermore, if all the p_i *are positive we have*

$$\nu(p_1, p_2, \ldots, p_n) \geq 2 - 2^{2-n}. \qquad (2.29)$$

These bounds are best possible.

Proof. The upper bound follows from (2.11) by noting that

$$\{2^m p_1\} + \{2^m p_2\} + \cdots + \{2^m p_n\} \leq \min(2^m, n-1) \qquad (2.30)$$

for all $m \geq 0$; the left-hand side of (2.30) is $2^m - \lfloor 2^m p_1 \rfloor - \lfloor 2^m p_2 \rfloor - \cdots - \lfloor 2^m p_n \rfloor$, an integer that is less than n. When $n = 6$ we can attain these bounds with the following binary numbers, for example:

$$
\begin{aligned}
p_1 &= (.001\,111110\,111110\,111110\ldots)_2, \\
p_2 &= (.001\,111101\,111101\,111101\ldots)_2, \\
p_3 &= (.001\,111011\,111011\,111011\ldots)_2, \\
p_4 &= (.000\,110111\,110111\,110111\ldots)_2, \\
p_5 &= (.000\,101111\,101111\,101111\ldots)_2, \\
p_6 &= (.000\,011111\,011111\,011111\ldots)_2.
\end{aligned}
$$

The same idea works for general n: If $q = \lceil \lg n \rceil$, we can let

$$
p_j = \begin{cases}
\dfrac{1}{2^q}\left(\dfrac{2^n - 1 - 2^{j-1}}{2^n - 1}\right) + \dfrac{1}{2^q}, & \text{if } 1 \leq j \leq 2^q + 1 - n; \\[2ex]
\dfrac{1}{2^q}\left(\dfrac{2^n - 1 - 2^{j-1}}{2^n - 1}\right), & \text{if } 2^q + 1 - n < j \leq n.
\end{cases} \qquad (2.31)
$$

Note that if $\theta = \lceil \lg n \rceil - \lg(n-1)$ we have $0 < \theta \leq 1$ and

$$\lceil \lg n \rceil + (n-1)/2^{\lceil \lg n \rceil - 1} = \lg(n-1) + \theta + 2^{1-\theta}.$$

The function $\theta + 2^{1-\theta}$ is ≤ 2 for $0 \leq \theta \leq 1$, so we have

$$\nu(p_1, p_2, \ldots, p_n) \leq \lg(n-1) + 2, \qquad (2.32)$$

with equality possible when $n - 1$ is a power of 2.

Let us now look for a formula for the lower bound. Clearly the lower bound can occur only when the DDG-tree has the smallest possible number of terminal nodes, namely n. In this case there are $n-1$ branch nodes, and it is known that the minimum value of $\nu(p_1, p_2, \ldots, p_n)$ occurs when the tree is degenerate (see [8, exercise 6.3–37], where an equivalent fact is stated without proof). Using the notation defined in the proof of Theorem 2.1, the optimum tree always has

$$\nu(p_1, p_2, \ldots, p_n) = \sum_{m \geq 1} m \frac{t(m)}{2^m}, \qquad (2.33)$$

by (2.15) and (2.8), and this equals

$$\sum_{m \geq 1} m \frac{2l(m-1) - l(m)}{2^m} = \sum_{m \geq 0} \frac{l(m)}{2^m}. \qquad (2.34)$$

Now $l(0) + l(1) + l(2) + \cdots = n - 1$, and (2.34) clearly takes its minimum value when $l(0) = l(1) = \cdots = l(n-2) = 1$. The probability distribution

$$p_j = 2^{-j + \delta_{jn}} \qquad (2.35)$$

achieves this lower bound.   ☐

When n is infinite we can readily construct probability distributions such that $\nu(p_1, p_2, \ldots) = \infty$, using Theorem 2.2. Perhaps the most interesting example of this kind is obtained when we set $p_1 = 0$ and

$$p_j = \frac{1}{2^{\lfloor \lg j \rfloor + 2\lfloor \lg \lg j \rfloor + 1}}, \qquad j \geq 2. \qquad (2.36)$$

It is amusing to verify that $\sum p_j = 1$ and $\sum \nu(p_j) = \infty$ in this case. Since each p_j is a reciprocal power of 2 the optimum DDG-tree can be constructed quite easily.

3. General Representation Systems

Before we turn to the study of continuous distributions, we will find it instructive to study a fairly general model for the representation of real numbers based on successive refinements of intervals.

Let R be a (possibly unbounded) interval of the real numbers. Furthermore let R be partitioned into one or more disjoint intervals, say

$$R = R[a] \cup R[a+1] \cup \cdots \cup R[b] \qquad (3.1)$$

where the indices a and b are integers or $\pm\infty$, with $a \leq b$, and where $R[i]$ lies strictly to the left of $R[j]$ for $i < j$. Furthermore let each $R[j]$ be partitioned into one or more disjoint intervals, say

$$R[j] = R[j, a_j] \cup R[j, a_j + 1] \cup \cdots \cup R[j, b_j] \tag{3.2}$$

in the same fashion; and furthermore let each $R[j_1, j_2]$ be similarly partitioned, and so on through countably many stages. The only requirement we shall place on these partitionings is that the lengths of the intervals eventually approach zero "in every direction"; formally, we require that the infinite intersection

$$R \cap R[j_1] \cap R[j_1, j_2] \cap R[j_1, j_2, j_3] \cap \cdots \tag{3.3}$$

should contain at most one point, for every infinite sequence of integers $j_1, j_2, j_3, \ldots$.

Such a tree of interval partitions will be called a *representation system* for R. It follows from the definitions that every real number $x \in R$ has a unique representation

$$x = \langle j_1, j_2, j_3, \ldots \rangle, \tag{3.4}$$

defined by the condition

$$x \in R[j_1, j_2, \ldots, j_r] \qquad \text{for all } r \geq 1. \tag{3.5}$$

If $x < x'$, the representation of x will always be lexicographically less than that of x'; in other words, if $x = \langle j_1, j_2, j_3, \ldots \rangle$ and $x' = \langle j_1', j_2', j_3', \ldots \rangle$, and $x < x'$, there will be some $m \geq 1$ such that $j_i = j_i'$ for $1 \leq i < m$ but $j_m < j_m'$.

Such representation systems include many familiar examples:

(a) Let $R = [0..1)$, and for $0 \leq j_1, j_2, \ldots, j_r < d$ let

$$R[j_1, j_2, \ldots, j_r] = [(j_1 d^{r-1} + j_2 d^{r-2} + \cdots + j_r)/d^r$$
$$.. (j_1 d^{r-1} + j_2 d^{r-2} + \cdots + j_r + 1)/d^r). \tag{3.6}$$

This, of course, is the standard radix-d number system in the unit interval.

(b) Let $R = (-\infty..\infty)$, and let

$$R[-1] = (-\infty..0), \qquad R[0] = [0..0], \qquad R[1] = (0..\infty),$$
$$R[-1, -i] = (-2^{i+1}.. -2^i], \qquad R[1, i] = [2^i .. 2^{i+1}), \tag{3.7}$$

for all integers i. These intervals are further subdivided by letting $R[0, \ldots, 0] = R[0]$ and

$$R[1, i, j_1, \ldots, j_r] = [2^i \times (1.j_1 \ldots j_r)_2$$
$$.. 2^i \times ((1.j_1 \ldots j_r)_2 + 2^{-r})),$$
$$R[-1, i, j_1, \ldots, j_r] = -R[1, -i, 1 - j_1, \ldots, 1 - j_r], \qquad (3.8)$$

for all $0 \leq j_1, \ldots, j_r \leq 1$. This is the *floating binary* number system.

(c) Let $R = (0..1]$, and for $j_1, j_2, \ldots, j_r \geq 1$ let the interval $R[-j_1, j_2, \ldots, (-1)^r j_r]$ be the set of all numbers between

$$\cfrac{1}{j_1 + \cfrac{1}{j_2 + \cdot \cdot \cdot_{\textstyle + \frac{1}{j_r}}}} \text{ (exclusive) and } \cfrac{1}{j_1 + \cfrac{1}{j_2 + \cdot \cdot \cdot_{\textstyle + \frac{1}{j_r + 1}}}} \text{ (inclusive).}$$

$$(3.9)$$

Furthermore let $R[-j_1, j_2, \ldots, (-1)^r j_r, 0, \ldots, 0]$, with one or more trailing zeros, be the single number $1/(j_1 + 1/(j_2 + 1/(\cdots + 1/(j_r + 1))\cdots))$. Thus, for example, $R[-3] = [1/4..1/3)$; $R[-3,1] = (1/4..2/7]$; $R[-3,0] = [1/4..1/4]$. This is the standard *continued fraction representation*, with slight perturbations to make sure that the lexicographic order of representation agrees with the usual order.

(d) Let $R = (-\infty..\infty)$, and for $x \in R$ let $x = n + \theta$ where n is an integer and $0 < \theta < 1$. There is a way to subdivide R repeatedly into pairs of subintervals so that, if $n > 0$, the representation of x will be $(n + 1)$ 1s followed by a 0 followed by the binary representation of θ, otherwise it will be $(-n)$ 0s followed by a 1 followed by the binary representation of θ. Thus,

$$\begin{aligned} R[0] &= (-\infty..0), & R[1] &= [0..\infty); \\ R[0,0] &= (-\infty.. - 1), & R[0,1] &= [-1..0); \qquad (3.10) \\ R[1,0] &= [0..1), & R[1,1] &= [1..\infty); \end{aligned}$$

and so on. This may be called the *unary-binary representation* of x. (We are making binary subdivisions at each stage, hence each stage contains infinite intervals; yet each of the infinite intersections (3.3) will still contain at most one point. There is a more "efficient" way to encode an arbitrary integer n as a sequence of 0s and 1s; this question has been pursued by Bentley and Yao [3].)

According to these conventions, the numbers $7/22$ and $1/\pi$ have the following representations.

	$7/22$	$1/\pi$
Radix 10:	$\langle 3,1,8,1,8,1,8,1,\ldots\rangle$	$\langle 3,1,8,3,0,9,8,8,\ldots\rangle$
Floating binary:	$\langle 1,-2,0,1,0,0,0,1,\ldots\rangle$	$\langle 1,-2,0,1,0,0,0,1,\ldots\rangle$
Continued fraction:	$\langle -3,6,0,0,0,0,0,0,\ldots\rangle$	$\langle -3,7,-15,1,-292,1,-1,\ldots\rangle$
Unary-binary:	$\langle 1,0,0,1,0,1,0,0,0,\ldots\rangle$	$\langle 1,0,0,1,0,1,0,0,0,\ldots\rangle$

Notice that representations (a), (b), and (d) have some sequences $\langle j_1, j_2, j_3, \ldots\rangle$ that correspond to valid intervals but do not represent any real number; this happens when the intersection (3.3) is empty. For example, $\langle 9,9,9,9,9,9,9,\ldots\rangle$ never occurs as a representation in the radix-10 system.

Whenever a partitioning step introduces more than two subintervals, we can replace it by a sequence of binary partitionings. For example, $R = R_1 \cup R_2 \cup R_3 \cup R_4$ can be replaced by $R = R' \cup R''$, $R' = R_1 \cup R_2$, $R'' = R_3 \cup R_4$; or by $R = R_1 \cup R'$, $R' = R_2 \cup R''$, $R'' = R_3 \cup R_4$. The unary-binary system in (3.10) illustrates how an infinite partition $R = \cdots \cup R_{-1} \cup R_0 \cup R_1 \cup \cdots$ can be broken into a sequence of binary partitions, so that each R_j is reached after a finite number of subdivisions.

If all partitions involve at most two parts, so that all indices j_i are restricted to the values 0 and 1, we shall call the resulting system a *binary-coded representation*. It follows from the previous paragraph that every given representation system can be "extended" to a binary coded representation in the following sense: For all finite sequences $\langle j_1, \ldots, j_r\rangle$ of integers there is a finite sequence $\langle j'_1, \ldots, j'_{r'}\rangle$ of 0s and 1 such that the interval $R[j_1, \ldots, j_r]$ in the given representation system is equal to the interval $R[j'_1, \ldots, j'_{r'}]$ in the binary-coded system that extends it. Furthermore this mapping $\langle j_1, \ldots, j_r\rangle \to \langle j'_1, \ldots, j'_{r'}\rangle$ preserves lexicographic order of the sequences.

We shall conclude this section by making a few definitions about the "frontiers" of a representation; this concept will prove to be helpful in Section 4. A frontier $\mathcal{F}$ of a representation is any set of disjoint intervals of that representation whose union is R. In particular, the set of all $R[j_1, \ldots, j_r]$ such that r has a fixed value k is always a frontier $\mathcal{F}$ that we may call the k-frontier. When a general representation maps into a binary-coded representation, its k-frontiers map into frontiers of the binary-coded representation. The image of the $(k+1)$-frontier is generally a finer partition than the image of the k-frontier.

A frontier $\mathcal{F}'$ in a binary-coded representation is said to be *covered* by another frontier $\mathcal{F}$ if $\mathcal{F}'$ is the same as $\mathcal{F}$ except that one of the intervals $I \in \mathcal{F}'$ has been split up into two intervals $I = I' \cup I''$, where $I', I'' \in \mathcal{F}$. Every frontier $\mathcal{F}$ of a binary-coded representation can be obtained from a sequence $\mathcal{F}_0, \mathcal{F}_1, \mathcal{F}_2, \ldots$ of frontiers where $\mathcal{F}_0 = \{R\}$ and $\mathcal{F}_{j+1}$ covers $\mathcal{F}_j$; if $\mathcal{F}$ is finite, this sequence is finite and ends with $\mathcal{F}$, otherwise the countably infinite frontier $\mathcal{F}$ is obtained in a natural way as the limit of a countably infinite covering sequence.

4. Generating Arbitrary Distributions

Let $F(x)$ be any monotone nondecreasing function on the reals such that $F(-\infty) = 0$, $F(+\infty) = 1$. Then F defines the distribution of a random real variable X under the conventions

$$\Pr(X \le x) = F(x+0); \qquad \Pr(X < x) = F(x-0). \qquad (4.1)$$

Here as usual we write

$$F(+\infty) = \lim_{n\to\infty} F(n), \qquad F(-\infty) = \lim_{n\to\infty} F(-n);$$
$$F(x+0) = \lim_{n\to\infty} F(x+\frac{1}{n}), \quad F(x-0) = \lim_{n\to\infty} F(x-\frac{1}{n}). \qquad (4.2)$$

If $F(x+0) \ne F(x-0)$, there is a nonzero probability that $X = x$, namely $F(x+0) - F(x-0)$. Thus, discrete distributions as well as continuous distributions fit this model, and we need not require that F be continuous from either the left or the right.

If I is an interval, we let $\Delta_F(I)$ be the probability that $X \in I$; thus,

$$\Delta_F\big((a\mathbin{..}b)\big) = F(b-0) - F(a+0),$$
$$\Delta_F\big((a\mathbin{..}b]\big) = F(b+0) - F(a+0),$$
$$\Delta_F\big([a\mathbin{..}b)\big) = F(b-0) - F(a-0),$$
$$\Delta_F\big([a\mathbin{..}b]\big) = F(b+0) - F(a-0). \qquad (4.3)$$

(We let $F(\infty - 0) = 1$ and $F(-\infty + 0) = 0$ in these formulas if a or b is infinite.) In this section we shall consider algorithms that generate a random variable X with arbitrarily high precision, as explained in

Section 1; furthermore we want to generate a representation of X in some specified representation system for R, as defined in Section 3. In particular, if $R[j_1, \ldots, j_r]$ is any nonempty interval of the representation system, we want to generate a representation beginning $\langle j_1, \ldots, j_r \rangle$ with probability $\Delta_F(R[j_1, \ldots, j_r])$. The DDG-trees of Section 2 show how to generate the probability distribution corresponding to an r-frontier for any particular r; now we want to see how to solve the problem for all r-frontiers simultaneously.

The basic idea is to *refine* a DDG-tree as we subdivide partitions. This can be understood as follows: Suppose we have an optimum DDG-tree for some set of probabilities p_1, p_2, $\ldots$, p_n; and suppose further that we wish to split the output x_1 into two different outputs x' and x'', with respective probabilities p' and p'' where

$$p_1 = p' + p''. \tag{4.4}$$

We will see that it is possible to refine any optimum DDG-tree for $(p_1, p_2, \ldots, p_n)$ by replacing all the $\boxed{x_1}$ terminal nodes by appropriate subtrees that generate x' and x'', in such a way that the refined DDG-tree is optimum for the new set of probabilities p', p'', p_2, $\ldots$, p_n. If such refinements are done repeatedly for all subdivisions of a binary-coded representation we will have grown a tree that is simultaneously optimum at all stages of the computation.

Before formalizing this idea, let us consider an example of the refinement process. Suppose $p = p_1$ in (2.16) is to be replaced by $p' + p''$ where

$$\begin{aligned}
p' &= 1/10 &&= (0.000110011001100\ldots)_2, \\
p'' &= p - p' &&= (0.001101111110001\ldots)_2, \\
p &= 1/\pi &&= (0.010100010111110\ldots)_2.
\end{aligned} \tag{4.5}$$

We are given the optimum DDG-tree of Figure 4, which has one $\boxed{A}$ node corresponding to each 1 in the binary representation of p; we want to replace these $\boxed{A}$ nodes by subtrees that have $\boxed{A'}$ and $\boxed{A''}$ nodes for each 1 in the respective binary representations of p' and p''. The fact that $p' + p'' = p$ will make this possible. We can scan the binary representations from left to right, gaining a node whenever we see a 1 in p and losing nodes whenever we see a 1 in p' or p''; when we are done with one level, we double the number of nodes on hand and move to the next level. Thus we obtain a refined optimum DDG-tree like that in Figure 5.

The optimum refinement algorithm can be formulated as follows, given $p = p' + p''$:

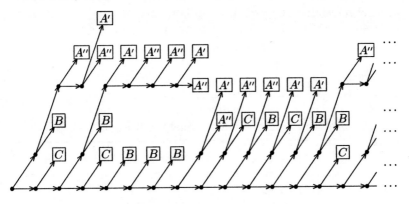

FIGURE 5. A refinement of Figure 4, using the probabilities
p' and p'' of (4.5) instead of p_1.

begin set of nodes S, T; **integer** m; **node** x;
 $m \leftarrow 0$; $S \leftarrow \emptyset$;
 while *true* **do**
  begin if $\varepsilon_m(p) = 1$ **then** insert the level-m $\boxed{A}$ node into S;
  if $\varepsilon_m(p') = 1$ **then** delete one node from S and
          change it to $\boxed{A'}$;
  if $\varepsilon_m(p'') = 1$ **then** delete one node from S and
          change it to $\boxed{A''}$;
  $T \leftarrow \emptyset$;
  for all $x \in S$ **do**
   begin replace x by the subtree $\begin{smallmatrix}\bullet\!\!\!\!<\end{smallmatrix}$;
   delete x from S;
   insert the two new children of x into T;
   end;
  $S \leftarrow T$; $m \leftarrow m + 1$;
  end;
 end;

There will never be more than three nodes in S at any time, so we
could actually replace the loop 'for all $x \in S$' by a simpler routine that
changes S from a one-element set to a two-element set. (The number
of elements in S at the time of this loop is the number of carries into
position m when p' is added to p''; hence it is always 0 or 1.) However, the algorithm has been presented in a slightly clumsy fashion to
show that it can be generalized easily to multiple refinement, where p
is replaced by any number of probabilities $p' + p'' + p''' + \cdots = p$. The

result of multiple refinement is essentially the same as repeated simple refinements, but we may prefer to do them simultaneously.

This refinement algorithm is nondeterministic since it does not specify which node of S is to be deleted and changed to $\boxed{A'}$ or $\boxed{A''}$. Thus we can in general find several ways to do the refinement. Conversely it is easy to see that *every* optimum refinement would be produced by some sequences of choices in the nondeterministic algorithm above.

The construction in Section 2 actually follows as a special case of the refinement process: We can refine $1 = p + (1 - p_1)$, then $(1 - p_1) = p_2 + (1 - p_1 - p_2)$, and so on. Even when there are infinitely many probabilities, these successive refinements produce an optimum DDG-tree as a "limit" in an obvious way.

Let us now apply the refinement idea to the generation of random deviates. Suppose we are given a binary-coded representation for some interval R, and a probability distribution F over R. (The probability that $F \notin R$ must be zero; that is, $\Delta_F(R)$ must be 1.) We shall define the concept of a DG-tree (distribution generating tree) for this distribution and this binary-coded representation: A *DG-tree* is a (usually infinite) binary tree containing nodes of two types:

i) Branch nodes, which have two sons, and which are labeled with a finite sequence (possibly empty) of 0s and 1s. The meaning of a branch node is, "Output this sequence of 0s and 1s as the next bits of the representation of X. Then flip a coin and go to the left or right child according as the result is 0 or 1."

ii) Terminal nodes, which have no children, and which are labeled with an infinite sequence of 0s and 1s. The meaning of a terminal node is, "Output this sequence of 0s and 1s as the remaining bits of the representation of X."

The algorithm specified by a DG-tree according to the meaning of its nodes is called a DG-tree algorithm.

The DG-tree must have the property that X has distribution F; this means that *if $R[j_1, \ldots, j_k]$ is any nonempty interval of the representation, and if $t(j_1, \ldots, j_k; m)$ is the number of nodes on level m of the tree such that the DG-tree algorithm has output the sequence $\langle j_1, \ldots, j_k \rangle$ and possibly further bits when it reaches this node, but the kth bit has been output at precisely this node (not before), then*

$$\sum_{m \geq 0} \frac{t(j_1, \ldots, j_k; m)}{2^m} = \Delta_F(R[j_1, \ldots, j_k]). \qquad (4.6)$$

This long-winded statement amounts to nothing more than the simple condition we need: The probability that our generated X has a representation beginning with $\langle j_1, \ldots, j_k \rangle$ is equal to the probability that a random variable with distribution F lies in the interval $R[j_1, \ldots, j_k]$, for all bit sequences $\langle j_1, \ldots, j_k \rangle$.

Figure 6(b) below shows an example of a DG-tree, corresponding to Algorithm C of Section 1. Here the distribution is $F(x) = x^2$ and the representation is the binary system over $[0..1)$. In this case there are no terminal nodes, and the string at each node consists of at most one bit.

It is possible for a DG-tree algorithm to output an invalid representation sequence such as the binary number $(0.1111\ldots)_2$; but this happens with probability 0. From a practical standpoint, of course, we never know that such an anomaly happens, since we never see all of the output.

Let $t_k(m)$ be the sum of all $t(j_1, \ldots, j_k; m)$ for $0 \le j_1, \ldots, j_k \le 1$. Then $t_k(m)/2^m$ is the probability that the DG-tree algorithm computes the kth bit of the representation of X after making precisely m flips of the coin. Since the sum of all $\Delta_F(R[j_1, \ldots, j_k])$ is 1, equation (4.6) implies that

$$\sum_{m \ge 0} \frac{t_k(m)}{2^m} = 1; \tag{4.7}$$

in other words, for every fixed k, the DG-tree algorithm will produce k or more bits of X, with probability 1.

The average running time of a DG-tree algorithm can be treated as in Section 2. Let

$$q_k(m) = \sum_{\mu > m} \frac{t_k(\mu)}{2^m} \tag{4.8}$$

be the probability that more than m flips of the coin are needed to compute the kth bit of X. The average number of coin flips is then $\sum_{m \ge 0} q_k(m)$, and we can extend Theorem 2.1 to DG-tree algorithms.

Theorem 4.1. *Let $F(x)$ specify a distribution of real numbers, and let a binary-coded representation system over R be given, where $\Delta_F(R) = 1$. Every DG-tree algorithm for this distribution and representation satisfies*

$$q_k(m) \ge \sum_{0 \le j_1, \ldots, j_k \le 1} \frac{\left\{ 2^m \Delta_F(R[j_1, \ldots, j_k]) \right\}}{2^m}. \tag{4.9}$$

Furthermore, there exists a DG-tree algorithm for which equality holds in (4.9) for all k and m.

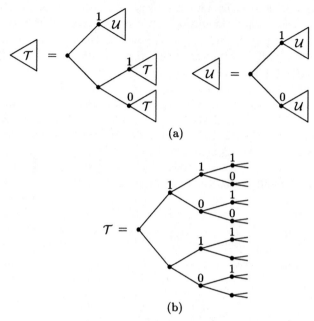

FIGURE 6. A DG-tree $\mathcal{T}$ corresponding to Algorithm C, for the distribution $F(x) = x^2$ in binary notation. The string associated with each node appears just above it. Part (a) shows a schema for generating the full tree, whose first few levels appear in (b).

Proof. Equation (4.9) is just a special case of (2.8), since the numbers $\Delta_F(R[j_1, \ldots, j_k])$ specify a discrete probability distribution. What we must prove is the existence of a DG-tree that attains this bound. By Theorem 2.1, this is equivalent to finding a DG-tree such that

$$t(j_1, \ldots, j_k; m) = \varepsilon_m\big(\Delta_F(R[j_1, \ldots, j_k])\big) \qquad (4.10)$$

for all $j_1, \ldots, j_k$, and m.

The DG-tree can be grown by induction on k, using the refinement algorithm on DDG-trees. First we begin with the DDG-tree for the trivial probability distribution $\Delta_F(R) = 1$; this tree, which consists simply of a single terminal node, is a DDG-tree for zero bits of output. Given a DDG-tree for k bits, we can refine each $\Delta_F(R[j_1, \ldots, j_k])$ into $\Delta_F(R[j_1, \ldots, j_k, 0]) + \Delta_F(R[j_1, \ldots, j_k, 1])$, thereby obtaining a DDG-tree for $k + 1$ bits. The terminal nodes for $\Delta_F(R[j_1, \ldots, j_k, 0])$ are marked with a 0, and the terminal nodes for $\Delta_F(R[j_1,\ldots,j_k,1])$ are marked with a 1.

The DG-tree is the limiting tree obtained by this construction as $k \to \infty$; the sequence of 0s and 1s associated with each node of the DG-tree is the sequence of marks attached to this node during the refinement process. (An example of DG-tree construction appears below.) Clearly condition (4.10) is satisfied, hence equality holds in (4.9). □

We shall say that a DG-tree algorithm is *optimum* if equality holds in (4.9) for all k and m. As in Theorem 2.1, we can characterize optimum trees in terms of a condition on k only:

Corollary. *Let A be a DG-tree algorithm for a specified distribution and binary-coded representation over R, and let $T_k(A)$ be the average number of random input bits needed by A to produce at least k bits of output. Then*

$$T_k(A) \geq \sum_{0 \leq j_1,\ldots,j_k \leq 1} \nu\big(\Delta_F(R[j_1,\ldots,j_k])\big). \tag{4.11}$$

Equality holds if and only if A is an optimum DG-tree algorithm. □

As an example of this corollary, let us look once again at Algorithm C of Section 1, which corresponds to the DG-tree in Figure 6. We know from (1.6) that $T_k(A) = k + 1 - 2^{-k}$. The lower bound (4.11) can be computed as follows, for this distribution and representation:

$$\sum_{0 \leq j_1,\ldots,j_k \leq 1} \nu\big(\Delta_F(R[j_1,\ldots,j_k])\big)$$

$$= \sum_{0 \leq j < 2^k} \nu\big(\Delta_F([j/2^k \ldots (j+1)/2^k)))\big)$$

$$= \sum_{0 \leq j < 2^k} \nu\big(((j+1)/2^k)^2 - (j/2^k)^2\big)$$

$$= \sum_{0 \leq j < 2^k} \nu\Big(\frac{2j+1}{2^{2k}}\Big)$$

$$= \sum_{0 \leq j_1,\ldots,j_k \leq 1} \nu\Big(\frac{j_1}{2^k} + \frac{j_2}{2^{k+1}} + \cdots + \frac{j_k}{2^{2k-1}} + \frac{1}{2^{2k}}\Big)$$

$$= \sum_{0 \leq j_1,\ldots,j_k \leq 1} \Big(\frac{kj_1}{2^k} + \frac{(k+1)j_2}{2^{k+1}} + \cdots + \frac{(2k-1)j_k}{2^{2k-1}} + \frac{2k}{2^{2k}}\Big)$$

$$= \frac{k}{2} + \frac{k+1}{4} + \cdots + \frac{2k-1}{2^k} + \frac{2k}{2^k}$$

$$= k + 1 - 2^{-k}. \tag{4.12}$$

Thus, we have proved our claim that Algorithm C is optimum.

It is instructive to consider the construction of an optimum DG-tree for the next harder case, $F(x) = x^3$, which corresponds to taking the maximum of *three* uniform deviates. For this problem we shall carry out the process outlined in the proof of Theorem 4.1, growing the DG-tree by superposing appropriate DDG-trees for $k = 1, 2, \ldots$. At the kth step there are 2^k intervals $[j/2^k \mathinner{..} (j+1)/2^k)$ for $0 \le j < 2^k$, and Δ_F applied to such an interval yields

$$\left(\frac{j+1}{2^k}\right)^3 - \left(\frac{j}{2^k}\right)^3 = \frac{3j^2 + 3j + 1}{2^{3k}}, \qquad 0 \le j < 2^k. \tag{4.13}$$

Our task is to construct a DDG-tree for this distribution by refining the distribution from the $(k-1)$st step; thus we are to use the facts that

$$\left[\frac{j}{2^{k-1}} \mathinner{..} \frac{j+1}{2^{k-1}}\right) = \left[\frac{2j}{2^k} \mathinner{..} \frac{2j+1}{2^k}\right) \cup \left[\frac{2j+1}{2^k} \mathinner{..} \frac{2j+2}{2^k}\right),$$

$$\frac{3j^2+3j+1}{2^{3(k-1)}} = \frac{3(2j)^2+3(2j)+1}{2^{3k}} + \frac{3(2j+1)^2+3(2j+1)+1}{2^{3k}}, \tag{4.14}$$

for $0 \le j < 2^{k-1}$.

When $k = 1$ the distribution is simply $(1/8, 7/8)$, so the first DDG-tree is

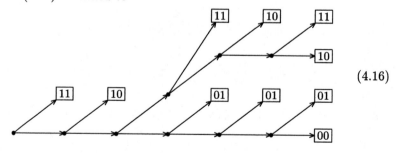

$$\tag{4.15}$$

Proceeding now to output level $k = 2$, (4.14) tells us to use the refinements $1/8 = 1/64 + 7/64$, $7/8 = 19/64 + 37/64$, namely

$$(.001)_2 = (.000001)_2 + (.000111)_2,$$
$$(.111)_2 = (.010011)_2 + (.100101)_2;$$

hence (4.15) is refined to

$$\tag{4.16}$$

by applying the refinement algorithm twice, once to the $\boxed{0}$ of (4.15) and once to the $\boxed{1}$s.

For $k \geq 3$ the tree begins to get uncomfortably large, so we shall study only its behavior up to level 3. The DDG-tree for $k = 3$ is

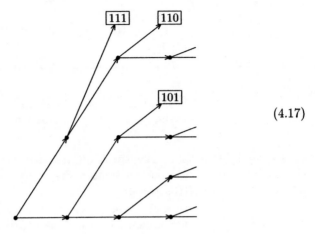

$$(4.17)$$

and for $k = 4$ it is

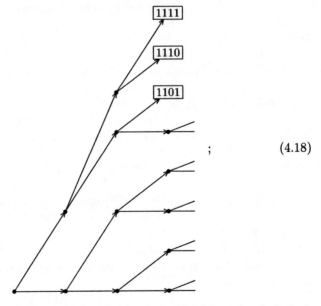

$$;\qquad(4.18)$$

by the time $k \geq 5$, all terminal nodes have vanished from levels 0, 1, 2, and 3. We obtain an optimum DG-tree by superposing these DDG-trees

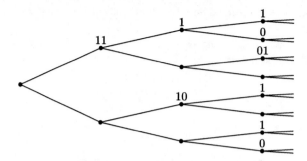

FIGURE 7. The first levels of an optimum DG-tree for the
distribution $F(x) = x^3$ in binary notation.

with appropriate output string specifications, as shown in Figure 7. Notice that two outputs occur on some nodes, since they were terminal
nodes in two of the DDG-trees.

In this example as well as the previous one, the DG-tree contains
no terminal nodes. Such nodes, with their associated infinite sequences
of 0s and 1s, occur if and only if the distribution F is discontinuous.

Let us conclude this section by observing that the optimum DG-
trees are optimum in a very strong sense. Given any DG-tree and any
frontier of the binary-coded representation, we can obtain a DDG-tree
for the probability distribution at the frontier in a straightforward manner by replacing a branch node and its descendants by a terminal node
marked $\langle j_1, \ldots, j_k \rangle$ whenever $R[j_1, \ldots, j_k]$ is an interval of the frontier and the branch node completes the output of j_1, ..., j_k. In these
terms, we have defined an optimum DG-tree as one for which the corresponding DDG-trees at each k-frontier are optimum for their discrete
distribution. But the k-frontiers include all nodes; hence each terminal node marked $\langle j_1, \ldots, j_k \rangle$ occurs the right number of times (namely
$\varepsilon_m(\Delta_F(R[j_1, \ldots, j_k]))$) on each level m, and it follows that the DDG-
trees obtained from an optimum DG-tree at *any* frontier of the binary-
coded representation are optimum. In particular, the optimum DG-tree
will yield an optimum algorithm for any representation system that maps
into the given binary-coded representation as discussed in Section 3.

Another consequence of this strong optimality is the fact that the
construction procedure of Theorem 4.1 produces *all* optimum DG-trees:

Theorem 4.2. *A DG-tree for a given distribution and binary-coded
representation is optimum if and only if the DDG-tree corresponding to*

every frontier $\mathcal{F}$ is an optimal refinement of the DDG-tree corresponding to every frontier covered by $\mathcal{F}$.

Proof. Suppose $\mathcal{F}$ covers $\mathcal{F}'$, where interval I of $\mathcal{F}'$ has been split into intervals I' and I'' in $\mathcal{F}$. The DDG-tree corresponding to $\mathcal{F}$, call it $\mathcal{T}(\mathcal{F})$, is obtainable from $\mathcal{T}(\mathcal{F}')$ by replacing all the terminal nodes corresponding to I by subtrees with terminal nodes corresponding to I' and I''. If $\mathcal{T}(\mathcal{F})$ is not an optimal refinement of $\mathcal{T}(\mathcal{F}')$ then $\mathcal{T}(\mathcal{F})$ and $\mathcal{T}(\mathcal{F}')$ cannot both be optimum DDG-trees.   □

5. The Optimum Average Running Time

Now that we have established the existence of (possibly infinite) algorithms that are optimum in a strong sense, let us see how good they really are. In relative terms, they minimize the average rth power of the running time for all r. And it turns out that they are always very good in absolute terms also, at least on the average: The output is produced at the same rate as the input, after a small initial delay, no matter what distribution we are considering.

Theorem 5.1. *For all $k \geq 1$ and for all distributions and binary-coded representations, an optimum DG-tree algorithm will output k bits of X after inputting fewer than $k + 2$ random bits, on the average.*

Proof. In fact, the average number of input bits is at most $k+2-2^{1-k}$, because we may set $n = 2^k$ in Theorem 2.3.   □

This theorem has similar variations in other representations; for example, in a radix-d number system we will be able to get k digits of output after fewer than $k \lg d + 2$ steps, on the average.

In a sense Theorem 5.1 is a very surprising result. For example, suppose you are asked to generate a random sequence of 0s and 1s in such a way that each bit takes the value 1 with probability $1/4$, independent of all other bits of the sequence. Intuitively it might seem that the best way to do this is the obvious approach, using the DG-tree

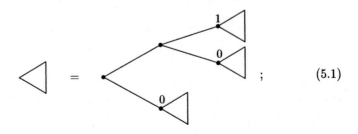

$$; \qquad (5.1)$$

but such a procedure requires an average of $\frac{3}{2}k$ steps to produce k outputs, so it must be far from optimal, according to the theorem. The DG-tree obtained from a more complex schema

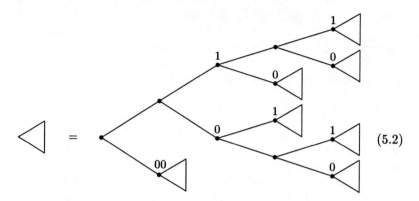

$$(5.2)$$

takes $\frac{9}{8}k$ steps, on the average, and an optimum DG-tree for this problem begins as follows:

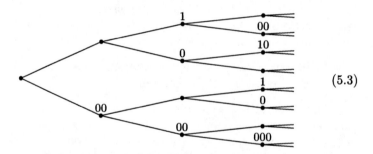

$$(5.3)$$

We have computed the average number of coin flips to get k bits of output in the case $F(x) = x^2$ for binary notation over $[0 \, . \, . \, 1)$, and the answer was $k + 1 - 2^{-k}$. (See (4.12).) If we try to use the same technique for the distribution $F(x) = x^3$, however, we soon run into grave difficulties; the sum

$$\sum_{0 \le j < 2^k} \nu\left(\frac{3j^2 + 3j + 1}{2^{3k}}\right) \tag{5.4}$$

does not appear to have any simple closed form as a function of k. Fortunately, there is a way out; the following theorem shows how to compute the asymptotic value in many cases of interest:

Theorem 5.2. *Let $F(x)$ be a distribution function over $[0..1)$, and assume that F has a continuous derivative $F'(x) = f(x)$, where $f(x)$ is bounded and the equation $f(x) = y$ has at most a bounded number of solutions x for each $y > 0$. Let $T_F(k)$ be the average running time (in terms of random flips of the coin) taken by an optimum DG-tree algorithm for F using binary notation. Then*

$$T_F(k) = k + d_F + O(k^2/2^k), \qquad (5.5)$$

where the asymptotic delay is

$$d_F = \sum_m \frac{m}{2^m} \int_0^1 \varepsilon_m(f(x)) \, dx. \qquad (5.6)$$

(The function $\varepsilon_m(x)$ is defined in (2.13); the integral $\int_0^1 \varepsilon_m(f(x)) \, dx$ is the measure of the set

$$\{x \mid \text{the } m\text{th bit in the binary representation of } f(x) \text{ is } 1\},$$

where by "mth bit" we mean the coefficient of 2^{-m}. The constant implied by the O in (5.5) depends only on the stated bounds for $f(x)$.)

Proof. We have $T_F(k) = \sum_{0 \le j < 2^k} \nu(A_{kj})$, where

$$A_{kj} = \Delta_F\left(\left[\frac{j}{2^k} .. \frac{j+1}{2^k}\right)\right) = \int_{j/2^k}^{(j+1)/2^k} f(x) \, dx; \qquad (5.7)$$

hence by (2.18),

$$T_F(k) = \sum_{m \ge 1} \sum_{j=0}^{2^k - 1} \frac{m}{2^m} \varepsilon_m(A_{kj}). \qquad (5.8)$$

Also $\sum_{m \ge 1} \varepsilon_m(A_{kj})/2^m = A_{kj}$, so

$$T_F(k) - k = \sum_{m \ge 1} \frac{m - k}{2^m} \sum_{j=0}^{2^k - 1} \varepsilon_m(A_{kj}) = \sum_{m \ge 1-k} \frac{m}{2^m} J_m(k), \qquad (5.9)$$

where

$$J_m(k) = \frac{1}{2^k} \sum_{j=0}^{2^k - 1} \varepsilon_{m+k}(A_{kj}). \qquad (5.10)$$

Let $\sup_{x \in [0..1]} f(x) = 2^\mu$; then $A_{kj} \le 2^{\mu-k}$, by (5.7), hence $J_m(k) = 0$ for all k when $m < -\mu$.

Now consider any fixed m. Our assumption about f implies that the following condition holds for all but $O(2^m)$ values of j in the range $0 \le j < 2^k$:

$$\lfloor 2^m f(x) \rfloor = \lfloor 2^m f(y) \rfloor \quad \text{for all } x, y \in \left[\frac{j}{2^k} \cdot \cdot \frac{j+1}{2^k}\right]. \tag{5.11}$$

For all such values of j we have

$$\varepsilon_{m+k}(A_{kj}) = \varepsilon_{m+k}\left(\int_{j/2^k}^{(j+1)/2^k} f(x)\,dx\right) = \varepsilon_m\bigl(f(y)\bigr),$$

for all $y \in \left[\frac{j}{2^k} \cdot \cdot \frac{j+1}{2^k}\right]$. Consequently

$$\frac{1}{2^k}\varepsilon_{m+k}(A_{kj}) = \int_{j/2^k}^{(j+1)/2^k} \varepsilon_m\bigl(f(x)\bigr).$$

It follows that

$$J_m(k) = \int_0^1 \varepsilon_m\bigl(f(x)\bigr)\,dx + O(2^{m-k});$$

and since $0 \le J_m(k) \le 1$ we have in fact

$$J_m(k) = \int_0^1 \varepsilon_m\bigl(f(x)\bigr)\,dx + O\bigl(\min(1, 2^{m-k})\bigr). \tag{5.12}$$

Using this value in (5.9) yields

$$T_F(k) = k + d_F + \sum_{-\mu \le m \le k} \frac{m}{2^m}O(2^{m-k}) + \sum_{m>k} \frac{m}{2^m}O(1)$$

and (5.5) follows immediately.   □

From this proof we can see that (5.5) holds also in other cases, for example when there are finitely many points $0 = x_0 < x_1 < \cdots < x_n = 1$ such that $F'(x) = f(x)$ exists and is bounded and monotonic on $(x_{i-1} \cdot \cdot x_i)$ for $1 \le i \le n$; such a distribution F may have jumps at the x_i, but "piecewise differentiability" in the stated sense is sufficient. On the other hand (5.5) is not true in general when there are *infinitely* many points where F fails to have a derivative, as we shall see later.

Let us first apply Theorem 5.2 to the distribution $F(x) = x^3$. The integral in (5.6) is

$$\int_0^1 \varepsilon_m(3x^2)\,dx = \int_0^3 \frac{\varepsilon_m(y)}{\sqrt{12y}}\,dy.$$

For $m = -1$ this is $\int_2^3 dy/\sqrt{12y} = 1 - \sqrt{2/3}$; for $m \geq 1$ it is

$$\sum_{j=1}^{3 \cdot 2^{m-1}} \int_{(2j-1)/2^m}^{2j/2^m} \frac{dy}{\sqrt{12y}} = \frac{h(3 \cdot 2^{m-1})}{2^{m/2}\sqrt{3}},$$

$$h(n) = \sum_{j=1}^n (\sqrt{2j} - \sqrt{2j-1}). \tag{5.13}$$

Let $g(n) = \sqrt{1} + \sqrt{2} + \cdots + \sqrt{n-1}$; then

$$h(n) = 2\sqrt{2}g(n) - g(2n) + \sqrt{2n}. \tag{5.14}$$

By Euler's summation formula

$$g(n) = \frac{2}{3}n^{3/2} - \frac{1}{2}\sqrt{n} + C + O(1/\sqrt{n}) \tag{5.15}$$

as $n \to \infty$, for some constant C (which turns out to equal

$$\zeta(-1/2) = -\frac{\zeta(3/2)}{4\pi}$$
$$\approx -0.20788\,62249\,77354\,56601\,73067\,25397\,04930\,22262\,68531,$$

see [8, exercise 6.1–8]); hence

$$h(n) = \sqrt{n/2} + (2\sqrt{2} - 1)C + O(1/\sqrt{n}). \tag{5.16}$$

For large m we have proved that $\int_0^1 \varepsilon_m(3x^2)\,dx = \frac{1}{2} + 2^{-m/2}c + O(2^{-m})$, where $c = (2\sqrt{2} - 1)C/\sqrt{3}$. We can develop this asymptotic expansion further, so that the term $O(2^{-m})$ becomes, for example, $2^{-m-4} - 2^{-3m-10} + 7 \cdot 2^{-5m-15} + O(2^{-7m})$, and we can evaluate

$$d_F = \sum_m \frac{m}{2^m} \int_0^1 \varepsilon_m(f(x))\,dx$$

$$= -2\left(1 - \sqrt{2/3}\right) + \frac{1}{\sqrt{3}} \sum_{m \geq 1} \frac{m}{2^{3m/2}} h(3 \cdot 2^{m-1}) \tag{5.17}$$

to any desired accuracy; it equals

$$0.46582\,55123\,10713\,08245\,65345\,56457\,55499\,21347-\,.$$

Note that the distribution $F(x) = x^3$ can therefore be generated more rapidly than the intuitively simpler distribution $F(x) = x^2$.

We shall now look at some rather pathological distributions. Let

$$F(x) = \begin{cases} \frac{1}{2}F(4x), & \text{if } 0 \le x < \frac{1}{4}; \\ \frac{1}{2}, & \text{if } \frac{1}{4} \le x < \frac{3}{4}; \\ \frac{1}{2} + \frac{1}{2}F(4x - 3), & \text{if } \frac{3}{4} \le x < 1. \end{cases} \qquad (5.18)$$

These function values can be easily understood in terms of binary notation: If α denotes an infinite string of 0s and 1s not ending with infinitely many ones, and if we regard $F(x)$ as such a string representing its radix-2 representation, we have

$$\begin{aligned} F(00\alpha) &= 0F(\alpha), \\ F(01\alpha) &= 1000\dots, \\ F(10\alpha) &= 1000\dots, \\ F(11\alpha) &= 1F(\alpha). \end{aligned} \qquad (5.19)$$

It is easy to see that $F(x)$ is a continuous nondecreasing function, which is differentiable almost everywhere in $[0\,.\,.\,1]$. The derivative fails to exist only at points whose binary expansion is generated by the extended regular expression $(00 + 11)^*010^\infty + (00 + 11)^\infty$; and everywhere the derivative exists, it is zero. Yet somehow this function manages to increase continuously from 0 to 1.

The optimum DG-tree for distribution (5.18) is actually very simple,

$$\qquad (5.20)$$

and the time to generate k bits of output is exactly $\lceil k/2 \rceil$, with zero variance.

We may also consider the related "Cantor ternary set" function, which is often used in textbooks as an example of a monotone, continuous function whose derivative vanishes almost everywhere:

$$F(x) = \begin{cases} \frac{1}{2}F(3x), & \text{if } 0 \le x < \frac{1}{3}; \\ \frac{1}{2}, & \text{if } \frac{1}{3} \le x < \frac{2}{3}; \\ \frac{1}{2} + \frac{1}{2}F(3x - 2), & \text{if } \frac{2}{3} \le x < 1. \end{cases} \qquad (5.21)$$

In this case the optimum DG-tree to generate the *ternary* (radix-3) representation of a random X is

$$\triangleleft \quad = \quad \begin{matrix} 2 \\ \\ 0 \end{matrix} \qquad ; \qquad (5.22)$$

hence on intuitive grounds we expect the binary representation to be generated in about $k/\lg 3$ flips per bit. This can be proved as follows: Let $l = \lfloor k/\lg 3 \rfloor$, so that $3^{-l-1} < 2^{-k} < 3^{-l}$. We divide the integers j such that $0 \le j < 2^k$ into $3^{l-1}+1$ classes numbered from 0 through 3^{l-1}, where class number n consists of those j such that $(3n-2)/3^l < j/2^k < (3n+1)/3^l$. There are at most nine values of j per class. The sum of the probabilities in class n is $F((3n+1)/3^l) - F((3n-2)/3^l)$, and it is not difficult to verify that this sum is always either 2^{-l} or 0 for all n. Hence it is nonzero for precisely 2^l values of n. For such n we have

$$\sum_{j \in \text{class } n} \nu(A_{kj}) = \sum_{j \in \text{class } n} \left(l A_{kj} + \frac{\nu(2^l A_{kj})}{2^l} \right) = \frac{l}{2^l} + \frac{1}{2^l} \sum_{j \in \text{class } n} \nu(2^l A_{kj})$$

by (2.21); and the latter sum is at most 5 by Theorem 2.3. We therefore have

$$\lfloor k/\lg 3 \rfloor \le T_F(k) \le \lfloor k/\lg 3 \rfloor + 5 \qquad (5.23)$$

for distribution (5.21).

Another distribution of this general type is $F(x) = F_0(x)$, where

$$F_j(x) = \begin{cases} \frac{1}{2} F_{j+1}(2^{2j+1}x), & \text{if } 0 \le x < 2^{-2j-1}; \\ \frac{1}{2}, & \text{if } 2^{-2j-1} \le x < 1 - 2^{-2j-1}; \\ \frac{1}{2} + \frac{1}{2} F_{j+1}(2^{2j+1}x - 2^{2j+1}+1), & \text{if } 1 - 2^{-2j-1} \le x < 1. \end{cases} \quad (5.24)$$

In this case the optimum DG-tree algorithm takes $\lceil \sqrt{k} \rceil$ steps to generate the kth bit; it produces $2j-1$ identical bits of output after the jth flip of the coin. Similarly we can construct continuous distribution functions whose running time as a function of k grows arbitrarily slowly.

All of our DG-tree examples so far have been for continuous $F(x)$; it is also interesting to consider the discontinuous distribution

$$F(x) = \begin{cases} \frac{1}{4} F(2x), & \text{if } 0 \le x < \frac{1}{2}; \\ \frac{3}{4} + \frac{1}{4} F(2x - 1), & \text{if } \frac{1}{2} \le x < 1. \end{cases} \qquad (5.25)$$

This might be called the "stuttering" function, since the binary representation of $F(x)$ is the binary representation of x but with each bit repeated twice. For example,

$$F\big((.010100010111\ldots)_2\big) = (.0011001100000011001111111\ldots)_2.$$

There is a jump of 2^{-2j+1} at each binary rational point of the form $x = q/2^j$, where q is odd. The function $F(x)$ is continuous except at the binary rationals, and it has zero derivative almost everywhere. There are certain irrational points where the derivative fails to exist; for example, one of the interesting points of this kind is

$$x_0 = 1 - 2^{-1} - 2^{-2} - 2^{-4} - 2^{-8} - 2^{-16} - \cdots = 1 - \sum_{j \geq 0} 2^{-2^j}. \quad (5.26)$$

If $\epsilon = 2^{-2^j}$, for any $j \geq 1$, we find

$$F(x_0 + \epsilon) - F(x_0) = 3\epsilon^2, \quad \text{but} \quad F(x_0 + 2\epsilon) - F(x_0) = 2\epsilon + 4\epsilon^2;$$

thus no derivative exists at x_0. (Incidentally, we have the curious identity $F(x_0) = 3x_0 - \frac{1}{2}$ at this point.)

The values $A_{jk} = \Delta_F\big([j/2^k \mathbin{..} (j+1)/2^k)\big)$ for $0 \leq j < 2^k$ include 2^{k-i} occurrences of $(2^{2i-1} + 1)/2^{2k}$, for $1 \leq i \leq k$, and one occurrence of $1/2^{2k}$. (Recall that $F(j/2^k - 0)$ must be used in this calculation, not $F(j/2^k)$.) Thus the average running time to generate k bits can be computed exactly, and it is

$$\sum_{j=0}^{2^k - 1} \nu(A_{jk}) = 3 - \frac{3}{2^k}. \quad (5.27)$$

The optimum DG-tree for distribution (5.25) turns out to be simply

$$(5.28)$$

Although the value x_0 in (5.26) has special properties with respect to F, it doesn't show up in this tree in any special way.

These examples show the necessity of at least some restrictive hypotheses about $F(x)$ in Theorem 5.2.

6. Monotone Generation Algorithms

In Section 1 we considered a square root method to generate random X for the distribution $F(x) = x^2$. The particular method we used required $2k$ input bits to get k bits of output, but it would have been possible to design a more complex square root routine that would have input only as many bits as absolutely necessary before producing the kth bit of output, for each k. For example, when $U = (.010\alpha)_2$, we always have $\sqrt{U} = (.100\ldots)_2$ regardless of the subsequent bits α.

This idea leads to a DG-tree that begins as shown in Figure 8. Intuitively we might think that this tree should be optimum; but the average time to generate the third bit of output turns out to be 4, while Algorithm C does the same job in only $3\frac{7}{8}$ steps. The reason is that our problem was not to generate the square root of a uniform deviate; the problem was to generate a random X that has the same *distribution* as the square root of a uniform deviate.

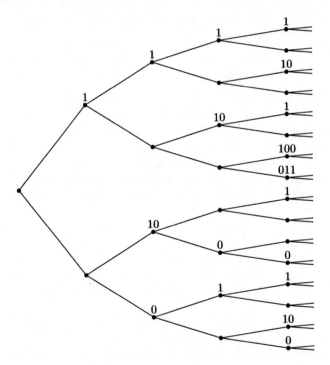

FIGURE 8. Optimum monotone DG-tree for the square root of a binary number between 0 and 1.

By comparing Figure 8 to Figure 6 we can see where Figure 8 loses: The output 101 occurs once on level 3 in Figure 6 but twice on level 4 in Figure 8. A moment's thought also explains why Figure 6 wins: Figure 8 is required to be a *monotone* DG-tree, in the sense that all the strings generated by paths on the left (lower) branch following each node must be lexicographically less than or equal to all the strings generated by paths on the right (upper) branch. Figure 6 is not subject to this requirement.

There is a unique optimum monotone DG-tree for every distribution and representation. Such trees are optimum for calculating $F^{[-1]}(U)$ from the binary representation of U; they are of general interest from the standpoint of computational complexity, whether or not we wish to generate random numbers. It appears to be difficult to compute the exact average running time for the optimum square-root tree, when we average over all possible inputs; however, we can show that the average number of bits input, before the kth bit of the square root can be output, is less than $k + 3$. In fact, a similar bound is true in general.

Theorem 6.1. *For any distribution and binary-coded representation, the optimum monotone DG-tree requires fewer than 2 more inputs than an optimum DG-tree does to generate k bits of output, on the average for all k.*

Proof. The average time for the kth output bit is $\sum L(v)/2^{L(v)}$ summed over all nodes v where the kth bit is output, where $L(v)$ denotes the level of v. Each node v is associated with some interval I of the kth level of the representation. For each I we shall prove below that there are at most two associated nodes v on any given level. This suffices to prove the theorem, since the cost associated with I can be written as

$$\nu(\Delta_I) + \nu(\Delta'_I), \qquad \text{where } \Delta_I + \Delta'_I = \Delta_F(I);$$

hence by (2.23) and (2.25) we have

$$\nu(\Delta_F(I)) \leq \nu(\Delta_I) + \nu(\Delta'_I) \leq \nu(\Delta_F(I)) + 2\Delta_F(I). \qquad (6.1)$$

Summing this inequality over all I, and noting that strict inequality occurs for some I, gives the result.

Consider the nodes v associated with an interval I; let $\Delta_F(I) = x - y$ where $x = F(b \pm 0)$ and $y = F(a \pm 0)$ as in (4.3). Assume that $x > y$. We are going to map all inputs that are $> y$ and $< x$ into the interval I. (The inputs *equal* to x or y are immaterial, as they have infinite precision so they occur with probability zero.) Consider, for example, values such as

$$x = (.01101001010011010101011\ldots)_2,$$
$$y = (.01101000110110101111010\ldots)_2;$$

then the $\boxed{I}$ nodes on the optimum monotone DG-tree all look like this, starting after the path for 0110100:

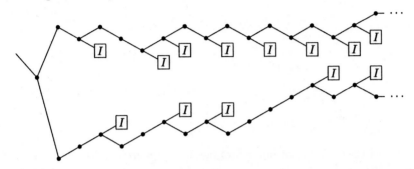

In general, after the first bit in which x and y differ, there will be an $\boxed{I}$ node for the 0 corresponding to each subsequent 1 bit of x, and an $\boxed{I}$ node for the 1 corresponding to each subsequent 0 bit of y. (A slight exception occurs if y is a terminating binary fraction; change '10^∞' at the end of y to '01^∞' to make the stated rule work in general.) Clearly there are at most two $\boxed{I}$ nodes per level, and at most one when $y = 0$, as claimed. $\square$

Corollary. Let $G(x)$ be any monotone increasing function from $[0 .. 1]$ into $[0 .. 1]$. It is possible to compute the kth bit of $G(x)$ accurately by reading fewer than $k + 4$ bits of x, on the average, assuming a uniform distribution of x values.

Proof. Let $F(x) = G^{[-1]}(x)$, with arbitrary values consistent with monotonicity when $G^{[-1]}(x)$ is undefined. Apply Theorems 5.1 and 6.1. $\square$

In particular, there is a way to compute weird functions such as $1/(2 - \exp(-\pi^2 \tan \sqrt{x}))$ nearly in "real time," given a sufficiently clever algorithm.

Let us now consider the optimum monotone DG-tree in a simple case for which the running time can be calculated explicitly: Suppose θ is a real number between 0 and 1, and suppose we want to compute $x + \theta$ in binary, given x in binary. In order to stay within the range $[0 .. 1]$, we shall compute $\frac{1}{2}(x + \theta)$, since it has the same binary digits (only shifted). The following algorithm for left-to-right addition gives its output as soon as possible, assuming that $x = (.x_1 x_2 x_3 \ldots)_2$ and that $\theta = (.\theta_1 \theta_2 \theta_3 \ldots)_2$ does not have a terminating binary representation.

```
begin integer j, m;
    m ← 1;  j ← 0;
    while true do
        begin
            if x_m + θ_m = 1 then j ← j + 1
            else begin
                if x_m + θ_m = 0 then output(01^j) else output(10^j);
                j ← 0;
            end;
            m ← m + 1;
        end;
end;
```

The average number of input bits before this algorithm produces k bits of output is $T_{k,0}$, where

$$T_{k,j} = \begin{cases} 0, & \text{if } k \le 0; \\ 1 + \tfrac{1}{2}T_{k-j-1,0} + \tfrac{1}{2}T_{k,j+1}, & \text{if } k > 0. \end{cases} \tag{6.2}$$

The solution that satisfies $0 \le T_{k,j} \le T_{k,0}$ is $T_{k,j} = \max(k+1-j, 2)$ for $k \ge 1$; thus the average is $k + 1$.

An optimum DG-tree for the corresponding distribution function $F(x) = 2x - \theta$, $\tfrac{1}{2}\theta \le x \le \tfrac{1}{2}(\theta + 1)$, can be shown to have running time $T_F(k) = k - 1 + 2^{2-k}$. (*Proof:* The nonzero numbers A_{kj} for $0 \le j < 2^k$ include the value 2^{1-k} exactly $2^{k-1} - 1$ times, plus two nonterminating binary fractions that sum to 2^{1-k}; thus $\sum \nu(A_{kj}) = 2^{1-k}\big((2^{k-1} - 1)(k - 1) + k + 1\big)$.) Therefore the constant 2 in Theorem 6.1 proves to be best possible even in this simple case.

7. Finite State Generators

We have seen that highly efficient generators exist for arbitrary distributions and representations, if "efficient" means that comparatively few random input bits need to be used. However, most of the algorithms that achieve these optimum bounds are very complex, requiring a tremendous amount of space (even infinite) to store the DG-trees. Therefore we would like to consider restricted classes of algorithms that have comparatively simple programs and require comparatively little space.

In this section we shall study algorithms that can be represented by a finite state automaton; Algorithm C of Section 1 is an optimum example of such an algorithm (see Figure 6). We shall obtain partial answers to the following questions: (i) What distributions can be generated by such algorithms? (ii) If a distribution F can be so generated, how close to the optimum running time $T_F(k)$ can we come?

Throughout this section we shall restrict attention to distributions $F(x)$ over $[0..1)$, in binary notation. A finite state generator (fsg) for F is a DG-tree algorithm for F whose tree has only finitely many non-isomorphic subtrees, where we regard two trees as isomorphic if they differ at most by interchanging left and right branches at branch nodes. For example, the infinite DG-tree in Figure 6(b) has only six nonisomorphic subtrees, as indicated in Figure 6(a); namely, $\mathcal{T}$ with or without a 0 or 1 at its root, $\mathcal{U}$ with a 0 or 1 at its root, and the other child of $\mathcal{T}$. (In practice only three of these six subtree types would correspond to distinct states of a computer program, since the output strings could be associated with transitions between states.)

The fsg model of computation is closely related to well-developed theories of probabilistic finite automata, and to the input-output realizability problem in Markov chains; see, for example, the book by Paz [9]. The connection of fsg's with random number generation provides a new direction for that theory.

In this section we shall show that each of the distributions $F(x) = x^n$ for $n \geq 3$ can be generated by an appropriate fsg, but none of these is an optimum DG-tree algorithm. On the other hand, given any $\epsilon > 0$ we shall construct an fsg for this polynomial $F(x)$ whose average running time to generate k bits is within ϵ of the optimum average running time $T_F(k)$. Finally we shall show that certain important distributions (such as the exponential and normal) cannot be generated by any fsg.

First, to generate $F(x) = x^n$ we can use a technique essentially like one that Ahrens and Dieter [1, Chapter 2] ascribe to G. Gaschütz. The idea is to simulate the operation of taking the maximum of n independent uniform deviates. The tree $\mathcal{T}_n$ begins by using a DDG-tree for the probabilities $\binom{n}{j}2^{-n}$ that the leading bits of the n simulated uniform deviates contain exactly j 1s. If $j = 0$, we output 0 and continue with tree $\mathcal{T}_n$; otherwise we output 1 (as soon as discovering that $j \neq 0$), and continue with $\mathcal{T}_j$. For example,

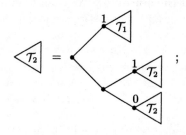

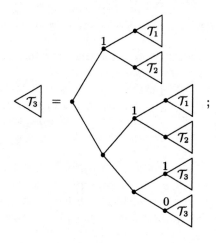

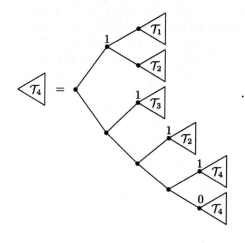

The average running time satisfies

$$
T_n(k) = \begin{cases}
2 - 2^{1-n}, & \text{if } k = 1; \\[2mm]
\displaystyle\sum_j \nu\!\left(2^{-n}\binom{n}{j}\right) \\[2mm]
\quad + \dfrac{1}{2^n}\left(T_n(k-1) + \displaystyle\sum_{j=1}^{n}\binom{n}{j}T_j(k-1)\right), & \text{if } k > 1.
\end{cases}
\tag{7.1}
$$

In particular, we have $T_1(k) = k$, $T_2(k) = k + 1 - 2^{-k}$, and $T_3(k) = k + \frac{5}{2} - \frac{3}{2}2^{-k} - 4^{1-k}$ for $k \geq 1$. The running time for each n has the form $k + d_n + O(2^{-k})$, where $d_n = O(\log n)^2$. (Recall that for $n = 3$ the optimum average running time is less than $k + .466 + O(k^2 2^{-k})$, according to our calculation in (5.17).)

Theorem 7.1. When $n \geq 3$, no fsg for $F(x) = x^n$ is an optimum DG-tree algorithm.

Proof. We will show that every optimum DG-tree has infinitely many nonisomorphic subtrees. If v is a node in any DG-tree, let $P(v)$ be the length of the longest "free path" leading from v, namely the longest distance that can be traveled from v to descendant nodes before an output occurs. If $P(v_1) \neq P(v_2)$ the subtrees rooted at v_1 and v_2 cannot be isomorphic; hence it suffices to show that, for all N, there exists a node v with $N < P(v) < \infty$. (It may seem paradoxical that the proof relies on long free paths, since free paths are intuitively inefficient, and our finite state generator for $F(x)$ contains no long free paths. Yet it is precisely the lack of long free paths that makes it nonoptimal, according to this proof.)

Recall from Theorem 4.2 that every optimum DG-tree is obtained by successive refinements. When $\boxed{v}$ is a terminal node of a DDG-tree at level k, the refinement to level $k+1$ replaces $\boxed{v}$ by a subtree $\mathcal{T}(v)$ whose terminal nodes are $\boxed{v'}$ or $\boxed{v''}$; the longest free path from v in the resulting DG-tree is the longest path from v in $\mathcal{T}(v)$. If $\mathcal{T}(v)$ contains a finite number, say $M(v)$, of terminal nodes $\boxed{v'}$ and $\boxed{v''}$, we must have $\lg M(v) \leq P(v) < M(v)$. To complete the proof, we need only exhibit nodes v such that $M(v)$ is an arbitrarily large finite number.

Consider first the case $n = 3$, since this makes the notation simpler. We shall use the integers

$$
b = \frac{4^{2t+1} - 4}{10}, \qquad j = 5 \cdot 2^m + b, \qquad k \geq m + 3, \tag{7.2}
$$

where t is very large but m is much larger, say $m \geq 100t$. Then our nodes v, v', v'' will correspond to the intervals

$$[j/2^k .. (j+1)/2^k) = [2j/2^{k+1} .. (2j+1)/2^{k+1})$$
$$\cup [(2j+1)/2^{k+1} .. (2j+2)/2^{k+1}).$$

The corresponding $\Delta_F(I)$, for $F(x) = x^3$, are respectively $p = p' + p''$ where

$$p' = (300 \cdot 2^{2m} + (12 \cdot 4^{2t+1} - 18) \cdot 2^m + 12b^2 + 6b + 1)/2^{3k+3},$$
$$p'' = (300 \cdot 2^{2m} + (12 \cdot 4^{2t+1} + 42) \cdot 2^m + 12b^2 + 18b + 7)/2^{3k+3}, \qquad (7.3)$$
$$p = (600 \cdot 2^{2m} + (24 \cdot 4^{2t+1} + 24) \cdot 2^m + 24b^2 + 24b + 8)/2^{3k+3}$$

When p' is added to p'', no carries occur between the parenthesized coefficients of $2^{2m-3k-3}$, 2^{m-3k-3}, and 2^{-3k-3} in these three binary fractions, since m is so large; hence the descendants v' and v'' of each node v corresponding to a bit in one of these three groups will also belong to the same group. The second group contains exactly four nodes v, together with 5 nodes v'' and $4t + 3$ nodes v'; hence one of the four nodes v will have at least $(5 + 4t + 3)/4 = t + 2$ of the nodes v' and v'' as descendants. Since t can be arbitrarily large, the proof is complete for $n = 3$.

The same sort of proof works for general $n \geq 3$, again choosing b, j, and k as in (7.2) and with m suitably large compared to t. The respective coefficients of $2^{m(n-2)-nk-n}$ will be $n(n-1)10^{n-3}(2 \cdot 4^{2t+1} - 3) + n(n-1)10^{n-3}(2 \cdot 4^{2t+1} + 7) = n(n-1)10^{n-3}(4 \cdot 4^{2t+1} + 4)$, and again we can produce a node v with arbitrarily many descendants when t is large enough.   □

A similar proof technique can be used to establish that the distribution $F(x) = q^2 x^2$, for $0 \leq x \leq 1/q$, cannot be optimally generated by any fsg when $q > 1$ is odd: The subdivision of $[j/2^k .. (j+1)/2^k)$, when $j = (2^t - a)/q^2$ is an integer and when $q^2/4 < a < q^2/2$, corresponds to the binary addition

$$(2^{t+2} + 3q^2 - 4a) + (2^{t+2} - (4a - q^2)) = 4(2^{t+1} + q^2 - 2a);$$

so it implies the existence of a node v with $P(v) \approx t$. Such integers t and a exist for arbitrarily large t, since we can let $a = 2^s$ and $t = rb + s$ where $2^r \bmod q^2 = 1$.

The next theorem shows that many distributions $F(x)$ that are polynomials with rational coefficients can be generated by an fsg.

Theorem 7.2. *Let $F(x)$ be a distribution function on $[0..1]$ whose derivative can be written as a finite sum of the polynomials*

$$f_{ab}(x) = x^a(1 - x)^b, \qquad 0 \le x \le 1, \qquad (7.4)$$

with positive rational coefficients. There is an fsg for distribution $F(x)$ whose average running time to generate k bits is $k + O(1)$.

Proof. Consider first the comparatively easy case

$$F(x) = p_1 x + p_2 x^2 + \cdots + p_n x^n, \qquad p_1 + p_2 + \cdots + p_n = 1, \qquad (7.5)$$

and where all p_j are rational and ≥ 0. The idea is to start with a DDG-tree for the discrete distribution $(p_1, p_2, \ldots, p_n)$: An optimum DDG-tree with finitely many nonisomorphic subtrees can be found, since each p_j has a periodic binary representation and we can use the least common multiple of the period lengths. Now wherever this DDG-tree has a terminal node, say for p_j, we substitute the fsg $\mathcal{T}_j$ defined above for distribution x^j. The average time for this method to generate k bits is at most $k + \max(d_1, \ldots, d_n)$, plus at most $\lg n + 2$ for the initial determination of j.

When $F(x)$ has negative coefficients but $F'(x)$ is a positive rational combination of the functions $f_{ab}(x)$ in (7.4), a similar argument applies: $F(x)$ will be a convex combination of the beta distributions

$$F_{ab}(x) = (a + b + 1)\binom{a + b}{b} \int_0^x t^a(1 - t)^b, \qquad 0 \le x \le 1 \qquad (7.6)$$

with rational coefficients p_{ab}, and it suffices to prove that each $F_{ab}(x)$ can be generated by an appropriate fsg. It is well known (see, for example, [8, exercise 5–7; exercise 5–9 in the second edition]) that $F_{ab}(x)$ is the distribution of the $(a + 1)$-st smallest of $a + b + 1$ independent uniform deviates; thus we need only generalize our previous construction for the maximum of n uniform deviates.

An fsg $\mathcal{T}_{n,t}$ for the tth largest of n uniform deviates can be constructed as follows: First proceed as in the construction of $\mathcal{T}_n$ to generate a random integer j with the binomial probability distribution $\binom{n}{j}2^{-n}$; then j represents the number of uniform deviates whose leading bit is 1. If $j \ge t$, output 1 and continue with the fsg $\mathcal{T}_{j,t}$; otherwise output 0 and continue with $\mathcal{T}_{n-j,t-j}$. (This construction reduces to the previous construction when $t = 1$; in other words, $\mathcal{T}_{n,1} = \mathcal{T}_n$.)

Since $F_{ab}(x)$ is generated by $\mathcal{T}_{a+b+1,b+1}$ in $k + O(1)$ steps, the proof is complete. ☐

The construction in this proof of the theorem yields an fsg whose running time is at most $k + D_n$, where the delay D_n depends only on the maximum degree n of the polynomials $F_{ab}(x)$ in the assumed decomposition of $F(x)$, not on the coefficients of this convex combination. However, the value of n is sometimes larger than the degree of $F(x)$ itself, when $F(x)$ has negative coefficients. For example, if $F'(x)$ is proportional to $1 - 3x + 3x^2$, we cannot obtain $F'(x)$ as a nonnegative linear combination of 1, x, $1 - x$, x^2, $x(1 - x)$, and $(1 - x)^2$, but we do have $1 - 3x + 3x^2 = (1 - x)^3 + x^3$.

It is possible to extend the construction of Theorem 7.2 to considerably more general polynomial distributions. For example, we can construct an fsg that simulates the evaluation of the tth largest of n independent random numbers uniformly distributed in $[p \mathinner{.\,.} q]$, where p and q are rational numbers with $0 \le p \le q \le 1$. Then we can generate $F(x)$ when $F'(x)$ is proportional to $(3x - 1)^2$, for example, by generating the ranges $[0 \mathinner{.\,.} 1/3]$ and $[1/3 \mathinner{.\,.} 1]$ separately. (This $F(x)$ does not meet the hypotheses of Theorem 7.2, since $F_{ab}(1/3) > 0$ for all a and b but $(3x - 1)^2$ vanishes at $x = 1/3$.) On the other hand, when $F'(x)$ has irrational roots (for example, if it is proportional to $(2x^2 - 1)^2$), there is no evident way to construct an fsg for $F(x)$.

We can now use Theorem 7.2 to deduce a stronger result of theoretical interest:

Theorem 7.3. *Let $F(x)$ be a polynomial distribution function in $[0 \mathinner{.\,.} 1]$, having the form (7.5) with nonnegative rational coefficients, and let $\epsilon > 0$. There is an fsg that generates $F(x)$ and whose average running time to generate k bits is less than ϵ more than the average running time of an optimum DG-tree algorithm, for all k.*

Proof. The idea is to use an optimum DG-tree algorithm to generate a large number of outputs, after which time most of the distribution will be generated by "uniform" subtrees (like T_1), while the residual part is polynomial so it can be generated quickly enough by fsg's using Theorem 7.2. This vague idea can be made precise by pursuing some of the ideas we used in the proof of Theorem 5.2.

Let m be a large integer. Since $F(x)$ satisfies the hypothesis of Theorem 5.2, we can conclude that all but $O(2^m)$ values of j in the range $0 \le j < 2^{2m}$ will satisfy (5.11); in other words there will exist an integer t_j such that

$$\frac{t_j}{2^m} \le f(x) < \frac{t_j + 1}{2^m}, \qquad \text{for all } x \in \left[\frac{j}{2^{2m}} \mathinner{.\,.} \frac{j+1}{2^{2m}}\right]. \qquad (7.7)$$

We will say that j is a "good" value when this holds. The probability $\Delta_F([j/2^m .. (j+1)/2^m))$ is

$$A_{(2m)j} = \int_{j/2^{2m}}^{(j+1)/2^{2m}} f(x)\,dx,$$

and for all $k \geq 0$ and all l between 0 and $2^k - 1$ we will therefore have

$$\frac{t_j}{2^{3m+k}} \leq A_{(2m+k)(2^k j + l)} < \frac{t_j + 1}{2^{3m+k}}. \tag{7.8}$$

In other words, the probabilities for all subdivisions of a good interval $[j/2^{2m} .. (j+1)/2^m)$ will have the same leading bits, given by t_j.

Let $p = p' + p''$ where p, p', and p'' have the same leading bits. That is, we assume that $\lfloor 2^s p \rfloor = \lfloor 2^{s+1} p' \rfloor = \lfloor 2^{s+1} p'' \rfloor$ for some integer s. Then it is easy to see what the refinement algorithm of Section 4 will do on the first s levels of the tree if the set S in that algorithm is treated as a queue (first in, first out): Every node $\boxed{v}$ on level s or less will be replaced by the subtree

Now *every* element of the subdivisions of a good interval will have the leading bit property; hence there is an optimum DG-tree in which every node v on level $\leq 3m$ belonging to a good interval will have the "uniform" subtree

$$\tag{7.9}$$

In other words, when we get to such a node v, all subsequent output is simply equal to the input. Thus, a large part of the optimum DG-tree is already an fsg, in the sense that the vast majority of its subtrees at the time we generate the $2m$th bit of output are isomorphic to the uniform subtree. To complete the proof, we will patch up the rest of the tree.

First consider a "bad" value of j. We can assume that the DDG-tree for output level $2m$ during the construction of the optimum DG-tree is a finite state DDG-tree, since all of the probabilities involved are rational numbers. (Indeed, the refinement algorithm transforms a finite state

DDG-tree into a finite state DDG-tree when p, p', and p'' are rational, if S is treated as a queue.) Every terminal node v of this DDG-tree, corresponding to a bad value of j, will now be replaced by an fsg for the polynomial distribution defined by

$$A_{(2m)j}F_j(x) = F\left(\frac{j+x}{2^{2m}}\right) - F\left(\frac{j}{2^{2m}}\right), \qquad 0 \le x < 1. \qquad (7.10)$$

Next, consider a "good" value of j. We replace each terminal node $\boxed{v}$ of the DDG-tree corresponding to such a j by the uniform subtree (7.9) if $\boxed{v}$ is on level $\le 3m$, otherwise we replace $\boxed{v}$ by an fsg for the polynomial distribution $G_j(x)$ with nonnegative rational coefficients defined by

$$\frac{t_j}{2^{3m}}x + \left(A_{(2m)j} - \frac{t_j}{2^{3m}}\right)G_j(x) = A_{(2m)j}F_j(x). \qquad (7.11)$$

The resulting tree, augmented by the output specifications for the DDG-trees from output levels $\le 2m$ as in the construction of optimum DG-trees in Theorem 4.1, is an fsg for $F(x)$. It remains for us to verify that its output time is sufficiently near the optimum.

The average time to output the kth bit for $k \le 2m$ is optimum, by construction. The average time to output the $(2m+k)$th bit exceeds the optimum by at most a bounded amount D_n (see Theorem 7.2) times the probability that an fsg for the polynomial distribution $F_j(x)$ or $G_j(x)$ is used. But the probability that an F_j is used is the probability that j is bad, namely $O(2^{-m})$; and the probability that a G_j is used is

$$\sum_{\text{good } j} \left(A_{(2m)j} - \frac{t_j}{2^{3m}}\right) < \sum_{j=0}^{2^{2m}-1} \frac{1}{2^{3m}} = 2^{-m}.$$

Hence the total average output time exceeds the optimum by at most $O(D_n/2^m)$, and for sufficiently large m this will be less than ϵ. $\quad\square$

Our final result in this section shows that the class of distributions realizable with an fsg is severely limited. We have seen in Section 5 that it is possible to generate some rather unusual continuous distributions with fsg's. However, it turns out that if $F(x)$ is a piecewise analytic function realizable by an fsg, then $F(x)$ must be a piecewise polynomial function.

We say that $F(x)$ is analytic on $[c \mathbin{..} d]$ if for all $x_0 \in [c \mathbin{..} d]$ there exists $\delta > 0$ and a sequence of coefficients $\langle a_0, a_1, a_2, \ldots \rangle$ such that

$$F(x) = \sum_{j \ge 0} a_j(x - x_0)^j \qquad (7.12)$$

for all $x \in [c \mathbin{..} d]$ with $|x - x_0| < \delta$.

Theorem 7.4. *If the distribution $F(x)$ over $[0 .. 1]$ is generated by an fsg, and if $F(x)$ is analytic on $[c .. d]$ for some c and d with $0 \le c < d \le 1$, then there exists a polynomial $p(x)$ with rational coefficients such that $F(x) = p(x)$ for all $x \in [c .. d]$.*

Proof. We shall make use of the following lemma, which is essentially a consequence of the theorem of Arbib [2] and Heller [4] about the reliability of stochastic systems. Since our model of computation is somewhat different from that of Arbib and Heller, we shall prove the result directly in our model.

Lemma. *Let $F(x)$ be generated by an fsg. Then there exists a finite set $\{G_1(x), G_2(x), \ldots, G_s(x)\}$ of functions on $[0 .. 1]$ with the following property: For each $k \ge 0$ and $0 \le j < 2^k$ such that F is continuous and not constant on $[j/2^k .. (j+1)/2^k)$, the function*

$$F_{kj}(x) = \frac{F\left(\frac{j+x}{2^k} - 0\right) - F\left(\frac{j}{2^k} - 0\right)}{F\left(\frac{j+1}{2^k} - 0\right) - F\left(\frac{j}{2^k} - 0\right)}, \qquad 0 \le x \le 1, \qquad (7.13)$$

is a convex combination of the G_i functions. In particular, any family containing more than s of the functions $F_{kj}(x)$ is linearly dependent over $[0 .. 1]$.

Proof. Since the fsg tree has finitely many nonisomorphic subtrees, there are finitely many distribution functions $\{G_1(x), G_2(x), \ldots, G_s(x)\}$ for the outputs following any bit that is output at any branch node. (The string at any branch node is finite, hence of bounded length. After we output each bit of the string, there will be a distribution $G_i(x)$ accounting for the remaining bits of that string and for the outputs at descendant nodes. By our definitions there is an fsg for the discontinuous distribution $F(x) = 0$ for $x < 1/\pi$, $F(x) = 1$ for $x \ge 1/\pi$, namely the trivial tree consisting of a single terminal node at which we output the infinite string of 0s and 1s corresponding to the binary representation of $1/\pi$. For this fsg there are infinitely many linearly independent distributions $F_{kj}(x)$. But the lemma actually holds also for discontinuous $F_{kj}(x)$, provided only that $F_{kj}(x)$ is not a "one-jump" step function, namely a distribution with $F_{kj}(x + 0) = F_{kj}(x - 0) + 1$ for some x.)

Given k and j, consider all nodes $v \in V_{kj}$ where the kth output has occurred and the first k outputs were the binary representation of $j/2^k$. Every such v occurs at some level $L(v)$ and specifies some

$G^{(v,k)}(x) \in \{G_1(x), \ldots, G_s(x)\}$, and we have

$$F_{kj}(x) = \sum_{v \in V_{kj}} \frac{1}{2^{L(v)}} G^{(v,k)}(x) = \sum_{i=1}^{s} \lambda_i G_i(x), \qquad (7.14)$$

for all $x \in [0 \mathbin{..} 1]$ and appropriate λ_i. This proves the lemma. $\quad\square$

Returning to the proof of the theorem, let us choose a point $x_0 = j/2^k$ such that $c < x_0 < d$. Then δ and $\langle a_0, a_1, a_2, \ldots \rangle$ exist satisfying (7.12). Replacing j by $2^t j$ and k by $k+t$ if necessary, we can assume that $1/2^k < \delta$ and $x_0 + 1/2^k < d$. By the lemma, there is a number s such that the functions $F_{(k+i)(2^i j)}(x)$ for $0 \le i \le s$ are linearly dependent; that is, there are nonzero numbers b_i such that

$$\sum_{i=0}^{s} b_i A_{(k+i)(2^i j)} F_{(k+i)(2^i j)}(x) = 0, \qquad 0 \le x \le 1. \qquad (7.15)$$

Now by (7.12) and (7.15) we have

$$A_{(k+i)(2^i j)} F_{(k+i)(2^i j)}(x) = \sum_{l \ge 0} a_l \left(\frac{x}{2^{k+i}} \right)^l, \qquad 0 \le x \le 1; \qquad (7.16)$$

hence (7.15) implies that

$$\sum_{i=0}^{s} \frac{b_i}{(2^{k+i})^l} = 0 \qquad (7.17)$$

for all values of l with $a_l \ne 0$. If at least $s + 1$ values of a_l are nonzero, (7.17) defines a system of linear equations whose determinant is a nonzero multiple of a nonzero Vandermonde determinant, hence all $b_i = 0$. It follows that $a_l = 0$ for all large l; that is, $F(x)$ is a polynomial $p(x)$ in the interval $[x_0 \mathbin{..} x_0 + 1/2^k)$. From the well-known theory of analytic functions, it follows that $F(x) = p(x)$ for all $x \in [c \mathbin{..} d]$.

It remains to be shown that the coefficients of $p(x)$ are rational. It suffices to prove that the A_{kj} for any fsg are rational numbers, since equation (7.16) for $x = 1$ and sufficiently many values of i will then determine the a_l as a rational combination of A_{kj}'s. Now A_{kj} is the probability of outputting a particular string of k 0s and 1s, so it can be represented as the sum of all entries in a row of the product of k transition matrices between "states" of the fsg. Here we refer to states in the conventional sense that exactly one output occurs as we enter each state of the device. Our fsg can readily be represented as a finite set of states with at most one output per state, if we simply split every node that produces two or more outputs into multiple nodes connected by transitions of probability 1. Now we can eliminate the states at which no output occurs, one by one, in the standard way. Namely, if v is such a state, with probability p_{vv} of going from state v to itself, we can eliminate v if, for every other pair of states u and w, we replace the probability p_{uw} of transition from u to w by

$$p_{uw} + \frac{p_{uv}p_{vw}}{1 - p_{vv}}. \tag{7.18}$$

A finite number of such transformations produces a finite state device with rational transition probabilities between each pair of states and with exactly one output produced at each state. It follows, as stated above, that each A_{kj} is a rational number.   □

It would be interesting to characterize those distributions for which an fsg is optimal. One important example is the distribution of $(U+V)/2$ when U and V are independent uniform deviates, namely

$$F(x) = \begin{cases} 2x^2, & \text{if } 0 \le x \le 1/2; \\ 1 - 2(1-x)^2, & \text{if } 1/2 \le x \le 1. \end{cases} \tag{7.19}$$

An optimal fsg for this distribution is obtained from the tree

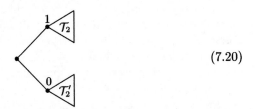

$$\tag{7.20}$$

where T_2' is the fsg $T_{2,2}$ defined in the proof of Theorem 7.2 (it corresponds to $\min(U, V)$). The reader may also verify that the distribution

$$F(x) = (x - p)/q, \qquad p \le x \le p + q \tag{7.21}$$

can optimally be obtained by an fsg, whenever p and q are rational numbers with $0 \le p < p + q \le 1$.

8. Generating the Exponential Distribution

Theorem 7.4 proves that the exponential distribution

$$F(x) = 1 - e^{-x}, \qquad x \geq 0, \qquad (8.1)$$

which is one of the most important distributions in practice, cannot be generated by an fsg. Clearly, therefore, fsg's are too restricted a model, while it is also clear that general DG-tree algorithms are too unrestricted a model. In this section we shall briefly discuss a simple algorithm for the exponential distribution, in hopes that it sheds some light on the general question of what kind of intermediate model might really be most relevant to practical problems.

The algorithm that follows is based on an elegant approach suggested by John von Neumann [11]. Many other methods are now known (see Ahrens and Dieter [1, Chapter 7]), but we shall work with von Neumann's approach since it is so easily programmed. The idea is to use the following method:

E1. [Initialize.] Set $c \leftarrow 0$.

E2. [Look for a rise.] Generate uniform deviates U_0, U_1, ... until finding the least $j \geq 1$ such that $U_{j-1} < U_j$.

E3. [Done?] If j is even, set $c \leftarrow c + 1$ and return to step E2; otherwise output $c + U_0$.   □

Our examples so far have been for distributions restricted to $[0 \mathinner{.\,.} 1]$, but exponential deviates can be arbitrarily large. Let us choose the unary-binary representation for real numbers, as discussed in Section 3 above, but without the initial '1' since all our numbers are positive. Thus a number $c + t$, where c is an integer and $t \in [0 \mathinner{.\,.} 1)$, is represented by c 1s, followed by a 0, followed by the binary representation of t. Then the exponential distribution can be generated by adapting von Neumann's method as follows:

begin integer f, p, s, t; **integer array** $a, b[1 : \infty]$;
    comment In this implementation of von Neumann's method,
        the variables have the following significance:
            $f = 1$ means $j = 1$, $f = 0$ means $j > 1$,
            p represents j mod 2,
            $a_1 \ldots a_s$ represents the leading bits of U_0,
            $b_1 \ldots b_t$ represents the leading bits of U_{j-1};
    while *true* **do**

```
                begin f ← 1;  p ← 1;  t ← 0;  comment j ← 1;
advance:   t ← t + 1;  bₜ ← flip;
                if f = 1 then begin s ← t;  aₜ ← bₜ end;
                if flip = 0 then go to advance;
inequality found: if bₜ = 1 then
                    begin comment Uⱼ₋₁ > Uⱼ;
                        f ← 0;  p ← 1 − p;  bₜ ← 0; comment j ← j + 1;
                        for i ← 1 step 1 until t do
                            if flip = 1 then
                                begin t ← i;  go to inequality found
                                end;
                        go to advance;
                    end else
                    begin comment Uⱼ₋₁ < Uⱼ;
                        if p = 1 then
                            begin output(0);
                                comment switching from unary to binary;
                                for i ← 1 step 1 until s do output(aᵢ);
                                while true do output(flip)
                            end else output(1);  comment c ← c + 1;
                    end
            end
        end;
```

This algorithm could clearly be performed by a stochastic Turing machine that operates in real time (that is, with one machine action per *flip* instruction), if the machine actions allow printing a symbol and positioning the head right one step or instantaneously resetting the head to the beginning of the tape. It does not seem possible to implement the algorithm on a stochastic pushdown automaton, even without the real time restriction.

The average running time of an optimum DG-tree algorithm for the exponential distribution with unary-binary representation can be estimated by extending the proof of Theorem 5.2. As in (5.9) we have

$$T_F(k) - k = \sum_{m \geq 1-k} \frac{m}{2^m} J_m(k); \qquad (8.2)$$

but for the unary-binary representation (modified for nonnegative numbers as above) we have

$$J_m(k) = \frac{1}{2^k}\left(\varepsilon_{m+k}\big(1 - F(k)\big) + \sum_{l=0}^{k-1} \sum_{j=0}^{2^{k-1-l}-1} \varepsilon_{m+k}\big(A_{kj}^{(l)}\big) \right), \qquad (8.3)$$

where

$$A_{kj}^{(l)} = F\left(l + \frac{j+1}{2^{k-1-l}}\right) - F\left(l + \frac{j}{2^{k-1-l}}\right). \tag{8.4}$$

Let m be fixed and $k \to \infty$. For all but $O(2^m)$ "bad" values of l and j, the density function $f(x) = F'(x)$ will have a constant value

$$t_{lj} = \lfloor 2^m f(x) \rfloor$$

for all x in the interval corresponding to $A_{kj}^{(l)}$; and for the "good" values, $2^{-k}\varepsilon_{m+k}(A_{kj}^{(l)})$ turns out to equal 2^{-1-l} times the integral of $\varepsilon_m(2^{-1-l}f(x))$ over that interval. Hence for the nonnegative unary-binary representation the analog of (5.12) is

$$J_m(k) = \sum_{l \geq 0} \frac{1}{2^{l+1}} \int_l^{l+1} \varepsilon_m\left(\frac{f(x)}{2^{l+1}}\right) dx + O(\min(1, 2^{m-k})). \tag{8.5}$$

Let $f(x) = e^{-x}$ and let J_m be the limiting value of (8.5) as $k \to \infty$. We find $J_1 = 0$, $J_2 = \frac{1}{2}\ln 2$, $J_3 = \frac{1}{2}\ln\left(\frac{4}{3}\frac{e}{2}\right)$, $J_4 = \frac{1}{2}\ln\left(\frac{8}{7}\frac{6}{5}\frac{4}{3}\right) + \frac{1}{4}\ln\left(\frac{4}{e}\right)$, etc. Numerical evaluation shows that the average running time for an optimum DG-tree algorithm will be $k + d_F + O(k^2/2^k)$ input bits for k outputs, where

$$d_F = 0.53854\,18997\,37707\,98213\,48307\,27471\,90948\,08837+. \tag{8.6}$$

It should be possible, and interesting, to analyze the average running time of the simple algorithm above, but at present we have only empirical results. After 1000 trials of the algorithm it appears that the time to produce k bits approaches $k + 5.4 \pm 0.2$, for large k.

9. Conclusions and Open Problems

We have discussed the rudiments of a new type of complexity theory, which combines mathematical and numerical analysis with the study of algorithms and automata in an interesting way, and which sheds some light on the problem of nonuniform random number generation. Although we have obtained the answers to several of the natural questions that arise in this theory, many further problems are suggested.

Perhaps the most interesting direction for further research is to study models intermediate between the finite state algorithms and the general tree algorithms; these models should relate in a natural way to the problem of generating exponential and normal and gamma distributions, etc., on a computer. How efficiently can we generate normal deviates from a sequence of random bits, using a reasonably simple algorithm?

Automata or algorithms that are allowed to "know" the binary representations of certain constants should certainly be considered in this connection. For example, the probability is $1/2^k$ that an exponential deviate exceeds $k \ln 2$, and one way to generate exponential deviates is to use this fact to reduce the problem to generating deviates in the range $[0 .. \ln 2)$; thus, the binary value of $\ln 2$ and perhaps its multiples would be helpful in such an algorithm.

Another interesting topic not pursued in this paper is the generation of important discrete distributions such as the Poisson distribution with parameter λ, or the binomial distribution with parameters (n, p). The interesting "count ones" approach of Ahrens and Dieter [1, Chapter 12] is a particularly noteworthy way to generate the binomial distribution; can one do substantially better?

Some of the other problems we have left unresolved are: (i) Can Theorem 5.2 be improved to cases where $F(x)$ has infinitely many points of discontinuity or nondifferentiability? How does the coefficient of k relate to properties of F? (ii) Determine the average running time of the simple method for exponential distributions presented in Section 8 above. (iii) Characterize all $F(x)$ for which an fsg is optimum. (iv) How large must the number of states be to generate $F(x) = x^3$ with an fsg that is within ϵ of optimum? (v) Which polynomial distributions $F(x)$ can be generated by an fsg? (vi) Do pushdown automata generate any interesting distributions? (vii) What if the source of independent random bits is biased towards 1 with probability p? (viii) What can be said about the *variance* of the running time of such algorithms?

This research was supported in part by the National Science Foundation, in part by the Office of Naval Research, and in part by IBM Corporation. Some of the calculations and formula manipulation were done with the MACSYMA system, a project supported by the Advanced Research Projects Agency.

References

[1] J. H. Ahrens and U. Dieter, *Non-Uniform Random Numbers* (Graz, Austria: Institut für Mathematische Statistik, Technische Hochschule Graz, 1974). [A planned book that was never completed.]

[2] Michael A. Arbib, "Realization of stochastic systems," *Annals of Mathematical Statistics* **38** (1967), 927–933.

[3] Jon Louis Bentley and Andrew Chi-Chih Yao, "An almost optimal algorithm for unbounded searching," *Information Processing Letters* **5** (1976), 82–87.

[4] Alex Heller, "On stochastic processes derived from Markov chains," *Annals of Mathematical Statistics* **36** (1965), 1286–1291.

[5] Donald E. Knuth, *Fundamental Algorithms*, Volume 1 of *The Art of Computer Programming* (Reading, Massachusetts: Addison–Wesley, 1968). Second edition, 1973; third edition, 1997.

[6] Donald E. Knuth, *Seminumerical Algorithms*, Volume 2 of *The Art of Computer Programming* (Reading, Massachusetts: Addison–Wesley, 1969). Second edition, 1981; third edition, 1997.

[7] Donald E. Knuth, "The Dangers of Computer Science Theory," *Logic, Methodology and Philosophy of Science* **4** (Amsterdam: North-Holland, 1973), 189–195. [Reprinted as Chapter 2 of the present volume.]

[8] Donald E. Knuth, *Sorting and Searching*, Volume 3 of *The Art of Computer Programming* (Reading, Massachusetts: Addison–Wesley, 1973). Second edition, 1998.

[9] Azaria Paz, *Introduction to Probabilistic Automata* (New York: Academic Press, 1971).

[10] Tom Stoppard, *Rosencrantz and Guildenstern are Dead* (London: Faber and Faber, 1967).

[11] John von Neumann, "Various techniques used in connection with random digits," notes by G. E. Forsythe, *National Bureau of Standards Applied Mathematics Series* **12** (1951), 36–38. Reprinted in von Neumann's *Collected Works* **5**, 768–770.

Addendum

Research problem (ii) was solved with an interesting analysis by Philippe Flajolet and Nasser Saheb, "The complexity of generating an exponentially distributed variate," *Journal of Algorithms* **7** (1986), 463–488. By studying related statistics about digital search trees (binary tries), they proved that $\lim_{k \to \infty} \big(T(k) - k \big)$ is the constant

$$e\left(2 - \frac{3}{e-1}\right) + \sum_{n \geq 0} \frac{1}{e^{1/2^n} - 1} \left(\frac{e}{4^n} + 1 - e^{1/2^n}\left(1 - \frac{1}{2^n}\right)\right)$$

$$= 5.67974\,69285\,27492\,09679\,20663\,26744\,85263\,19308 - .$$

Preliminary results on problems (v) and (vi) were obtained by Andrew C. Yao, "Context-free grammars and random number generation," in *Combinatorial Algorithms on Words*, edited by Alberto Apostolico and Zvi Galil (Springer, 1984), 357–361. He showed in particular that polynomial distributions for which $F'(x)$ has an irrational root cannot be generated by an fsg; pushdown automata do have the ability to generate certain polynomial distributions with irrational algebraic cofficients, but they cannot generate analytic nonpolynomial distributions.

Conversely, if $F(x)$ is a polynomial distribution with rational coefficients for which $F'(x)$ has no irrational roots, Guy Kindler and Dan Romik have shown that $F(x)$ *can* be generated by an fsg; this completes the solution of problem (v). ["On distributions computable by random walks on graphs," *SIAM Journal on Discrete Mathematics* **17** (2004), 624–633.]

Practical programs for the efficient generation of discrete distributions are often based on "Walker's alias method" (see [6, second or third edition, Section 3.4.1A]). When this method is represented as a DDG-tree it is not always optimal, but B. B. Pokhodzeĭ proved that its average running time is at most the upper bound (2.28) of Theorem 2.3. [See "Сложность метода Уолкера для моделирования конечных распределений," *Vestnik Leningradskogo Universitata* **19**, 1 (1986), 58–63; English translation, "Complexity of Walker's method for generating finite discrete distributions," *Vestnik Leningrad University: Mathematics* **19**, 1 (1986), 70–76.] The Walker alias method for simulating a single die is, for example,

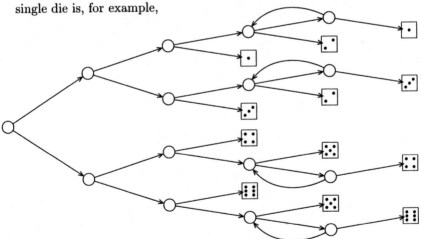

with average running time $4\nu(1/6) + 4\nu(1/12) = 4$.

Index